Second Edition

ATHLETIC INJURIES TO THE HEAD, NECK, AND FACE

SECOND EDITION

Athletic Injuries to the Head, Neck, and Face

Joseph S. Torg, M.D.
Professor of Orthopaedic Surgery
University of Pennsylvania
Director, University of Pennsylvania Sports Medicine Center
Philadelphia, Pennsylvania

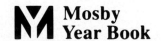
Mosby
Year Book

St. Louis   Baltimore   Boston   Chicago   London   Philadelphia   Sydney   Toronto

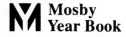
**Mosby
Year Book**

Sponsoring Editor: James D. Ryan
Assistant Editor: Joyce-Rachel John
Associate Managing Editor, Manuscript Services: Deborah Thorp
Production Project Coordinator: Karen Halm
Proofroom Manager: Barbara Kelly

1 2 3 4 5 6 7 8 9 0 CL MV 95 94 93 92 91

Library of Congress Cataloging-in-Publication Data
Athletic injuries to the head, neck, and face / [edited by] Joseph S.
  Torg.—2nd ed.
      p.   cm.
    Includes bibliographical references and index.
    ISBN 0-8151-8846-3
    1. Head—Wounds and injuries.   2. Neck—Wounds and injuries.
  3. Face—Wounds and injuries.   4. Sports—Accidents and injuries.
  I. Torg, Joseph S.
    [DNLM: 1. Athletic Injuries.   2. Facial Injuries.   3. Head
  Injuries.   4. Neck—injuries.   WE 706 A871]
  RD521.A83   1991
  617.1'027—dc20
  DNLM/DLC   91-13658
  for Library of Congress   CIP

To my wife Barbara, whose organizational skills, editing abilities, and efforts were responsible for making this edition a reality.

CONTRIBUTORS

Wayne M. Alves, Ph.D.
Assistant Professor
Division of Neurosurgery
University of Pennsylvania School of
  Medicine
Philadelphia, Pennsylvania

Doris Bixby-Hammett, M.D.
Member, American Medical Equestrian
  Association
Safety Committee of the United States Pony
  Club, Inc.
Philadelphia, Pennsylvania

William H. Brooks, M.D.
Clinical Assistant Professor
Division of Neurosurgery
University of Kentucky
Chief of Neurosurgery
Central Baptist Hospital
Lexington, Kentucky

Alexander J. Brucker, M.D.
Associate Professor of Ophthalmology
Chief, Retina and Vitreous Service
Scheie Eye Institute
Department of Ophthalmology
University of Pennsylvania School of
  Medicine
Philadelphia, Pennsylvania

Leonard A. Bruno, M.D.
Clinical Associate Professor of Surgery
Temple University School of Medicine
Chief, Department of Neurosurgery
Germantown Hospital
Philadelphia, Pennsylvania

Albert H. Burstein, Ph.D.
Professor of Applied Biomechanics (in
  Surgery)
Cornell University Medical College
Senior Scientist
Department of Research
Director, Department of Biomechanics
Hospital for Special Surgery
New York, New York

Robert C. Cantu, M.D., F.A.C.S.
Chief Neurosurgery Service
Chairman, Department of Surgery
Director, Service of Sports Medicine
Emerson Hospital
Concord, Massachusetts

Kenneth S. Clarke, Ph.D.
Former Dean
College of Applied Life Studies
University of Illinois
Urbana, Illinois

Myles R.J. Coolican, M.D.
Visiting Medical Officer
The Royal North Shore Hospital
St. Leonards, Australia

Michael D.F. Deck, M.D.
Vice Chairman of Radiology
Professor of Clinical Radiology
Cornell University Medical College
Chief, Division of Neuroradiology
New York Hospital
New York, New York

Michael Easterbrook, M.D., F.R.C.S.(C)., F.A.C.S.
Associate Professor
Department of Ophthalmology
University of Toronto
Chairman, Task Force of Canadian Standards
  Association Committee on Eye Protection
  in Racquet Sports
Toronto, Canada

Colleen M. Fay, M.D.
Staff Attending Physician
White Plains Hospital Center
Assistant Adjunct Attending Physician
Bronx Lebanon Hospital Center
White Plains, New York

Thomas A. Gennarelli, M.D.
Professor of Neurosurgery
Department of Neurosurgery
University of Pennsylvania School of
  Medicine
Philadelphia, Pennsylvania

Roger M. Glaser
Professor and Acting Chairman
Department of Rehabilitation Medicine and
  Restorative Care
Professor of Physiology and Biophysics
Wright State University School of Medicine
Dayton, Ohio

Steven G. Glasgow, M.D.
Professor of Orthopaedic Surgery
Sports Medicine Center
University of Pennsylvania
Philadelphia, Pennsylvania

Martin S. Greenberg, D.D.S.
Assistant Professor and Chairman School of
  Dental Medicine
University of Pennsylvania
Philadelphia, Pennsylvania

Steven D. Handler, M.D.
Associate Professor
Department of Otorhinolaryngology
University of Pennsylvania School of
  Medicine
Associate Director
Department of Otorhinolaryngology
Children's Hospital of Philadelphia
Philadelphia, Pennsylvania

Elliott B. Hershman, M.D.
Staff, Nicholas Institute of Sports Medicine
  and Athletic Trauma
Associate Orthopaedic Surgeon
Department of Orthopaedic Surgery
Lenox Hill Hospital
New York, New York

Voigt Hodgson, Ph.D.
Director, Gurdjian-Lissner Biomechanics Lab
Department of Neurosurgery
Wayne State University
Detroit, Michigan

Caren Jahre, M.D.
Assistant Professor of Radiology
Department of Radiology
Albert Einstein College of Medicine
Attending Neuroradiologist
Montefiore Medical Center
Bronx, New York

Robert J. Johnson, M.D.
Emeritus Professor of Anatomy and Surgery
University of Pennsylvania School of
  Medicine
Philadelphia, Pennsylvania

David M. Kozart, M.D.
Associate Professor of Ophthalmology
Scheie Eye Institute
University of Pennsylvania School of
  Medicine
Philadelphia, Pennsylvania

Marvin R. Leventhal, M.D.
Assistant Professor of Orthopaedic Surgery
University of Tennessee
Active Staff
Campbell Clinic
Memphis, Tennessee

Frederick O. Mueller, Ph.D.
Professor of Physical Education
Department of Physical Education
University of North Carolina
Chapel Hill, North Carolina

Charles W. Nichols, M.D.
Associate Professor of Ophthalmology and
  Pharmacology
University of Pennsylvania School of
  Medicine
Deputy Chief of Ophthalmology
Hospital of the University of Pennsylvania
Philadelphia, Pennsylvania

James C. Otis, Ph.D.
Associate Professor of Biomechanical
  Engineering in Surgery
Cornell University Medical College
Senior Scientist
Department of Biomechanics
Research Laboratories
Hospital for Special Surgery
New York, New York

Dan Patterson, J.D.
Auburn, California

Helene Pavlov, M.D.
Professor of Clinical Radiology
Department of Radiology
Cornell University Medical College
Attending Radiologist
Hospital for Special Surgery
New York, New York

Irving M. Raber, M.D.
Clinical Assistant Professor of
    Ophthalmology
University of Pennsylvania School of
    Medicine
Clinical Assistant Professor of
    Ophthalmology
Thomas Jefferson University School of
    Medicine
Philadelphia, Pennsylvania

David C. Reid, M.D.
Professor of Orthopaedic Surgery
Adjunct Professor of Rehabilitation Medicine
Honorary Professor of Physical Education
University of Alberta
Director, Glen Sather University of Alberta
    Sports Medicine Clinic
Edmonton, Alberta, Canada

Allan J. Ryan, M.D.
President and Director
Sports Medicine Enterprise
Edina, Minnesota

Linda A. Saboe, M.C.P.A., B.P.T.
Physical Therapist
University of Alberta
Edmonton, Alberta, Canada

Carson D. Schneck, M.D.
Professor of Anatomy and Diagnostic Imaging
Department of Anatomy and Cell Biology
Temple University School of Medicine
Philadelphia, Pennsylvania

Philip S. Springer, D.M.D.
Clinical Assistant Professor of Oral Medicine
School of Dental Medicine
University of Pennsylvania
Assistant Chairman for Academic Affairs
Department of Dental Medicine
Hospital of the University of Pennsylvania
Philadelphia, Pennsylvania

Charles H. Tator, M.D., Ph.D., F.R.C.S.(C.)
Chairman and Professor
Division of Neurosurgery
University of Toronto
Director, Canadian Sports Spine and Head
    Injuries Research Center
Toronto Western Hospital
Toronto, Canada

Thomas K.F. Taylor, M.D.
Professor of Orthopaedics and Traumatic
    Surgery
Department of Orthopaedic Surgery
The University of Sydney
The Royal North Shore Hospital
St. Leonard's, Australia

Joseph S. Torg, M.D.
Professor of Orthopaedic Surgery
University of Pennsylvania
Director, University of Pennsylvania Sports
    Medicine Center
Philadelphia, Pennsylvania

Joseph J. Vegso, M.S., A.T.C.
Administrator, Miami Rehabilitation Institute
Coral Gables, Florida

PREFACE

Richard Schneider, former Professor and Chairman of Neurosurgery at the University of Michigan, succinctly noted that "the football fields of our nation have been a vast proving ground or laboratory for the study of tragic neurologic sequelae of head and neck trauma in man." His practical applications of this observation resulted in a series of major contributions that included descriptions of the "acute anterior spinal cord injury syndrome," and the "acute central cervical cord injury syndrome." In addition, his laboratory model for impacting the anesthetized primate resulted in the development of the double-crowned pneumatic football helmet used today. He must also be given credit for having been the first to conclude that "fractured cervical spines with tetraplegia could be avoided by enforcing a rule that outlawed spearing and stick-blocking." His true genius was perhaps best demonstrated by his position in 1972, that in the face of cervical spine fracture with spinal cord injury "the early administration of steroids . . . seems as effective or perhaps even better than surgery." Recently, some 18 years later, *The New England Journal of Medicine* reported a major multi-center study regarding the use of steroids in acute spinal cord injury, with similar conclusions.

Although material in this book takes issue with Dr. Schneider's concept of the role of the helmet in cervical spine injury, i.e., the proposed guillotine mechanism, and questions his concept of the "teardrop fracture," he is acknowledged as *the* pioneer in the academic pursuit of dealing with the problems presented by head and neck injuries in the athlete.

With the exception of the Dr. Schneider and the efforts and contributions of Drs. Joseph Marrone and Robert Cantu in this country and Charles Tator in Canada, the concern of the neurosurgical community with neurologic problems confronting those who participate in recreational and competitive athletics can best be described as underwhelming. As one prominent neurosurgeon admitted, "If it's not a brain tumor, we are not really interested."

With a few exceptions, the performance of the orthopaedic sports medicine community in dealing with these problems has been equally inadequate. Dr. John Albright clearly understood the scope of the problem of cervical spine injury in American football. His article, "Nonfatal Cervical Spine Injuries in Interscholastic Football," published in JAMA in September 1976—although it seems to me to have been neither appreciated nor understood—represented the first scientific attempt to define the problem of cervical spine injuries in this particular group.

More recently, the efforts of Dr. Robert Watkins to address the issue of risk criteria following cervical spine injury are noteworthy, as is the fact that his efforts were motivated by concerns of physicians caring for professional football teams. These physicians have developed significant discomfort due to both a lack of creditable data and workable principles to deal with cervical spine injuries and the demands and pressures brought to bear upon them by team owners, coaches, and players, in what can be best described as litigiously hostile environment.

Why have the orthopaedic sports medicine mavens failed to direct attention to the problems presented by cervical spine injuries in the athlete? Or more pointedly, why has the orthopaedic sports medicine leadership completely failed to recognize the cervical spine as an area demanding recognition, concern, and attention? To this observer, the answer is quite obvious. Just as a neurosurgeon is not "really interested unless the patient has a brain tumor," the sports medicine orthopaedist is not really interested unless the patient has torn his or her anterior cruciate ligament. The anterior cruciate ligament has become the focus of an obsession that has dominated the interest, efforts, and resources of the orthopaedic sports medicine community, a phenomenon dramatically demonstrated by the fact that during the five-year period 1985 through 1989, the *American Journal of Sports Medicine* published 90 articles dealing with the anterior cruciate ligament and only one dealing with the cervical spine.

Although this material represents the latest word regarding these matters, it certainly should not be the last. It is intended that this edition will fill the void that currently exists with regard to available information pertaining to the definition of the problem, prevention, treatment, and rehabilitation of athletic injuries to the head, neck, and face.

JOSEPH S. TORG, M.D.

CONTENTS

Problems and Prevention

CHAPTER 1

Anecdotal Observations

Joseph S. Torg, M.D.

A tremendous increase in active participation in recreational and competitive physical activities has occurred during the past several decades. With more leisure time, affluence, and media attention to sports, Americans by the millions are flocking to the playing fields, courts, and trails. Recent estimates place the number of individuals who run and jog on a regular basis to be in the order of 25 million.[6] Another 110 million Americans swim, 65 million bicycle, 26 million play softball, and 25 million ice-skate. In addition, 1,300,000 youngsters participate in interscholastic football programs each season.

Associated with large numbers participating in many forms of physical activity, many of which involve body contact, has been a variety of injuries and health problems. It has been estimated that about 17 million Americans seek medical care each year because of such athletic- and recreation-related problems.[5] Because of that need, an area of medical interest referred to as sports medicine has developed. Sports medicine is multidisciplinary in nature. The basic goal is to provide total health care for the athlete through a team effort directed toward injury prevention, treatment, and rehabilitation (Fig 1–1).

The majority of sports-related injuries involve the musculoskeletal system, and therefore the orthopaedic surgeon has assumed a visible and prominent role. Sports medicine is an area requiring multidisciplinary input and cooperation, however. It necessarily involves the participation of individuals with medical as well as nonmedical backgrounds. Specifically, sports medicine requires the expertise, knowledge, and cooperation of the physical educator, athletic trainer, exercise physiologist, kinesiologist, biomechanical engineer, and epidemiologist, as well as the pediatrician, family practitioner, radiologist, neurosurgeon, and many other specialists.

Prevention and management of athletic injuries of the head, neck, and face exemplify the interdisciplinary approach to a group of problems confronting the recreational and competitive athlete.

Fortunately, serious athletic injuries to the head, neck, and eyes do not occur often. In many activities, however, their occurrence is persistent and demands the attention of those involved with the administration and care of athletes. In some activities the consequences of these injuries require that they be given a high priority, with particular regard to prevention as well as to improvement of methods of medical care. Examples of this group include fatal head injuries resulting from boxing and football; cervical spine injuries with associated neurologic involvement occurring in water sports, use of the trampoline,[2, 9] and football;[13, 14]

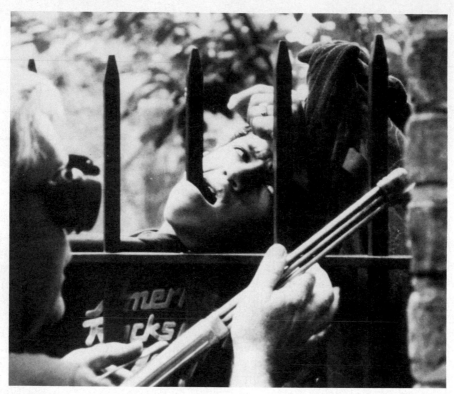

FIG 1–1.
A 15-year-old baseball player was impaled on an iron fence spike while attempting to catch a baseball. Although a bizarre injury, it not only emphasizes the multidisciplinary nature of athletic injuries to the neck and face, but also, more importantly, underlines the importance of preventive measures. In this instance such hazardous objects should not have been present in or near the playing environment. (AP/Wide World Photos. Used by permission.)

and disabling face and eye injuries in racquet sports and ice hockey.[7, 8, 16]

Head injuries resulting from athletic participation are not a new problem. Gonzales[3] reported that 104 fatal injuries occurred in competitive sports in New York City during the 32-year period from 1918 to 1950. Head injuries accounted for 27 of the 43 deaths that resulted from baseball. Of the 21 deaths that resulted from boxing, the majority were due to closed head injuries.

BOXING

Unterharnscheidt,[15] in his monograph on injuries occurring in boxing, noted that "this sport deserves special attention because, by its intentional destructiveness, it stands apart from all other athletic activities in which injuries are normally of an accidental nature" (Fig 1–2). The validity of this observation has been emphasized by five boxing deaths that occurred in a 7-month period from November 1979 to June 1980. On Nov 28, 1979, Willie Classen died from head injuries sustained in a professional bout in Madison Square Garden. On Jan 1, 1980, Tony Thomas, a 20-year-old professional, died in Spartanburg, Va, from head injuries sustained in a bout on Dec 22, 1979. On Jan 9, 1980, Charles Newell, a 26-year-old professional fighter, died in Hartford, Conn, from injuries sustained in a fight on Jan 1, 1980. On Jan 18, 1980, Cleveland Denny died as a result of a

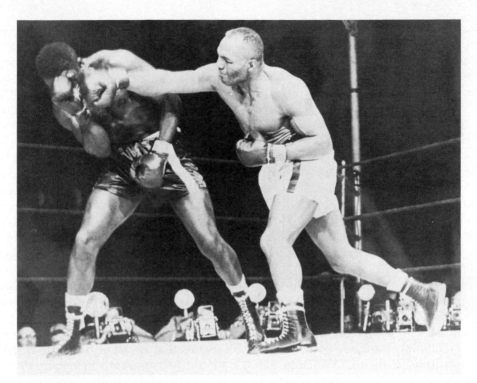

FIG 1–2.
A picture being worth a thousand words, the intentional destructiveness of boxing is vividly demonstrated by such telling blows to the head and, consequently, the brain of the opponent. (Photo by Sam Psoras, *Philadelphia Daily News*. Used by permission.)

"massive brain injury" sustained in a fight on June 20 in Montreal, Canada.

Unterharnscheidt[15] has also described the acute and chronic clinical manifestations of boxing injuries, a description that is simple, lucid, and worthy of consideration:

Clinically, boxing injuries can be grouped into acute and chronic. The first group includes, for example, cases in which the blow has sufficiently accelerated the head so as to produce cerebral concussion . . . or sudden falls like those in which the boxer is hit much above his center of gravity and is literally knocked off his feet, hitting his occiput in a rapid deceleration trauma.

The chronic brain lesions of boxers produce a condition known as punch-drunkenness, or chronic progressive traumatic encephalopathy of the boxer. This progressive clinical syndrome becomes noticeable only after a number of years. Frequently, this point coincides with the end of a boxer's career, or may occur a little later. Clinically the boxer exhibits a combination of extrapyramidal disturbances and cerebellar signs such as disturbed gait and coordination, tremor of the hands and body, and slurred speech.

Although specific head injury fatality rates have not been determined for boxing, in view of the comparatively few participants and the number of deaths reported in the press, it would appear that they are unacceptably high. Recent published reports indicate that supervision of boxing activities by the state boxing commissions leaves much to be desired.[4] It is necessary to establish and implement criteria as to when a fighter may return after having been rendered unconscious. Also, it is necessary to establish and enforce ringside standards by experienced medical personnel to protect the boxer who has been injured and impaired. As will be emphasized in other chapters, more current diagnostic and treatment methods for the critically head-injured fighter appear to be in order.

FOOTBALL

An annual survey of fatalities that resulted from tackle football has been conducted since 1931. Blyth and Arnold[1] indicated that head and face injuries account for 66% of all football fatalities, while those involving the spine account for 19%.

Consideration of severe head injuries occurring in football should include the total number of direct fatalities, intracranial injuries with associated hemorrhage, and intracranial injuries with hemorrhage resulting in death. Available data permit a nonstatistical comparison of these entities for two 5-year periods: 1959–1963 and 1971–1975.

For the 5 years 1959–1963, when 820,000 youths were exposed each year, the annual football fatality survey recorded 86 deaths as a direct result of football. During the period from 1971 to 1975, when 1,275,000 players were exposed annually, 77 deaths occurred. When compared on an exposure basis, these figures represent a reduction in the total number of documented direct fatalities. Schneider[10] recorded 139 lesions in which intracranial hemorrhage was a component during the 1959–1963 period. The National Football Head and Neck Injury Registry has recorded 72 similar lesions during the 1971–1975 period.[14] These figures indicate a decrease in injuries in which intracranial hemorrhage was a component.

Schneider[10] reported 65 intracranial injuries that resulted in death during the 1959–1963 period. Between 1971 and 1975, fifty eight similar fatal lesions were registered. When compared on an exposure basis, an apparent decrease in re-

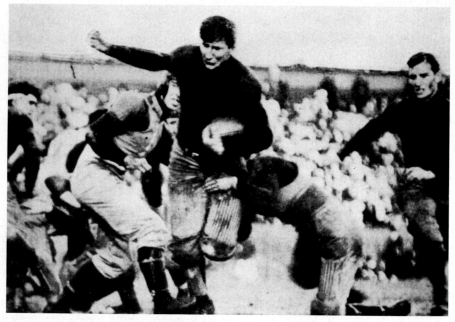

FIG 1–3.
Action photograph of a 1905 Swarthmore-Penn football game. Noteworthy is the absence of protective headgear. The 1905 college season was characterized by 18 deaths and 159 serious injuries, and resulted in President Theodore Roosevelt's order to "adjust rules to eliminate the injury risk."

ported deaths had occurred during the more recent 5-year period.

Although improvements in the quality of available medical care have played a role, the increased protective capabilities of the helmet–face mask protective system appear to be the major cause of the observed decrease in these three categories. It would appear that a further reduction could be obtained by continuing the enforcement of helmet standards, enforcing rules to preclude the use of the head as a primary point of contact in blocking and tackling, and implementing more advanced diagnostic and treatment techniques.

The design of protective head coverings for football has evolved during the past 70 years. In 1905, protection was afforded by a full head of hair (Fig 1–3). The first "helmet" appeared soon after, and was essentially a pair of heavy-duty leather earmuffs. By 1918 the cranial component, consisting of an outer leather cover and an inner felt lining, was developed. In 1932 a more modern helmet appeared that included a primitive suspension webbing. Modest improvements in the design and quality of the suspension system occurred in the early 1940s. The plastic shell, which displayed a significant improvement in design and construction, appeared in 1950.

Early face protectors were improvised to protect a nose that had already been fractured (Fig 1–4). It was not until the early 1950s that the single-bar and, subsequently, the double-bar mask were adopted to prevent injuries.

Today the helmet–face mask protective system consists of a bird cage attached to a polycarbonate shell with a variety of pneumatic, hydraulic, and web suspension systems (Fig 1–5).

Today's helmet–face mask system provides an extraordinary degree of protection to the head and face. As a result, in recent years coaching methods and playing techniques have developed in

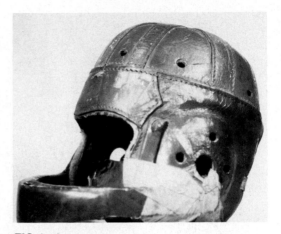

FIG 1–4.
A leather football helmet, vintage 1934. The improvised "single-bar face mask" was constructed by the Temple University trainer-equipment man to protect the fractured nose of a player. Although the single-bar face mask did not become common until 1950, the first such device originated at Temple University 15 years earlier.

which the head and helmet are utilized as a weapon—as a battering ram in blocking and tackling, and for "butting" when running with the ball (Fig 1–6).

Analysis of severe neck injuries that occur in football requires consideration of two parameters: cervical spine fracture

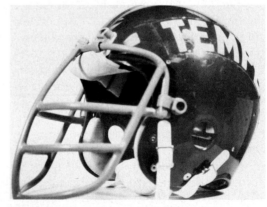

FIG 1–5.
The evolution of the helmet–face mask protective system resulted in a device that effectively protects the head and face from direct-blow injuries. The modern helmet afforded such a high degree of protection that it permitted the head to be used as a battering ram, placing the cervical spine at significant risk of injury.

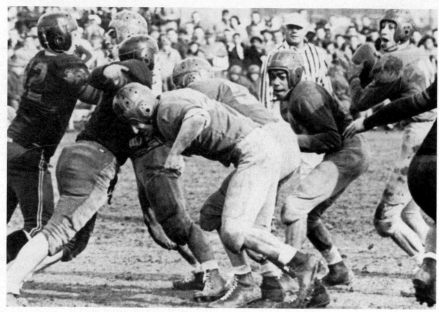

FIG 1–6.
A high school football game in the early 1950s in which all participants were wearing leather helmets without face masks. Notice the "picture-perfect" shoulder block being performed by the offensive lineman. Cervical spine injuries were not a problem when such playing techniques were employed.

or dislocation and cervical spine fracture or dislocation with quadriplegia. Available data permit a comparison of these entities for the two 5-year periods 1959–1963 and 1971–1975.

Between 1959 and 1963, Schneider[10] documented 56 injuries to the cervical spine involving fractures and dislocations. For the 5-year period 1971–1975, the National Football Head and Neck Injury Registry documented 259 similar lesions.[14] These figures demonstrate an increase in documented cervical spine fracture-dislocations during the more recent period.

Schneider[10] documented 30 cases of permanent quadriplegia during the 1959–1963 period, while the Registry documented 99 such lesions that occurred between 1971 and 1975. When compared on an exposure basis, these figures represent an increase in documented injuries that resulted in quadriplegia during the more recent 5-year period.

Thus between these two 5-year peri-ods there have been decreases in the total number of fatalities, the total number of closed head injuries associated with intracranial hemorrhage, and the total number of head injuries resulting in death. However, significant increases have occurred in both the number of documented fractures or dislocations involving the cervical spine and cervical spine fractures or dislocations associated with quadriplegia. This is attributed to the protective capabilities of the modern helmet–face mask system that adequately protects the head and face, but has encouraged the use of the head as a primary point of contact in blocking, tackling, and head butting. Thus the head and face are protected by equipment permitting the use of techniques that place the cervical spine at risk for catastrophic injury resulting from axial loading (Fig 1–7; also see Fig 1–6).

Collision injuries caused by spring-loaded dummies have presented an unusual situation from the standpoint of in-

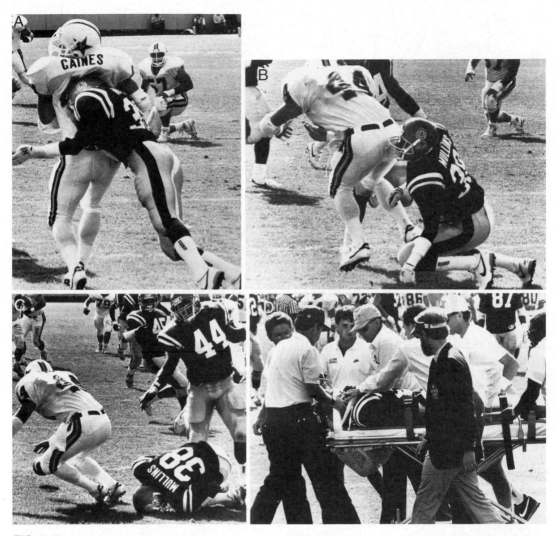

FIG 1–7.
A, with the advent of the polycarbonate helmet–face mask protective device, use of the top or crown of the helmet as the initial point of contact in blocking and tackling became prevalent. Contact is made, the head abruptly stops, the momentum of the body continues, and the cervical spine is literally crushed between the two. In this instance the fracture-dislocation transected the spinal cord. **B,** the injured player collapses, having been rendered quadriplegic. **C,** further collapse is noted. **D,** the player is evacuated on a spine board and stretcher. (Photos by Randy Green, Vanderbilt Student Communications.)

jury mechanism and prevention.[12] The involved devices were manufactured by an independent commercial firm and marketed throughout the United States without having been subjected to any form of safety control. Both tackling (Fig 1–8) and blocking (Fig 1–9) dummies are spring-loaded devices that travel on a suspended railing. Although the dummy itself is made of sponge rubber, the inner core consists of a 3 in. diameter steel pipe. The impact force can be adjusted by changing the springs to strike the subject with either 100, 200, or 300 pounds of force. The object is for the player to "attack" the dummy after it has been released and neutralize its force by striking it with his head and face, or arms and chest.

As a result of a collision with one of

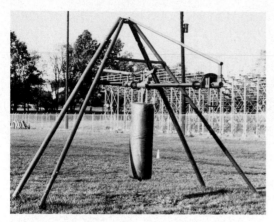

FIG 1–8.
A spring-loaded tackling dummy that was developed and marketed without safety evaluation. Depending on how it is spring-loaded, it can strike with 100, 200, or 300 pounds of force. This device has caused severe neck injuries, including one case of quadriplegia.

these devices, a 17-year-old high school player sustained comminuted fractures of C3, C4, and C5. Fortunately the youngster did not have neurologic involvement and recovered with conservative management. Another 17-year-old high school player was not so fortunate. After having been struck on the head with a spring-loaded blocking dummy, he immediately lost consciousness. Two days after the injury, he died. Autopsy revealed hemorrhages in the brain stem and pons, as well as evidence of subarachnoid bleeding.

In response to the apparent danger presented by these devices, the National Collegiate Athletic Association (NCAA) Committee on Competitive Safeguards and Medical Aspects of Sports issued a position statement "advising against the use of self-propelled mechanized blocking and tackling apparatus because of the apparent undue risk of head or neck injury." These devices are no longer used, and it is hoped that this particular problem has been solved. An issue raised by these injuries is why such an apparently dangerous device was not adequately evaluated from the safety standpoint before distribution and use, however.

WATER SPORTS

The frequency of cervical cord injuries in football has been well publicized.

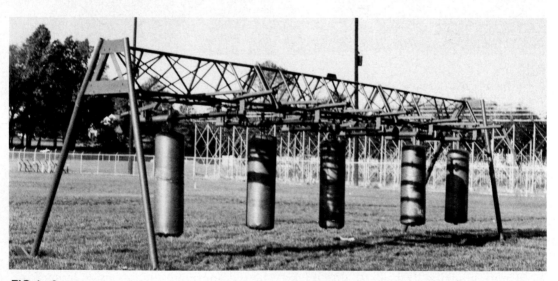

FIG 1–9.
Spring-loaded blocking dummies function on the same principle as the spring-loaded tackling device. The players are expected to meet the moving dummy and neutralize its impact by blocking it with the face, forearm, chest, and shoulders. This particular device was responsible for a brain stem injury resulting in death.

However, a report by Shields et al.[11] indicates that the majority of injuries to the cervical cord occur during water-related activities. Between June 1, 1964, and Dec 31, 1973, 1,600 patients were admitted to the Spinal Injury Service at Rancho Los Amigos Hospital. Of these, 152, or 9.5%, of the patients had been injured in recreational activities. During that period, 118, or 73%, of the 152 patients were injured in water-related sports. Diving accidents were the leading cause of injury, and occurred because the patient misjudged the depth and safety of the water at the time of incidence. Most of these patients were injured by diving into shallow water or striking a submerged object. The average depth of the water in which neck injuries occurred was five feet. Football accounted for only 16 of the 152 sports-related injuries, or 10% of all sports-related cervical cord injuries, and 1.0% of cervical cord injuries from all causes.

ICE HOCKEY

Injuries to the head and face are prevalent in ice hockey. Those to the intraocular structures present a major problem.

Pashby et al.,[7,8] soliciting information from the Canadian Ophthalmological Society, attempted to document eye injuries in Canada during the 1972–1973 and 1974–1975 seasons. For the first period, 287 injuries were reported, the majority of which were caused by sticks. Notable is the fact that 13.7% of these injuries resulted in blindness in the injured eye. During the 1974–1975 season, a total of 253 injuries were reported, and again the majority were caused by sticks. Of these, 16% resulted in blindness in the injured eye. Pashby et al. observed that "the number of blinding injuries was a shocking revelation which demanded action." Because of their efforts great strides have been made in the development of stan-

dardized face protectors for forwards and defensemen.

The early development of protective equipment in ice hockey, as well as in most other sports, has been the product of the efforts of various players, coaches, trainers, and craftsmen, with little if any engineering or mechanical input. Jacques Plante, a former great goaltender from Montreal, was responsible for helping to develop the protective face mask. During the early years of his career, Plante suffered four separate fractures of his nose, fractures of both cheekbones, and two separate fractures of his mandible. In addition, he sustained a number of facial lacerations that required more than 250 stitches. In 1956, while playing goalie for Montreal, he experimented with a wire face mask. Because of the distorted optical relationship caused by the wire and the feeling of "dizziness" that he experienced when wearing the mask, he discarded it. Philip Burchmore, a Canadian who worked with fiberglass, suggested to Plante, in 1957, the feasibility of constructing a fiberglass face mask. Two years later, after he had stopped several more pucks with his face, Plante pursued Burchmore's suggestion. In the spring of 1959 a fiberglass mask was constructed from a plaster mold taken of Plante's face.

Because of strenuous objections from the Montreal coach, the mask was not worn. The coach believed it would obstruct Plante's vision, and, equally important, he told Plante that the scars he was accumulating would be "trophies" to be cherished in his later years. Plante acquiesced to the coach's objections. On Nov 1, 1959, in a game in Madison Square Garden between Montreal and New York, the Rangers' winger Andy Bathgate shot a puck at Plante from a sharp angle. It struck Plante above his upper lip, ripping part of his nose from his face. At that time the teams carried only one goalie, and Montreal was vying for an advantaged position in the Stanley Cup Playoff. Plante was taken to the locker room, and the laceration was hastily sutured. He agreed to return to the game only if he could wear his fiberglass mask; this time the coach relented. Montreal won the game 4 to 1. While wearing the mask, Plante led Montreal on an 11-game winning streak, and the Canadians swept Chicago and Toronto to win the Stanley Cup in eight games. In addition, for the fifth time in his career, Plante won the Vezina trophy as the National Hockey Leagues' outstanding goalie. However, it was not until 1964, when Detroit Redwings' goalie, Terry Sawchuck, started wearing the fiberglass mask that it became generally accepted.

Plante's performance as a goaltender is documented in the record book. For future generations of hockey players, however, Plante's lasting contribution to the game will be that of a pioneer in protective equipment. Without the benefit of biomechanical, biomaterial, medical, or scientific testing expertise, he helped develop a protective mask that eventually every goalkeeper from the amateur through the professional levels wore.

Unfortunately the fiberglass goalie mask did not prove to be invulnerable. Bernie Parent, the premiere goalie for the Philadelphia Flyers, sustained a career-ending intraocular injury during the 1978–1979 season when the tip of a hockey stick penetrated the visual aperture in his mask, striking him in his eye. Apparently a similar injury had happened to Buffalo's Gerry DesJardin. What is surprising is not that these injuries occurred to Parent and DesJardin, but rather that they have not occurred more frequently. Inspection of the molded fiberglass protective goalie mask reveals that the contour of the device is such that the periocular area has a funnel-like configuration that tends to deflect the ends of sticks and pucks directly into contact with the eye, which lies flush against the aperture (Fig 1–10).

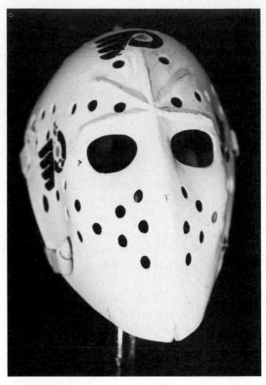

FIG 1–10.
The molded fiberglass protective goalie mask appears invulnerable. Severe eye injuries resulted, however, from stick ends penetrating the visual aperture.

The work of Pashby and his coworkers in Canada and of Vinger in the United States has contributed to the further development and establishment of standards for size, position, visual resolution, prismatic deviation, haze, luminous transmittance, peripheral vision, and penetration for protective masks for goalies as well as for line players (Fig 1–11).

"AN OUNCE OF PREVENTION"

For those responsible for dealing with athletic injuries, whether they occur to the head, neck, face, or other areas of the body, the adage, "an ounce of prevention is worth a pound of cure," is well taken. The logical sequence in this regard is to first identify the problem by applying sound epidemiologic principles. Once the problem has been identified, ei-

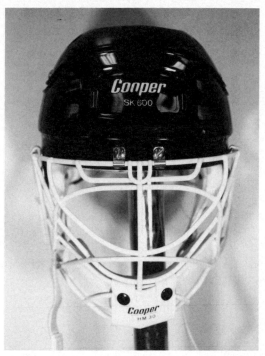

FIG 1–11.
The wire protective goalie mask provides better vision and ventilation, and is firmly attached to the helmet. Presumably, its configuration makes the eye less vulnerable to direct-blow injury.

ther with regard to the severity of the sequelae or the frequency of occurrence of the injury, appropriate modifications of conditioning methods, protective equipment, playing technique, and rules modifications should be implemented on the basis of sound scientific methodology. Available expertise in engineering, materials, and medicine precludes an anecdotal approach to these problems. Existing regulatory and administrative bodies for the many amateur, interscholastic, intercollegiate, and professional athletic activities should establish, support financially, and be guided by injury-prevention research commissions. These commissions should consist of experts from both industry and the academic communities working independently to deal with the matter of injury prevention.

The National Operating Committee on Standards for Athletic Equipment (NOCSAE) is the existing prototype for such research commissions. Established in 1970 in response to a concern about the safety of protective equipment used in competitive sports, NOCSAE is a non-profit corporation. The charter members were the NCAA, the National Federation of State High School Associations (NFSHSA), the National Junior College Athletic Association, the Sporting Goods Manufacturers Association, the American College Health Association, and the National Athletic Trainers Association. Subsequently, the National Sporting Goods Dealers Association, the National Athletic Equipment Reconditioners Association, and the National Association for Intercollegiate Athletics were added to the membership. Consisting of representatives from each of these organizations, the group authorized and sponsored in-depth experimentation of protective equipment conducted by the Gurdjian-Lissner Biomechanics Laboratory at Wayne State University in Detroit. The objectives of this organization have been to promote, conduct, and foster research and to study, analyze, and collect data and statistics relating to athletic equipment, with the view of encouraging the establishment of safety standards. They also disseminate information and promote, conduct, and further activities designed to increase knowledge and understanding of safety, comfort, utility, and the legal aspects of athletic equipment. NOCSAE provides a forum with which individuals and organizations may consult and cooperate in considering problems related to athletics. All activities of the organization are for charitable, educational, and scientific purposes.

REFERENCES

1. Blyth CS, Arnold DC: The forty-seventh annual survey of football fatalities: 1931–1978. *Athletic Training* 1979; 4:234.

2. Committee on Accident and Poison Prevention of the American Academy of Pediatrics. *Am Acad Ped News and Comment* 1977; 28:5.

3. Gonzales TA: Fatal injury in competitive sports. *JAMA* 1951; 146:1506.

4. Kirshenbaum J: Time for reform. *Sports Illustrated* 1980; 52:Feb 18, 12.

5. Nicholas JA: *Hippocrates, the Father of Sports Medicine.* Institute of Sports Medicine and Athletic Training, Lenox Hill Hospital, 1975.

6. Nicholas JA: What sports medicine is about. *Community Med* 1978; 42:4.

7. Pashby TJ: Eye injuries in Canadian amateur hockey. *Am J Sports Med* 1979; 7:254.

8. Pashby TJ, Pashby RC, Chisholm LD: Eye injuries in Canadian hockey. *Can Med Assoc J* 1975; 113:663.

9. Rapp GF, Nicely PG: Trampoline injuries. *Am J Sports Med* 1978; 6:269.

10. Schneider RC: *Head and Neck Injuries in Football.* Baltimore, Williams & Wilkins, 1973.

11. Shields CL Jr, Fox JM, Stauffer ES: Cervical cord injuries in sports. *Phys Sportsmed* 1978; 6:71.

12. Torg JS, et al.: Collision with springloaded football tackling and blocking dummies. *JAMA* 1976; 236:1270.

13. Torg JS, et al.: Severe and catastrophic neck injuries resulting from tackle football. *J Am Coll Health Assoc* 1977; 25:224.

14. Torg JS, et al.: The National Football Head and Neck Injury Registry: 14 Year Report on Cervical Quadriplegia, 1971–1984. *JAMA* 1985; 254:3439–3443.

15. Unterharnscheidt FJ: Injuries due to boxing and other sports. *Handbook Clin Neurol* 1975; 23:527.

16. Vinger PF, Tolpin DW: Racquet sports: An ocular hazard. *JAMA* 1978; 239:2575.

CHAPTER 2

An Epidemiologic View

Kenneth S. Clarke, Ph.D.

The purpose of this chapter is to characterize, with available epidemiologic data, the current picture of athletic injuries to the head, neck, and face. Attention is given to the degree of severity of these injuries in descending order: fatalities, nonfatal catastrophic injuries (e.g., quadriplegia), and potentially catastrophic neurotrauma (e.g., concussion).

EPIDEMIOLOGY

Epidemiology is concerned with studying the distribution of disease or injury within a population and its environment. Its method is to follow frequencies and patterns of distribution in the search for causative agents (determinants). The goals are to remove or negate the influence of an alleged determinant, and then to observe whether the distribution of that disease or injury has been altered accordingly.

While addressing itself to cause and effect, the epidemiologic model must deal with associations. One must appreciate that a documented association between a hypothesized determinant, for example, a defectively designed helmet, and a particular type of injury, such as cerebral neurotrauma, does not constitute proof of cause and effect. A stable lessening of the problem after removing the alleged agent would be strong confirmation of that hypothesis, but a more powerful argument obtained with epidemiologic data is that of "disconfirmation." If, for example, a particular helmet is alleged to be the cause of serious cerebral neurotrauma because of its defective design, a strong association between the use of that helmet and such injuries *must* be found, or the cause-effect relationship is disconfirmed.

To evaluate injury patterns (frequencies and associations), comparison must be made. Whether the comparison is year to year, sport to sport, squad to squad, helmet to helmet, or male to female, one must have both a reasonable rationale and sufficient data to permit a fair comparison. The epidemiologic model requires a merging of population data, exposure data, injury data, and injury scenario data for that purpose. We first need to characterize the population at risk and then to reasonably establish the opportunity for them to contract the disease, that is, the opportunity for them to receive an injury. The experiences recorded as injuries can then be put in perspective with the use of "rates."

For example, 50 athletes attending 5 practices constitute 250 athlete-exposures, that is, the opportunity for 250 injuries. If 2 were injured, the rate would be 2 cases per 250 athlete-exposures, or 80/10,000 athlete-exposures. If variation in length of season between squads is not substantial, a rate of 2 cases per 50 athletes, or 4/100 athletes, would also be a legitimate expression. More precise measures of exposure may be warranted for particular detailed investigations.

Other types of rates may be used to help understand a problem. The number of athletes per case, for example, one football fatality for every 175,000 athletes, gives a probability figure that can be used for describing and comparing an individual's risk in sport. The number of squads per case gives a probability figure helpful to a sponsoring institution's understanding of its relative risk of experiencing a case.

Injury scenario data (related circumstances) are necessary to examine associations of the many potentially preventive or injurious factors, individually and in combination, with the injuries experienced.

The bottom line in epidemiology is knowing the incidence of the problem (frequency of new cases within a population). Without a baseline, the effectiveness of preventive measures cannot be evaluated. But without identifying patterns within the aggregate of injuries as well, there is no beacon for foreseeing the relative merits of suggested preventive measures.

FATALITIES

Football is the only school-college sport for which sufficient mortality incidence data are available since 1931.[2] The data first received epidemiologic treatment in the mid-1960s.[4] In that study, the football fatality data had been reported by the Metropolitan Life Insurance Company.[11] Table 2–1 presents relative risk obtained when the epidemiologic consideration of population-at-risk to raw totals is added.

The purpose of that study, however, was to demonstrate the epidemiologic te-

TABLE 2–1.

Average Annual Fatality Rates in Selected Competitive Sports, 1960–1964*

Sport	Fatalities	Fatality Rate/100,000 Participants
Football	26	3.9
Power boating	1	16.7
Auto racing	30	120.0
Horse racing	2	133.3
Motorcycling	5	178.6

*From Clarke K: JAMA 1966; 197:894. Used with permission.

net of exposure, as well as population, for evaluating the actuarial question of football deaths. The resulting statistical rationale yielded a 1:1 ratio when the fatality rate from football among football players aged 15 to 24 was compared with the fatality rate among all male individuals in that age group from all accidental causes. In other words, when an athlete stepped on the football field in 1964, one of the worst years in modern football in terms of fatalities, he was no higher an insurance risk for traumatic death than his nonparticipating peers. This exercise also yielded a ratio, again controlled for population and exposure, of one football-related fatality for every nine auto-related fatalities among male individuals in that age group, automobile driving being the only alternative activity for which sufficient data were available to permit such a comparison.

The same rationale was applied 10 years later with use of 1974 data.[8] Not only did the actuarial picture for football remain favorable, but also the football-auto fatality ratio now was 1:27. During the intervening decade deaths in football had decreased, while participation (population and exposure) had increased.

Putting these data in another perspective, in high school and college football, one fatality occurred during Fall 1974 for every 6 million athlete-exposures. In 1964 it had been one fatality for every 1.5 million athlete-exposures; since 1977 it has been one fatality for every 10 million athlete-exposures.

Head and Neck Injury Fatalities

From the 1950s through the present, approximately nine of every ten football deaths from traumatic injury have involved the head or neck. By distinguishing between head and neck injuries, different frequency patterns are seen, however (Fig 2–1). The development of the modern helmet and face mask in the 1950s and 1960s was associated with changes in blocking and tackling techniques, that is, the helmeted head was brought into contact more purposefully. It is apparent that these changes were accompanied by a substantial increase in deaths from head injuries, while deaths from cervical cord injury remained infrequent yet persistent through the years. The trend in head-related fatalities was not only reversed by the early 1970s, but after 1976 it also dropped down to the "infrequent yet persistent" level of neck injuries. Several determinants were undoubtedly responsible.

In the late 1960s the National Operating Committee on Standards for Athletic Equipment (NOCSAE) initially formed to develop standards against which all football helmet models were to be tested successfully before being marketed. By 1974 these standards were being utilized by all manufacturers, even though the wearing of helmets, which had passed NOCSAE standards, was not to be mandatory until 1978 at the college level and until 1980 at the high school level.

Also, by the late 1960s, an educational campaign against spearing had been intensified by the American Medical Association (AMA), National Federation of State High School Associations (NFSHSA), National Collegiate Athletic Association (NCAA), and others.[1] Then in January 1976, high school rules, college rules, and coaching ethics were formally adopted to prohibit tackling-block-

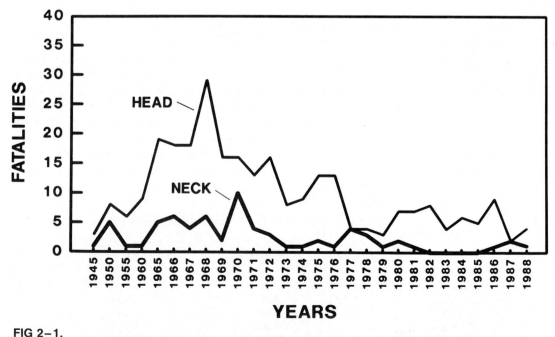

FIG 2–1.
Intracranial and cervical spine injury fatalities, 1945–1988. Data presented were prepared by the author from the AFCA Annual Football Fatality Reports.

ing techniques in which the helmeted head received the brunt of the initial impact. The primary reason for these rules was the vulnerability of the athlete's cervical spine when he struck his opponent with the top or the crown of the helmet (e.g., NCAA Rule 9–1–2–n and NFSHSA Rule 9–3–1). However, the phrasings and intent were also intended to preclude the deliberate use (and the teaching) of face mask and brow contact (e.g., NCAA Rule 9–1–2–1 and NFSHSA Rule 9–3–2–k). The contention was that by leading with the head the player cannot always be sure of achieving the desired football position of "head up, neck bulled" at the moment of contact, and improper execution could put his head or neck in a vulnerable position. When the player was not leading with his head, improper execution was not considered as potentially devastating, and the rule was thereby adopted. In 1978 an organized approach to the coach's education of the athlete concerning the athlete's shared responsibility in this regard was initiated by the NCAA.[13]

To sum up, one can make several observations with respect to fatalities:

1. The advent of conscious attention to helmet standards in the late 1960s and early 1970s was associated with a distinct decrease in deaths related to head injuries.

2. The advent of rule changes in 1976 that prohibited leading with the head for contact was associated with another distinct drop in deaths related to head injuries.

3. The emergence of the face mask in the 1950s and its subsequent continuous use was not accompanied by a sustained increase in the relative frequency of deaths related to neck injuries.

NONFATAL CATASTROPHIC INJURIES

Equivalent trend-line data were not available for nonfatal catastrophic injuries until recently. In 1976 I[6] surveyed retrospectively (1973–1975) spinal cord injuries among the varsity programs of all high schools and colleges in the nation and found gymnastics had the highest average annual injury rate of all the sports (Table 2–2). Of the others, only football and wrestling showed an annual persistence of such injuries. Of these three sports, only gymnastics and football displayed describable patterns.

Gymnastics

The patterns of injury among all gymnastic events revealed that the permanent spinal cord injuries were primarily associated with the trampoline as a training device, but not to the exclusion of other gymnastic apparatuses (Table 2–3). The vast majority of these injuries occurred when the athlete came down incorrectly

TABLE 2–2.

Average Annual Incidence of Spinal Cord Injury in School-College–Sponsored Sports, 1973–1975*

Sport	Athletes/Case	Programs/Case
Gymnastics, men	7,000	281
Gymnastics, women	24,000	1,113
Football	28,000	403
Wrestling	62,000	1,781
Baseball	177,000	6,254
Basketball, men	793,000	23,024

*From Clarke K: J Safety Res 1977; 9:140. Used with permission.

TABLE 2–3.

Adjusted Proportion of Permanent Spinal Cord Injuries by Type of Event in School-College– Sponsored Gymnastics, 1973–1975*

Event	Men (%)	Women (%)
Trampoline	33	71
Minitramp	11	—
Horizontal bar	22	—
Rings	11	—
Floor exercise	22	14
Uneven parallel bars	—	14

From Clarke K: J Safety Res 1977; 9:140. Used with permission.

on the trampoline. This finding, coupled with a subsequent finding that the stricken trampolinist had invariably been attempting a somersault, resulted in national consensus guidelines in 1978 on the controlled use of the trampoline and minitramp.[15, 18]

Another offshoot of this survey was the advent, in July 1978, of a National Registry of Gymnastic Catastrophic Injuries patterned after the American Football Coaches Association (AFCA) Football Fatality Report.[3] In its first 4 years (through June 1982), 20 gymnastic injuries, which resulted in cervical neurotrauma, occurred across the nation: 17 of these persons developed permanent quadriplegia, and 3 died. As shown in Table 2–4, most injuries were to skilled performers while practicing.

The results of the study suggest that catastrophic injuries in gymnastics have lessened substantially since the mid-1970s. Injury control in gymnastics is a reasonable expectation if supervision and training controls are in place.

Football

In Fall 1975, while I was preparing the retrospective survey of spinal cord injuries in school sports and physical education,[6] Torg et al.[17] were establishing a National Football Head and Neck Injury Registry patterned after the clinical case-finding method used by Schneider[12] in

TABLE 2–4.

National Incidence of Gymnastic Catastrophic Injuries, July 1978 through June 1982*

Event	Sex	Person	Circumstances	Injury
1. Trampoline	M	Skilled teenager	Practice, Gymnastics Club	Quadriplegia
2. Trampoline	M	Young boy	Backyard recreation	Death
3. Trampoline	M	Skilled young adult	Backyard game of "Horse"	Quadriplegia
4. Trampoline	M	Advanced beginner teen	Military base recreation	Quadriplegia
5. Trampoline	M	College asst. instructor	P.E. class demonstration	Quadriplegia
6. Minitramp	M	College cheerleader	Warmup for football game	Quadriplegia
7. Minitramp	M	High school gymnast	Practice for pep rally	Quadriplegia
8. Tumbling	F	High school cheerleader	Cheerleader practice	Death
9. Trampoline	M	College gymnast	Practicing Hi-Bar dismount	Quadriplegia
10. Unevens	F	High school gymnast	Practicing routine	Quadriplegia
11. Minitramp	M	College cheerleader	Unscheduled practice	Quadriplegia
12. Minitramp	F	High school gymnast	Practice for competition	Quadriplegia
13. Trampoline	M	Skilled young adult	Backyard recreation	Quadriplegia
14. Minitramp	M	Skilled college student	Intramural activity	Quadriplegia
15. Unevens	F	College gymnast	Practice for competition	Quadriplegia
16. Trampoline	M	College P.E. instructor	Demonstration in class	Quadriplegia
17. Vault	F	Skilled H.S. student	Physical education class	Quadriplegia
18. Trampoline	M	College student	Physical education class	Quadriplegia
19. Unevens	F	Unskilled Jr. H.S. student	Physical education class	Death
20. Rings	M	Semiskilled H.S. student	Physical education class	Quadriplegia

From Christensen C: Fourth Annual Gymnastics Catastrophic Injury Report. Washington, D.C., U.S. Gymnastics Safety Association, 1984. Used with permission.

TABLE 2–5.

Proportion of Quadriplegic Cases in School-College Football Associated With Tackling

	Torg* (%) (1971–1975)	Clarke* (%) (1973–1975)
High school	72	83
College	78	83

Data from Torg J, et al: JAMA 1979; 241:1477; Clarke J: J Safety Res 1977; 9:140.

1963. Initially, Torg et al. solicited retrospective documentation of catastrophic cases experienced during the 1971 through 1975 seasons, in order to have a 5-year period comparable to that of Schneider (1959–1963). In cooperation with the AFCA system, Torg et al. continued to maintain the Registry as a continuous surveillance system, but extended the survey to injuries other than fatalities. In 1985 they completed a survey review of the status of all athletes in the Registry, making some minor changes in the original data that had been published earlier. Tables 2–5 and 2–6 compare their findings for catastrophic injury patterns in football during 1971–1975 with my findings for 1973–1975. The high degree of compatibility lends credence to the principal injury scenario of a defensive back coming up to make an open-field tackle.

Tables 2–7 and 2–8 display the different patterns of serious neurotrauma in high school–college football during the

TABLE 2–6.

Proportion of Quadriplegic Cases in School-College Football Associated With Selected Positions

	Torg* (%) (1971–1975)	Clarke* (%) (1973–1975)
Defensive back		
High school	52	50
College	73	67
Linebacker		
High school	10	29
College	0	0

Data from Torg J, et al: JAMA 1979; 241:1477; Clarke J: J Safety Res 1977; 9:140.

TABLE 2–7.

Comparison of Permanent Cerebral Injuries Nationally in High School–College Football

	Schneider* (1959–1963)	Torg* (1971–1975)
Total cases reported	112	72
High school–college cases	87 (est.)	65
Average annual incidence/100,000 athletes	2.6 (est.)	1.0
Fatal cases	41%	81%

Data from Schneider R: Clin Neurosurg 1965; 12:226; Torg J, et al: JAMA 1979; 241:1477.

1959–1963 and the 1971–1975 eras. Essentially, both the frequency of, and mortality from, serious cerebral injuries decreased. Serious cervical cord injuries, on the other hand, had increased. Their predominantly nonfatal nature had precluded detection of this trend via the annual fatality report.

As seen in Table 2–9, however, Torg et al.'s Registry reveals a distinct drop in quadriplegia after 1976.[16] The incidence in 1977 and 1978 was half that of 1975 and 1976. Since the rule changes in 1976 required profound adjustments of the athlete, coach, and official to new expectations and different techniques, the 1-year lag in its impact was not unexpected. Further, the incidence continued to drop once the success of the rule change became appreciated, and new

TABLE 2–8.

Comparison of Permanent Cervical Spinal Cord Injuries Nationally in High School–College Football

	Schneider* (1953–1963)	Torg* (1971–1975)
Total cases reported	38	99
High school–college cases	30 (est.)	95
Average annual incidence/100,000 athletes	0.9 (est.)	1.5
Fatal cases	42%	8%

Data from Schneider R: Clin Neurosurg 1965; 12:226; Torg J, et al: JAMA 1979; 241:1477.

TABLE 2–9.

Number of Nonfatal Permanent Cervical Neurotrauma Nationally in School–College Football, 1975–87*

	1975	1976	1977	1978	1979	1980	1981
High school	21	23	11	11	8	11	6
College	6	8	1	0	3	2	2
Total	27	31	12	11	11	13	8

	1982	1983	1984	1985	1986	1987
High school	7	9	4	5	6	7
College	1	1	0	2	0	0
Total	8	10	4	7	6	7

From Torg J: Cervical neurotrauma in football. Unpublished presentation, American Orthopaedic Society for Sports Medicine. Annual Meeting, July 1989, and subsequent personal communications.

football players, who learned the proper technique from the outset, became the population at risk.

Calculated as rates, the current incidence of permanent cervical cord injury, nonfatal and fatal combined, was one per 100,000 athletes in 1977 and 1978, the same as that during the period of the Schneider study[12] (see Table 2–8).

Thus the various efforts in the late 1960s toward the development of mandatory helmet standards, and in the teaching and practice of blocking-tackling techniques, eventually resulted in a decline in the frequency of both fatal and nonfatal catastrophic neurotrauma. This does not mean that all helmets in use at that time were substandard; it means that all helmet models being sold had not yet been subjected to performance tests that would provide confidence that they were not substandard. Similarly, this does not mean that coaches were necessarily teaching an improper technique; it means that improper execution of certain techniques constituted a highly serious hazard.

The Torg versus Schneider data initially suggested that a tradeoff was occurring: the quest for helmet standards was associated with both lowered cerebral injury frequencies and increased cervical cord injuries. To some this meant that the modern helmet was literally causing these injuries (back of helmet forcibly im-

pinging on the spine) instead of, or in addition to, prompting the well-protected athlete to "stick his head-neck in places where he never used to." The distinct drop in the frequency of cervical cord injuries since 1976 disconfirms the implication of the helmets as causative agents, however. The premise for the 1976 rule changes was that helmets can neither cause nor prevent the serious neck injury; it is principally a matter of the blocking-tackling technique. The available epidemiologic data are consistent with that contention.

As was the case for fatalities alone, the trends in relative frequency of all cervical neurotrauma, which by 1978 had returned to that of 1960, do not support an indictment of the face mask as a causative agent.

Intracranial Hemorrhage

Torg et al.'s Registry obtains information about the annual incidence of nonfatal intracranial hemorrhage, as well as quadriplegia, from football.[16] Whether permanent neurologic deficit resulted from the hemorrhage is not, unfortunately, obtained consistently by the Registry, and this remains a problem that would benefit from more intensive follow-up prerogative. From 1976 through 1987, of the 99 such injuries that were reported (about 8 per year), three fifths of those injured were known to have returned to normal, and about one per year (on the average) was known to have had some residual deficit. The remaining one fourth of reported cases were of unknown outcome.

POTENTIALLY CATASTROPHIC INJURIES

We cannot ignore severe injuries because they are infrequent, nor can we focus only on these injuries. The National Athletic Injury/Illness Reporting System (NAIRS) has been following all athletic injuries in various sports since 1975, including the potentially serious head injuries called concussions.[5]

Concussions

In the NAIRS system, a reportable concussion is any disorientation caused by trauma that required cessation of play to examine the athlete, no matter how momentary the symptoms nor the subsequent disposition of the athlete with respect to participation. The rate of reportable concussions among the collegiate athletes followed by NAIRS is found in Table 2–10. One concussion in football result-

ed in death; none of the others produced perceptible permanent brain damage. By both population and exposure, football clearly is the sport most frequently associated with these injuries. Adjusted for exposure, however, the data reveal a difference between Spring football and Fall football. They also show strikingly uniform rates among the other sports.

NAIRS is also able to retrieve injury data by degrees of severity. Customarily, preference for analysis is given the *significant* injuries, that is, those keeping the athlete out of participation for at least 1 week. Table 2–11 reveals that the year-to-year rates of both reportable and significant concussions in football were stable.[9] Since the 1976 rule changes, however, the proportion of significant concussions resulting from tackling has dropped steadily.

Football Helmets.—While cerebral concussion is an infrequent occurrence in football, the next concern is whether particular helmets may be contributing to more than their share of these injuries. If a particular helmet is sufficiently defective in design to account for a disproportionate number of these injuries, the rate of concussions would be lowered if that helmet were removed from use.

TABLE 2–10.

Average Annual Incidence of Reportable Concussions in Selected College Sports, 1975–1977*

	Average Number of Teams	Cases/10,000 Athlete-Exposures	Cases/ 100 Athletes
Football, Spring	26	11.1	2.2
Football, Fall	49	7.3	6.1
Lacrosse	5	4.1	1.9
Ice hockey	8	3.5	3.7
Softball (women)	10	3.5	1.7
Wrestling	20	3.0	2.5
Basketball (women)	21	2.7	2.2
Soccer	13	2.7	1.6

*From the National Athletic Injury/Illness Reporting System. The Pennsylvania State University, 1979. Used with permission. NAIRS data bearing no reference to other published work were prepared by me with the assistance of the NAIRS staff for inclusion in this chapter.

TABLE 2–11.

Average Annual Rate (Cases/100 Athletes) of Concussions in Collegiate Football Accompanied by Proportion of Significant Concussions Associated With Tackling*

Concussions	1975	1976	1977	1978
Reportable	5.8	6.4	6.0	7.0
Significant	0.6	0.7	0.6	0.6
(while tackling)	58%	40%	30%	23%

From the National Athletic Injury/Illness Reporting System. The Pennsylvania State University, 1979. Used with permission.

NAIRS data were examined for this possibility, with Table 2–12 displaying the findings for significant concussions per 1,000 athlete-exposures per type and brand of helmet for the seasons of 1975 through 1977.[9] Clearly, these injuries were distributed randomly through the population proportionate to the frequency of use of each helmet.

NAIRS data also were examined for the association of particular helmets with major cervical spine fractures.[9] These data are presented in view of the conten-

tion of some that the back edge of certain helmets can produce a "karate chop" injury to the spine, causing quadriplegia. The data are presented in Table 2–13 in terms of manufacturer only instead of type and brand, because shell configuration did not vary within brand. Rates were expressed per 100,000 athlete-exposures because of the rarity of these occurrences. The criterion of *major* injury used was more than 3 weeks' absence from participation.

Only six major vertebral injuries occurred during the three seasons in which there were more than one million athlete-exposures, with only one resulting in neurologic deficit.

The vast number of helmet contacts in a season (giving ample opportunity for a defective design to operate), the infrequency of this type of injury, and the proportionate distribution of these injuries commensurate with the number of helmets being worn epidemiologically disconfirmed the allegation that the helmet causes cervical injury.

TABLE 2–12.

Average Annual Rate (Cases/1000 Athlete-Exposures) of Significant Concussions by Type and Brand of Helmet in School-College Football, 1975–1977*

	All Helmets	Helmet												
		#1	#2	#3	#4	#5	#6	#7	#8	#9	#10	#11	#12	#13
Rate	0.1	0.1	0.1	0.1	0.1	0.1	0.1	0.1	0.0	0.1	0.0	0.0	0.1	0.0
Cases	92	7	19	6	24	2	5	19	0	3	3	0	3	0
% Use	100	6.5	22.7	9.9	15.2	2.7	5.8	19.7	3.2	2.7	5.9	0.1	2.1	0.5

From Clarke K, Powell J: Med Sci Sports 1979; 11:138. Used with permission.

TABLE 2–13.

Average Annual Rate (Cases/100,000 Athlete-Exposures) of Major Cervical Spine Fractures by Brand of Helmet in School-College Football, 1975–1977*

	All Helmets	Helmet						
		#1	#2	#3	#4	#5	#6	#7
Rate	0.5	0.0	0.5	0.0	1.4	2.4	0.0	0.0
Cases	6	0	4	0	1	1	0	0
% Used	100	8.6	60.7	6.6	5.9	3.5	2.9	10.2

From Clarke K, Powell J: Med Sci Sports 1979; 11:138. Used with permission.

TABLE 2–14.

Annual Rate (Cases/1000 Athlete Exposures) of Significant Concussions by Type of Playing Surface in College Football, 1975–1977*

	1975	1976	1977
Natural grass			
Athlete-exposures	171,386	157,665	318,040
Concussion rate	0.1	0.1	0.1
Astroturf			
Athlete-exposures	95,803	87,382	155,027
Concussion rate	0.0†	0.1	0.1
Tartanturf			
Athlete-exposures	35,300	28,652	43,161
Concussion rate	0.0†	0.1	0.1

*From Clarke K, Alles W, Powell J: An epidemiologic examination of the association of selected products with related injuries in football, 1975–77. Final Report, U.S. Consumer Product Safety Commission, Contract #CPSC-C-77–0039, 1978. Used with permission.
†Not zero but less than 0.05.

Playing Surface.—NAIRS data also made it possible to examine the effect of playing surface on the incidence of selected injuries in college football.[7] The results clearly reveal no undue association of any playing surface with significant concussions, when analyzed on an equivalent exposure basis (Table 2–14). Further, none of the six cervical fractures in Table 2–13 had occurred during participation on an artificial surface, while 35% of the athlete-exposures had been on an artificial surface.

Brachial Plexus ("Burner") Injuries

With the rule changes in 1976 requiring a return to shoulder-blocking and tackling techniques, concern is frequently expressed about an increase in brachial plexus injuries from these changes. The potential for this had been acknowledged by those encouraging the 1976 changes, but the tradeoff between "burners" and quadriplegia presented no argument.

Interestingly, NAIRS data reveal no shift in frequency of reportable or significant brachial plexus injuries after 1976 (Table 2–15). The slight rise in 1978 is not significant, since it is well within the range of normal variation.

Table 2–15 also permits examination of this concern by the proportion of such injuries resulting from tackling (the principal activity associated with this injury). A steady increase in this association is seen among significant brachial plexus injuries from 1975 to 1977 (31% to 47%). In 1978, however, this trend was clearly reversed. It is plausible to assume that the new coaching techniques for tackling have evolved into improved methods, or that better neck-conditioning practices have been implemented. Again, the patterns associated with this injury continue to be followed by NAIRS.

Facial Injuries

In Table 2–16, the frequency of various facial injuries can be compared in different sports. While ice hockey leads

TABLE 2–15.

Rate (Cases/100 Athletes) of Brachial Plexus Injuries in Collegiate Football Accompanied by Proportion of Such Injuries Associated With the Act of Tackling*

	1975	1976	1977	1978
Reportable cases	2.2	2.2	2.2	2.4
(while tackling)	45%	47%	43%	38%
Significant cases	0.5	0.5	0.5	0.7
(while tackling)	31%	40%	47%	27%

*From the National Athletic Injury/Illness Reporting System, The Pennsylvania State University, 1979. Used with permission.

TABLE 2–16.

Average Annual Rate (Cases/100 Athletes) of Facial Injuries in Selected Collegiate Sports by Category of Injury, 1975–1978*

	Eye-Orbit	Maxillofacial	Mouth-Teeth	Total
Ice hockey	3.8	14.3	9.3	27.4
Wrestling	2.8	2.9	2.0	7.7
Basketball	1.3	2.1	2.7	6.1
Field hockey (W)	1.1	1.7	2.4	5.2
Basketball (W)	1.4	1.0	2.1	4.5
Football, Spring	1.1	2.1	1.1	4.3
Soccer	0.3	1.1	1.1	2.5
Football, Fall	0.3	1.2	0.5	2.0

From the National Athletic Injury/Illness Reporting System, The Pennsylvania State University, 1979. Used with permission.

all other sports in frequency of facial injuries, most of this dominance is related to injuries that have few neural implications. Injuries to the eye and orbit are infrequent, yet pose a persistent threat to an athlete participating in any sport. This is one injury category in which Fall football is in last place among the injury-producing sports.

Noncatastrophic injuries with a potential for neurologic impairment can be evaluated only from 1975 to the present. Within this time span, the frequency of these injuries has remained stable at what can be considered a tolerable level. Further, patterns within these frequencies do not implicate a particular type or brand of helmet or playing surface. Much additional analysis of other potential factors is warranted if further practicable preventive measures are to be identified for implementation and evaluation.

CONCLUSIONS

Catastrophic neurotrauma in organized sports is infrequent, yet consistently associated with gymnastics, football, and wrestling. Such injuries occur periodically in other sports, such as baseball and basketball, but not with the persistence that would enable epidemiologic analysis.

From the catastrophic data at hand, fatal and nonfatal, the recent definitive measures adopted by those sharing responsibility for school and college sports have been followed by a substantial lessening of the problems that had been identified:

1. The 1978 clarification of guidelines for the controlled use of the trampoline and minitramp in school and college programs has been followed with a drop in catastrophic injuries from these activities.

2. The decision to promulgate uniform testing standards for football helmets in the late 1960s was accompanied by a downward trend in serious cerebral trauma.

3. The decision, in 1976, to outlaw by rule and ethic the use of the helmeted head as the initial point of contact in blocking and tackling was followed by both another drop in fatal cerebral injuries and a substantial drop in cervical spinal cord injuries. Moreover, these latter changes have not caused (to date) an anticipated increase in another neurologic type of injury, that to the brachial plexus.

In addition, analysis of recent epidemiologic data disconfirmed the possibility that a particular type or brand of helmet or playing surface was a determinant in cerebral or spinal injuries in football.

Further, continuous use of the face mask during the period of evaluation was not associated with any trends that would suggest its involvement as a determinant in serious neck injuries. This is corroborated by Torg et al.'s clinical analysis of each case reported to their Registry, and by Shield's analysis of the 16 patients with football quadriplegia who were admitted to Rancho Los Amigos Hospital from 1964 through 1973. Of these, only one was labeled as hyperextensive.[14, 16]

Before 1978, no quadriplegia from hockey had been recorded; in 1987 the number of occurrences of permanent neurotrauma in hockey was estimated to be about 4 per year.[10] As in football, the advent of better helmets and face masks caused a change in the athlete's use of the head. In this instance, players began letting their helmeted head take the impact of going into the boards when checked from the rear, that is, they "speared" the boards, causing quadriplegia. As a result, amateur hockey rules were changed in 1988 to permit checking from the rear to be a major penalty, and coaches were advised to prohibit checking from the rear in practice and to educate their athletes as to this problem. Torg et al.'s Registry is now following this sport as well as football.

In football, as in gymnastics and ice hockey, and probably in wrestling and other sports in which reliable data are not available, the problem of neurotrauma is principally a matter of player technique and conditioning (conditioning should be considered part of "technique"). Education of coaches, athletes, and officials about the catastrophic hazards of improper techniques should continue to be emphasized in preventive efforts.

A catastrophic injury, however, is only one outcome on an injury spectrum of graded severity stemming from a particular etiologic mechanism. It is advisable to monitor continuously any injury pattern that is associated with the threat of permanent impairment.

REFERENCES

1. AMA Committee on the Medical Aspects of Sports: Spearing and Football, in *Tips on Athletic Training*. X. Chicago, American Medical Association, 1968.

2. Blyth C, Arnold D: *The Forty-seventh Annual Football Fatality Report*. Chapel Hill, NC, The American Football Coaches Association, 1979.

3. Christensen C: *Fourth Annual Gymnastics Catastrophic Injury Report*. Washington, DC, U.S. Gymnastics Safety Association, 1984.

4. Clarke K: Calculated risk of sports fatalities. *JAMA* 1966; 197:894.

5. Clarke K: Premises and pitfalls of athletic injury surveillance. *Am J Sports Med* 1975; 3:292.

6. Clarke K: Survey of spinal cord injuries in schools and college sports, 1973–75. *J Safety Res* 1977; 9:140.

7. Clarke K, Alles W, Powell J: An *Epidemiological Examination of the Association of Selected Products With Related Injuries in Football, 1975–77. Final Report*. U.S. Consumer Product Safety Commission, Contract No. CPSC-C–77–0039, 1978.

8. Clarke K, Braslow A: Football fatalities in actuarial perspective. *Med Sci Sports* 1979; 10:94.

9. Clarke K, Powell J: Football helmets and neurotrauma—an epidemiological overview of three seasons. *Med Sci Sports* 1979; 11:138.

10. Clarke K: Critical role of epidemiological studies in assessing the frequency and causative factors in sports related injuries, in *Safety in Hockey Symposium Proceedings*, American Society for Testing of Materials, 1981.

11. Competitive sports and their hazards. *Stat Bull Metrop Insur Co* 1965; 46:1.

12. Schneider R: Serious and fatal neurosurgical football injuries. *Clin Neurosurg* 1965; 12:226.

13. *Shared Responsibility for Sports Safety*. A statement of the Committee on Competitive Safeguards and Medical Aspects of Sports. Shawnee Mission, Kan, National College Athletic Association, 1978.

14. Shields C, Fox J, Stauffer E: Cervical cord injuries in sports. *Phys Sportsmed* 1978; 6:21.

15. *The Use of Trampolines and Minitramps in Physical Education*. A policy statement of the American Alliance for Health, Physical Education, Recreation, and Dance. Washington, D.C., 1978.

16. Torg J: *Cervical Neurotrauma in Football*. Unpublished presentation, American Orthopaedic Society for Sports Medicine, Annual Meeting,

July 1979, and subsequent personal communications.

17. Torg J, et al.: The National Head and Neck Injury Registry—report and conclusions, 1978. *JAMA* 1979; 241:1477.

18. *Use of the Trampoline for the Development of Competitive Skills.* A policy statement of the National Collegiate Athletic Association Committee on Competitive Safeguards and Medical Aspects of Sports. Shawnee Mission, Kan, 1978.

CHAPTER 3

Impact Standards for Protective Equipment*

Voigt R. Hodgson

The object of impact Standards is to minimize injuries through the efforts of protective equipment designers to meet at least a minimum level of protection performance. The level of protection performance is based on a criterion referred to the best available human tolerance data in tests that, in conformity with human performance and practical considerations, are designed to simulate rarely exceeded field collisions. Head protection in sports can be divided grossly into helmets designed to protect against blunt surface and concentrated surface (e.g., missile) impacts. The National Operating Committee on Standards for Athletic Equipment (NOCSAE) football helmet (blunt surfaces) and baseball batter's helmet Standards will be discussed as typical.

When a serious injury to the head, neck, or face occurs in competitive sports, the protective equipment or the standard with which it complied (or both) is often brought into question. It is important before describing the formulation of standards for protective equip-ment,† and what is expected to be accomplished by them, to list some of the factors that limit the expectations:

1. Increased protection for one area can adversely affect other areas of the body.

2. We are limited in terms of our knowledge concerning injury mechanisms, injury criteria, range of human tolerance, impact environment, making surrogates, measurement technique and accuracy, impact environment simulation, and epidemiology, for example.

3. Parts of the body where equipment with improved impact protection is worn may be used more aggressively.

4. Players are getting bigger, faster, more specialized, and, therefore, becoming more skilled and punishing performers.

5. There are practical limitations in size, weight, cost, mobility, appearance, and construction of protective equipment.

6. With so much money and acclaim now available for those who excel in

*Funded in part by the National Operating Committee on Standards for Athletic Equipment, Wayne State University Patton Hammers-Neurosciences Fund, and the Neurotrauma Prevention Fund.

†National Operating Committee on Standards for Athletic Equipment (NOCSAE): *Standard Method of Impact Test and Performance Requirements for Football Helmets*, revised 1988; ditto *Baseball Batter's Helmet*, revised July 1987.

sports, safety for self and others is often a low priority item.

Despite all of these limitations on injury reduction, the combination of art and science that goes into standards for protective equipment is challenging and has led to some very worthwhile results that are discussed in the following sections.

HEAD PROTECTION

Mechanical injury to the brain can apparently result from one or a combination of the following physical phenomena acting to cause excessive stress at some location in brain tissue or vasculature: (1) linear acceleration, (2) angular acceleration, and (3) excessive pressure under the impact site.

The first two are usually associated with diffuse injuries such as concussion[1] and diffuse axonal injury.[2]

The third results in a focal injury under the impact site if the energy level and concentration of forces overwhelm the helmet and produce excessive deflection or disruption of the skull sufficient to cause injury to the brain surface or vasculature. If the impact force is distributed over a sufficiently small or weak area, focal injury can occur with relatively low head acceleration. The temple area is particularly vulnerable to focal injury forces because of the thin bone and the meningeal artery branches coursing between the bone and the dura mater in this region.

Focal injuries such as subdural hematomas (SDH) remote from the impact site, resulting from rupture of a bridging vessel, can also be caused by the sudden relative motion between skull and brain, most likely due to angular acceleration but possibly to linear acceleration also. Because of the potentially catastrophic nature of cerebrovascular injuries, high-

est priorities of protection should be assigned to prevent SDH. Knowledge of how they occur (either the head motion causing them, or low-tolerance individuals, or a combination of both) is rare. For this reason we cannot accumulate enough evidence to be certain of what can be done practically within limitations of performance in a sport such as football.

It appears at this point that for the vast majority of players concussion is the threshold injury. Equipment designed to meet standard test methods and criteria that minimize this injury will also minimize other injuries. In a recent study of three levels of National Collegiate Athletic Association (NCAA) football, Zemper[3] reported the number of concussions for the 1982, 1983, 1986, and 1987 seasons to be 134/4998, 112/4383, 73/3431, and 69/2798 concussions/players, respectively, the majority being of the grade 1 or dazed variety. If these rates were projected across the approximately 1,500,000 high school and college players, they would equate to an average of more than 36,000 concussions annually. The number of reported cerebral injuries, mostly SDHs that resulted in no permanent disability, permanent disability, or death, has fluctuated between 8 and 13 annually for all levels of play during the 1984–1987 seasons.[4, 5]

Protection against concussion in terms of numbers and severity among players appears, from experience, to be best accomplished in the following manner. Make the shell and the liner combine to absorb energy over the widest range of impact intensity anticipated. Energy absorption should be sufficient to maintain the magnitude and rate of onset of forces acting on the head (as judged by head acceleration response) below those levels that exceed tolerable limits for the maximum number of players. Uncertainties about human tolerance have made this a difficult goal to achieve, but a recent advance in the state of the art of evaluating serious head injury risk versus head injury criterion (HIC)* or Gadd severity index (SI)† levels has helped to reduce some of the guesswork. Mertz and Weber[6] devised a way to evaluate the probability of risk of serious head injury to the population, associated with head injury criterion levels derived from cadaver drop tests that in general produced either more or less than that necessary to cause a threshold injury only.

Prasad and Mertz[7] evaluated data from all available cadaver drop tests in which HIC was computed consisting of those tests (1) attempting to produce linear skull fracture and (2) attempting to produce a simulated cerebrovascular accident. They found that the risk curves that they developed from the cadaver tests associated with either the linear skull fracture or vascular ruptures fell so close to each other that they were plotted as one (Fig 3–1). The solid line is the best estimate, and the dash curves to the left and right are the 5th and 95th percentile estimates, respectively. For example, the best estimate predicts that a HIC of 1,000 would put 15% to 16% of the population at risk of a serious head injury (abbreviated injury scale [AIS][8] of 3 or more). There would be a 95% probability of seriously injuring 3% to 4%, and a 5% probability of seriously injuring about 28% at this level of intensity.

Assuming the results to be the most reliable available, it is now possible to choose the level of risk for which a hel-

met is to be designed for a particular impact environment. It should be kept in mind, however, that the data apply to the entire adult population. According to a government report, the incidence of cerebrovascular disease for 18-year-old and 60-year-old men is 1/100,000 and 100/100,000, respectively,[9] and a similar relationship probably exists for susceptibility to cerebrovascular accidents due to impact. Consequently it is reasonable to assume that Figure 3–1 is somewhat conservative for midteen to mid–20-year-old players.

Validation of the graph by means of surrogate simulation of live injuries is not known to me, but a drop test simulation of a two-player head-to-head impact fatal to both players lends some credibility to it.[10] The first drop onto a rigid flat plate* with an impact velocity of 7.15 m/sec (16 mph) produced 1,500 HIC (1,770 SI), with best estimate that 55% of the population would be at risk of serious injury. At this point the helmet energy-absorbing capability was apparently near saturation, and increasing the speed to only 7.6 m/sec (17 mph) produced a HIC in excess of 2,500 (>3,000 SI), estimated to put more than 99% of the population at risk of a serious brain injury.

Head Model

The most important feature of the test system is the head model. Saczalski et al.[11] have shown how important it is that the surrogate match human response. There is so much interplay between the mechanical properties of the helmet and those of the head, and so little room for error, that unless helmets are tested with a surrogate having the weight, shape, mass distribution, and deformation qualities similar to those of the head, the most efficient use of helmet space to minimize

$$*HIC = \left(t_2 - t_1 \right) \left[\frac{1}{t_2 - t_1} \int_{t_1}^{t_2} a(t)dt \right]^{2.5} \Bigg|_{max}$$

(See references 6 and 7.)

$$\dagger SI = \int_o^T A^{2.5}\, dt \leq 1{,}500,\, where$$

$A = acceleration\ in\ G's$
$2.5 = weighting\ factor$
$t = time\ interval\ in\ seconds$
$T = pulse\ duration\ in\ seconds$
$0.0025 < T < 0.050$

(See references 15, 16, and 19.)

*It was assumed that as reported, at least one of the two dropped straight down as though having run into a rigid wall.

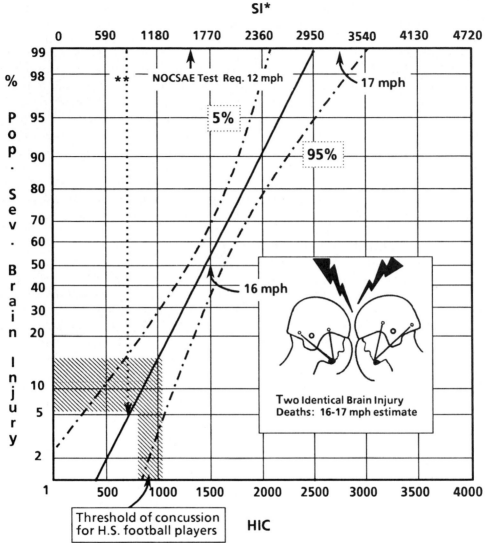

FIG 3–1.
Percent population severe brain injury vs. SI or HIC level.

* The SI relation to HIC values is not constant, but depends on the shape of acceleration -time history of head response. All SI values on this chart have been assumed 18 percent higher than the corresponding HIC.
**Average of first 60 inch drop for all size helmets, all locations on all Standard recertification tests:

	SI	Sdv	G	Sdv	Year
	776	174	146	21	1987
	730	206	142	27	1988
	Best estimate: 5% risk				

stress on the brain during impact will not be achieved. Results obtained from helmets tested on a head form lacking biofidelity of response to the human head cannot be referred to the plot in Figure 3–1. This leaves a greater degree of uncertainty in estimating helmet perfor-mance in the field than by use of a Standard model that attempts to simulate the characteristics of the human head that have been discussed.

Because of cost, helmets are currently made in either two or three shell sizes, with variations in liner thickness to accommodate a range of head sizes in each shell size. In the case of a drop test the largest size in each shell is critical since its liner is thinnest. The requirements of a size 8 helmet, which must decelerate a 6.0 kg (13.2 lb) head, are greater than those of a size 6 ⅝ helmet, which must protect a 4.2 kg (9.3 lb) head in the Standard test. Conversely, in a missile impact test, helmets that fit the small head are generally hardest to pass because, other things being equal, the smaller mass of the small head is accelerated to higher levels than the larger head models when struck. Three sizes of head models, 6 ⅝, 7 ¼, and 7⅝, are currently used in the NOCSAE system. It is difficult to maintain a completely comprehensive line of head model sizes. Critical helmet sizes change as the manufacturers learn on existing sizes that a shift of head size into a larger shell (e.g., size 7¼ changed from medium to large shell) would benefit a large group of players (approximately 65% are size 7¼).

FOOTBALL HEAD PROTECTION— METHODS

Number of Impacts

Football is a multiple-impact sport in which impacts are delivered anywhere on the helmet. Although it is highly unlikely, repetitive blows that significantly deform the liner can occur at or near the same spot. Resilient materials recover their original shape at varying rates. Usually the stiffest and most efficient recover slowest of all, but at the same time cannot be compressed as thin as softer materials to make maximum use of the shell head energy-absorbing space before forces become excessive. To assure protection from repetitive blows, two impacts on each of six locations are required as follows: front, front boss, side, rear boss, rear, and crown. These impacts are delivered at any one location within

75 ± 15 seconds of each other. On front and side locations, two additional incremental drops from lower levels are required to determine the helmet performance as it varies over a range of energy. It is important to screen out a helmet having performance characteristics that increase exponentially and score just under the limit of the minimum requirement. The least slip in quality control of material or construction, change in temperature, or odd-shaped head and the margin of performance below the Standard requirement vanishes.

Impact Surface

Examination of rare films, which are clear enough to display injury impacts, reveals that the primary hazards to the head are impact with other heads, driving knees, padded elbows, or the turf. All four are relatively firm, blunt surfaces. A flat, firm, rubber pad,* 1.3 mm (0.5 in.) thick, mounted on a rigid base is used to simulate these injury surfaces. It is durable, consistent, and avoids unrealistic damage to nylon and metal rivets and fittings on the exterior of the shell, and to shells themselves, which would be caused by a rigid surface. A resilient impact surface is a very important consideration because the Standard test system is used for safety quality control of new and used helmets, not feasible with a destructive test against a rigid surface.

Impact Speed

The fastest football players can run 36.6 m (40 yd) in 4.4 seconds, 8.2 m/sec (27 ft/sec) average speed, evidently reaching maximum speeds of around 10.7 m/sec (35 ft/sec). If a player wearing a helmet runs into a brick wall with his head

---

*With use of the standard system of rating resiliency of rubber and rubberlike materials, the pad is 38 durometer (D) on the Shore A scale.

TABLE 3–1.

Energy Level in NOCSAE Football Helmet Impact Standard for Each of Three Head Models Over Range of Standard Drop Heights, J (ft-lb)*

	Head Model Size		
	Small	Medium	Large
Head weight, kg (lb)	4.2 (9.3)	4.8 (10.5)	6.0 (13.2)
Head and carriage, kg (lb)	6.4 (14)	7.0 (15.3)	8.2 (18.0)
Drop height, cm (in.)			
91 (36)	57 (42)	62 (46)	73 (54)
122 (48)	76 (56)	83 (61)	98 (72)
152 (60)	95 (70)	104 (77)	122 (90)

Joule = ft-lb/1.356.

at this speed, serious injury or death would most likely result. Since it is impossible for what is now considered a helmet of practical size to protect at a 1,500 SI level (approximately 225 G) or less, under these extreme conditions the standard test speed is less than this. Also, football helmets must withstand countless numbers of impacts. For this application, resilient foams that revert to their original shape after impact are the most practical, although not as efficient as crushable foams. By comparison, higher-velocity-performing fiberglass shell crash helmets are designed to self-destruct, primarily for one massive impact, and can be fitted with a rigid foam that crushes at a certain load level. Originally a survey of the performance of representative helmets helped to arrive at a helmet drop

height of 152 cm (60 in.), which produces an impact speed of 5.5 m/sec (17.9 ft/sec). This has not been changed, but the energy level of the test has been raised by increasing the drop weight.

The kinetic energy level at impact for the three head models when dropped from the various heights used in the Standard are given in Table 3–1. It is presently being proposed for all sizes of helmets to meet the Standard performance requirements at a uniform level of energy of 108 J (80 ft-lb), corresponding to an impact speed of 5.6 m/sec (18.2 ft/sec), to go along with a proposal to reduce the SI requirement level described under Performance Requirements. Comparison of energy levels and performance requirements of other helmet standards is given in Table 3–2.

TABLE 3–2.

Comparison of Energy Levels and Approximate Performance Requirements of NOCSAE Football Helmet Impact Standard vs. Crash Helmet Standards for Flat Surface Drops[1]

Standard—Size	Head and Carriage Weight, kg (lb)	Energy Drop,[1] J (ft-lb)	Energy Drop,[2] J (ft-lb)	Total Energy 2 Drops, J (ft-lb)	Allowable G
NOCSAE-L	8.2 (18.0)	122 (90.0)	122 (90.0)	244 (180)	225[2]
NOCSAE-M	7.0 (15.3)	104 (76.5)	104 (76.5)	208 (153)	225[2]
NOCSAE-S	6.4 (14.0)	95 (70.0)	95 (70.0)	190 (140)	225[2]
MVSS218-C(12)	5.0 (11.0)	89 (66.0)	89 (66.0)	178 (132)	300
ANSI Z90.1–1979-C(13)	5.0 (11.0)	119 (88.0)	89 (66.0)	209 (154)	300
SNELL-1985(14)	5.0 (11.0)	149 (110.0)	111 (82.0)	260 (192)	314[3]

[1]The crash helmet flat surface is rigid. The NOCSAE surface is a ½ in. 38 D rubber pad on a rigid surface.
[2]Performance criterion for NOCSAE is 1,500 SI, approximately, accompanied by 225 G. This is a triaxial resultant, whereas the others are uniaxial measurements. Also, drops of 91 cm (36 in.) and 122 cm (48 in.) on the front and side location precede the 152 cm (60 in.) drops in the NOCSAE Standard.
[3]Arithmetic average of nine impacts shall not exceed 285 G, and no single impact shall exceed 314 G.

Weather Factors

It is essential for a standard to reject equipment that deteriorates seriously in impact performance because of the weather extremes of football. Heat is the primary environmental factor that degrades most helmets by softening the liner and some shell materials. As a result they bottom out more easily and thus absorb less energy at high temperatures than at lower temperatures over the range from $-17.78°$ C ($0°$ F) to $32.2°$ C ($90°$ F) at which football is played (including August in the South and playoff games in the North). It is the purpose of the Standard to eliminate those potential liner and shell materials that deteriorate unsafely. Therefore the helmet is dropped twice from a height of 152 cm (60 in.) on the right frontal boss immediately after soaking for 4 hours at $49°$ C ($120°$ F), and it must meet the same criterion as in the ambient temperature tests. This location exercises all three channels of the triaxial accelerometer.

Generally materials get stiffer and performance improves as the temperature drops. If helmets are tested at temperatures as low as $-29°$ C ($-20°$ F), normally resilient materials will sometimes suffer brittle failure, although in rupturing, energy is absorbed and acceleration is attenuated below normal values. This is not a realistic situation, because even though the game is sometimes played in sub-freezing weather, head temperatures warm up the lining material enough to prevent it from becoming brittle. Some standards employ a moisture environmental condition, but football helmet materials are either impermeable to moisture, or if they absorb moisture, their ability to absorb energy improves. Consequently this condition was dropped from the NOCSAE Standard.

Mechanical Test Setup

A test system must be repeatable within narrow limits to ensure that helmet compliance tests are conducted fairly. Also, if the same system is to be used for research, development, and quality control, reproducibility and ruggedness are desirable features to ensure that different laboratories are in reasonable agreement and the system is able to withstand a large number of impacts without mechanical breakdown.[12-14] The essential mechanical parts of the NOCSAE test system are the head model mounted on a lightweight aluminum carriage with nylon bearings, a position adjuster for controlling impact location, and stainless steel strand guide wires. The system is propelled by gravity (Fig 3–2).

Performance Requirements

When the NOCSAE football helmet Standard was originated in 1973, a 1,500 SI was considered to be the threshold

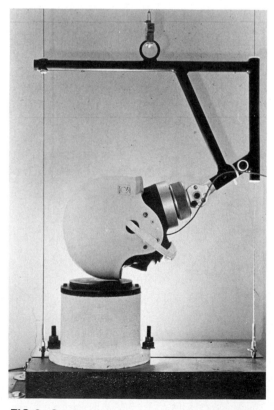

FIG 3–2.
NOCSAE football helmet drop test system featuring head models with near-human impact response.

concussion level for distributed impact for the average individual, based on the research of Gadd et al.[15, 16] According to Figure 3−1 this SI level is now considered to put 35% to 40% of the adult population at risk of a serious head injury, but is probably lower for healthy young men.

Figure 3−3 is shown to provide some insight into the kinematics associated with a 1,500 SI level. The accelerations and duration combinations that produce 1,500 SI are superimposed on a kinematics chart that plots the relationship between displacement, pulse duration, and velocity change for uniform acceleration in discrete increments. Any impact experienced by the human head surrogate that produces an acceleration or deceleration time history in which the effective average acceleration area under the acceleration-time oscillogram divided by baseline

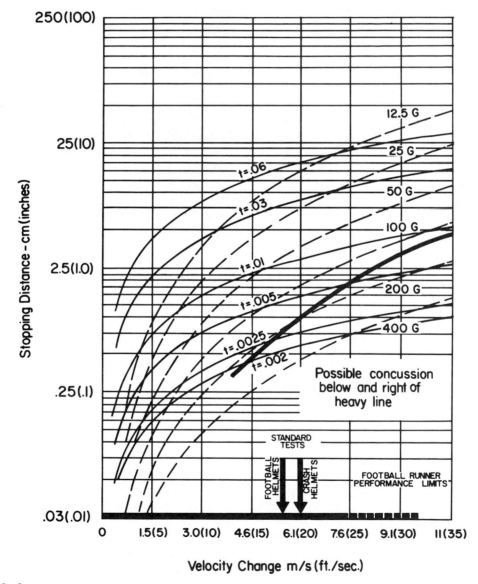

FIG 3−3.
Kinematics chart on which a cerebral concussion tolerance curve is superimposed, corresponding to a 1,500 SI for distributed impact (no fracture hazard).

time and time duration ordinate-abscissa combination, which when plotted lies below the curve, is expected to produce a concussion. When the acceleration and time are plotted, the corresponding velocity change and stopping distance can be compared with the impact velocity and helmet liner thickness, respectively, to evaluate the helmet effectiveness.

With the assumed ideal stopping (or starting) uniform acceleration (square wave), the stopping distance would equal the liner thickness, and velocity change would equal impact velocity. Actually, the stopping distance for impact against a rigid surface is always less than liner thickness, and velocity change is always greater than impact velocity. Although in mechanical handling systems uniform stopping is preferable for economy of time, space, and materials, some recent evidence indicates that materials with crush characteristics approaching uniform acceleration on impact are not desirable for the head. According to one biologic materials property study, the parasagittal bridging veins between brain and sagittal sinus are strain rate sensitive,[17] although a finite element study found this effect to be minimal.[18]

Use of the SI as a performance requirement makes it more difficult to hold tight tolerances among several laboratories because of the 2.5 weighting factor; for example, a 15% increase in a half-sine-shaped pulse peak acceleration from 200 to 230 G, $t = .005$ sec, can result in a 42% change in SI. Use of the SI is justified, however, because the exponent flies a warning flag that reveals undesirable rapid changes in helmet performance as energy is increased slightly (approach of bottoming out) more sensitively than measuring peak accelerations alone. Head injury is not something that gradually gets a little worse with each increment of acceleration. Rather, the threshold of concussion (unconscious level) is usually sudden and usually reversible,

but farther up the intensity scale irreversible changes occur and a concussion is potentially lethal. Cerebrovascular accidents also occur suddenly at no known level of impact intensity in a widely varying individual case and cause irreversible damage.

The HIC has supplanted the SI in U.S. government Standards. It has become apparent on the basis of experimental surrogate and volunteer air bag and seat belt tests that head injury does not occur for impacts lasting longer than 15 ms.[19, 20] Dummy head impacts in car crash tests often last much longer than 15 ms. The SI, which is defined for the interval 0.0025 to 0.050 second, can integrate to a large value, much of which is artifactual under these circumstances, whereas helmet drop tests are typically in the 0.007 to 0.012 second range. Since it is not certain which is the best predictor of physiologic injury in the sports helmet impact time regime, SI has continued to be used for the reasons that follow. For theoretic half-sine and triangular pulses, the HIC is 9.4% and 13.8% lower than SI, the triangular shape representing a more destructive physical impact, other things being equal. For football helmet drop tests, the HIC is about 15% lower than SI. Some complex waveforms such as might occur when there is a sudden "oil canning" of a helmet shell, followed by inertia loading of the impact surface by the head model, can further widen the difference. For these reasons, the SI tends to be more conservative than HIC if used in the 0.0025 to 0.015 second range, and consequently SI has continued to be used for NOCSAE helmet tests. This may change as more head injury—related data on volunteers, cadavers, and surrogates are generated as a function of HIC or other criteria.

Acceleration-time pulses that integrate to 1,000 SI equate approximately to the original Wayne State University curve, which was based in its short duration on results obtained from cadaver skull fractures due to rigid, flat-surface impact on the forehead.[21] Gadd, the originator of the SI,[22] has pointed out many instances of distributed (nonfracturing) impact in which volunteers experienced a much higher SI without concussion.[15, 16] Accordingly he recommended, and the NOCSAE Standard adopted, an SI of 1,500 for distributed impacts in which the fracture hazard is absent. Since skull fractures in modern football have been virtually eliminated, football helmets fall into this category.

As Figures 3–1 and 3–3 illustrate, the use of a calibrated humanoid surrogate makes it possible to extrapolate from mechanical kinematics to human tolerance criteria. This approach helps the designer to estimate a proposed helmet HIC or SI performance relative to a risk of injury level.

The NOCSAE Standard was intended to force helmet designers to employ either slightly denser, stiffer, resilient foams or slightly larger helmets than many of those on the market before the Standard. Range of player tolerance to head impact uncertainties precedes drastic changes because what may be good for preventing concussion at high levels of impact intensity for some individuals may be too stiff or put too much leverage on the heads of others prone to SDH in lower-intensity situations. Also, to be effective, helmets have to be worn as purchased and not tampered with for comfort's sake. There are practical constraints of size and comfort beyond which it is not fruitful to force the design of helmets.

Despite the higher than originally assumed serious head injury risk estimated by Figure 3–1 for a 1,500 SI level, this value has remained as the Standard performance requirement since 1973. The reason for this has been to avoid confusion, because several changes affecting the SI and energy level have been taking place and the fatal head injuries have been declining.

Since the risk curve of Prasad and Mertz was first published in a Society of Automotive Engineers (SAE) paper in 1985,[7] changes have been made in the head models to bring their specific gravity up to a humanlike 1.1, which prior petroleum-based material limitations had held down to 0.9. Consequently the test severity has increased to be on a par with the most demanding crash helmet Standards (see Table 3–2).

Also, as shown below Figure 3–1, improvements by manufacturers had lowered average recertified helmet scores well below the 1,500 level as one of the positive spinoffs of having a Standard and the Standard test equipment. Because of this improvement, guidelines were included in the Appendix of the 1985 revision to show that although 1,500 was the limit, because of variation in used helmets the average test SI + 3 SD* should not exceed 1,500 for a given model, size, and location, for good assurance in sample testing that all recertified helmets meet the Standard.

Now under consideration are Standard proposals to have uniform drop energy at levels just above those of the medium head (108 J [80 ft-lb] max; see Table 3–1); and an SI reduction to the equivalent of 1,000 HIC. Concurrent with these proposals are studies to determine the effects of helmet size on head angular acceleration and neck forces and bending moments.

RESULTS

Since the NOCSAE football helmet impact Standard was enacted in 1973, the present five manufacturers and 39

*SD = standard deviation: 3 SD above the average SI provides assurance that 99% of all helmets in the population from which the sample was randomly chosen would not exceed that level.

helmet reconditioners have installed the Standard test equipment and use it for quality control of impact-attenuating characteristics among new and used helmets.

Standard research has shown the limitations of a helmet, that is, that: (1) it can be overwhelmed by some impact situations; (2) it can reduce but not eliminate rotational accelerations; (3) helmets do not cause neck injury by a guillotine mechanism; (4) most paralyzing neck injuries are due to head-down orientation in tackling, blocking, and ball carrying; (5) the inertia of the body compresses and bends the flexed neck to fracture-dislocation; and (6) the helmet can do little to prevent neck injury in this attitude.

Figure 3–3 shows that fatal head injuries, primarily due to acute SDH, declined by 65%, comparing pre- and post-Standard periods for high school players. It cannot be shown that this very significant injury reduction is altogether due to improved helmets, since rules changes against head hitting and warnings may have also had effects.

Mueller and Blyth[4] found that SDHs with permanent disability were 7, 4, 2, and 2 in the 1984–1987 seasons. Concussion studies have been limited. Earlier figures indicated a steady decline among high school players, post-Standard during the 1970s, but no further information is available from this source.[23]

The National Sports Injury Surveillance System reported by Zemper[3] showed concussion rates during 1982–1983 seasons among the three NCAA College Divisions to be running at 0.32/1,000 athlete-exposures (A-E)* and 0.31/1,000 in 1986. Zemper included only concussions that kept a player from participation for one day or more. Gerberich et al.[24] reported a higher incidence of 19/100 players, but included players not only

*A-E = one athlete, one game or practice exposed to the possibility of injuries.

with a mild concussion characterized by loss of consciousness but also with a loss of awareness experience, among 103 secondary school football teams in Minnesota. Neither of these studies found a relation to helmet model.

BASEBALL BATTER'S HELMET STANDARD—TEST METHOD

Number and Location of Impacts

In contrast to the multiple impacts received on the helmet by the more head-intensive sport of football, baseball batter's helmet impacts by a ball are relatively rare. This is due in part to the fact that the head is not in the strike zone and to a self-preservation instinct among virtually all players to avoid being struck on the head by a high-speed pitch, even if wearing a helmet. Consequently, to encourage the use of the most efficient energy-absorbing slow- or low-recovery foams, only one impact at any one site should be required. Generally speaking, six impact sites (including front, front boss, side, rear, rear boss, and one randomly chosen location to coincide with an apparent weak spot or gap in shell or liner) are sufficient to evaluate comprehensively the impact attenuation characteristics of a helmet at ambient temperature. One impact after exposure to high temperature on the side location of a new helmet, together with a repeat of these tests on two other helmets, should suffice for the total number of impacts required for each head model.

Impact Surface

Initially the NOCSAE baseball batter's helmet Standard was designed around baseball impact protection.[25] This was because, even though the same helmets are used for baseball and softball, it was generally assumed that baseball impacts were the worst. Subsequent research has shown that which ball is most hazardous to head injury depends on the speed, type of helmet, ball size, weight, and stiffness. There are so many combinations of variables available that it is difficult to sort them out. Consequently, the Standard was changed in July 1987. Helmets are now required to meet Standard requirements for impacts with both baseballs and softballs, the hardest and liveliest of each type chosen as the worst impacts.

Stitched seams in official league–sanctioned types of balls can introduce variable head accelerations to the head model at the same ball speed with or without a helmet. Therefore, Standard seamless balls with similar characteristics in hardness and liveliness to the worst-impact types of baseballs and softballs are to be preferred for testing. Preferably such seamless balls would also be more durable; that is, maintain their shape and playing characteristics longer than regular stitched balls, thus avoiding change of test balls, with the possible introduction of ball-to-ball variation in impact characteristics.

Impact Speed

The NOCSAE Standard ball speed requirement is 60 mph.* Since measurements are usually conducted at around 62 mph to assure compliance with Standard requirements, this represents a 50% increase above the average pre-Standard helmet kinetic energy absorption capabilities. This was achieved by some manufacturers with material changes, while others added new shell sizes to accommodate more uniform liner thickness over a wider range of head sizes. A ball speed of around 60 mph produces a head acceleration response in the medium-

sized Standard head model equivalent to about that for a 75 mph impact to the head of a Hybrid III dummy. The dummy response is probably more typical of a live batter with eyes on the ball, head, neck, and body coupled alertly, whereas the head model tends to represent a relaxed person hit without seeing the ball.

With a combination of added shells with more hemispheric shapes, some helmets now can exceed the minimum Standard ball speed of 60 mph by at least 10 mph on the critical side location of the head model, and should be able to meet the Standard requirements on the Hybrid III dummy for ball speeds greater than 80 mph.

Further improvements in helmets to meet requirements at higher ball speeds may come about as the result of proposed changes to the Standard. As an incentive for higher protective performance, it has been proposed to open both baseball and softball Standards up into four tiers of ball speed, that is, 60–70, 71–80, 81–90, 91–100 mph. Manufacturers that meet minimum performance requirements in any range could advertise their helmet thusly. Cost, size, weight, stability, durability, and level of play may dictate the type of helmet selected by the consumer.*

Weather Factors

Generally speaking, baseball and softball are played at temperatures in the range of 10° C (50° F) to 38° C (100° F). The protective characteristics of most traditional shell and liner materials tend to decline at elevated temperatures. Consequently, one way to evaluate this characteristic is to heat the helmet to a temper-

---

*Ball speed in miles per hour (mph) has become so generally accepted that conversion to SI units has been eliminated in this section; 1 mph = 0.447 m/sec.

*Included is also a proposal to separate the Standard into separate baseball and softball Standards. Furthermore, since baseballs and softballs come in many degrees of stiffness and liveliness, it has also been proposed to allow balls to meet Standard requirements for impacts to the unprotected head model in any of the proposed ball speed tiers.

ature slightly above the highest level anticipated, allow it to stabilize, and test it under this condition. The NOCSAE Standard uses 49° C (120° F) for 4 hours' soak; heat flows out of the helmet to between 43° C (110° F) and 38° C (100° F) when tested. A helmet hotter than this would not be tolerated on the head.

Wet conditions generally improve the energy absorption capabilities of materials such as foams, if open celled, or even on the surface of closed-cell forms as sweat. Moisture on a shell's outer surface improves glance protection.

Cold shells tend to distribute the force of impact over more liner material, which in turn generally improves as energy absorbers at the lower end of the playing temperature scale.

Balls on the other hand tend to become more stiff and therefore more hazardous at lower temperature. If the proposal to admit balls to meet the NOCSAE Batter's Helmet Standard for impacts to the unprotected head is adopted, one of the requirements will most likely be low temperature tests.

Mechanical Test Setup

Because of the relatively high speed, small mass, and rigidity of a baseball/softball used in batter's helmet tests, measurement accuracy is much more difficult than a drop test of a helmeted head model. A drop test is rather forgiving because it is a slow-speed (⅕ rate at which balls are propelled at helmets) impact distributed over a large area, 3,870 mm² (6.00 in.²) compared with a baseball impact of more than 323 mm² (1.0 in.²). Furthermore, a ball must be flung or shot out of a tube with accurate aim at a location on a head model that is repeatable on any one head model and reproducible on others.

All of these require head model clones tested in identical test systems with careful control of ball velocity and

line of action as well as location of impact. Shown in Figure 3–4 is the setup for testing batter's helmets.

Performance Requirements

The same 1,500 SI requirement used for the football helmet drop test is used

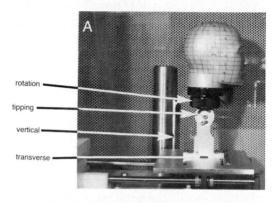

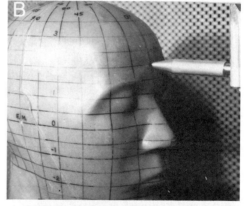

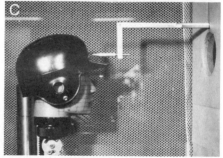

FIG 3–4.
Baseball batter's helmet test setup. **A,** head model on slide table showing rotation, tipping, vertical, and transverse position adjustments. **B,** locator tip aligned with center line of air cannon pointing at reference head model. **C,** head model wearing helmet.

for baseball/softball impacts at present, even though concussions, considered a diffuse injury, are the most common head injury to be prevented in football, while prevention of focal injuries is the main concern in baseball. Focal injuries in football are usually SDH,[4, 5] but are assumed to be most often remote from the impact site as a result of rupture of, for example, a bridging vein into the sagittal sinus due to a head impulse that usually is too mild to cause a concussion. Such focal injuries as these are difficult to eradicate. The baseball focal injury, on the other hand, is assumed usually to be directly under the impact site. Consequently, the problems of understanding the mechanics of the injury process and how to minimize the risk for most players are at least theoretically simpler and should be solved sooner than the SDH football injury problem. The SI appears to be a good indicator of helmet saturation in either the distributed (football) or localized (baseball) impact environment. Because of the 2.5 power attached to head acceleration, it waves a "red flag" of danger before acceleration measured by itself.*

Some form of pressure measurement under the impact site that does not significantly affect the response of the head would be desirable for high-speed hardball and bat impacts to see how well SI and pressure correlate under extreme concentrated force conditions, but none is currently available.

RESULTS

Serious head injuries in baseball/softball are rare, and there are no injury data available to compare players injured while wearing certified or noncertified

helmets or comparing pre- and post-Standard helmet injury records.

A report by the U.S. Consumer Product Safety Commission examined the injury rate among youngsters 5 to 14 years of age for the 1973–1983 period (there were 86,500 hospital emergency room–treated injuries in 1983). In organized baseball during that period, one batter was killed who was not wearing a helmet.[26] Most of the helmets worn would have been pre-Standard.

An NCAA study of baseball/softball injuries showed the following records for head injury (degree of cerebral concussion) during the 5/15/88–5/15/89 period for softball and 6/19/88–6/19/89 period for baseball[27]:

	Degree of Concussion	No. of Injuries	Rate/1,000 Athlete-Exposures
Baseball	1	12	0.07
	2	2	0.01
	3	1	0.01
Softball	1	5	0.08
	2	1	0.02
	3	1	0.02

Wearing or not wearing a helmet data were not made available, nor were the positions played. Studies such as these and more in-depth investigations in the next few years may shed light on whether the proposed helmet and ball Standard modifications are effective in reducing the already low head injury rates in these games.

Acknowledgments

Jamie Mayes was responsible for the typing and construction of charts and graphs.

---

*The proposed SI reduction for football helmet drop test performance, if adopted, would apply to the baseball and softball Standards as well.

REFERENCES

1. Gurdjian ES: *Impact Head Injury*. Springfield, Ill, Charles C Thomas, Publisher, 1975, p 257.

2. Gennarelli TA, Thibault LE: Biomechanics of acute subdural hematoma. *J Trauma* 1982; 22:680–686.

3. Zemper ED: *Cerebral Concussion Rates in Various Brands of Football Helmets*. International Institute for Sport and Human Performances, 1989.

4. Mueller FO, Blyth CS: *National Center for Catastrophic Sports Injury Research, Fifth Annual Report, 1982–1987*. Research funded by a grant from the National Collegiate Athletic Association, American Football Coaches Association and the National Federation of State High School Associations.

5. Mueller FO, Schindler RD: *Annual Survey of Football Injury Research 1931–1987*. Prepared for American Football Coaches Association, National Collegiate Athletic Association, and the National Federation of State High School Associations.

6. Mertz HJ, Weber DA: *Interpretations of the Impact Responses of a Three Year Old Child Dummy Relative to Child Injury Potential*. Proceedings of the 9th International Technical Conference of Experimental Safety Vehicles, Kyoto, Japan, November 1982.

7. Prasad P, Mertz HJ: *The Position of the United States Delegation to the ISO Working Group 6 on the Use of HIC in the Automotive Environment*. Prepared for the Society of Automotive Engineers Technical Paper Series No. 851246, May 20–23, 1985.

8. *The Abbreviated Injury Scale*. Prepared for the American Association of Automotive Medicine, 1980.

9. Siekert RG (ed): *Cerebrovascular Survey Report*. Prepared for Joint Council Subcommittee on Cerebrovascular Disease, National Institute on Neurological and Communicative Disorders and Stroke and National Heart and Lung Institute. Rochester, Minn, January 1976.

10. *Verbal Report From Fred Mueller*. Department of Physical Education, University of North Carolina, Chapel Hill, NC.

11. Saczalski KJ, et al: *A Critical Assessment of the Use of Non-Human Responding Surrogates for Safety System Evaluation*, in Twentieth Stapp Car Crash Conference Proceedings. New York, Society of Automotive Engineers, October 1976.

12. *Federal Safety Standard*. MVSS 218, Motor Vehicle Safety Standard No. 218, Motorcycle Helmets—Helmets Designed for Use by Motorcyclists and Other Motor Vehicle Users, effective March 1, 1974.

13. *American National Standard Specifications for Protective Headgear for Vehicular Users*. American National Standards Institute, Inc., New York, NY, 1972.

14. *1985 Standard for Protective Headgear*. Snell Memorial Foundation, Wakefield, RI, 1985.

15. Gadd CW: *Report to SAE Performance Criteria Subcommittee, March 8, 1972*. Vehicle Research Department, General Motors Research Laboratories, G.M. Technical Center, Warren, Mich.

16. Haut RC, Gadd CW, Madeira RG: *Nonlinear Viscoelastic Model for Head Impact Injury Hazard*. Proceedings of the Sixteenth Stapp Car Crash Conference, 1972.

17. Lowenhielm P: Dynamic properties of the parasagittal bridging veins. *Z. Rechtsmed* 1974, 74:55–62.

18. Lee MC, Haut RC: Biomechanics of traumatic subdural hematoma due to failure of the parasagittal bridging veins, in *Head Injury Prevention Past and Present Research*. Wayne State University, Department of Neurosurgery, Detroit, Mich, 1988.

19. Hodgson VR, Thomas LM: *Effect of Long-Duration Impact on Head*. Proceedings of the Sixteenth Stapp Car Crash Conference, 1972.

20. Mertz HJ. Chm: *SAE Human Biomechanics and Simulation Standards Committee*. Personal communication.

21. Gurdjian ES, Lissner HR, Patrick LM: Protection of the head and neck in sports. *JAMA* 1962; 182:509–512.

22. Gadd CW: *Use of a Weighted-Impulse Criterion for Estimating Injury Hazard*, in Tenth Stapp Car Crash Conference Proceedings. New York, Society of Automotive Engineers, November 1966.

23. Hodgson VR: *Reducing Serious Injury in Sports (Table 3–2)*. Prepared for National Federation of State High School Associations, vol. 7, no. 2, Winter 1980.

24. Gerberich SG, Priest JD, Boen JR, et al: Concussion incidence and severity in secondary school varsity football players. *Am J Public Health* 1983; 73:1370–1375.

25. The NOCSAE Baseball Helmet Task Force for National Operating Committee on Standards

for Athletic Equipment: *Standard Method of Impact Test and Performance Requirements for Baseball Batters' Helmets, 1982.*

26. Rutherford GW, Kennedy J, McGhee L: *Baseball and Softball Related Injuries to Children*

5–14 Years of Age. Washington, D.C., U.S. Consumer Product Safety Commission, June 1984.

27. NCAA *Baseball Injury Surveillance System.* NCAA, Shawnee Mission, Kan.

CHAPTER 4

Standards for Protective Eye Guards

Michael Easterbrook M.D., F.R.C.S.(C)

The purpose of this chapter is to review the history and method of certification of safe sports eye protection, using squash and racquetball as examples.

It has been apparent for many years to ophthalmologists in North America that the racquetball ball, the squash ball (Fig 4–1), and the badminton shuttlecock (Fig 4–2) readily penetrate the orbital rim. Also, in a confined space squash, racquetball, and handball are played with speeds as high as 140 mph. Many retrospective and prospective studies[1–49] have demonstrated significant eye injury in these racquet sports.

Any racquet player of any experience knows someone who has sustained a significant eye injury in squash, racquetball, badminton, or tennis.

As the risk of eye injury became known among those who play racquet sports, an attempt by manufacturers was made to introduce eye guards to prevent eye injury from a badminton shuttlecock, racquetball ball, or squash ball or racquet. The first eye guard commercially available was the Champion eye guard (Fig 4–3), which seemed to be of some value in preventing injuries from the racquet in squash (60% of eye injuries in

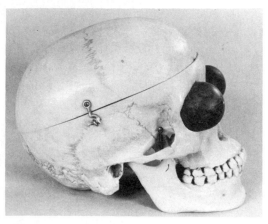

FIG 4–1.
70+ squash ball in right orbit; international ball in left orbit.

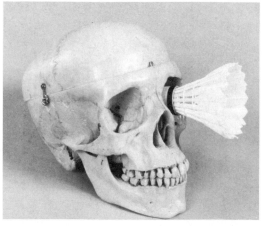

FIG 4–2.
Badminton shuttlecock readily penetrates orbit.

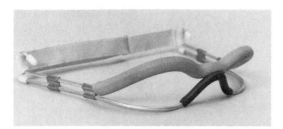

FIG 4–3.
Champion wire open eye guard, first used in handball.

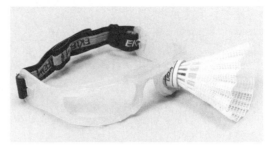

FIG 4–5.
Open eye guard (Ektelon), readily penetrated by shuttlecock.

squash are caused by the racquet) but was of little or no use in racquetball, in which 95% of the injuries are caused by the ball.[25] With the advent of plastic eye protectors, Protec and Ektelon introduced unbreakable open eye guards (Fig 4–4). In the late 1970s, however, we began to receive reports that the ball had penetrated these open eye guards, causing ocular injury.[17] Also, players informed us that they were playing with a false sense of security because they believed that they were being adequately protected. It could be argued, however, that these open eye guards, because they are unbreakable, do nothing but channel a compressible missile, such as a squash or racquetball ball, directly into the orbit, thus *increasing* the risk of ocular injury. Figures 4–5 and 4–6 demonstrate that the open eye guard is readily penetrated by a squash ball, racquetball ball, and bad-

minton shuttlecock. No sophisticated testing is required to realize the ready penetration of the open eye guard. In Canada we received 80 reports of eye injuries to players who were wearing the open eye guard (Table 4–1). I phoned each player. Sixty-nine of them told me that the ball penetrated the open eye guard. Eleven patients stated that the eye guard was too narrow and rotated up into the eye. Further testing by Bishop et al.[30] and Fiegelman et al.[36] with high-speed film proved conclusively that open guards did not protect the eye from a squash or a racquetball ball (Figs 4–7 and 4–8).

It became apparent then that eye guards were being sold with little or no testing of their ability to prevent eye injury. In the late 1970s, however, little was known about specific speeds of squash and racquetball balls; therefore, work was commissioned in Canada with Patrick Bishop, M.D., and in the United

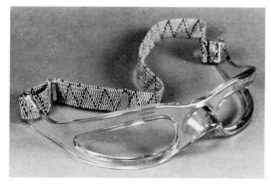

FIG 4–4.
Open eye guards distributed widely by Protec and Ektelon.

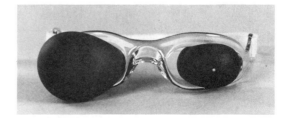

FIG 4–6.
Racquetball ball and squash ball easily penetrate open eye guards.

TABLE 4–1.

Injuries With Open Eye Guards in 80 Players

Injury	
Lid hemorrhage	11
Lid lacerations	3
Corneal abrasions	10
Iritis	8
Hyphemas	56
Cause of injury	
Ball	77
Racquet	3
Ball penetrated eye guard	69
Eye guard displaced	11

Type of Eye Guard	Sport	
	Squash	Racquetball
Protec	14	22
Ektelon	1	15
Rainbow	5	2
Voit	2	13
Solari	1	2
Champion	1	—
Duraguard	0	2
	24	56

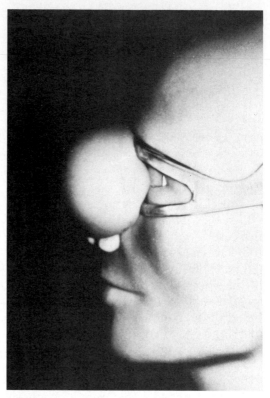

FIG 4–7.
High-speed film demonstrates penetration of open eye guard by racquetball ball. *(Courtesy of M. Elman.)*

States with C.A. Morehouse, Ph.D., to ascertain speeds in squash and racquetball (Table 4–2).

COLLECTION OF DATA OF EYE INJURY IN RACQUET SPORTS

In the late 1970s Thomas Pashby, M.D. sent questionnaires to all members of the Canadian Ophthalmological Society asking them to report eye injuries. I sent questionnaires to racquetball clubs and Canadian squash clubs for distribution, asking for eye injury reports from those players who had received eye injuries (Fig 4–9). The initial surveys demonstrated a significant incidence of eye injuries, with loss of vision in many players (Table 4–3). These questionnaires revealed that the experienced "A" player was at least at much at risk of an eye injury as the novice player.[44] Also, the risk of players wearing street wear glasses on the court became apparent because we had many reports of street wear prescription glasses, whether plastic, glass, or hardened glass, breaking when struck by a ball or a racquet in any of the racquet sports.

TABLE 4–2.

Ball and Racquet Velocities*

Type of Ball/Racquet	Speeds (mph)
Racquetball	
Ball	85–110
Racquet	85–90
Squash	
Ball	130–140
Racquet	95–110
Tennis ball	90–110
Handball	60–70
Badminton shuttlecock	130–135

From C. A. Morehouse, American Society for Testing and Materials, Philadelphia.

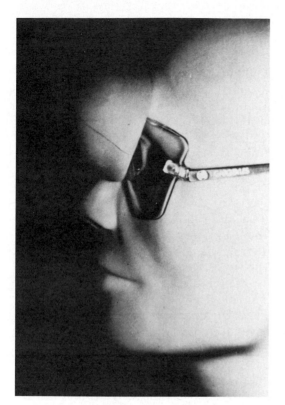

FIG 4-8.
Closed polycarbonate protector prevents eye contact.
(Courtesy of M. Elman.)

STANDARDS AND CERTIFICATION OF EYE GUARDS FOR RACQUET SPORTS

In 1980 a Canadian Standards Association (CSA) committee, composed of manufacturers, opticians, ophthalmologists, optometrists, and representatives of consumer groups, was formed to write a standard for racquet sport eye protectors. In 1982 the CSA passed a preliminary standard Z400, which was revised in 1985 and 1986. In 1983 the American Society for Testing and Materials (ASTM) passed a standard F803 for racquet sports in the United States, which was updated in 1985, 1986, 1987, and 1988. These standards are performance rather than design standards: eye guards that pass will prevent eye contact of a squash or

CANADIAN OPHTHALMOLOGICAL SOCIETY

CANADIAN RACKET SPORTS INJURY QUESTIONNAIRE

Player

Name:

Address:

Phone: Home _____ Business _____ Age _____ Sex _____

Date of injury _____ Years played _____

Class of player: A _____   B _____   C _____   D _____

Class of opponent: A _____   B _____   C _____   D _____

Hit by racket: Volley _____ Follow-through _____ Forehand _____ Backhand _____

Playing: Soft ball _____   Hard ball _____

Hit by ball: Direct shot _____   Off wall _____

Wearing: Regular glass _____ Hardened glass _____ Plastic _____

Wearing eye protection made for racket sports: Yes _____   No _____

Wearing contact lens: Soft _____ Semi-soft _____ Hard _____

Lens or contact: Broken _____   Lost _____

Ophthalmologist

Name:

Address:

Remarks/Suggestions

May I get in touch with your family doctor or ophthalmologist for more details of your injury?
Yes _____ No _____

Signature _____ Date _____

Please return to:

FIG 4-9.
Questionnaire sent to squash and racquetball clubs.

TABLE 4-3.
Canadian Racquets Survey (1978-1987)

Injury	No. of Patients	
	Squash	Racquetball
Lid hemorrhage	57	42
Lid laceration	36	19
Subconjunctival hemorrhage	31	14
Corneal abrasion	44	32
Corneal lacerations requiring surgery	6	2
Iritis	26	26
Iris tear or dialysis	10	8
Angle recession	18	4
Hyphema	114	106
Secondary hemorrhage	5	4
Cataract	8	6
Vitreous/retinal hemorrhage	17	21
Macular scar	8	5
Retinal detachment	10	3
Orbital fracture	3	1
Total	393	293

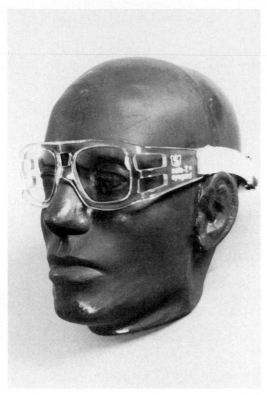

FIG 4–10.
Alderson head form used in Canada by CSA and in the United States by Detroit Testing Laboratories.

racquetball ball at speeds of 90 mph (40 m/s) when impacted from the front and from the side (Figs 4–10 and 4–11). Optical quality and fields of vision were specified.

In November 1986 after several years of testing, six racquet sports eye protectors have been certified by the CSA (Table 4–4). In the United States ASTM set standards but does not certify protective equipment. By the fall of 1987 five eye guards (Table 4–5) met the 1985 or 1986 ASTM requirements in tests by an independent laboratory (Detroit Testing Laboratories, Detroit, Mich).

Manufacturer representatives, ophthalmologists, physicians, and racquet sports organizations in the United States have formed a Sports Certification Council, under the auspices of the National Society to Prevent Blindness, in an attempt to certify eye protection for general use by racquet players in the United States. No significant eye injury has been reported to date in a squash or racquetball player wearing CSA-approved eye guards or eye guards that meet the ASTM United States standard.

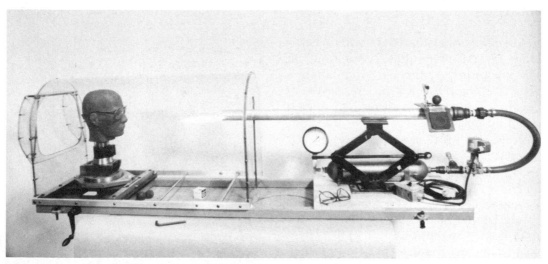

FIG 4–11.
CSA testing eye guards.

TABLE 4–4.

CSA-Approved Eye Guards (1989)

Model	Cost (Canada)	Manufacturer/Distributor	Address (Canada)	Address (United States)
1. Defender 600	$26.00	Peepers	Peepers Inc. P.O. Box 951, Station "A" 150 Chatham Steel Hamilton, Ontario L8N 3P9 416-525-3369	Peepers International 417 Fifth Ave. New York, NY 10016 212-696-9797
2. CRS 300	$29.95	CRS Sports	CRS Sports International Inc. 10021 169th St. Edmonton, Alberta T5P 4M9 403-483-5149	CRS Sports International Inc. 10021 169th St. Edmonton, Alberta T5P 4M9 403-483-5149
3. Sports Scanners	$35.40	American Optical	AOCO Limited 80 Centurian Dr. Markham, Ontario L3R 5Y5 416-479-4545	American Optical Mechanic Optical Southbridge, MA 01550 617-765-9711
4. Safe-T Eye-Gard	$30.00	Imperial Optical	Imperial Optical Canada 21 Dundas Square Toronto, Ontario M5B 1B7 416-595-1010	Embassy Creations P.O. Box 143 234 Holmes Rd. Holmes, PA 19043 215-586-9640
5. Albany	$22.00	Leader	International Forums Inc. (Leader Sports) 1150 Marie Victoria Longuevil, Quebec J4G 1A1 514-651-2300	LST Leader Sports Products Inc. P.O. Box 271 Main St, Route 22 Essex, NY 12936 518-963-4268
6. New Yorker	$27.50	Leader	Same as no. 5	Same as no. 5

SUMMARY

Surveys of ophthalmologists in Canada and the United States in the late 1970s demonstrated a significant risk of eye injury in squash, tennis, badminton, and racquetball. It became apparent that eye protectors on the market in the late 1970s and early 1980s were permitting eye contact and were associated with significant eye injuries.

Performance standards, both in Canada and in the United States, involve testing an eye guard on a head form. Certified protectors must withstand squash or raquetball balls at speeds of 90 mph.

Although protectors have not been certified in the United States, the National Society to Prevent Blindness does have an active certification council that seeks manufacturers' support to provide players of racquet sports good protection from eye injury.

Acknowledgments

I acknowledge the insight, example, and dedication of Thomas Pashby, M.D., in Canada and Paul Vinger, M.D., in the United States, who unselfishly instigated and guided the certification of eye protection in hockey and racquet sports for the

TABLE 4–5.

United States ASTM: Passed to 1985 and/or 1986 Standard

Model	Cost (U.S.)	Manufacturer/Distributor	Address (Canada)	Address (United States)
1. Action Eyes	$30.00	Viking Sports	Black Knight Enterprises 3792 Commercial St. Vancouver, British Columbia V5N 4G2 604-872-3123	Viking Sports 5355 Sierra Rd. San Jose, CA 95132 408-923-7777
2. Albany	$20.00	Leader	International Forums Inc. (Leader Sports) 1150 Marie Victoria Longuevil, Quebec J4G 1A1 514-651-2300	LST Leader Sports P.O. Box 271 Main St., Route 22 Essex, NY 12936 518-963-4268
3. New Yorker	$25.00	Leader	Same as no. 2	Same as No. 2
4. Sierra	$20.00	Ektelon	Paris Glove of Canada Ltd. 9200 Rue Meilleur St. #101 Montreal, Quebec B2N 2A8 514-381-8611	Ektelon 8929 Aero Dr. San Diego, CA 92123 619-560-0066
5. Court Goggles	$20.00	Ektelon	Same as no. 4	Same as no. 4

benefit of recreational and professional athletes.

REFERENCES

1. Editorial: A ball in the eye. *Br Med J* 1973; 195–196.

2. North IM: Ocular hazards of squash. *Med J Aust* 1973; I: 165–166.

3. Ingram DV, Lewkonia I: Ocular hazards of playing squash racquets. *Br J Ophthalmol* 1973; 57:434–438.

4. Chandran S: Ocular hazards of playing badminton. *Br J Ophthalmol* 1974; 58:757–760.

5. Blonstein JL: Eye injury in sport. *Practitioner* 1975; 215:208–209.

6. Sabiston D: Squash and eye injuries. *NZ J Sports Med* 1976; 4:3–5.

7. Seelenfreund MH, Freilich DS: Rushing the net and retinal detachment. *JAMA* 1976; 235:2723–2726.

8. Moore MC, Worthley DA: Ocular injuries in squash players. *Aust J Ophthalmol* 1977; 5:46–47.

9. Berson BL, Passoff TL, Nagelberg S, et al: Injury patterns in squash players. *Am J Sports Med* 1978; 6:323–325.

10. Keates RH, Easterbrook M, Vinger PF, et al: Eye protection for athletes (round table). *Phys Sportsmed* 1978; 6:44–60.

11. Vinger PF, Toplin DW: Racquet sports: An ocular hazard. *JAMA* 1978; 239:2575–2577.

12. Easterbrook M: Eye injuries in squash: A preventable disease. *Can Med Assoc J* 1978; 118:298–305.

13. Rose CP, Morse JO: Racquetball injuries. *Phys Sportsmed* 1979; 73–78.

14. Chapman-Smith JS: Eye injuries: A twelve-month survey. *NZ Med J* 1979; 640:47–49.

15. Rousseau AP: Ocular trauma in sports, in Freeman HM: *Ocular Trauma.* East Norwalk, Conn, Appleton-Lange, 1979, pp 353–361.

16. Rose CP, Morse JO: Racquetball injuries. *Phys Sportsmed* 1979; 7:72–78.

17. Easterbrook M: Eye injuries in racquet sports: A continuing problem. *Can Med Assoc J* 1980; 123:268.

18. Clemett RS, Fairhurst SM: Head injuries from squash: A prospective study. *NZ Med J* 1980; 92:1–3.

19. Fowler BJ, Seelenfreund M, Newton JC: Ocular injuries sustained playing squash. *Am J Sports Med* 1980; 8:126–128.

20. Doxanas MT, Soderstrom C: Racquetball as an ocular hazard. *Arch Ophthalmol* 1980; 98:1965–1966.

21. Vinger PF: Sports related eye injury: A preventable problem. *Surv Ophthalmol* 1980; 25:47–51.

22. Easterbrook M: Eye injuries in racquet sports, in Vinger P (ed): *Ocular Sports Injuries. Int Ophthalmol Clin,* Winter 1981; 21:87–119.

23. Maberley, AL: Retinal detachments and athletic eye injuries. *Br Columbia Med J* 1981; 23:70–73.

24. Easterbrook M: Eye protection for squash and racquetball players. *Phys Sportsmed* 1981; 9:79–82.

25. Easterbrook M: *Prevention of Injuries in Squash and Racquetball.* Proceedings of the Third International Symposium on the Effective Teaching of Racquet Sports, University of Illinois at Urbana-Champaign, June 10–13, 1981; 43:45.

26. Vinger PF: Sports eye injuries—a preventable disease. *Ophthalmology* 1981; 88:108–113.

27. Vinger PF: The incidence of eye injuries in sports, in Vinger P (ed): *Ocular Sports Injuries. Int Ophthalmol Clin,* Winter 1981; 21:33.

28. Barrell GV, Cooper PJ, Elkington AR, et al: Squash ball to eye ball: The likelihood of squash players incurring an eye injury. *Br Med J* 1981; 283:893–895.

29. Bell JA: Eye trauma in sports: A preventable epidemic (editorial). *JAMA* 1981; 246:256.

30. Bishop PJ, Kozey J, Caldwell G: Performance of eye protectors for squash and racquetball. *Phys Sportsmed* 1982; 10:63–69.

31. Easterbrook M: Eye injuries in squash and racquet players: An update. *Phys Sportsmed* 1982; 10:47–56.

32. Easterbrook M: Eye injuries in squash and racquetball players: An update. *Phys Sportsmed* 1982; 10:47–56.

33. Diamond GR, Queen GE, Pashby TJ, et al: Ophthalmologic injuries, in Cohen BE (ed): *Clin Sports Med* 1982; 1:469–482.

34. Pashby TJ, Bishop PJ, Easterbrook M: Eye injuries in Canadian racquet sports. *Can Fam Phys* 1982; 23:967–971.

35. Vinger P, Easterbrook, M: Prevention of eye injuries in racquet sports (editorial). *JAMA* 1983; 250:3322.

36. Feigelman MJ, Sugar J, Rednock N, et al: Assessment of ocular protection for racquetball. *JAMA* 1983; 250:3305–3309.

37. Diamond GR, Quinn GE, Pashby TJ, et al: Ophthalmological injuries. *Primary Care* 1984; 11:161–174.

38. Feigelman M, Sugar J, Rednock N, et al: Assessment of ocular protection for racquetball. *JAMA* 1984; 250:3305–3309.

39. Easterbrook M: Sports injuries; mechanisms, prevention and treatment. in Schneider RC, et al: *Injuries in Racquet Sports.* Baltimore, Williams & Wilkins, 1985, pp 553–564.

40. Kennerley Bankes JL: Squash rackets: A survey of eye injuries in England. *Br Med J* 1985; 291:1539–1540.

41. Vinger P: The eye and sports medicine, in Duane T (ed): *Clinical Ophthalmology.* Philadelphia, Harper & Row, 1985:1–51.

42. Locke AS: Squash rackets: A review—deadly or safe? *Med J Aust* 1985; 143:565–567.

43. Gregory PTS: Sussex Eye Hospital sports injuries. *Br J Ophthalmol* 1986; 70:748–750.

44. Easterbrook WM: Eye protection in racquet sports: An update. *Phys Sportsmed* 1987; 15:180–186.

45. Clemett RS, Glogau TH, Jackson BR, et al: Eye protectors for squash players. *Aust NZ J Ophthalmol* 1987; 15:151–156.

46. Labelle P, Mercier M, Podtetenev M, et al: Eye injuries in sports: Results of a five-year study. *Phys Sportsmed* 1988; 16:126–138.

47. Easterbrook M: Eye protection in racquet sports, in Lehman RC (ed): *Racquet Sports: Injury, Treatment and Prevention. Clin Sports Med* 1988; 7:253–266.

48. Easterbrook M: Assessing ocular trauma in athletes. *Can J Diagnosis* 1988; 5:43–49.

49. Easterbrook M: Ocular injuries in racquet sports. *Int Ophthalmol Clin* 1988; 28:232–237.

APPENDIX 4A

Eye Injuries and Eye Protection in Sports: A Position Statement from the International Federation of Sports Medicine (*Sports Med Bull** 1989; 24:11-12)

The International Federation of Sports Medicine calls attention to the fact that, while eye injuries in sports can be relatively frequent, they are almost completely preventable. Loss of sight, even in one eye, involves changes in life-style for the individual and serious financial and social consequences both for the individual and for society as a whole. It is imperative that sports eye injury risk be reduced to as low a level as possible by enforcement of existing safety rules or by rules changes, where applicable. All athletes should be prescribed eye protectors where appropriate to the sport.

Sports can be classified on the basis of low risk, high risk, and extremely high risk for eye injury. Most sports that pose risk for unprotected eyes can be made quite safe with the use of appropriate protective devices. Eye examination and counseling should play an important part in the screening physical examination for every athlete before sports participation. The athlete deserves a careful explanation of the risk of eye injury, both with and without various types of eye protectors in the proposed sport. Athletes who are functionally one-eyed must have their status diagnosed and appropriate eye protection prescribed.

Glass lenses, ordinary plastic lenses, and open (lensless) eye guards do not provide adequate protection for those involved in active sports. In many situations their use can increase the risk for, and the severity of, eye injury. Because contact lenses do not protect the athlete from serious eye injury, they should be

*A publication of the American College of Sports Medicine. Reprinted with permission.

worn only in combination with recommended sport eye protectors.

Eye Injury Risk in Sports

Eye injury risk is almost totally related to the particular type of sport.[10, 11, 13] Low-risk sports do not involve a thrown or hit ball, a bat or a stick, or close aggressive play with body contact. Examples include track and field, swimming, gymnastics, and rowing. Sports with high risk of eye injury (when protective devices are not being worn) involve a high-speed ball (or puck), the use of a bat or stick, close aggressive play with intentional or unintentional body contact and collision, or a combination of these factors. Examples include hockey (ice, field, and street), the racquet sports (racquetball, squash, tennis, badminton), lacrosse (men's and women's), handball, baseball, basketball, football (United States, Canada, Australia), soccer, and volleyball.[3, 9, 11, 14] The incidence of serious eye injury in these sports is a source of great concern, but adequate eye protective devices are available.[1, 2, 4, 5, 8]

Sports involving extremely high risk for eye injury are the combative sports, such as boxing and full-contact karate,[7, 11, 12] for which effective eye protective devices are not available. The functionally one-eyed athlete should be strongly advised against participation in such sports.

Other Risk Factors

It is suspected but not yet proved that risk for eye injury may also be related to physical development, skill level, and existing visual impairment. It is believed that a beginner is more prone to injuries than are intermediate or advanced players because beginners have not yet learned or refined the necessary skills to master the sport. In sports such as hockey, squash, and racquetball, however, highly skilled athletes play a faster game with more aggressiveness, and, thus, may be subject to a higher eye injury risk than other participants.

Any eye condition that could be made worse if the eye were to be struck places the athlete at increased risk of serious eye injury. Athletes with retinal degenerations, thin sclera, prior eye surgery (including cataract surgery, retinal detachment surgery, and radial keratotomy), prior serious eye injury, or eye disease should seek consultation with an ophthalmologist before participating in a sport.

The Functionally One-Eyed Athlete

Sports participants with only one good eye are at particular risk since a serious injury to the good eye could leave the person with a severe visual handicap or permanently blind. Any person with good vision in only one eye should consult with an ophthalmologist on whether to participate in a particular sport. If a decision is made to participate, the person should wear maximum protection for the particular sport for all practice sessions and for competition.

A person is functionally one eyed when loss of the better eye would result in a significant change in lifestyle because of poorer vision in the remaining eye. There is no question that a person with 6/60 (20/200) or poorer best-corrected vision in one eye is functionally one eyed since loss of the good eye would result in legal or total blindness, with its attendant burden both to the individual and to society. On the other hand, ophthalmologists believe that most persons with one eye function quite well with 6/12 (20/40) or better vision in that eye.

Every athlete who tests less than 6/12 (20/40) with glasses, if worn, on the screening examination should be evaluated by an optometrist or an ophthalmologist to determine if the subnormal vision is simply due to a change in refraction. If the best-corrected vision in either eye is less than 6/12 (20/40) after refraction, ophthalmologic evaluation to obtain a definitive diagnosis of the visual deficit is indicated. If the athlete is functionally one eyed, the potential serious, long-term consequences of injury to the better eye should be discussed in detail.

Eye Protectors

Most eye (and face) injuries could be prevented or, at least, the effects of such injuries minimized by using protective eyewear. Normal "street wear" eyeglass frames with 2 mm polycarbonate lenses give adequate, cosmetically acceptable protection for routine use by active people. Such protective glasses are recommended for daily wear by the visually impaired or functionally one-eyed athlete. They are also satisfactory for athletes in competition who wear eyeglasses and participate in low-risk sports.

Molded polycarbonate frames and lenses (plano/nonprescription protective eyewear) are suggested for contact lens wearers and athletes who ordinarily do not wear glasses but participate in moderate to high-risk, noncontact sports (e.g., racquet sports, baseball, basketball). In high-risk contact or collision sports, they can be used in combination with a face mask or helmet with face protection for additional protection. Such protective glasses are recommended to the functionally one-eyed athlete who does not require prescription protective eyewear in the good eye to be used in combination with a face mask and helmet for higher-risk contact sports. Face masks or helmets with face protection are required for use in the high-risk contact or collision sports (e.g., ice hockey, U.S. football). The face mask may consist of metal wire, coated wire, or a transparent polycarbonate shield.

When protective eyewear has been employed in racquet sports and face protection devices employed in hockey, eye injuries have been eliminated.[6, 8]

Routine Examination

General practitioners providing medical screening for athletes should have facilities for vision testing and basic eye examination at their disposal and be aware of both the basic principles of eye protection in sports and the available protective eyewear. It is recommended that athletes have their vision tested and eyes examined on a regular basis. Vision or eye problems are best corrected by an eye care specialist when detected early. An examination also offers an opportunity to discuss any sports vision needs and the most appropriate type of protective eyewear.

REFERENCES

1. American Society for Testing and Materials: *Standard Safety Specification for Eye and Face Protective Equipment for Hockey Players (F513-86)*. Philadelphia, Penn, 1986.

2. American Society for Testing and Materials: *Eye Protection for Use by Players of Racket Sports (F803-88)*. Philadelphia, Penn, 1988.

3. Burke MJ, Sanitato JJ, Vinger PF, et al: Soccer-ball induced injuries. *JAMA* 1983; 249:2682–2685.

4. Canadian Standards Association: *National Standard of Canada (CAN 3-Z262.2-M83). Face Protectors for Ice Hockey and Box Lacrosse Players*. Rexdale, Ontario, 1983.

5. Canadian Standards Association: *National Standard of Canada (P400-M 1982). Racket Sports Eye Protection Preliminary Standard*. Toronto, Ontario, 1982.

6. Easterbrook M: Eye protection in racket sports: An update. *Phys Sportsmed* 1987; 15:180–192.

7. Giovinazzo VJ, Yannuzzi LA, Sorenson JA, et al: The ocular complications of boxing. *Ophthalmology* 1987; 94:587–596.

8. Pashby TJ: Eye injuries in Canadian hockey: Phase III. Older players now at risk. *Can Med Assoc J* 1979; 121:643–644.

9. Pashby TJ: Eye injuries in boxing. *Int Ophthalmol Clin* 1981; 21:59–86.

10. Portis JM, Vassallo SA, Albert DM: Ocular sports injuries: A review of cases on file in the Massachusetts Eye and Ear Infirmary Pathology Laboratory. *Int Ophthalmol Clin* 1981; 21:1–20.

11. Schnell D: Augenverletzungen, Verletzungsfolgen und andere Affektionen wahrend sportlicher Betatigung, in Rieckert H (ed): *Sportmedizin-Kursbestimmung*. Berlin/Heidelburg, Springer, 1987.

12. Smith DJ: *Ocular Injuries in Boxers*. Proceedings of the Research to Prevent Blindness, Inc., Science Writers Seminar, pp 17–18, 1987.

13. Vinger PF: The incidence of eye injuries in sports. *Int Ophthalmol Clin* 1981; 21:21–46.

14. Vinger PF, Tolpin DW: Racket sports: An ocular hazard. *JAMA* 1978; 239:2575–2577.

CHAPTER 5

Intracranial Injuries Resulting From Boxing

Allan J. Ryan, M.D.

Injuries to the head may result in immediate or subsequent fatalities when the brain, or its coverings, or both are damaged. The category *head injury* has some significance to the epidemiologist of sports injuries because it indicates for a particular sport the relative degree of risk to that part of the body. It can include a broken nose, a fractured tooth, a corneal abrasion, or a lacerated ear. These are painful and unsightly injuries that may result in some permanent deformity but do not cause fatalities. The extent to which the brain has been damaged as the result of an injury to the head is most commonly unknown and often, unfortunately, ignored. This is partly because the brain is not seen directly, except in the case of a compound skull fracture, partly because the symptoms and objective findings of such an injury may be confusing, minimal, or delayed, and partly because, if the victim remains conscious and appears to be able to function within normal limits, there is a reluctance on the part of the victim as well as other observers to believe that anything of "serious consequence" has happened.

Fatal brain injuries may occur in a number of sports, including automobile racing, hang gliding, diving, and horseback riding. There is concern about preventing these fatalities, and protective headgear has been developed and is available for three of these sports, but the head is not seen as the principal body site at risk, except in diving where the head and neck share this place. Boxing is viewed differently because for the past 125 years, since the introduction of the boxing glove, the head has been the principal target of attack. Also, it is the repeated target of attack, perhaps 50 or more times in the course of a 10-round bout, and does not simply require protection against one accidental but potentially damaging blow.

For this reason boxing is periodically attacked and banned because of the public perception, for which there is certainly justification given current trends, that the chief purpose of boxing is to disable your opponent, and the best way to do this is to attack his brain through punching his head so that he is not able to function effectively or at all. Despite inflammatory statements made by fighters for publicity or psychologic purposes and understandable rivalries and jealousies, boxers for the most part do not wish to injure their opponents seriously. Many of them are friends and close associates who realize as professionals how dependent they are on each other to earn a living. One psychologic study of boxers indicated that they tend to be self-punitive rather than sadistic.[13] When one has been the cause of the death of another in the ring, it has had a profound effect on the survivor's future ring career, in some instances precipitating retirement.

The history of boxing goes back at least three thousand years. It was a pre-eminent sport among the ancient Greeks, involving probably as many as 100,000 men and boys during one thousand years of Olympic, Nemean, Pythian, and many other championships. It seems clear that the loser in these contests was the one who was unwilling or unable to continue and there was no time limit. Despite many surviving detailed descriptions of championship contests, we know definitely of only two fatalities. Although such scholars as Plato and Aristotle took boxers to task as being lazy, gluttonous, and intemperate, there was no mention of abolishing boxing because of its brutality. In the case of the pancratium, a form of wrestling in which kicking and punching were allowed, however, there were frequent references to its deadly character.

PROTECTIVE BOXING EQUIPMENT

The concern that the ancient Greek boxers had to prevent breaking their hands led them to wear leather straps (*himantes*), wrapped around their knuckles and held in place by 1 in. wide thongs attached to straps laced across the back of the hand and tied up on the forearm. For training they wore padded gloves that they called "spheres." Theseus is supposed to have invented the cestus, which had spikes over the knuckles, but this was used only for a type of gladiatorial combat and never for sport. The use of hand protection by a glove, which was resumed for exhibitions of sparring by Jack Broughton, the English champion from 1734 to 1750, led to the development of the modern boxing glove.

The difficulties that have beset pro-fessional boxing in recent years arise from a multitude of different sources, creating a tangled web that may not be disentangled in our lifetimes. These troubles are chronic, but they are brought to a focus periodically to create a crisis whenever there is a death of a notable fighter in the ring. Fatalities in recent years have been responsible for the ban on professional boxing in the state of Connecticut and the countries of Czechoslovakia, Sweden, and Poland.

It is ironic that the principal cause of these fatalities has been the equipment that was originally introduced for the purpose of making the sport safer and more acceptable to the public at large—the boxing gloves. Jack Broughton was the boxing champion of England from 1734 to 1750. He has been given credit for introducing scientific boxing and the art of deception into the ring. In 1743 he wrote a code of rules that governed boxing in England until 1838. He also introduced the first boxing gloves in sparring exhibitions.

Broughton announced in 1747 that instruction would be given at his boxing academy in Haymarket, "With the utmost tenderness and regard to the delicacy of the frame and constitution of the pupil. For which reason mufflers are provided that will effectively secure them from the inconvenience of black eyes, broken jaws and bloody noses." The "mufflers" were lightly padded leather gloves. The purpose, of course, was to attract the gentry and their sons, who supported boxing by their patronage and were eager to learn the art but afraid of facial disfigurement.

At that time, and later on, the fencing masters were also teaching boxing to satisfy the new demand. They wished to be as careful of their hands and faces as their pupils, so that the use of gloves became very popular among the amateurs. Gloves were still not used generally by professionals for many years thereafter.

The use of gloves was not required

under the London Prize Ring Rules, which succeeded those of Broughton and continued to govern boxing bouts generally, with some modification, until 1892. Butting, kicking, and gouging were forbidden under these rules, measures designed to appeal to the supposedly more refined tastes of the gentry and the growing conservatism of the new age.

Although these changes were generally conceded to be an improvement, it is a remarkable fact that there is no record of any contestant fighting under Broughton's rules losing an eye, despite the fact that gouging was perfectly permissible. This situation might be contrasted with the record of the modern era when all fighters wear gloves, and yet many have had to be retired because of serious permanent damage to one or both eyes, and some, like Kid Gavilan, have been blinded from repeated injuries. The gloved thumb is very easily poked into the eye by its wearer, who would never think of sticking his naked thumb there, and, in fact, would be forbidden by the rules from so doing. Almost every professional fighter has had his eyes burned or stung at some time by the rubbing of glove laces across them or from some substance being carried onto them by the glove. Rosin is now forbidden in the ring because of the eye damage it caused. The referee's rubbing of a fighter's gloves on his trousers after a knockdown is a gesture to the past and not of much practical effect.

The rules proposed by the Marquis of Queensberry did specify the use of gloves when they were presented in 1865, but were applied in their entirety for the first time at a tournament in London in 1872. Two simple statements covered the subject: "Rule 8. The gloves to be fair-sized boxing gloves of the best quality and new. Rule 9. Should a glove burst, or come off, it must be replaced to the referee's satisfaction." In the meantime, however, British boxers had been using padded gloves in exhibitions abroad as early as 1818.

Gloves were apparently introduced into the American ring by the English pugilists who came over in numbers in the 1850s and 1860s. When John L. Sullivan knocked out Paddy Ryan in nine rounds in Mississippi City in 1882, he became the last of the bareknuckle champions. He had had considerable previous experience in fighting with gloves and had found that although boxing was still illegal it was frequently tolerated by the police under these conditions. He had also discovered that he could hit with more damaging force with the gloves than without.

The weight of boxing gloves gradually became standardized at 8 oz for ordinary bouts and 6 oz for championship bouts, with some exceptions. Gloves weighing 10 oz were used for intercollegiate and many other amateur competitions. This weight, together with the weight of the gauze and tape, gave the boxer a club weighing about a pound on the end of a long lever, his forearm and arm. To this weight was still to be added that additional amount of water absorbed by the gloves from the sweat of the fighters and the water dashed on them by their seconds between rounds. On one occasion when a pair of 8 oz gloves was weighed directly after being removed from a fighter who had completed a 10-round bout, each glove had *doubled* its original weight.

In a move aimed at greater safety, the New York State Athletic Commission has been experimenting since 1963 with 10 oz gloves. They were apparently unaware that between 1945 and 1960 three college boxers died of head injuries sustained in bouts where 10 oz gloves were used, and where they were also wearing prescribed "protective" headgear. Cleveland Williams attracted some publicity in 1964 by paying $155 a pair for specially constructed 24 oz gloves. His manager claimed that Cleveland hit so hard (49 knockouts to his credit) that it was necessary to use these "pillows" to keep his sparring partners from quitting. Significantly, the sparring partners continued to complain of being hurt by the punches.

Since 1945, *Ring* magazine has published annually the total of deaths recorded in amateur and professional boxing around the world. The average for the 24-year period has been about 12 deaths a year. The overwhelming majority of these deaths are due to brain injury. There has been no decline in the number of deaths despite the fact that there has been a significant decrease in the number of participants in many countries, such as the United States, in recent years. It was estimated that there were 5,000 professional and 10,000 amateur boxers in training in this country in 1962. It would not be surprising to find that there are one-third to one-half less this number at the present time. Russia is said to have 50,000 amateur boxers in training, but it is difficult to confirm these figures and to decide how many of these devote a substantial part of their time to boxing as a sport.

A tremendous amount of research relating to brain injury has been carried out in the past 20 years. Most of it has been motivated by the desire to reduce the number of deaths in automotive accidents rather than in sports, but the findings that have resulted are applicable to both. The brain may be severely damaged when the skull remains intact if the head is accelerated or decelerated rapidly enough to cause it to come into violent contact with the inside of the skull or if the vessels that connect it with the general circulation are torn. Momentary or sustained loss of consciousness may result. "Knockout" may apparently also occur without such direct contact if the motion of the brain is so violent that the surge of spinal fluid through and around the brain acts as a blow might on the sensitive cortex of the brain.

There is no way of determining when a fighter is knocked down by a punch to the head and then strikes his head on the ring flooring or on the ropes, causing a second deceleration, which blow is responsible for the damage found in the operating room or at autopsy. Enough patients in whom no second violent blow was sustained have been examined, however, for us to know that the most severe type of damage to the brain may occur as the result of punching alone. When more than one punch has been landed on the head before the final one, it is also impossible to judge exactly the effect of repeated blows.

Not only does boxing face the continuing occurrence of death in the ring, but, for every boxer who dies, how many live on with severe, permanent brain damage that makes them not only unfit to box but also to earn a respectable living in any way except possibly through manual labor? Despite the denials of a small group of neurologists who have based their opinions on electroencephalograms performed directly after prizefights, the evidence has piled up in recent years to prove that the "punchdrunk" syndrome is a function of the number and frequency of bouts fought and is not decided by the skill of the fighter in being able to evade or parry punches. Whether it is due to the gradual accumulation of relatively minor brain injuries or to a greater number of more serious ones is not known. Paradoxically, the device that was used to protect the hands, and later the face, became a principal cause of increasing assault on the boxer's brain. The long history of bare-knuckle boxing with the rare fatalities contrasts with the much shorter modern period and its many deaths, the great majority of which have been due to brain damage. The hand has been converted to a club because of the added weight of the gauze, tape, and the glove, which holds the bones together to attack the head with relative impunity. Hand fractures do occur despite the glove, but usually from hooking and not from punching straight ahead.

To protect the forehead, orbits, eyes, and parts of the face and scalp from abrasions and lacerations in training, fighters began in the 19th century to wear a knotted handkerchief or padded leather straps, which developed into the sparring helmet. This development had been anticipated by the ancient Greeks, who had originated a protective boxing helmet made of leather studded with iron knobs and padded, called the *amphotides*. A modern helmet, at first padded with horsehair but now with foam, to protect the head and face is required in the United States at most levels of amateur boxing, but is not worn in international or Olympic boxing.

The helmet currently used has some ability to decelerate blows, but it serves mainly to prevent hematomas of the ears and lacerations of the forehead and scalp. It can do nothing to affect the torsion caused by blows to the side of the head, and by its weight may actually increase the effect of the torsion. Brain injuries, some of which have resulted in fatalities, have occurred in boxers wearing the older and the modern helmets.

OCCURRENCE OF BRAIN INJURIES IN BOXERS

The occurrence of permanent disability or fatality as a result of participation in any recreational or sport activity attracts public and professional attention because it seems to be so inappropriate. Injuries sustained in sports activities are not reportable under public law as are communicable diseases. For this reason we lack information about the frequency of their occurrence except as collected and reported by some individuals or groups who are treating or attempting to prevent these injuries. In such experiences the collected injuries may range in severity from trivial to disabling, and criteria such as time lost from participation may be used to evaluate their impact. Fatalities make a sharp end point for evaluation of the relative risk of a sport or recreational activity when they are related to the numbers of participants. When they can be directly related to the particular activity in which the individual was involved, they can provide useful and striking guidelines to measures for safety and protection for such activities in the future.

In many reports of the occurrence of intracranial injuries in boxers during the past 70 years, there are mentions and descriptions of nonfatal injuries as well as fatalities (Fig 5–1). It is only among the latter that we have reasonably accurate numbers, since virtually all of the victims have been examined by a physician and have been reported in one way or another. In the case of the former, the less serious are never attended by a physician or brought to his attention, and even the more serious come to medical care only after their late effects became manifest, months or years after the initial injury, or as the result of an accumulation of similar injuries in continuing boxing experience.

It is possible to say with reasonable accuracy as of this writing that 655 fatalities resulting from boxing injuries have been recorded from January 1918 to January 1989 (Table 5–1), an average of less than 10 a year.[28] Of this number, 193 (30%) were amateurs. Despite what is probably more complete reporting in the 44-year period from January 1945 to January 1989, there does not appear to be any increase in the number of fatalities for this period, which is 363, an average of only 8.2 per year.[25] These figures include my continuing personal collection.[33] This shows also that with 50 deaths from 1970 to 1981 and 38 from 1979 to 1988, there is a continuing decrease in the average number of fatalities per year.

Of the 38 that occurred from 1979 to

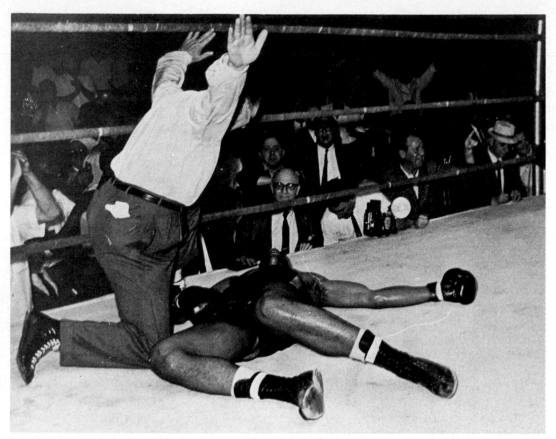

FIG 5–1.
Lucian "Sonny" Banks lies unconscious as he is counted out by the referee at the Philadelphia Arena on May 10, 1965. He subsequently died as a result of a closed head injury. (Photo by Sam Psoras, *Philadelphia Daily News.* Used by permission.)

1988, the weight classes were reported for 26 (Table 5–2). There were two heavyweights, three light heavyweights, two middleweights, eight welterweights, 6 lightweights, two featherweights, two bantamweights, and one flyweight. All but nine of these deaths occurred in the United States, with three in South Africa and one each in Scotland, the Philippines, Nigeria, France, Japan, and Venezuela.

There have been many case reports and descriptions of clinical series concerning boxers who sought medical assistance because of psychiatric and neurologic symptoms. The clinical spectrum of posttraumatic encephalopathy that they exhibit has been summarized by Roberts[30] as ranging from dysarthria to dysequilibrium, disabling ataxia, spasticity, extrapyramidal tremors, and psychiatric disturbances. There have been three studies reported, however, dealing with samples of boxers or ex-boxers. One was done by Roberts,[30] which gives a better idea of what might be expected in the case of the typical boxer.

Roberts examined 224 of 250 boxers who had been identified as a 1.5% random sample of 18,781 who had boxed professionally in the United Kingdom between 1929 and 1955 (Table 5–3). Twenty-five were dead or could not be located. Thirty-seven (17%) had chronic neurologic sequelae, of whom 13 showed characteristic posttraumatic encephalop-

TABLE 5-1.

Fatalities in Boxing From 1918 to 1989*

January 1918–January 1989 Average, 9.3 per year	5 fatalities; 193 amateurs
January 1945–January 1989 Average, 8.2 per year	363 fatalities
January 1970–December 1981 Average, 4.2 per year	50 fatalities
January 1979–January 1989 Average, 3.8 per year	38 fatalities; 10 amateurs

*Data from Putnam P: Sports Illustrated 1983; 58:23–46; Ryan AJ: Personal collection, 1989.

TABLE 5-3.

Random Sample (1.5%) of 18,781 Men Who Had Boxed Professionally in the United Kingdom Between 1929 and 1955*

Total names selected	250
Dead or not located	25
Total number examined	224
Chronic neurologic sequelae	37 (17%)
Posttraumatic encephalopathy	13
Frank dementia	2
Associated factors	
Older age when examined	
No. of bouts fought	
Heavier fighting weights	

*Data from Roberts AH: Brain Damage in Boxers. London, Pitman Publishing, 1969.

athy. Two were suffering from frank dementia. Age, number of bouts, and heavy weights were factors associated with an increased frequency of neurologic sequelae.

Jedlinski et al.[14] studied 60 amateur Polish boxers who had more than 100 bouts (Table 5–4). Thirty-three (55%) showed positive neurologic signs, although frank encephalopathy was manifested in only 21.7%, and severe damage, including dementia, was found in only 8.4%. Those who were heavier and had fought more bouts were more likely to exhibit these signs and symptoms.

Thomassen et al.[37] studied 33 former champion amateur Danish boxers and compared them with 53 former First Di-

vision soccer players. He found no difference in the frequency and severity of neurologic symptoms and signs between the two groups. The Danish boxers, however, had averaged only half as many fights as the Polish boxers.

These studies suggest that the occurrence and severity of neurologic signs and symptoms in former boxers are a function of the number and frequency of bouts they have fought, and that boxers in the heavier weight classes are most likely to exhibit these findings. Whether this is because of the gradual accumulation of relatively minor brain injuries or a greater number of more serious ones is not known.

TABLE 5-2.

Boxing Fatalities by Weight Class (1979–1988)*

Weight classes reported	
Heavyweights	2
Light heavyweights	3
Middleweights	2
Welterweights	8
Lightweights	6
Featherweights	2
Bantamweights	2
Flyweight	1
Total	26

*Data from Putnam P: Sports Illustrated 1983; 58:23–46, Ryan AJ: Personal collection, 1989.

TABLE 5-4.

Study of 60 Amateur Polish Boxers With More Than 100 Bouts Fought*

Positive neurologic signs	33 (55%)
Frank encephalopathy	13 (21.7%)
Dementia	5 (8.4%)
Associated factors	
No. of bouts fought	
Heavier fighting weights	

*Data from Jedlinski J, Gatarski J, Szymusik A: Acta Med Pol 1971; 12:443.

OCCURRENCE AND EFFECTS OF ACUTE BRAIN INJURIES

Some of the confusion that surrounds the diagnosis and management of the person who has suffered an acute brain injury or who manifests the chronic effects of repeated acute brain injuries arises from the proper definition of the term *cerebral concussion*. It is neither a symptom nor a diagnosis but is a clinical syndrome describing a temporary state of the brain that may occur from stimulation of the reticular activating system in the medulla. It is characterized by a loss of awareness of the surroundings, varying changes in pulse rate and blood pressure, generalized weakness of the skeletal musculature, and loss of the head's ability to maintain the body in the erect posture. Its use as a symptom causes a tendency to overlook the fact that an injury to the brain has occurred. Its use as a diagnosis raises, without answering, the question as to whether any pathologic change has taken place in the brain. Classifying concussion by degrees of from 1 to 3 or 1 to 5 suggests that lesser or greater injury to the brain has occurred without specifying the location or character of the injury, and has led to the use of nonspecific terms such as *serious* and *not serious*. All this makes it difficult to establish whether there may be cumulative effects of acute brain injuries that do not manifest overt and gross changes, and leaves guidelines for appropriate management up in the air.

The work of Rimel et al.[29] has established on clinical grounds that persons who have suffered head (brain) injuries that were classified as "minor" and who were not given specific management frequently produce symptoms and functional deficiencies that are apparent 6 months or more later. Even among those classified as "moderate," such deficiencies may become permanent (Tables 5–5 to 5–8).

Delayed recovery of intellectual function and the cumulative effects of concussion were described by Gronwall and Wrightson.[11, 12] They found that patients who have suffered concussions are unable for a period of time afterwards to process information at a normal rate. The time taken to recover is related to the severity of the injury, and after uncomplicated concussion it is usually less than 35 days. In those who experience persistent headache and other postconcussion syndromes, it often persists beyond 35 days. Those who have suffered a second concussion take longer to recover information processing skills. The implications for boxers, who frequently suffer many more concussions, are obvious.

Since the state of cerebral concussion occurs commonly in boxers in sparring as well as in formal bouts, whether or not they have been temporarily rendered unconscious, the question of the nature and

TABLE 5–5.

Minor Head Injury Study Population*

Total number of patients with minor head injury	538
No. of patients assessed after 3 mo	424
No. of patients assessed after 3 mo who had been gainfully employed before injury	310
No. of patients administered the neuropsychologic battery	69
No. of patients administered the 3-mo outcome family psychologic assessment who had been gainfully employed before injury	59

*Data from Rimel RW, et al: Neurosurgery 1981; 9:221–228.

TABLE 5–6.

Information About Accident (*n* = 538)*

Mechanism of Injury	Patients (%)	Blood Alcohol Level (mean, 0.08 g/dL)	Patients (%)
Vehicular accidents	46	Negative	39
Falls	23	0.01–0.09 g/dL	8
Sports (including bicycling)	18	0.10–0.20 g/dL > 0.20 g/dL	16
Assaults	10	Not done	18
Other	3		

Data from Rimel RW, et al: Neurosurgery 1981; 9:221–228.

location of the brain injury that is associated with it becomes extremely important in terms of the immediate and long-term management of the boxer. Electroencephalograms (EEGs) are not immediately helpful in this regard, and the mandatory computed tomography (CT) or magnetic resonance imaging (MRI) scans now taken after knockouts in some states will reveal only major intracranial or extracranial damage or hemorrhage. Certain psychologic tests are more sensitive but require serial monitoring; although they may localize the damage to certain brain areas, they do not indicate precisely the extent or permanency of the damage. Boxers and their managers certainly resist permanent retirement from the ring while they feel they are still physically capable of fighting, but the persistence of

symptoms and signs of chronic brain injury should provide adequate justification.

There are principally two mechanisms involved in the occurrence of disabling and fatal brain injuries. The first is the direct transmission of force through the skull to the brain and its coverings, often accompanied by a contrecoup effect. The second is sudden acceleration and deceleration of the brain within the skull, resulting in a similar action of the body as a whole in any direction, or a sudden torsion of the head or the neck. Since sports such as boxing are characterized by vigorous motion, often accompanied by sudden starting and stopping and frequent changes in direction, there is no

TABLE 5–7.

Outcome at 3 Months—Subjective Complaints (*n* = 424)*

Complaint	Patients (%)
Persistent headaches	78
Memory deficit	59
Difficulty with household chores (activities of daily living)	14
Change in transportation	15
Number of complaints	
0	16
1 complaint	79
≤2 complaints	5

Data from Rimel RW, et al: Neurosurgery 1981; 9:221–228.

TABLE 5–8.

Outcome at 3 Months—Objective Measures (*n* = 424)*

Objective Measure	Patients (%)
Positive neurologic findings	2
Pupillary	1
Cranial nerve deficit	0.1
Seizures	1
Reported change in financial status	49
Change in marital status	0.1
Total patients unemployed	24
Unemployed patients gainfully employed before injury (*n* = 310)	34
Change in employment due to injury	3

Data from Rimel RW, et al: Neurosurgery 9:221–228.

way to prevent such actions without drastically changing the nature of the sport and perhaps eliminating important elements that make this sport attractive and exciting. Preventive measures then must be directed toward improvement of factors in general body conditioning, such as strength, flexibility, balance, and position sense, which can help the individual to minimize the effects of collisions, impacts, and sudden directional changes. Rules that discourage or prevent actions in which excessive or uncontrolled force can be applied to the head in a damaging way may also be effective.

Where the concussed individual has fallen as the result of a blow to the head, as in boxing or as the result of a severe acceleration followed by sudden deceleration, the fall is not simply the result of a momentary loss of consciousness. Instead, the individual throws himself/herself to the ground from the activation of the righting reflex as a result of overloading of the reticular system from the combined effects of impact on the brain and overloading impulses from the vestibular coordinating system. This has been determined by measuring on film the time of descent to the standing surface and by showing that an unopposed free fall from the same height would have taken longer.[9] Landing hard as the result of the reflex in a semiconscious or unconscious state may cause further injury to the brain.

There is good evidence to indicate that repeated brain injury, even though each individual injury produces minimal or unobservable immediate effects, causes chronic brain damage with degeneration and atrophy. The ability of undamaged brain tissue to take over or compensate for the loss of damaged tissue is limited. Damaged central nervous system tissue does not regenerate. It is therefore incumbent on those charged with the medical supervision of athletes to identify brain injury when it occurs, even

when signs and symptoms may be minimal or absent, and to allow the athlete to recover from that injury as much as possible before resuming sports competition. This may help to prevent a rapid summing up of the effects of acute brain injury. The persistence of signs and symptoms of brain injury may also call for the physician to recommend retirement from a sport where there is grave danger of reinjury to the brain before disabling chronic brain injury occurs.

OCCURRENCE OF CHRONIC BRAIN INJURIES IN BOXERS

The nature of chronic brain injury in boxers and its results in terms of the individual's behavior and longevity have been the subjects of many studies and publications since 1952. The term *punch-drunk* is a popular one of long standing. It was used as the title of an article by Martland,[23] a medical examiner, who described a series of autopsies of persons who died with chronic brain injuries, but none of whom were boxers. Because he related his findings to the experiences of some notable boxers who were said to have been afflicted with symptoms and behavior that might be related to chronic brain injuries, this article has been mistakenly cited as the beginning of modern studies of chronic brain injuries in boxers.

In fact, the credit for the first such publication in English must go to Busse and Silverman,[4] who compared EEGs of boxers who had been knocked out in the ring with some taken on a control group of the same ages. There was a 37% occurrence of abnormal findings among the boxers. No correlation was found between the changes observed in different individuals. Kaplan and Browder,[18] working with the New York State Boxing Commission between 1950 and 1954, studied 1,043 professional fighters, including all divisions and types, recording a total of 1,400 EEGs. Forty of these EEGs were made in an anteroom off the ringside within 10 minutes after losing a fight. They observed the styles of the fighters at ringside, estimated the relationship of physical fitness and experience to their performance in the ring, and watched for the apparent effects of blows delivered to the head. Sixteen-millimeter, regular speed, and slow-motion films of the fights were made for later study. The defeated fighters were also given a gross neurologic examination in the dressing room immediately after the fight. The EEGs were analyzed to divide them into 12 categories. Thirty-four percent of the fighters had EEG patterns that fell within the normal range. When the fighters were divided according to age, number of previous fights, style (slugger or boxer), ring rating, weight, number of bouts lost, and number of knockouts (10 second or technical), there were no significant differences between them based on disorganization of their EEGs. One hundred ninety-seven had from one to six repeat EEGs within the next 4 years, and one-quarter showed some change from their previous pattern. The only conclusion from this study was that those with the lower ring ratings had a higher percentage of disorganized electroencephalograms.

Johnson[16] examined 15 professional boxers about 22 years after their careers had ended and found that 11 showed diffuse pathologic EEG changes. Each boxer had had from 200 to 300 fights. Air encephalography showed chronic brain damage in all but 3.

OCCURRENCE AND EFFECTS OF ACUTE BRAIN INJURIES

Larsson et al.[20] examined 75 junior boxers whose ages ranged from 17 to 25 years, competing in the Swedish junior championships (JM) in 1950 and 1951 and in the Swedish championships (SM) in 1951. Sixty-three were from the junior match (JM) and 12 from the senior match (SM). A detailed medical history, a history of school and work achievements, and a history of previous boxing experience were taken before the bouts, and a neurologic examination (which proved to be normal in all cases) was made. They appeared to be a generally healthy young group. EEGs were made on 44 before and immediately after their matches. These were also made on 31 who had not had this examination before their match after they had experienced a hard bout, and some of these were tested more than once. All boxers were evaluated after their matches for their orientation to time and place and for possible amnesia as possible evidences of having sustained a concussion.

Among the entire 75 boxers, 35 had been knocked down in their bouts, and 14 had been knocked out. Of the 44 examined before and after bouts, 13 had been knocked down and 5 knocked out. Pronounced periods of amnesia and disorientation occurred in 14 of the 75, and there were 9 who had slight symptoms of the same type. In 12 who had been knocked down or out, there was no disorientation or amnesia. One boxer who had been knocked down early in his match won it despite complete amnesia for the match and 20 minutes thereafter.

Of the total of 75 boxers, 48 showed no changes in EEGs after their matches. Nine showed a general aptitude decrease, 4 a decrease plus slow activity, and 3 slow activity only. Where the group of those tested before and after was divided between those who had sustained severe head blows in their matches[17] from those who had not,[47] the suggestive EEG changes were found in 30% of the former and in only 13% of the latter. Among those tested only after matches because of a relatively severe injury,[25] pathologic or borderline EEG changes were found in 52%. The conclusion of Larsson et al. was that slight cerebral injuries probably occurred frequently in junior matches and that even if the changes demonstrated are largely reversible, there is a risk of permanent and more significant cerebral lesions as the result of cumulative damage from repeated matches, even without knockouts. The rate of serious mental and emotional disturbance was high.

Kaste et al.[19] found EEG abnormalities in the brains of 6 of 14 Finnish boxers, although 12 of the 14 showed no neurologic deficit. Sironi et al.[35] found EEG abnormalities in 3 of 10 young Italian boxers (ages 18 to 24), and they were all in boxers who had been knocked out more than twice. Casson et al.[5] found two abnormal EEGs in 10 boxers (aged 20 to 31) who had been knocked out. Both were in fighters whose clinical findings were normal, but one of them showed a cavum septi pellucidi on his CT scan. Ross et al.[32] examined 38 ex-boxers and 2 current boxers with use of neurologic examinations,[24] EEGs,[24] CT scans,[38] and a questionnaire concerning performance and medical history. Findings in only 7 of the 24 EEGs were positive. Of the 11 boxers who had less than 50 bouts, 2 (18%) had positive findings, of 6 with 50 to 100 bouts, 1 (17%) had positive findings, and of the 7 with more than 100 bouts, 4 (57%) had positive findings. Beaussart and Beaussart-Boulenge,[1] who performed EEGs before and within 15 minutes after bouts, found no evidence of pathologic changes even in boxers who had been knocked out. They failed to find any correlation between EEG changes and the severity of postconcussion syndrome in 3,100 cases of the latter.

Evaluation of chronic brain damage by other means, in some instances including EEG examination, began with Sercl and Jaros,[34] who studied 1,582 boxers from 1957 to 1961 and compared their neurologic findings with those in 100 nonboxers. They found signs of chronic encephalopathy in 9% of the former compared with 4% of the latter. This study was preceded by isolated reports of a few cases of former boxers who had died and whose brains were examined postmortem. Brandenberg and Hallervorden[2] found changes characteristic of Alzheimer's disease in a 51-year-old former middleweight champion who had boxed as an amateur for 10 years and had begun to show clinical signs and symptoms of encephalopathy at the age of 38. Grahmann and Ule[10] found brain atrophy and neurofibrillary tangles, with large lateral ventricles and a cavum septi pellucidi, in a former amateur and professional boxer who died at the age of 48 with clinical evidence of chronic encephalopathy. Neuberger et al.[26] found cerebral atrophy with considerable gliosis throughout the cerebral cortex in the brains of two former boxers with clinical chronic encephalopathy. Spillane[36] found septal abnormalities in pneumoencephalograms of four of five boxers with symptoms of chronic encephalopathy.

Mawdsley and Ferguson[24] examined 10 ex-boxers and obtained a postmortem examination of the brain in one. Lumbar pneumoencephalography in the other nine showed abnormal findings in eight, specifically evidence of enlarged lateral ventricles, cavum septi pellucidi, or evidence of cerebral and cerebellar atrophy. The examined brain showed all of these. Only one man showed a significantly abnormal EEG. All showed historical or clinical evidence of chronic encephalopathy, or both historical and clinical evidence.

Constantinides and Tissot[6] examined the brain of a 58-year-old boxer who had been fighting from 17 to 24 years of age and died after a long history of chronic encephalopathy with occasional epileptic seizures. They found neurofibrillary damage throughout the brain, cerebral atrophy, and a cavum septi pellucidi. Brennan and O'Connor[3] found, among amateur boxers who were Air Force personnel between 1963 and 1966, two deaths and one boxer who became a permanent invalid. Neuberger et al.[26] found, in a cerebral biopsy of the frontal lobe of an ex-boxer who had suffered 30 knockouts in his career, senile plaques and miniature scars in the gray matter, and in the brain of another boxer who had chronic encephalopathy and died at the age of 53, enlarged ventricles and brain atrophy with miniature scars in the gray matter.

The report of the Royal College of Physicians, London, Committee on Boxing on the medical aspects of boxing was published by Roberts[30] in *Brain Damage in Boxers*. This was a study of a 1.5% random sample of 16,781 men who had boxed professionally in the United Kingdom from 1929 to 1955. Only 224 were examined because 25 were dead or could not be located and 1 refused to participate. Thirty-seven (17%) demonstrated chronic neurologic symptoms or findings based on neurologic, psychometric, or electroencephalographic tests. Of these, 13 demonstrated classic chronic encephalopathy, and 2 had frank dementia. Older age, number of bouts, and heavier weights were all positively associated with these changes.

The most complete and elaborate study of the brains of deceased boxers is found in *The Aftermath of Boxing* by Corsellis et al.[7] Brains of 15 ex-boxers (12 professionals, 3 amateurs) were collected during a 16-year period. Their lives were investigated in retrospect through visits to relatives and friends by a psychiatric social worker, hospital records were obtained, and boxing journals were culled for information about their ring careers, which extended during the period from 1900 to 1940. Two had been world champions, and six national or regional champions. Ages at death ranged from 57 to 91. Two of the boxers died after ventricu-

lar hemorrhage, and in both the leaves of the septum were torn and separated, possibly as the result of the hemorrhage, so that they were excluded from further analysis. There was a striking difference between the septa of the 13 boxers and 500 controls. All but one of the boxers had a cavum septi pellucidi; in 10 of 12 it was fenestrated. Only 28% of the controls had a cavum septi pellucidi, and in only 3% of the 500 was it accompanied by fenestration. The average width of the cavum septi pellucidi in the boxers was three times that in the nonboxers. Five of the 15 nonboxers with a cavum septi pellucidi and fenestration had firm clinical or other pathologic evidence of past head injury. Examination of the cerebellum showed cortical scarring on the inferior surface of the lateral lobes and significant losses of Purkinje cells on the ventral surface. Both of these findings would be consistent with the cerebellum having been forced into the foramen magnum by the shock of impact. These findings are similar to those of Unterharnscheidt[38] in cats whose brains were damaged experimentally. Degeneration and loss of pigmented cells in the substantia nigra and the presence of many neurofibrillary tangles, both of which are common findings in parkinsonism, were also noted in the majority of these boxers' brains.

The historical and clinical findings in the boxers in this study appeared to confirm and reinforce the pathology noted in their brains. Four had had other single head injuries, none of which appeared serious. Many had been alcohol drinkers at one time or another, and ten were reported to have drunk to excess. Four had cerebrovascular disease resulting in hemiplegia, and one had been treated successfully for tabes dorsalis. None of these conditions could have been responsible for the findings in their brains. The majority had memory defects beginning for the most part early in life. For all but three their memory disorders merged imperceptibly into a state of dementia. Some of the men remained addicted to violence long after they had stopped boxing.

Cruikshank et al.[8] reported the cases of two young boxers who suffered acute intracranial hemorrhage not identified until 2 weeks and 2 months later. The first had a hematoma occupying the left lateral ventricle, the head of the caudate nucleus, and the splenium of the corpus callosum. After the surgical evacuation of the hematoma, his recovery was good. The second had a right parieto-occipital subdural hematoma that was evacuated through burr holes, resulting in complete recovery.

In noncontrast CT scans of ten boxers, performed within 1 week of their being knocked out, Casson et al.[5] reported normal findings in five. The others showed cerebral atrophy and one a cavum septi pellucidi. They ranged in age from 18 to 22, and only one had a minimally abnormal EEG. Four had had 20 or more professional bouts.

Sironi et al.[35] found abnormal CT scans in six of ten young (18 to 24 years of age) professional boxers. Four showed enlargements of the convexity of the central sulci, and two showed widening of the lateral and third ventricles. These were in boxers who had been knocked out more than twice.

Oleman et al.[27] reviewed the reports of all personnel of the Army of the United Kingdom admitted to hospitals of the Royal Army Medical Corps during the years 1969 to 1980 and the reports of those who died or were medically discharged between 1952 and 1980. There were 437 admissions for boxing injuries, of which 296 (67.7%) were head injuries. Of these, 115 (39%) were for concussions and 69 (23%) for "intracranial injury of other and unspecified nature." There were 2 cases (0.68%) of cerebral laceration and contusion (one resulted in a medical discharge) and 3 (1%) of subdural hemorrhage (all of which resulted in

medical discharges). There were no deaths during this period. The only estimate of the population at risk is based on a random sample of 3,185 Army personnel made in 1962 that found 113 engaged in boxing for an average of 4.9 hours per month each. If these ratios remained constant from 1969 to 1980, there would have been about 5,700 men boxing, each of them for about 59 hours a year. With an average of 35 injuries a year serious enough for hospital admission, there would have been 150 boxers admitted per year, or one serious injury for every 9,000 man hours of boxing.

Among ex-boxers examined by Ross et al.,[32] of the 38 who had CT scans, 24 also had a complete neurologic examination. Based on evaluation of the CT scans graded on a scale of 0 to 4 for evidence of cerebral atrophy and ventricular enlargement, there was a significant relationship between the number of bouts fought and the composite CT score, but this was due more to the presence of ventricular enlargement than evidence of gyral atrophy. This was particularly striking since 25 had less than 100 bouts and only 5 had more than 150 bouts. The standard neurologic examination was of little value in detecting chronic cerebral damage, since only 25% of the boxers showed positive findings. No psychometric tests were administered.

It is difficult to evaluate the results of Rodriguez et al.,[31] who found regional cerebral blood flow to be significantly below normal in seven professional boxers. This would have to be correlated with EEG recordings, CT scans, and possibly postmortem brain examinations to determine how it might relate to boxing injury.

A study by the New York State Athletic Commission of acute boxing injuries suffered in the professional ring in New York from Aug 1, 1982, to July 1, 1984, and reported by Jordan and Campbell,[17] identified 377 that occurred in 3,110 rounds of boxing (Table 5–9). Of these,

TABLE 5–9.

Acute Boxing Injuries in 3,110 Rounds of Boxing Reported by New York State Athletic Commission, Aug 1, 1982, to July 1, 1984*

Head injuries other than lacerations or eye injuries	262
Lacerations and eye injuries	8
Requiring hospitalization	4
Postconcussion syndrome	2
Fatalities	1
Musculoskeletal injuries	100
Total	377

Data from Jordan BD, Campbell EA: Acute Boxing Injuries Among Professional Boxers in New York State: A Two-Year Survey. American College of Sports Medicine, 32nd Annual Meeting, 1986.

262 were described as injuries to the head other than lacerations and eye injuries, of which there were 8. Four of these fighters required hospitalization, and 1 of them died. Two, not necessarily of those who were hospitalized, suffered from a postconcussion syndrome. There was no follow-up regarding how many of the hospitalized or postconcussion fighters returned to the ring later.

EVIDENCE OF APPARENT ABSENCE OR PRESENCE OF CHRONIC BRAIN DAMAGE IN VETERAN BOXERS

Reports of clinical examination of former boxers, including neurologic, radiologic, and electroencephalographic testing, and of postmortem examination of some former boxers' brains by Roberts,[30] Mawdsley and Ferguson,[24] Corsellis et al.,[7] and others indicate a relatively high occurrence of chronic brain damage, often associated with serious behavior disorders, chronic mental and physical disability, and perhaps decreased longevity. Since the principal correlation with these disorders appears time and again to be the number of bouts fought, it is surprising to learn that there are former boxers with records of many bouts who have apparently lived a normal lifespan without marked disability.

Liebling[22] reported in 1950 meeting 90-year-old Billy Ray, who described himself as "the last surviving bare knuckle fighter" and admitted to 140 fights before his retirement. He was apparently physically fit and in full command of his senses. Liebling had been a boxer himself, knew everyone in the fight game, and was a man not easily deceived. H. R. Tuttle, who fought as a lightweight and welterweight many times from 1925 through 1932, died in 1988 at age 84 without ever showing evidence of chronic brain damage. Henry Armstrong, who held world titles in featherweight, lightweight, and welterweight boxing all at the same time in 1937 to 1938, died at age 75 in 1988. He was a Baptist minister for many years after his retirement. Johnny Paychek, one-time national Golden Gloves heavyweight champion and later a professional heavyweight contender, died at age 74 in 1988.

Among well-known fighters who have died or are still living with chronic brain disease, however, there has been a uniform reluctance on their part or that of their relatives to admit that it had anything to do with boxing. Mickey Walker died at age 72, Sid Terris at 70, Max Rosenbloom at 71, and Steve Belloise at 66. Walker and Terris were said to have Parkinson's disease, Rosenbloom, Paget's disease, and Belloise, Alzheimer's disease. Ray Robinson, who recently died at 68, was completely disabled, supposedly because of Alzheimer's disease. Muhammad Ali and his medical consultants have attributed his quite apparent neurologic disorder to Parkinson's disease, or household pesticide poisoning, or both.

CONTINUING OBSERVATIONS AND DEVELOPMENTS

The question of whether wearing a glove increases the numbers of blows to the boxer's head compared with fighting without them has been answered to some extent by a study of contestants in the Danish karate championships from 1983 to 1986 by Johannsen and Noerregaard.[15] Knuckle protection was mandatory in 1983 and 1986 (290 matches, 0.26 injuries per match) and prohibited in 1984 and 1985 (620 matches, 0.25 injuries per match). Head injuries were more common in the tournaments in which fist pads were used, but the severity of head injuries decreased.

Short-term neurobehavioral deficits were evaluated during a 6-month period in 13 young amateur boxers compared with a matched group of 13 amateur athletes who were not boxers.[21] The neuropsychologic tests evaluated cognition, memory, and motor speed. Baseline scores showed no significant intergroup differences except for faster reaction time in boxers. Improvement in test performance was noted in both groups at 6-month follow-ups, but there were still no significant intergroup differences. MRI findings at follow-up were normal in all boxers.

The continued use of brain scans, both CT and MRI, has resulted in fighters being temporarily banned from the ring pending later reevaluation in the United States and the United Kingdom. Apparently only two boxers have been permanently retired because of findings on brain scans, Thomas Kopcke of the Federal Republic of Germany in 1978 and Graeme Brooke of Australia in 1987.

Metallic ring ropes covered only with velvet were eliminated in the 1960s. Since 1983 the 1 in. thick rope of manila hemp has been replaced with one that is 1½ in. thick and covered with shock-absorbent foam under velvet corduroy.

The U.S. Naval Academy, which has maintained boxing as a training method after it had been abandoned as an accepted intercollegiate sport, suspended boxing for a short period in 1988 after a sparring session necessitated surgery for removal of a blood clot from the head of a plebe. Boxing was reinstated there in 1989 after what was described as more protective headgear was ordered.

REFERENCES

1. Beaussart M, Beaussart-Boulenge L: Experimental study of cerebral concussions in 123 amateur boxers by clinical examination and EEG before and immediately after fights. *Electroencephalogr Clin Neurophysiol* 1970; 29:529–530.

2. Brandenburg W, Hallervorden J: Dementia pugilistica mit anatenischem befund. *Virchows Arch [B]* 1954; 325:680–709.

3. Brennan TN, O'Connor PJ: Incidence of boxing injuries in the Royal Air Force in the United Kingdom 1953–1966. *Br J Industr Med* 1968; 25:326–329.

4. Busse EW, Silverman AJ: Electroencephalographic changes in professional boxers. *JAMA* 1952; 149:1522–1525.

5. Casson RI, Sham R, Campbell EA, et al: Evaluation of knocked-out boxers. *J Neurol Neurosurg Psychiatry* 1982; 45:170–174.

6. Constantinides JN, Tissot R: Lesions neurofibrillaires d'Alzheimer generalisees sans plaques seviles, *Arch Suisses Neurol, Neurochirurg Psychiatr* 1967; 100:117–130.

7. Corsellis JAN, Bruton CJ, Freeman-Browne D: The aftermath of boxing. *Psychol Med* 1973; 3:270–303.

8. Cruikshank JK, Higgens CS, Gray JR: Two cases of intracranial hemorrhage in young amateur boxers. *Lancet* 1980; 1:626–627.

9. Govons SR: Brain concussion and posture—the knockdown blow or the boxing ring. *Confin Neurol* 1968; 30:77–84.

10. Grahmann H, Ule G: Beitrag zur Kenntnis der chronischen cerebralen Krankheitsbilder bei Boxern. *Psychiatr Neurol* 1957; 134:261–283.

11. Gronwall D, Wrightson P: Delayed recovery of intellectual function after minor head injury. *Lancet* 1974; 2:605–609.

12. Gronwall D, Wrightson P: Cumulative effect of concussion. *Lancet* 1975; 995.

13. Hussman BF: Aggression in boxers and wrestlers as measured by protective techniques. *Res Quart Am Assoc Health Phys Educ Rec* 1985; 26:421–425.

14. Jedlinski J, Gatarski J, Szymusik A: Encephalopatha Pugilistica (punch drunkenness). *Acta Med Pol* 1971; 12:443.

15. Johannsen HV, Noerregaard FOH: Prevention of injury in karate. *Br J Sports Med* 1988; 22:115–118.

16. Johnson J: Organic psychosyndromes due to boxing. *Br J Psychiatry* 1969; 115:45–53.

17. Jordan BD, Campbell EA: *Acute Boxing Injuries Among Professional Boxers in New York State: A Two-Year Survey*. American College of Sports Medicine, 32nd Annual Meeting, 1986.

18. Kaplan HA, Browder J: Observations on the clinical and brain wave patterns of professional boxers. *JAMA* 1954; 156:1138–1144.

19. Kaste M, Vilkki J, Sainio K, et al: Is chronic brain damage in boxing a hazard of the past? *Lancet* 1982; 2:1186–1188.

20. Larsson LE, Melin KA, Nordstrom-Ohrberg G, et al: *Acute Head Injuries in Boxers*. Swedish Neurological Society, 1954, p 42.

21. Levin HS, Lippold SC, Goldman A: Neurobehavioral functioning and magnetic resonance imaging findings in young boxers. *J Neurosurg* 1987; 67:657–667.

22. Liebling AJ: *The Sweet Science*. New York, Viking Press, 1956, p 4.

23. Martland HS: Punch drunk. *JAMA* 1928; 91:1103–1107.

24. Mawdsley C, Ferguson FR: Neurological disease in boxers. *Lancet* 1983; 2:795–801.

25. Moore M: The challenge of boxing: Bringing safety into the ring. *Phys Sportsmed* 1980; 8:101–105.

26. Neuberger KT, Sintar DW, Denst J: Cerebral atrophy associated with boxing. *Arch Neurol Psychiatry* 1959; 81:403–408.

27. Oleman BJ, Rose CME, Arlow KJ: Boxing injuries in the army. *JR Army Med Corps* 1983; 129:27–32.

28. Putnam P: Going-going-gone. *Sports Illustrated* 1983; 58:23–46.

29. Rimel RW, Giordani B, Barth JT, et al: Disability caused by minor head injury. *Neurosurgery* 1981; 9:221–228.

30. Roberts AH: *Brain Damage in Boxers*. London, Pitman Publishing Co, 1969.

31. Rodrigues G, Ferrillo F, Montano V, et al: Regional cerebral blood flow in boxers. *Lancet* 1983; 2:858.

32. Ross RJ, Cole C, Thompson JS, et al: Boxers computed tomography, EEG, and neurological evaluation. *JAMA* 1983; 249:211–213.

33. Ryan AJ: Personal collection.

34. Sercl M, Jaros O: The mechanisms of cerebral concussion in boxing and their consequences. *World Neurology* 1962; 3:351–358.

35. Sironi VA, Scotti G, Ravagnati L, et al: CT-scan and EEG findings in professional pugilists: Early detection of cerebral atrophy in young boxers. *J Neurosurg Sci* 1982; 26:165–168.

36. Spillane JD: Five boxers. *Br Med J* 1962; 2:1205–1210.

37. Thomassen A, Juul-Jensen P, Olivarius B, et al: Neurological electroencephalographic and neuropsychological examination of 53 former amateur boxers. *Acta Neurol Scand* 1979; 60:352–362.

38. Unterharnscheidt FJ: Injuries due to boxing and other sports, in Viuken PJ, Bruyra GW (eds): *Handbook of Clinical Neurology*, vol 23. Amsterdam. North-Holland Publishing Co, 1975, pp 527–593.

CHAPTER 6

Position Statement of the American Medical Association on Boxing: Analysis and Perspective

Robert C. Cantu, M.D.

Today there is excellent unequivocal evidence that repeated brain injury of concussive or even subconcussive force results in characteristic patterns of brain damage and a steady decline in the ability to process information efficiently.[1-6] Furthermore, the effects of repeated head injury are cumulative; this can be shown immediately at the time of the second injury, not years later. A recent study showed an alarmingly high degree of morbidity 3 months after what appeared to be seemingly insignificant head injuries.[7] While some blows to the head may be more severe than others, none is trivial and each has the potential to be lethal.

Blunt head trauma causes shearing injury to nerve fibers and neurons in proportion to the degree the head is accelerated, and these acceleration forces are imparted to the brain.[8-10] Blows to the side of the head tend to produce greater acceleration forces than those to the face, while those to the chin, which acts as a lever, produce maximal forces. Falls may impart similar deceleration forces. Shearing of blood vessels may lead to subdural and intracerebral hematomas with rapid death.[11] Experiments indicate that by thickly padding gloves or wearing well-padded headgear the force of brain acceleration can be lessened but the length of time during which it is applied is increased.[11] While this seems to lessen the chance of a fatal blood clot, it increases the amount of nerve fiber and axonal shearing.[12, 13] Thus extra padding may reduce the chance of death, but will not prevent brain damage due to tearing of brain substance.

Martland[14] introduced the term *punch drunk* into the medical literature in 1928. While described in boxers, this traumatic encephalopathy may occur in anyone subjected to repeated blows to the head from any cause.

In 1957 Critchley[13] reported on his experience with 69 cases of chronic neurologic disease in boxers. The characteristic symptoms and signs of the punch drunk state include slow appearance of a fatuous or euphoric dementia with emotional lability, with the victim displaying little insight into his deterioration. Speech and thought become progressively slower, while memory deteriorates considerably. There may be mood swings, intense irritability, and sometimes truculence leading to uninhibited violent behavior. Simple fatuous cheerfulness is, however, the most common prevailing mood, although sometimes there is depression with a paranoid coloring. From the clinical standpoint, the neurologist may encounter almost any combination of pyramidal, extrapyramidal, and cerebellar signs. Tremor and dysarthria are two of the most common findings.

In Critchley's experience, the syndrome was more common among professionals than among amateurs, and also in second-rate performers, particularly those looked upon as "sluggers," notorious for their ability to "take it."

In the same article, Critchley describes what he calls the "groggy state," which he regards as being midway between normal performance and a knockout and which he characterizes as "mental confusion with subsequent amnesia, together with an impairment in the speed and accuracy of the motor skill represented by the act of boxing." Using the definitions of concussion found in Chapter 20, Critchley is actually describing a grade 1 concussion. Martland's[14] now famous 1928 essay in the *Journal of the American Medical Association (JAMA)* describes Gene Tunney's grade 3 concussion suffered in training for the second Dempsey fight that was responsible for Tunney retiring from the ring while still heavyweight champion:

I went into a clinch with my head down, something I never do. I plunged forward, and my partner's head came up and butted me over the left eye, cutting and dazing me badly. Then . . . he stepped back and swung his right against my jaw with every bit of his power. It landed flush and stiffened me where I stood. . . . That is the last thing I remembered for two days. They tell me that I finished the round, knocking the man out.

In conclusion he said:

From that incident was born my desire to quit the ring forever, the first opportunity that presented itself . . . But most of all I wanted to leave the game that had threatened my sanity before I met with an accident in a real fight with six ounce gloves that would permanently hurt my brain.

In the 1957 article, Critchley[13] reviews the published electroencephalographic experience[15, 16] (brain wave measurements) of that decade and concludes that the electroencephalographic (EEG) record at that time was a "less sensitive index of punch drunkenness than . . . the clinical evidence" as he had observed symptoms and signs in subjects with normal EEG records.

During the next decade, additional case reports accumulated documenting further evidence of chronic degeneration in mental function.[17–32]

In 1969, at the behest of the Royal College of Physicians of London, Roberts published a monograph reviewing the medical literature and presented studies of British professional boxers (see reference 11 in Appendix 6A). Roberts described the clinical features of the punch drunk syndrome in its mildest form as consisting of some or all of several features: (1) dysarthria, that is, problems with muscular control resembling those of Parkinson's disease; (2) spasticity, that is, a jerky form of impaired muscle control; (3) tremor or shaking; and (4) dementia, or a reduction in intelligence.

The following year, Unterharnscheidt[11] published a massive review of the historical and medical aspects of boxing in which, in addition to the exhaustive review of the medical literature published at that time, he reported original scientific measurements of forces applied to the head in boxing with gloves of varying weights. He commented that "every boxer must expect permanent traumatic damage which is greater the earlier he begins to box, the more frequently he participates, and the longer his career. . ."

It remained for Corsellis et al.[33] to describe the postmortem findings in the brains of men who had been boxers. They described a characteristic pattern of cerebral change that appeared not only to be the result of the boxing but also to changes in the septum pellucidum, a partition in the middle of the brain that may shear into two layers or even be shredded by the distortions of the brain that follow blows to the head. They found destruction of the limbic system, a portion of the brain that governs emotion and has a role in memory and learning. There was a characteristic loss of cells from the cerebellum, a part of the brain that governs balance and coordination. Finally, there was an unusual microscopic change widespread throughout the brain resembling changes that occur with Alzheimer's disease, which caused progressive loss of intelligence, but sufficiently different (neurofibrillary tangles only and no senile plaques) to be regarded as a distinct, different entity unique to subjects suffering repeated blows to the head.

Structural changes in the brains of boxers were identified during life as early as 1962 when Spillane[32] drew particular attention to the cavum septi pallucidi, which he had outlined in pneumoencephalograms of four of his five patients. Pneumoencephalograms involve the injection of air into the spinal fluid compartment that surrounds the brain. At that time they were the only means of showing the shape of the brain on x-ray films. The tests were painful, generally required hospitalization, and had some potential for harm. As a result they were not widely done. With the advent of the computed tomographic (CT) scanner and more recently magnetic resonance imaging (MRI), there is now an innocuous, painless, outpatient means to identify the same changes that used to be diagnosed by means of pneumoencephalography. Utilizing the CT scan, recent reports have documented characteristic changes in currently practicing boxers. One report[34] concludes that the "data show that boxers with even a moderate number of bouts may suffer cerebral atrophy" (loss of brain tissue). Furthermore, the authors found that the degree of cerebral atrophy corresponded with the number of bouts in which the subject had been a participant. The second article, which reported on ten professional boxers, confirmed these findings.[35] The third report, which gave less detail than the others, also indicated changes in four of six professional boxers studied.[27]

Through the 1962 statement of the AMA Committee on the Medical Aspects of Sports "Statement on Boxing," the American Medical Association (AMA) long ago addressed the issue of the medical risks of boxing.[36] It was the Jan 14, 1983, issue of *JAMA* that sparked a debate resulting in extensive major network television coverage, newspaper articles and editorials, magazine stories, an AMA-sponsored conference on the medical aspects of boxing, a Congressional hearing on boxing, and the embarrassing position of the AMA appearing to support both sides of the debate simultaneously.

In that issue of *JAMA* were published two major articles on boxing,[34, 37] neither calling for the abolition of boxing based on moral, ethical, and medical grounds.[39, 40] It is ironic that the AMA's Council on Scientific Affairs study on the safety issue of boxing, a study and recommendations already approved by the House of Delegates at the 1982 annual meeting and thus the official policy of the AMA (see Appendix 6A), appears in the same issue as the conflicting editorial opinion. The council, after deliberation of the medical evidence, concluded that "boxing is a dangerous sport and can result in death or long-term brain injury" but to ban boxing would not be a "realistic solution of the problem of brain injury." It called for establishing a national registry for all amateur and professional boxers, mandating the use of uniform protective equipment and standardizing ringside safety and medical procedures.

At odds with these recommendations were the editorial by Lundberg[38] who concluded, "Boxing seems to me to be less sport than is cockfighting; boxing is an obscenity. Uncivilized man may have been bloodthirsty. Boxing, as a throwback to uncivilized man, should not be sanctioned by any civilized country."[39] Furthermore, a second editorial by Van Allen[39] chimed in: "Is now not the time to suppress exposure of this fragment of our savagery by the mass media and leave boxing to those who enjoy privately staged dogfights."[40]

While the controversy sparked by the Jan 14, 1983, *JAMA* issue raged, the AMA conference on the medical aspects of boxing was held in February 1983. The panel, which included among others professors of neurology and neurosurgery, after reviewing all the medical evidence did not call for a ban on boxing, but rather made eight recommendations to improve boxing safety: (1) establish a national registry of boxers; (2) authorize the ring physician to stop a bout at any time to examine a contestant and to terminate the bout; (3) hold frequent medical training seminars for all ring personnel; (4) provide adequate ringside life support systems and evacuation plans; (5) hold bouts only where proper neurosurgical facilities are nearby; (6) establish mandatory safety standards for ring equipment; (7) upgrade and enforce medical evaluations of boxers by all state boxing commissions; and (8) eliminate "tough man" contests.[37, 41]

At the June 1983 AMA annual meeting in Chicago, the 351-member house of delegates, by voice vote, adopted a resolution (see Appendix 6B) calling for the "elimination of boxing from amateur scholastic, intercollegiate, and government athletic programs" because it is deleterious to health. This June resolution represents the first time the AMA officially opposed boxing and does conflict with previous endorsement of the coun-

cil report. The AMA, apparently not for the first time, was endorsing conflicting policies. When asked of the dilemma, an AMA spokesperson responded that "he didn't know whether the June resolution accurately represented the feeling of most physicians" and that "the Board of Trustees traditionally endorses reports of its scientific committee".[41]

Professional boxing is not sport but big business entertainment. Certainly the more successful champions are not paid so much for winning, but how they win and how many spectators they can draw to the live gate and television audience. As long as the participants understand the risks they are taking and are of sound mind and body when they make that judgment, we must question the right of anyone to prevent them from the possibility of achieving economic benefits they might otherwise never attain. If society condones and supports motorcycle, car, and horse racing, pursuits with more than a tenfold greater chance of fatality than boxing, and football which may contribute more than 250,000 concussions annually[40] and more than 95% of all catastrophic sports injuries,[42, 43] then it appears inappropriate to unilaterally call for the abolition of professional boxing.

Amateur boxing is another situation. Despite all the amateur boxing enthusiasts' protestations that the aim is to score points and reward defense, the fact remains that boxing is the only amateur sport in which purposefully inflicted face, eye, or brain injury is rewarded and thus used as an aid to winning.

At this point in time it is strongly suggested that the following be implemented:

1. All amateur boxers should be required to wear custom-fitted head protection meeting certified standards such as those required for football helmets.

2. The level of competence of amateur boxers should be certified similar to

various belts in karate or rankings in tennis, and only boxers of a like degree of competence should be allowed to compete against each other.

3. Boxing gloves and headgear are presently archaic, with little change in the past 40 years, and the need for improvement with use of space age technology and materials is urgent.

4. Research is required to either improve existing techniques or to determine new ones so that early permanent brain damage can be detected.

5. Boxing participants should be required to sign a waiver indicating that they fully understand that they will likely inflict and receive brain damage by boxing.

There is no question that forceful acceleration blows to the head are not beneficial. Based on present hard scientific evidence, however, there is no proof that the risk of head injury in boxing is higher than in other collision sports. On the other hand, the sociologic significance attached to boxing is profound. The sport affords especially the small, short, low-weight athlete in low socioeconomic levels a chance to "be somebody." A study in keeping with this[44] found that amateur boxers were better educated and worked in a higher-level occupation than their parents or siblings.

To date a total of ten epidemiologic studies have been reported on amateur boxers.[44-50] All but one were retrospective and cross-sectional in design. Thus it is not known if neuropsychologic abnormalities are attributable to factors other than boxing, such as drug abuse, alcoholism, or accidents. These studies are further limited by the absence of an appropriate control or comparison group, that is, age- and sex-matched siblings with similar education who do not box. Presently there is a prospective study on the health risks associated with amateur boxing without the design flaws of prior ones being conducted by a group at Johns Hopkins Medical School. It will be several years before the study is concluded. Thus it appears appropriate to await the results of such research based on strict scientific methodology, for only with this knowledge can subjective bias be eliminated and appropriate decisions be made as to whether there is a basis for banning boxing.

REFERENCES

1. Gronwall D, Wrightson P: Delayed recovery of intellectual function after minor head injury. *Lancet* 1974; 2:605–609.

2. Gronwall DMA: Paced auditory serial-addition task: A measure of recovery from concussion. *Perpetual and Motor Skills* 1977; 44:367–373.

3. Gronwall D, Wrightson P: Duration of post-traumatic amnesia after mild head injury. *J Clin Neuropsychol* 1980; 2:51–60.

4. Gronwall D, Wrightson P: Memory and information processing capacity after closed head injury. *J Neurol, Neurosurg Psychiatry* 1981; 44:889–895.

5. Gronwall D, Wrightson P: Cumulative effect of concussion. *Lancet* 1975; 2:995–997.

6. Symonds C: Concussion and its sequelae. *Lancet* 1962; 1:1–5.

7. Rimel RW, Bruno-Giordani NP, Barth JT, et al: Disability caused by minor head injury. *Neurosurgery* 1981; 9:221–228.

8. Gennarelli TA, Segawa H, Wald U, et al: Physiological response to angular acceleration of the head, in Grossman RG, Gildenberg PL (eds): *Head Injury: Basic and Clinical Aspects.* New York, Raven Press, pp 129–140.

9. Peerless SJ, Rewcastle NB: Shear injuries of the brain. *Can Med Assoc J* 1967; 96:577–582.

10. Strich SJ: Shearing of nerve fibers as a cause of brain damage due to head injury. *Lancet* 1961; 2:443–448.

11. Unterharnscheidt F: About boxing: Review of historical and medical aspects. *Texas Rep Biol & Med* 1970; 28:421–495.

12. Gennarelli TA, Thibault LE: Biomechanics of acute subdural hematoma. *J Trauma* 1982; 22:680–685.

13. Critchley M: Medical aspects of boxing, partic-

ularly from a neurological standpoint. *Br Med J* 1957; 1:357–362.

14. Martland HS: Punch drunk. *JAMA* 1928; 91:1103–1107.

15. Busse EW, Silverman AJ: Electroencephalographic changes in professional boxers. *JAMA* 1952; 149:1522–1525.

16. Kaplan AJ, Browder J: Observations of the clinical and brain wave patterns of professional boxers. *JAMA* 1954; 156:1138–1144.

17. Betti OO, Ottino CA: Pugilistic encephalopathy. *Acta Neurol Latino Americana* 1969; 15:47–51.

18. Blonstein JL, Clarke E: Further observations on the medical aspects of amateur boxing. *Br Med J* 1957; 1:362–364.

19. Brayne CEG, Dow L, Calloway SP, et al: Blood creatinine kinase isoenzyme BB in boxers. *Lancet* 1982; 2:1308–1309.

20. Brennan TNN, O'Connor PJ: Incidence of boxing injuries in the Royal Air Force in the United Kingdom, 1953–1966. *Br J Ind Med* 1968; 25:326–329.

21. Colmant HJ, Dotzauer G: Analyse eines todlich ausegangenen Boxkampfes mit ungewohnlich schweren cerebralen Schaden. *Recthsmedizin* 1980; 84:263–278.

22. Courville CB: The mechanism of boxing fatalities. *Bull Los Angeles Neurol Soc* 1964; 29:59–69.

23. Govons SR: Brain concussion and posture, the knockdown blow of the boxing ring. *Confinia Neurol* 1968; 30:77–84.

24. Jedlinksi J, Gatarski J, Szymusik A: Chronic posttraumatic changes in the central nervous system in pugilists. *Polish Med J* 1970; 9:743–752.

25. Jedlinksi J, Gatarski J, Szymusik A: Encephalopathia pugilistica (punch drunkenness). *Acta Med Pol* 1971; 12:443–451.

26. Johnson J: Organic psych-syndrome due to boxing. *Br J Psychiatry* 1969; 115:45–53.

27. Kaste M, Vilkii J, Sainio K, et al: Is chronic brain damage in boxing a hazard of the past? *Lancet* 1982; 2:1186–1188.

28. Khosla T, Hitchens RAN: Johnny Owen's ill-fated fight. *Lancet* 1980; 2:1254–1255.

29. Mawdsley C, Ferguson FR: Neurological disease in boxers. *Lancet* 1963; 2:795–801.

30. Paul M: A fatal injury at boxing (traumatic de-

cerebrate rigidity). *Br Med J* 1957; 1:364–366.

31. Payne EE: Brains of boxers. *Neurochirurgia (Stuttg)* 1968; 11:173–188.

32. Spillane JD: Five boxers. *Br Med J* 1962; 2:1205–1210.

33. Corsellis JAN, Bruton DJ, Freeman-Browne D: The aftermath of boxing. *Psychol Med* 1973; 3:270–303.

34. Ross RJ, Cole M, et al: Boxers—computed tomography, EEG and neurological evaluation. *JAMA* 1983; 249:211–213.

35. Casson IR, Sham R, Campbell EA, et al: Neurological and CT evaluation of knocked-out boxers. *J Neurol, Neurosurg Psychiatry* 1982; 45:170–174.

36. AMA Committee on the Medical Aspects of Sports "Statement on Boxing." *JAMA* 1962; 181:242.

37. Council on Scientific Affairs report: Brain injury in boxing. *JAMA* 1983; 249:242–257.

38. Lundberg GC: Boxing should be banned in civilized countries. *JAMA* 1983; 249:250.

39. Van Allen MW: The deadly degrading sport. *JAMA* 1983; 249:250–251.

40. Ryan AJ: AMA Conference on Medical Aspects of Boxing. *Phy Sportsmed* 1983; 11:145–146.

41. Cantu RC: Head injury in sports, in Grana WA, Lombardo JA (eds): *Advances in Sports Medicine and Fitness, vol 2.* St Louis, Mosby–Year Book, 1988.

42. Cantu RC: Catastrophic injuries in high school and collegiate athletes: A five year experience 1982–1987. *Surgical Rounds for Orthopaedics*, vol 2, 1988; 11:62–66.

43. Kaste M, Vilki J, Sainio K, et al: Is chronic brain damage in boxing a hazard of the past? *Lancet* 1982; 2:1186.

44. Blonstein JL, Clarke E: Further observations on the medical aspects of amateur boxing. *Br Med J* 1957; 1:362.

45. Blonstein JL, Clarke E: The medical aspects of amateur boxing. *Br Med J* 1954; 2:1523.

46. Casson IR, Siegel O, Sham R, et al: Brain damage in modern boxers. *JAMA* 1984; 251:2663.

47. Corsellis JAN, Bruton CJ, Freeman-Browne D: The aftermath of boxing. *Psychol Med* 1973; 3:270.

48. Johnson J: Organic psychosyndromes due to boxing. *Br J Psychiatry* 1969; 115:45.

49. Serel M, Jarso O: The mechanisms of cerebral concussion in boxing and their consequences. *World Neurology* 1962; 3:351.

50. Thomassen A, Juul-Jensen P, Olivarius B, et al: Neurological electroencephalographic and neuropsychological examination of 53 former amateur boxers. *Acta Neurol Scand* 1979; 60:352.

APPENDIX 6A

Council on Scientific Affairs Report (*JAMA* 1983; 249:254)*

A resolution regarding brain injury in boxing was introduced to the House of Delegates of the American Medical Association by the American Association of Neurological Surgeons. The sponsor of the resolution noted that brain damage, as evidenced by dementia, memory loss, slurred speech, tremor, and abnormal gait, is seen in perhaps 15% of professional boxers. The sponsor further noted that death is an occasional consequence of the sport in which the ultimate goal is to reduce the opponent to a state of total and complete helplessness.

The resolution was referred to the Board of Trustees with the request that the board "study the matter of brain injury in boxing and report the results of the study, along with such remedies as may be appropriate." The Board of Trustees referred the matter to the Council on Scientific Affairs.

The Council on Scientific Affairs concurs with the findings in the following report, which was prepared by its expert Advisory Panel on Brain Injury in Boxing.

Boxing is a collision sport that stimulates extreme emotion from both proponents and opponents. Proponents claim that the sport requires rigorous training, strict discipline, tolerance to pain, resolution, alertness, courage, and endurance. These are desirable qualities that may contribute to the physical and social development of youth. Furthermore, boxing has been proposed as a controlled outlet for aggressive human instincts. Under properly controlled and supervised circumstances, proponents claim that the risk of serious head injuries is no greater than for other collision sports.

Opponents of boxing use the adjectives "suicidal," "brutal," and "murderous" to describe action in the sport, and further point out that it is the only sport in which, within the rules, each contestant deliberately tries to inflict severe physical injury on his opponent and render him senseless through a "knockout" blow. Accordingly, they claim boxing to be morally indefensible. They further state that no present equipment can completely protect the brain from short-term or long-term injury. The benefits and intangible values attributed to boxing can be derived as well from other less dangerous individual sports.

The AMA has previously addressed the issue of the dangers of boxing through the statement of the AMA Committee on the Medical Aspects of Sports "Statement on Boxing" (*JAMA* 1962; 181:242).

Boxing Activity in the United States

Amateur Boxing.—Approximately 15,000 boxers between the ages of 10 and 15 years are registered with the National Amateur Athletic Union (NAAU) Junior Olympic boxing program (Dusenberry JR: Written communication, May 11, 1981). Each boxer will average between 10 and 30 bouts a year for a period of 5 to 6 years. The incidence of knockouts is calculated at approximately 5% for the 14- to 15-year-old age group, and knockouts are extremely rare among the younger age groups.

Current estimates indicate that an additional 12,500 amateur boxers participate in the Golden Gloves Association of

*Reprinted with permission.

America boxing program (Gallup S: Written communication, June 4, 1981). Each boxer averages approximately 20 bouts per year for 3 to 5 years. Less than 5% of these amateur boxers sustain a knockout blow during their careers.

In recent years "tough man" and woman boxing contests have been promoted and staged in various sections of the country. These contests usually involve poorly conditioned, unlicensed amateurs, and are not sanctioned by appropriate state boxing commissions. The potential for serious injury is high in any such unlicensed boxing bouts. In at least three reported instances, a "tough man" contest has resulted in brain injury and, in two instances, death.

The National Collegiate Athletic Association (NCAA) does not recognize boxing as a varsity sport. There are several colleges where boxing is a club sport. Intramural boxing contests continue to be held under close supervision at the service academies, however.

Professional Boxing.—Boxing is regulated by state or local boxing commissions established under law in 46 states, 5 territories, and the District of Columbia. The states of Georgia, Oklahoma, South Carolina, and Wyoming have no boxing statutes. There may be as many as 5,000 licensed professional boxers in this country, although the precise number is unknown. Licensed boxers frequently move between states for scheduled bouts. There are reports that some boxers perform under different names in several states. The various boxing commissions provide medical standards for the physical examination and licensure of boxers and medical supervision of boxing bouts. There appears to be incomplete and fragmentary exchange of information between many state boxing commissions regarding the routine identification and medical conditions of injured boxers, however.

A report from the New York State Athletic Commission indicated that 856 boxers with an average age of 22.3 years were licensed in New York between 1976 and 1981.[1] These boxers participated in approximately 677 bouts per year, fighting an average 2,907.4 rounds of boxing. During the 5-year period there were 544 suspensions of licensed boxers.

The principal professional boxing governing bodies are the World Boxing Council (WBC) and the World Boxing Association (WBA). Each organization provides ratings for individual boxers under its control and sponsors championship matches in the various weight divisions. Neither organization routinely accepts the ring ratings of the other. Other active boxing associations with ring ratings and individual champions include the United States Boxing Association (USBA) and the North American Boxing Federation (NABF). A majority of the state or local boxing commissions are voluntary members of one or more of the various boxing associations. The large sums of money involved in professional boxing encourage accusations of fraud and corruption, which has been the subject recently of several articles published in major sports magazines.

Boxing Deaths.—According to Moore[1] 335 deaths occurred among amateur and professional boxers worldwide during the 35-year period between 1945 and 1979. Calculation of mortality rates for the sport is imprecise, since the exact number of amateur and professional boxers in the world is unknown. The fatality rate for boxing has been calculated as 0.13 death per 1,000 participants, however.[2] The following are calculated fatality rates per 1,000 participants for other sports during the same period: college football, 0.3; motorcycle racing, 0.7; scuba diving, 1.1; mountaineering, 5.1; hang gliding, 5.5; skydiving, 12.3; and horse racing (jockeys and sulky drivers),

12.8. The advisory panel had no information on how these statistics were compiled and cannot attest to their validity or reliability. The studies by Refshauge[3] and Gonzales[4] suggest low mortality rates in boxing compared with other sports.

A study by Payne[5] indicated also that the usual cause of boxing fatalities was subdural hemorrhage and its complications. The mechanism of the fatal injury is related to rotational acceleration of the head from a forceful blow, with rupture of bridging or connecting veins. Such hemorrhage may result from the direct effects of the blow or from subsequent impact of the head against the floor or ring posts.

Cerebral Concussion.—A *knockout* and, in many instances, a *technical knockout* (TKO) indicate that the boxer has suffered a cerebral concussion. The recent incidence of knockouts in professional fights in New York State has been reported to be 43/677 bouts (Folk, Frank S, M.D.: Written communication, September 1981). More than 90% of the knockouts occur during the first three rounds. Blonstein and Clarke[6] assessed boxing injuries encountered in 3,000 London Amateur Boxing Association contests during 1955 and 1956. Only 29 boxers (0.58%) had severe concussions or were knocked out more than once. The results of neurologic and EEG examinations were normal in all boxers examined.

In their report of the brain wave patterns of professional boxers, Kaplan and Browder[7] mention that the EEG examinations performed on 40 boxers within 10 minutes after losing the fight by a decision or a TKO (a number of them had been dazed by a blow to the head, which in many instances led to a TKO) showed no constant change from their prefight tracing. They also mention that "detailed examinations" after the fight failed to disclose any abnormal neurologic signs, even in those boxers who were knocked out.

Busse and Silverman[8] carried out routine EEG studies on boxers who had been knocked out in the ring and compared them with those of a control group. Although they reported a high incidence of abnormalities (37%), they were unable to correlate the degree of electrical abnormality with the knockout.

A cerebral concussion may be associated with other brain injuries, such as a subdural hematoma. The number of nonfatal acute intracranial hemorrhages sustained in boxing is not known. Two cases in young amateur boxers were recently reported by Cruikshank et al.[9]

Long-Term Neurologic Sequelae of Boxing.—The greater portion of the literature on the chronic neurologic sequelae of boxing has dealt with the "punchdrunk syndrome." This term, first introduced by Martland in 1928,[10] describes boxers who were ataxic, had a broad-based gait, slurred speech, and dementia. Roberts[11] performed examinations on 224 of 16,731 professional boxers registered with the British Boxing Board of Control between 1929 and 1955. Boxers were given physical examinations, psychiatric interviews, and a number of memory tests. The study indicated that 17% of those who had boxed for 6 to 9 years displayed brain damage, and one third showed signs of punchdrunk syndrome. The extent of the damage was related to the number of bouts fought.

Sercl and Jaros[12] reported the incidence of chronic boxer's encephalopathy to be 9%. Johnson[13] reviewed the cases of 15 professional fighters about 22 years after their careers ended. Each boxer had experienced from 200 to 300 fights. Half of this group were found to have neurologic signs compatible with traumatic encephalopathy. All but three boxers showed damage to the brain evident by air encephalography. Eleven boxers had diffuse EEG abnormalities. Mawdsley and Ferguson[14] studied ten retired boxers who displayed neurologic abnormalities. The neurologic dysfunctions included dementia and extrapyramidal and cerebellar signs, with pyramidal dysfunction being less frequent. Air encephalography disclosed evidence of cerebral and cerebellar atrophy, and cavum septi pellucidi was common. They concluded that boxing is sometimes the cause of progressive neurologic disorder.

There are other isolated case reports describing similar neurologic abnormalities in boxers. Harvey and Davis[15] reported the syndrome in a 25-year-old middleweight boxer. Of interest is that Corsellis[16] reported the conditions resembling the punchdrunk state in rugby football players, professional wrestlers, a parachute jumper, and steeplechase jockeys.

Corsellis et al.[17] examined the brains of 15 retired boxers and interviewed relatives and friends about the boxers' lives. From these investigations, they concluded that in some boxers a neurologic disorder developed that correlated with "cerebral damage or degeneration that is concentrated on the septal regions, on the deep temporal gray matter, and on certain neurons along the cerebellar and nigral pathways."

Many boxing physicians believe that the incidence of the punchdrunk syndrome has been sharply reduced because of increased medical supervision. This is perhaps substantiated by Thomassen et al.,[18] who performed neurologic, EEG, and neuropsychologic examination on a total of 53 former champion amateur boxers. Only minor neuropsychologic disturbances were found in the boxers, and were most pronounced in impaired motor function of the left hand. The EEG studies of Kaplan and Browder,[7] as well

as those of Busse and Silverman,[8] show an increased incidence of abnormalities in boxers; however, a cause-and-effect relationship has been questioned.

Other potential long-term neurologic sequelae from boxing, such as posttraumatic epilepsy and traumatic cranial nerve palsies, have not been adequately documented.

Comment

The advisory panel has carefully reviewed studies of deaths from boxing injuries and reported instances of brain injury in boxing. It has been reasonably well established in the medical literature that there was a punchdrunk syndrome that had adversely affected boxers in past years and may be a specific long-term occupational hazard of the sport. A traumatic encephalopathy resulting from repeated blows to the head has affected unspecified numbers of boxers. This progressive and disabling disorder is seen less often now, and may be prevented by sound medical and administrative measures in the sport.

Evaluation for the possible confounding effects of excessive alcohol use, sexually transmitted disease, and the aging process on the brain has been lacking in previous investigations, and reports frequently have not included suitable control populations. In addition, there has not been a comprehensive medical study of boxers since many medical surveillance measures were instituted in the 1950s. Earlier investigations included boxers who had fought in the 1920–1940 period when medical supervision was infrequent, and when boxers had a greater number of bouts and generally longer careers in the ring.

In recent years medical supervision of boxing has improved in some boxing jurisdictions. Improvements have been noted in the following areas: (1) basic standards and requirements for the medical examination of boxers, (2) adequate medical supervision and equipment for the boxer at ringside, and (3) periodic examination and evaluation of poor medical and boxing risks. Such precautions minimize and may even prevent acute intracranial hemorrhage and death.

The activities of the New York State Athletic Commission provide one example of improved medical supervision of professional boxers. After the death of a boxer in 1979, the Athletic Commission made a series of changes in its boxing rules and practices. A boxer must have a "passport" to fight in New York, and all medical and previous boxing data are checked by computer before he receives clearance for a fight. The state assigns two physicians at ringside before the start of any boxing program; each physician can enter the ring at any time and stop the fight for medical reasons. A boxing match is never started until an ambulance and emergency equipment are on the premises. If he sustains lacerations of the face, a boxer may receive a suspension of 60 days, while TKOs for minor injuries entail a suspension of 30 days and those for head injuries, 45 days. Boxers with immediate response to a knockout receive a 60-day suspension, while those with a slow response receive a 90-day suspension plus CT scan and EEG within 24 hours.

Conclusion

Boxing is a dangerous sport and can result in death or long-term brain injury. Other sports may also result in accidental death or brain injury for participants, however.

Amateur boxing is fairly well supervised in this country through several national organizations. Professional boxing is less well controlled, since the supervision of the sport is carried out worldwide through numerous uncoordinated national, state, and local boxing commis-

sions. Therefore, it is difficult to determine the medical chronology of injuries in boxers.

No reliable test exists to identify boxers at risk for sudden death or impending brain injury. To reduce this risk, central administrative regulations and strict medical supervision should be required for the sport of boxing.

Recommendations

Some would favor banning boxing completely, but this is not a realistic solution to the problem of brain injury in boxing. Moreover, the sport does not seem any more dangerous than other sports presently accepted by society. The Advisory Panel on Brain Injury in Boxing does see a need for specific improvements in administrative and medical standards, and the Council on Scientific Affairs recommends that the AMA implement the following measures:

1. Encourage the establishment of a "National Registry of Boxers" for all amateur and professional boxers, including "sparring mates," in the country. The proposed functions of a computer-based central registry would be to record the results of all licensed bouts, including TKOs, knockouts, and other boxing injuries, and to compile injury and win-lose records for individual boxers.

2. Plan and conduct a conference with representatives of the American Association of Ringside Physicians, medical representatives, medical representatives of the various state and local boxing commissions, and representatives of organized professional and amateur boxing organizations, to review criteria for the physical examination of boxers, to determine other comprehensive medical measures necessary for the prevention of brain injury in the sport, and to develop specific criteria for the discontinuance of a bout for medical reasons.

3. Recommend to all boxing jurisdictions that the ring physician should be authorized to stop any bout in progress, at any time, to examine a contestant, and, when indicated, to terminate a bout that might, in his opinion, result in serious injury for either contestant.

4. Urge state and local commissions to conduct frequent medical training seminars for all ring personnel.

5. Recommend to all boxing jurisdictions that no amateur or professional boxing bout should be permitted unless (1) the contest is held in an area where adequate neurosurgical facilities are immediately available for skilled emergency treatment of an injured boxer; (2) advanced life-support systems are available at ringside; and (3) a comprehensive evacuation plan for the removal of any seriously injured boxer to hospital facilities is ready.

6. Inform state legislatures that unsupervised boxing competition between unlicensed boxers in "tough man" contests is a most dangerous practice that may result in serious injury or death to contestants, and should be condemned.

7. Urge state and local boxing commissions to mandate the use of safety equipment, such as plastic safety mats and padded cornerposts, and encourage continued development of safety equipment.

8. Urge state and local boxing commissions to extend all safety measures to sparring partners.

9. Urge state and local boxing commissions to upgrade, standardize, and strictly enforce medical evaluations for boxers.

REFERENCES

1. Moore M: The challenge of boxing: Bringing safety into the ring. *Phys Sport Med* 1980; 8:101–105.

2. Some high risk sports. *Sporting News,* Aug 16, 1980.

3. Refshauge JGH: The medical aspects of boxing. *Med J Aust* 1963; 1:611–613.

4. Gonzales TA: Fatal injuries in competitive sports. *JAMA* 1951; 146:1506–1511.

5. Payne EE: Brains of boxers. *Neurochirurgia* 1968; 11:173–189.

6. Blonstein JL, Clarke E: Further observations on the medical aspects of amateur boxing. *Br Med J* 1957; 1:362–364.

7. Kaplan HA, Browder J: Observations on the clinical and brain wave patterns of professional boxers. *JAMA* 1954; 156:1138–1144.

8. Busse EW, Silverman AJ: Electroencephalographic changes in professional boxers. *JAMA* 1952; 149:1522–1525.

9. Cruikshank JK, Higgens CS, Gray JR: Two cases of acute intracranial haemorrhage in young amateur boxers. *Lancet* 1980; 1:626–627.

10. Martland HS: Punch drunk. *JAMA* 1928; 91:1103–1107.

11. Roberts AH: Brain Damage in Boxers. London, Pitman Publishing Co, 1969.

12. Sercl M, Jaros O: The mechanisms of cerebral concussion in boxing and their consequences. *World Neurology* 1962; 3:351–358.

13. Johnson J: Organic psychosyndrome due to boxing. *Br J Psychiatry* 1969; 115:45–53.

14. Mawdsley C, Ferguson FR: Neurological disease in boxers. *Lancet* 1963; 2:799–801.

15. Harvey PKP, Davis IN: Traumatic encephalopathy in a young boxer. *Lancet* 1974; 2:928–929.

16. Corsellis JAN: Brain damage in sport. *Lancet* 1976; 1:401–402.

17. Corsellis JAN, Bruton CJ, Freeman-Browne D: The aftermath of boxing. *Psychol Med* 1973; 270–303.

18. Thomassen A, Juul-Jensen P, Olivarius B, et al: Neurological electroencephalographic and neuropsychological examination of 53 former amateur boxers. *Acta Neurol Scand* 1979; 60:352–362.

APPENDIX 6B

American Medical Association House of Delegates Resolutions

On June 23, 1983, the House of Delegates of the American Medical Association passed the following resolution:

RESOLVED, That the American Medical Association: 1. Publicize the deleterious effects of boxing on the health of participants; 2. Encourage the elimination of boxing from amateur scholastic, intercollegiate and governmental athletic programs as detrimental to the health of participants; 3. Develop model legislation seeking to curtail the utilization of boxing as a public spectacle to the extent feasible.

In December 1984, the AMA House of Delegates passed Substitute Resolution 26, which stated as follows:

RESOLVED, That the American Medical Association: 1. Encourage the elimination of both amateur and professional boxing, a sport in which the primary objective is to inflict injury; 2. Communicate its opposition to boxing as a sport to appropriate regulating bodies; 3. Assist state medical societies to work with their state legislatures to enact laws to eliminate boxing in their jurisdictions; and 4. Educate the American public, especially children and young adults, about the dangerous effects of boxing on the health of participants.

CHAPTER 7

Trampoline-Induced Cervical Quadriplegia

Joseph S. Torg, M.D.

Cervical spine injuries resulting from participation in gymnastics have become synonymous with the trampoline and the minitrampoline. Numerous reports in the world's literature have documented an alarming number of catastrophic injuries resulting in cervical quadriplegia, and clearly indicate a real danger in the use of these devices. Controversy exists concerning whether the trampoline and the minitrampoline should be banned from use in recreation, supervised physical education, and competition, or whether, with implementation of manufacturing standards and enforcement of safety guidelines, their use can be made safe. It should be noted that the American Academy of Pediatrics (AAP) lifted its 1977 ban[1] on the use of the trampoline in March 1981. The AAP[2] now advocates ". . . a revision of the Academy's position to allow for a trial period of limited and controlled use by schools. . . . However, careful assessment of the incidence and severity of injury must continue during this trial period." In neither statement has the AAP taken a position about the use of the minitrampoline. The soundness of this change in policy is questioned.

The purpose of this chapter is to (1) examine the world's literature documenting cervical spine injuries; (2) attempt to determine common factors regarding patient characteristics, environment, injury mechanisms, and pathology; (3) review policy statements and safety guidelines of both the AAP and athletic administrative bodies; and (4) evaluate what effect, if any, these policies and guidelines have had on documented injuries.

In 1946 Zimmerman[20] was the first to mention cervical spine injuries that occurred on trampolines. In a retrospective study, 167 injuries were reported, only four of which involved the cervical spine. No associated neurologic involvement is mentioned in any of these four cases.

Four years later Ellis et al.[8] published a "communication designed to warn the medical profession of the hazards involving the use of the trampoline." They reported on five patients who incurred serious neurologic injuries, three as a result of cervical spine injuries (Table 7–1). They concluded that these injuries resulted from attempts at difficult maneuvers before the fundamentals had been mastered, and proposed a set of ten regulations designed to minimize serious injuries in trampoline amusement areas.

In 1967 Witthaut[19] reported on six patients with trampoline injuries, which included two with cervical spine injuries. Witthaut pointed out that cervical

TABLE 7–1.

Patient Data*

Patient	Attempted Stunt	Mechanism of Injury	Roentgenograms	Pathology	Neurologic Status
19-yr-old university team gymnast	Back drop on trampoline	Compression-flexion	Anterior dislocation, C5–6	Fracture, C-5; intact anterior and posterior longitudinal ligaments	Quadriplegic, died
38-yr-old former high school gymnast	Backward somersault on amusement area trampoline	Hyperflexion	1 cm anterior subluxation, C5–6	Ligamentous disruption, C5–6	Quadriplegic
17-yr-old high school physical education class member	Backward somersault on commercially operated trampoline	Compression-flexion	Comminuted compression fracture, C-5; anterior displacement, C4–5	Fracture, C-5	Quadriplegic

*Data from Ellis WP, Green D, Holzaepfel NR, et al: JAMA 1960; 174:1673–1676.

spine injuries incurred on the trampoline ". . . either resemble those which occur when swimmers dive into shallow water or those which occur during high dives into deep water when the neck is forcefully hyperextended."

Three cervical spine injuries were reported in Swedish literature by Frykman and Hilding[10] in 1970 (Table 7–2). These three injuries have several points in common. All of them occurred in young, well-trained gymnasts performing difficult stunts. Although the nature and severity of the lesions differed somewhat in each case, all lesions occurred at the C5–6 level. Finally, all three patients experienced a "blackout" or period of unconsciousness just before their injuries. Frykman and Hilding[10] suggested that

the blackouts experienced by these patients might be due to brief concussions or pathologic conditions similar to Wallenberg's syndrome (occlusion of the posteroinferior cerebellar artery). They recommended that trampolines be banned from school gymnastics and that continuing investigation into these cervical spine injuries be undertaken.

In the German literature, Steinbruck and Paeslack[17] reported 25 cases of cervical quadriplegia due to trampoline- and minitrampoline-related injuries. Between 1967 and 1977, they treated eight of these patients at the Heidelberg Center for Spinal Cord Injuries (Table 7–3). Most of these injuries occurred in patients younger than 20 years; most resulted from a fall onto the bed of the trampo-

TABLE 7–2.

Patient Data*

Patient	Mechanisms	Roentgenograms	Neurologic Status
27-yr-old male trampoline athlete	Hyperflexion, "blacked out"	Dislocation, C5–6	Quadriplegic
23-yr-old male expert	Hyperflexion, "blacked out"	Anterior subluxation, C5–6; fracture, arches of C-5	Quadriplegic
30-yr-old male elite gymnast	Hyperflexion, "blacked out"	Anterior subluxation, C5–6	Quadriplegic

*Data from Frykman G, Hilding S: Lakartidningen 1970; 67:5862–5864.

TABLE 7–3.

Patient Data*

Patient	Apparatus	Stunt	Anatomic Lesion	Neurologic Lesion
26-yr-old male competitive athlete†	Trampoline	Forward somersault	Fracture-dislocation, C5–6	Complete quadriplegia below C-5
18-yr-old man†	Trampoline	Forward somersault	Fracture dislocation, C5–6	Complete quadriplegia below C-5
16-yr-old male student†	Trampoline	Forward somersault	Compression fracture, C4–5; fracture, left vertebral arch, C-4	Complete quadriplegia below C-5
14-yr-old boy†	Minitrampoline	Flying roll	Fracture-dislocation, C4–5	Complete quadriplegia below C-4
17-yr-old male experienced trampolinist†	Trampoline	Double forward somersault	Fracture-dislocation, C6–7	Complete quadriplegia below C6–7
56-yr-old man†	Trampoline	Backward somersault	Fracture-dislocation, C5–6	Slight motor and sensory deficit below C-5
14-yr-old male experienced trampolinist†	Trampoline	Forward somersault	Fracture-dislocation, C4–5	Complete quadriplegia below C-4
15-yr-old boy†	Minitrampoline	Jump over a chest	Dislocation, C5–6	Quadriplegia below C4–5; can move legs slightly
19-yr-old woman	Minitrampoline	Somersault	Fracture-dislocation, C5–6	Complete quadriplegia below C5–6; died after 4 days
30-yr-old man	Trampoline	Practice jump	Fracture-dislocation	Complete quadriplegia below C4–5; died after 6 days
34-yr-old man	Minitrampoline	Forward somersault	Fracture-dislocation	Complete quadriplegia below C5–6; died after 6 days
66-yr-old man in good physical condition	Trampoline	Forward somersault with roll	Fracture-dislocation	Complete quadriplegia below C4–5; died after 14 days
19-yr-old man	Trampoline	Forward somersault	Fracture-dislocation	Complete quadriplegia below C4–5
21-yr-old man	Trampoline	Forward somersault	Fracture-dislocation	Incomplete quadriplegia below C4–5
26-yr-old man	Minitrampoline	Somersault	Fracture-dislocation	Incomplete quadriplegia below C-5
29-yr-old man	Trampoline	Practice jump for jackknife roll	Fracture-dislocation	Incomplete quadriplegia below C4–5
16-yr-old girl	Trampoline	Forward somersault	Dislocation	Quadriplegia below C4–5

*Data from Steinbruck K, Paeslack V: MMW 1978; 120:985–988.
†Patients treated at Heidelberg Center for Spinal Cord Injuries.

line; most injuries were fracture-dislocations that were caused by either hyperextension or hyperflexion of the cervical spine; and most occurred during attempts to do a forward somersault. Steinbruck and Paeslack[17] attribute these injuries to (1) little or no assistance; (2) failure to secure the trampoline; (3) fatigue, loss of concentration, and carelessness; and (4) poor technique. They made a number of recommendations to prevent the injuries.

Evans[9] reported a fracture-dislocation

TABLE 7–4.
Patient Data*

Patient	Apparatus	Stunt	Blackout	Safety Mat	Spotters	Lesion	Neurologic Lesion
30-yr-old male expert gymnast, 5 yr minitrampoline experience	Minitrampoline	Forward somersault	Yes	10–12 cm thick	Present	Anterior dislocation, C-4 on C-5	Complete quadriplegia
20-yr-old male army draftee, no trampoline experience	Minitrampoline	Forward somersault	No	30 cm thick	Present	Fracture, body of C-6; rupture of disk, C6–7	Complete quadriplegia
25-yr-old male trampoline instructor	Minitrampoline	Forward double somersault	No	30 cm thick	Present	Anterior dislocation, C-4 on C-5	Complete quadriplegia
40-yr-old male trained athlete, sports physician, no trampoline experience	Trampoline	Back drop	No	—	—	Rupture of disk, C6–7; large tear, posterior longitudinal ligament; free disk compression 7th cervical nerve root	None after excision of disk and extruded disk
18-yr-old male elite gymnast, 8 yr experience on trampoline and minitrampoline	Minitrampoline	Forward somersault	Yes	30 cm thick	Present	Anterior dislocation, C-5 on C-6; posterior dislocation, C-6 on C-7	Incomplete spastic quadriplegia
17-yr-old male student, 2 yr experience on minitrampoline	Minitrampoline	Forward somersault	Yes	30 cm thick	Present	Compression fracture, body of C-6	Undefined residual neurologic lesion
16-yr-old female student, 1 yr minitrampoline experience	Minitrampoline	Forward somersault	No	30 cm thick	Present	Asymmetric rotatory dislocation, C-4 on C-5; compression fracture	Complete quadriplegia
15-yr-old female student, 1 yr trampoline experience	Minitrampoline	Extended leg jump	Yes	30 cm thick	Absent	Fracture, right posterior arch, C-1; hypoplasia, posterior arch, C-1	None after conservative treatment

*Data from Hammer A, Schwartzback A-L, Darre E, et al.: Ugeskr Laeger 1981; 143:2970–2974.

of the cervical spine resulting in quadriplegia in a 13-year-old girl who had been performing on a trampoline.

Hammer et al.[12] in Denmark reported eight trampoline-related accidents that resulted in severe neurologic damage (Table 7–4). In seven cases the accidents occurred on minitrampolines, and in six of these seven accidents a very thick mat (30 cm) was used and spotters were present. Only two of the eight patients had little experience with the trampoline. Four of them experienced momentary blackouts immediately preceding their accidents. From their findings and those in the literature, Hammer et al.[12] concluded that (1) these neurologic injuries were associated with the trampoline and were independent of the milieu in which it was used; (2) the use of preventive measures (good-quality safety mats, spotters) did not help to prevent these accidents; (3) although these injuries can occur in any kind of jump, they occurred most commonly in jumps with a rotation movement; (4) a short blackout could have been a contributing cause to these accidents and may be a reason why such accidents cannot be prevented; and (5) these accidents were independent of the jumper's experience. Whereas seven of the eight accidents in this series occurred on the minitrampoline, it is pointed out that when all of the reported cases of such injuries are reviewed, the large trampoline and the minitrampoline accounted for about equal numbers of the accidents.

During the early and mid-1970s, a number of reports appeared in the American literature on the occurrence of cervical quadriplegia resulting from trampoline-related injuries (Table 7–5). These articles called attention to a possible problem with the use of the trampoline as a cause of cervical spine injuries in the United States. A review of these articles, however, reveals that almost all of them are retrospective "head counts" that do not document the cases and that add to the confusion regarding the scope of the problem because of cross-reporting. On the basis of a National Electronic Injury Surveillance System (NEISS) survey,

TABLE 7–5.

Quadriplegia Resulting from Trampoline-Related Injuries, United States

Source	No. of Patients	Other Documentation Data
Stolov, cited in Kravitz[13] and Rapp and Nicely[15]	7	Department of Rehabilitation, University of Washington 1972–1977
Jackson, cited in Rapp and Nicely[15]	6	Craig Rehabilitation Hospital, Englewood, Colo., 1972–1977
Rapp and Nicely[15]	1	Personal case
Rapp and Nicely[15]	20	Personal communications and review of literature
Kravitz[13]	5	Chicago survey, 1975
Rutherford et al.[16]	5	Spinal injury and paralysis in 5- to 14-year-old children
Rutherford et al.[16]	6	Deaths in 5- to 14-year-old children
Clarke[7]	9	Retrospective National Athletic Injury/Illness Reporting System survey

Kravitz[13] estimated that 50 cases of severe injuries to the spinal cord occurred yearly. This paper[13] actually documents seven cases of quadriplegia resulting from trampoline use (Stolov W: Personal communication, 1978). These same seven cases reported by W. Stolov were also reported by Rapp.[14] On the basis of this information, Kravitz[13] states, "It is our judgment that trampolining should be abolished as a sports activity in all schools."

In 1976 Rapp and Nicely[15] reported on 34 cases of quadriplegia resulting from trampoline accidents in the United States. Twenty-nine of these injuries had occurred in the preceding 6 years. Three injuries resulted in death. Of these 34 cases, Rapp and Nicely had personal experience with only one; they included the seven cases reported by Stolov, six cases reported by Jackson at the Craig Rehabilitation Hospital at Englewood, Colo., and another 20 cases "from personal communications and a review of the literature." On this basis they proposed a 16-point safety program.[15] Among these 16 points were suggestions that somersaults should be eliminated from physical education classes and should be done only by advanced gymnasts with an overhead spotting device; that 2¾ forward and backward somersaults should be banned except for advanced gymnasts; that the poorly designed minitrampoline not be used for complicated tricks; and that recreational "jump centers" be closed.

In an attempt to reduce the hazards associated with use of the trampoline, the American Society for Testing and Materials (ASTM)[5] published a standard in 1974 entitled "Standard Consumer Safety Specifications for Components, Assembly, and Use of a Trampoline." This statement of trampoline specifications, materials, and general requirements for usage is voluntary rather than compulsory, but presumably would help improve the safety of the equipment.

The U.S. Consumer Product Safety Commission[18] also became concerned about trampoline accidents, and, in 1976, published a fact sheet dealing with features to be considered when purchasing such an apparatus. The placement, maintenance, and use of trampolines are also discussed. Their information is largely based on the standard issued by ASTM.[5]

One of the most influential articles in the recent American literature is that of Clarke,[7] who, in 1975, did a retrospective survey of sports-related spinal cord injuries. Questionnaires were sent to 18,085 high schools, 683 2-year colleges, and 1,125 4-year colleges to ascertain the incidence of permanent paralysis resulting from sports participation that occurred during the period 1973 to 1975. There were 15 such gymnastic injuries for which the activity is specified, eight of which occurred on the trampoline and one on the minitrampoline. Not all of these injuries were suffered by varsity athletes. From this study it was concluded that competent trampoline teachers are necessary to prevent gymnastic students from attempting maneuvers for which they are not prepared. Clarke also advocated that a spotter be present for off-apparatus landings.

A result of this paper was the issuance of a policy statement by the AAP Committee on Accident and Poison Prevention[1]:

Trampoline accidents have resulted in a significant number of cases of quadriplegia. In many cases, these accidents have occurred while the victims were participating in supervised physical education activities. A recent national survey of sports injuries in high schools and colleges conducted by the National Athletic Injury/Illness Reporting System (NAIRS) showed that between 1973-1975 spinal cord injuries with permanent paralysis resulted more frequently from trampolines than any other gymnastic sports. Next to football, trampolines were found to be the highest cause of permanent paralysis in this survey.

Therefore, the Committee on Accident

and Poison Prevention of the American Academy of Pediatrics recommends that trampolines be banned from use as part of the physical education programs in grammar schools, high schools, and colleges, and also be abolished as a competitive sport.

It should be noted that no mention is made of the minitrampoline, although it appears to account for about the same number of catastrophic injuries as the large trampoline.[12]

In 1978 the American Alliance for Health, Physical Education, and Recreation (AAHPER) issued two statements. The first position statement, which dealt with the use of trampolines in physical education, did not advocate a ban on the use of the trampoline. Instead, it recommended that use of the trampoline in physical education programs be made optional and voluntary. All athletes were to be helped to appreciate the risks involved in using the trampoline and measures that could be taken to minimize those risks. These measures included supervision by an instructor competent to use the trampoline; the use of trained spotters; the wearing of a safety harness while practicing new skills involving the somersault; locking up of the apparatus to prevent unsupervised use; erection, inspection, and maintenance of the trampoline in accordance with the manufacturer's recommendations; preplanning policies for emergency care in case of accident; and keeping and analyzing records on trampoline participation and accidents. Additional guides for use of the minitrampoline specified that (1) no multiple somersaults should be attempted, and (2) single somersaults should be performed only if the intended result is a foot-landing, the student has proved competence to do the maneuver while wearing a safety harness, spotters are able to control a safety harness, the minitrampoline is set up in such a way as to prevent slippage, and an appropriate mat is used.[3]

The second statement,[4] which dealt with the use of the trampoline to develop competitive skills in sports, such as diving, gymnastics, and pole vaulting, emphasized the necessity for wearing a safety harness to prevent serious neck injury and quadriplegia. It acknowledged, however, that at times the competitive athlete "requires freedom from the safety harness to refine and ready his/her skills for competition in another sport."

Also, in 1978, the National Collegiate Athletic Association Committee on Competitive Safeguards and Medical Aspects of Sports issued a series of guidelines for the trampoline that were identical to those of the American Alliance for Health, Physical Education, and Recreation's first statement.[11]

After the AAP issued its 1977 policy statement on trampolines, most school districts eliminated the use of the trampoline from their physical education programs, either voluntarily, as a result of parental pressure, or because liability insurance became difficult or impossible to obtain. By 1979 the Nissen Corporation, the largest trampoline manufacturer in the United States, had stopped selling trampolines and replacement parts as a result of a sharp decrease in sales and a marked increase in liability lawsuits.[11]

Because of this strong reaction against the use of the trampoline in schools, the U.S. Gymnastics Safety Association and a group of trampoline manufacturers sponsored the establishment of the National Gymnastic Catastrophic Injury Registry at the University of Illinois in 1978. The purpose of this Registry was to collect reliable data for accurate characterization of the patterns and relative frequency of catastrophic head, neck, and spinal injuries occurring in gymnastics and cheerleading. Estimation of national participation in gymnastics was a secondary objective of the Registry. Under the directorship of Kenneth Clarke and, more recently, Charlene Christensen,[6] this Registry has issued four annual reports that document 20 catastrophic gym-

TABLE 7–6.

Catastrophic Gymnastic Injury (Trampoline) Data

Date	Age (yr)	Sex	Skill Level	Equipment	Stunt	Lesion	Sequelae
9/9/78	19	M		Minitrampoline	Forward somersault	Neck fracture	Quadriplegia
9/13/78	16	M		Minitrampoline	Double front flip	Neck fracture	Quadriplegia
9/19/78	16	M	Highly skilled	Trampoline	Full twisting 1½ forward somersault	Neck fracture	Quadriplegia
9/29/78	?	M		Trampoline	"Playing"	Neck fracture	Death
10/29/78	14	M		Trampoline	Knee drop + forward somersault	Neck fracture	Quadriplegia
12/23/78	35	M	Highly skilled	String bed trampoline	Backyard game of horse	Neck fracture	Quadriplegia
5/21/79	20	M	Highly skilled	Trampoline	Triple front somersault	Neck fracture	Quadriplegia
12/6/79	19	M	Skilled	Trampoline	Front somersault, half twist, back somersault	Neck fracture	Quadriplegia
2/21/80	20	M	Skilled	Minitrampoline	?	Neck fracture	Quadriplegia
8/16/80	20	M	Skilled novice	Trampoline	Double back somersault	?	Permanent paralysis from chest down
12/29/80	16	F	Skilled novice	Minitrampoline	Dive forward roll	Cervical spinal cord damage	Permanent paralysis
2/4/81	20	M	Skilled	Minitrampoline	Over-rotation after landing	Neck fracture	Permanent paralysis
3/23/81	23	M	Expertly skilled	Trampoline	1¼ front somersault	Fracture C5–6	Incomplete quadriplegia
4/30/81	21	M		Trampoline	Incorrect landing with head between mat and support bar	?	Incomplete quadriplegia, sensory disturbances

*Data from Christensen C (with assistance of Clarke KS): Fourth Annual National Gymnastic Catastrophic Injury Report 1981–82. Urbana-Champaign, Ill. College of Applied Life Studies, University of Illinois, April 1982, pp 1–35.

nastics injuries, 14 of which occurred on the trampoline (Table 7–6). The large trampoline was implicated in nine and the minitrampoline in five of these injuries. Most of the maneuvers leading to these injuries were somersaults, but one trampolinist incurred his injury when he landed on his head between the mat and the support bar. Another suffered a neck fracture when he landed incorrectly during a backyard game of "horse." One fatal injury occurred in a young boy who was playing on a backyard trampoline and fractured his cervical spine.

From July 1978 to June 1982, the frequencies of cervical cord injuries due to trampoline use were as follows: 1978 to 1979, seven injuries; 1979 to 1980, two injuries; 1980 to 1981, five injuries; and 1981 to 1982, no injuries. Christensen and Clarke[6] comment that, "In the four annual reports, the cases reported do not reflect annually persistent patterns," and they caution against any generalization on the state of the problem from a single year's experience. A distinct decrease was observed, however, in all catastrophic gymnastic injuries occurring in U.S. school and college programs since 1978 and, more specifically, a decrease in injuries resulting from use of trampolines and minitrampolines.

From a study of trampoline-related head and neck injuries in children between 5 and 14 years of age who were treated in hospital emergency rooms, the Consumer Product Safety Commission[16] estimated the annual frequency of such injuries from 1975 to 1980. Commenting on these statistics, Christensen and Clarke[6] observed:

Trampoline injuries for the 5 to 14 age group account for almost 50 percent of the trampoline injuries treated in hospital emergency rooms each year. Head and neck injuries account for an average of 19 percent of those injuries incurred in the 5 to 14 age group. It should be noted, however, that the estimated frequency of head/neck injuries associated with trampolines reported through NEISS has declined by almost two-thirds since 1978 (from 1,755 to 600) [Table 7–7]. This may be a result of the removal of trampolines from many athletic programs in the schools. . .

Head and neck injuries due to other forms of gymnastics have not shown a similar decline: rather they have remained relatively constant showing a slight increase. In gymnastic activities (including trampolines) there is no specific protection for the head or neck. The participant must rely on his/her abilities and those of a spotter. The use of harnesses in teaching various stunts and techniques is essential to prevent impacts to the head or neck from falls.

Presumably on the basis of the Consumer Product Safety Commission report indicating an almost two thirds decline

TABLE 7–7.

Estimated Frequency of Head/Neck Injuries to 5- to 14-Year-Old Children Treated in Hospital Emergency Rooms for Selected Sports Activities*, †

Sport	1975	1976	1977	1978	1979	1980
Gymnastics injuries						
No.	2,662	2,778	2,846	2,451	3,286	3,842
%	8.0	8.0	8.5	7.6	9.8	10.3
Trampoline-related injuries						
No.	1,843	1,754	1,823	1,755	1,019	600
%	16.3	17.6	15.2	17.2	11.9	21.8

*Data from Rutherford GW, Miles RB, Brown VR, et al: Overview of Sports-Related Injuries to Persons 5–14 Years of Age. Washington, D.C., U.S. Consumer Product Safety Commission, December 1981, pp 1–47.
†Only those injuries coded to the head or neck are included here; face, mouth, ear, and eye injuries are not included.

in head and neck injuries resulting from use of the trampoline and a decline in catastrophic injuries resulting in quadriplegia observed by the National Gymnastic Catastrophic Injury Report, the AAP Committees on Accident and Poison Prevention and on Pediatric Aspects of Physical Fitness, Recreation, and Sports reassessed their position on the use of the trampoline.[2] Their 1981 statement is as follows:

In September 1977, the Academy published a statement calling for a ban on the use of trampolines in schools because of the high number of quadriplegic injuries caused by this apparatus.[1] A considerable amount of thought and action resulted. The Academy does not endorse trampoline use, but a revision of the Academy's position to allow for a trial period of limited and controlled use by schools seems appropriate. However, careful assessment of the incidence and severity of injury must continue during this trial period.

The trampoline is a potentially dangerous apparatus, and its use demands the following precautions:

1. The trampoline should not be a part of routine physical education classes.
2. The trampoline has no place in competitive sports.
3. The trampoline should *never* be used in home or recreational settings.
4. Highly trained personnel who have been instructed in all aspects of trampoline safety must be present when the apparatus is used.
5. Maneuvers, especially the somersault, that have a high potential for serious injury should be attempted only by those qualified to become skilled performers.
6. The trampoline must be secured when not in use, and it must be well maintained.
7. Only schools or sports activities complying with the foregoing recommendations should have trampolines.

It should be noted that the AAP presents no data or rationale to explain or justify its change in position "to allow for a trial period of limited and controlled use" of the trampoline. Perhaps the committees responsible for this statement overlooked the well-documented cases in the European literature that clearly establish the unpreventable nature of these trampoline accidents. Like its predecessor, the September 1977 Trampoline statement,[1] Trampolines II[2] does not deal with use of minitrampolines. On the basis of available facts and observations, it appears that the advisability of permitting even limited use of the trampoline or minitrampoline is to be seriously questioned.

DISCUSSION

Starting with the report of Ellis et al.[8] 30 years ago, this review of the world's literature has identified 114 catastrophic cervical spine injuries with associated quadriplegia resulting from use of the trampoline and the minitrampoline. Unfortunately, it is not possible to present these injuries on a rate or exposure basis.

Because of the magnitude of the human and economic consequences of quadriplegia, however, we firmly believe that the trampoline and the minitrampoline have clearly been established as very dangerous devices.

No firm conclusions can be drawn from the literature regarding any clearly definable pathology patterns. In those 58 cases in which the level of the lesion is determined, however, the distribution is as follows: C-1, two cases; C2−3, one case; C3−4, no cases; C4−5, 21 cases; C5−6, 31 cases; C6−7, one case; and C-7 to T-1, two cases.

With regard to pathology type, a variety of lesions have been reported: vertebral body compression-burst fractures; facet dislocations and subluxations without fractures; fracture-dislocations; and fracture-dislocations associated with intervertebral disk herniations. It appears that irreversible injury to the spinal cord can occur with various injury patterns at any level of the cervical spine.

Just before their injuries, all three of the Swedish children and four of the eight Danish children blacked out.[10, 12] The pathophysiology of this brief interval of unconsciousness before the injury requires explanation and further study.

Most noteworthy are observations on the skill levels of well-documented cases.[6, 10, 12] Specifically, Frykman and Hilding[10] reported that their patients involved experienced, expert, and elite trampolinists, respectively. Of the eight Danish patients, five had from 1 to 8 years' experience, and one was a trampoline instructor.[12] As noted, the 14 cases of Christensen and Clarke[6] involved one expertly skilled, three highly skilled, two skilled trampolinists, and two skilled novices. Most of these cases fall into a pattern. While attempting to perform a forward or backward somersault, a highly skilled and experienced trampolinist sustains an injury to the cervical spine resulting in quadriplegia. This set of circumstances certainly calls into question the widespread assumption that catastrophic trampoline injuries can be prevented with equipment standards, better-trained instructors and spotters, and safety harnesses.

Since 1977, when the first trampoline position paper was published by the AAP,[1] there has been a decrease in both noncatastrophic head and neck injuries[16] and in catastrophic neck injuries due to the use of the trampoline and the minitrampoline.[6] We believe that the decrease in trampoline-related injuries is the direct result that this statement had on the use, manufacture, and distribution of these devices. Unfortunately, prompted by the success of its own efforts, the AAP has chosen to soften its stand on this matter. Item 5 of the Trampoline II position paper states: "Maneuvers, especially the somersault, that have a high potential for serious injury should be attempted only by those qualified to become skilled performers." Judging from well-documented evidence in the literature that has been cited, it is the "skilled performer" attempting difficult maneuvers and somersaults who is at risk of sustaining a cervical spine injury resulting in quadriplegia.

On the basis of this review, we believe that the AAP was ill advised in altering its position on the use of trampolines. It is our opinion that both the trampoline and the minitrampoline are dangerous devices when used in the best of circumstances, and their use has no place in recreational, educational, or competitive gymnastics.

REFERENCES

1. American Academy of Pediatrics: Committee on Accident and Poison Prevention: *Trampolines*. Evanston, Ill, American Academy of Pediatrics, September 1977.

2. American Academy of Pediatrics: Committee on Accident and Poison Prevention and Committee on Pediatric Aspects of Physical Fitness, Recreation, and Sports: Trampolines. II. *Pediatrics* 1981; 67:438.

3. American Alliance for Health, Physical Education, and Recreation: The use of trampolines and minitramps in physical education. *J Phys Educ Recreation* 1978; 49:14.

4. American Alliance for Health, Physical Education, and Recreation: The use of the trampoline for the development of competitive skills in sport. *J Phys Educ Recreation* 1978; 49:14.

5. American Society for Testing and Materials: Standard consumer safety specification for components, assembly, and use of a trampoline, F381-77, in *Annual Book of ASTM Standards*. Philadelphia, American Society for Testing and Materials, 1977, part 46, pp 586–589.

6. Christensen C (with assistance of Clarke KS): *Fourth Annual National Gymnastic Catastrophic Injury Report 1981–82*. Urbana-Champaign, Ill, College of Applied Life Studies, University of Illinois, April 1982, pp 1–35.

7. Clarke KS: A survey of sports-related spinal cord injuries in schools and colleges, 1973–1975. *J Safety Res* 1977; 9:140–146.

8. Ellis WB, Green D, Holzaepfel NR, et al: The trampoline and serious neurological injuries: A report of five cases. *JAMA* 1960; 174:1673–1676.

9. Evans RF: Tetraplegia caused by gymnastics (letter). *Br Med J* 1979; 2:732.

10. Frykman G, Hilding S: Hopp pa studsmatta kan orsaka allvarlige skador. *Laekartidningen* 1970; 67:5862–5864.

11. Hage P: Trampoline: An "attractive nuisance." *Phys Sportsmed* 1982; 10:118–122.

12. Hammer A, Schwartzbach A-L, Darre E, et al: Svaere neukrologiske skader some folge af trampolinspring. *Ugeskr Laeger* 1981; 143:2970–2974.

13. Kravitz H: Problems with the trampoline: I. Too many cases of permanent paralysis. *Pediatr Ann* 1978; 7:728–729.

14. Rapp GF: Problems with the trampoline: II. Safety suggestions for trampoline use. *Pediatr Ann* 1978; 7:730–731.

15. Rapp GF, Nicely PG: Trampoline injuries. *Am J Sports Med* 1978; 6:269–271.

16. Rutherford GW, Miles RB, Brown VR, et al: *Overview of Sports-Related Injuries to Persons 5–14 Years of Age.* Washington, DC, US Consumer Product Safety Commission, December 1981, pp 1–47.

17. Steinbruck K, Paeslack V: Trampolinspringen—ein gefahrlicher Sport? *Munchen Med Wochenschr* 1978; 120:985–988.

18. US Consumer Product Safety Commission: Fact Sheet 85: *Trampolines.* Y3,C76/3:11/85, Washington, DC, February 1976, pp 1–3.

19. Witthaut H: Verletzungen beim Trampolinturnen. *Monatsschr Unfallh* 1969; 72:25–29.

20. Zimmerman HM: Accident experience with trampolines. *Res Quart* 1956; 27:452–455.

CHAPTER 8

The Epidemiologic, Biomechanical, and Cinematographic Analysis of Football-Induced Cervical Spine Trauma and Its Prevention

Joseph S. Torg, M.D.

Athletic injuries to the cervical spine resulting in damage to the spinal cord are infrequent but catastrophic events. Accurate descriptions of the mechanism or mechanisms responsible for a particular injury transcend simple academic interest. Before preventive measures can be developed and implemented, identification of the mechanisms involved in the production of the particular injury is necessary. Because of the inability of the nervous system to recover significant function after severe trauma, prevention assumes a most important role when considering these injuries.

Injuries resulting in spinal cord damage have been associated with football,* water sports,† gymnastics,[48, 47] wrestling,[7, 68] rugby,‡ trampolining,[13, 19, 53, 58] and ice hockey.[54, 56] Torg et al.,[59, 61, 62] through the use of epidemiologic data, biomechanical evidence, and cinematographic analysis, have (1) defined the in-

*References 10, 14, 24, 25, 28, 47–50, 60–62, and 64.
†References 1–4, 8, 9, 11, 15, 16, 18, 23, 24, 29, 31, 35, 37, 39, 42, and 45.
‡References 6, 30, 33, 41, 43, 44, 46, 51, and 67.

volvement of axial load forces in cervical spine injuries occurring in football, (2) demonstrated the success of appropriate rule changes in the prevention of these injuries, and (3) emphasized the need for employment of epidemiologic methods to prevent cervical spine and similar severe injuries in other high-risk athletic activities.

During the 1975 season, twelve football players in Pennsylvania and New Jersey sustained severe cervical spine injuries. Eight of these injuries resulted in permanent cervical quadriplegia. Analysis of the injuries determined that all twelve occurred during a headfirst tackle or block.[60] In order to ascertain whether the local increase in catastrophic football neurotrauma reflected a national trend, the National Football Head and Neck Injury Registry was established.[59, 61, 62] Consideration of the head and neck injuries by the Registry included four parameters: (1) intracranial hemorrhages, (2) intracranial injuries resulting in death, (3) cervical spine fractures, subluxations, and dislocations, and (4) cervical spine trauma resulting in permanent quadriplegia. The total number of head and neck injuries was cal-

TABLE 8–1.

Comparison of Occurrence and Rate of Head and Neck Injuries in American Football in Two 5-year Periods

Source (yr)	Intracranial Hemorrhages	Craniocerebral Deaths	Cervical Spine Fractures/Subluxations/ Dislocations	Permanent Cervical Quadriplegia
Schneider and Kahn[50] 1959–1963	139 (3.39)	65 (1.58)	56 (1.36)	30 (0.73)
National Football Head and Neck Injury Registry, 1971–1975	72 (1.15)	58 (0.92)	259 (4.14)	99 (1.58)

culated retrospectively from 1971–1975 and compared with the values compiled by Schneider and Kahn[50] in a similar study during the years 1959–1963. A 66% decrease in rate of intracranial hemorrhages and a 42% decrease in the rate of craniocerebral deaths between the two periods is noted. More significantly, the rate of cervical spine fractures, subluxations, and dislocations increased 204%, and the rate of cervical spine injuries associated with permanent quadriplegia increased 116% (Table 8–1).

Comparison of head injury data from the period 1959–1963 with that obtained by the Registry for the years 1971–1975 demonstrated that both intracranial hemorrhages and intracranial deaths had decreased (see Table 8–1). Schneider and Kahn[50] found 139 lesions (3.39/100,000) in which intracranial hemorrhages were a component and 65 deaths (1.58/100,000) from craniocerebral injuries. The Registry documented 72 intracranial lesions (1.15/100,000) and 58 craniocerebral deaths (0.92/100,000) occurring between 1971 and 1975. These rates represent a 66% decrease for hemorrhages and a 42% decrease in craniocerebral deaths.

With regard to cervical spine injuries, Schneider and Kahn[50] reported 56 injuries (1.36/100,000) that involved a fracture or dislocation (or both) and 30 with associated permanent cervical quadriplegia (0.73/100,000). The Registry documented 259 injuries (4.14/100,000) involving a fracture or dislocation (or both) of the cervical spine and 99 cases (1.58/

100,000) of cervical quadriplegia. These rates represented a 204% increase for cervical spine fractures/subluxations/dislocations and a 116% increase for cases of cervical quadriplegia. While the rates of head injuries had decreased, the rates of cervical spine injuries with or without quadriplegia had increased dramatically from the data reported by Schneider and Kahn (see Table 8–1).

Three conclusions were made based on these findings: (1) the improved protective capabilities of modern helmets accounted for the decrease in head injuries between the two studies; (2) the improved protection of the head led to the development of playing techniques that used the top or crown of the helmet as the initial point of contact; and (3) these headfirst techniques placed the cervical spine at risk for serious injury. It was postulated that execution of headfirst techniques increased the risk of neck injury by exposing the athlete's cervical spine to excessive axial loads, a force to which the cervical spine appears to be particularly susceptible.

These preliminary observations were reported at the annual meeting of the National Collegiate Athletic Association (NCAA) Football Rules Committee in January 1976. As a result, the following rules were instituted beginning with the 1976 season: (1) no player shall intentionally strike a runner with the crown or top of the helmet; (2) spearing is the deliberate use of the helmet in an attempt to punish an opponent; and (3) no player shall deliberately use his helmet to butt or ram an opponent (NCAA Football Rule Changes and/or Modifications, Jan 23, 1976, Rule 2, Section 1, Articles 2-L, 2-N). Similar rules were also adopted by the National Federation of High School Athletic Associations (NFHSAA) during the same year. The goal of these rule changes was to bring about changes in coaching and playing techniques to eliminate the use of the head as the initial point of contact in blocking and tackling.

Axial loading has been implicated as the primary mechanism producing severe cervical spine injuries in tackle football through review of epidemiologic, biomechanic, and cinematographic data compiled by the National Football Head and Neck Injury Registry. In the course of a contact activity, such as tackle football, the cervical spine is repeatedly exposed to potentially injurious energy inputs. Fortunately, however, most forces are effectively dissipated by the energy-absorbing capabilities of the cervical paravertebral musculature and the intervertebral disks through controlled spinal motion. However, the vertebra, intervertebral disks, and supporting ligamentous structures can be injured when contact occurs on the top or crown of the helmet with the head, neck, and trunk positioned in such a way that forces are transmitted along the vertical axis of the cervical spine. In this situation in which the cervical spine assumes the physical characteristics of a segmented column, motion resulting in energy dissipation is precluded in response to axial-directed impacts, and the forces are directly transmitted to the spinal structures.

When viewed from the lateral perspective, with the neck in the neutral position, the normal alignment of the spine is one of extension because of the normal lordotic curve (Fig 8–1). It is with 30 degrees of neck flexion that the cervical spine is straightened (Fig 8–2). With impact exerted along the longitudinal axis of a straight spine, loading of a seg-

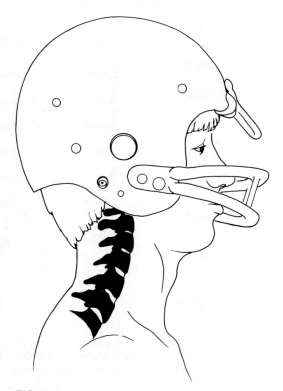

FIG 8–1.
When the neck is in a normal, upright, anatomic position, the cervical spine is slightly extended because of natural cervical lordosis. (From Torg JS, et al: *Am J Sports Med* 1990; 18:50–57. Used by permission.)

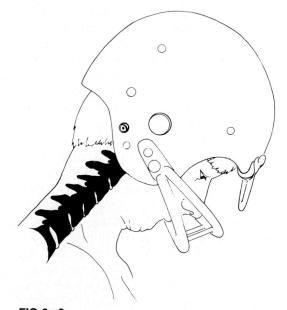

FIG 8–2.
When the neck is slightly flexed to approximately 30 degrees, the cervical spine is straightened and converted into a segmented column. (From Torg JS, et al: *Am J Sports Med* 1990; 18:50–57. Used by permission.)

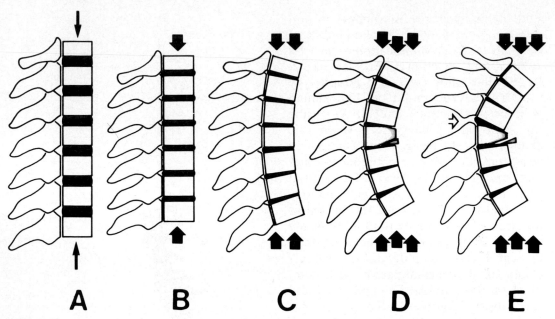

FIG 8–3.
Biomechanically, the straightened cervical spine responds to axial loading forces like a segmented column. Axial loading of the cervical spine first results in compressive deformation of the intervertebral disks (**A** and **B**). As the energy input continues and maximum compressive deformation is reached, angular deformation and buckling occur. The spine fails in a flexion mode (**C**), with resulting fracture, subluxation, or dislocation (**D** and **E**). Compressive deformation to failure, with a resultant fracture, dislocation, or subluxation, occurs in as little as 8.4 msec. (From Torg JS, et al: *Am J Sports Med* 1990; 18:50–57. Used by permission.)

mented column occurs (Fig 8–3,A and B). At first energy inputs are absorbed by the intervertebral disks, and compressive deformation occurs. When maximum deformation is reached, continued energy input results in angular deformation and buckling, with failure of the intervertebral disks or bony elements, or both. This results in subluxation, facet dislocation, or fracture-dislocation at one spinal level(Fig 8–3,C–E).[12]

Axial loading of the cervical spine occurs when the neck is slightly flexed, normal cervical lordosis is straightened, and the spine is converted into a segmented column. Assuming the head, neck, and trunk components of a composite injury model to be in motion, rapid deceleration of the head occurs when it strikes another object, such as an opposing player, and results in the fragile cervical spine being compressed by the force of the oncoming trunk. Essentially,

the head is stopped, the trunk is still moving, and the spine is crushed between the two. As mentioned, if the compression force is not dissipated by controlled motion in the spinal segments, fracture, or dislocation, or both result.

To obtain data on football-related injuries with associated neurologic sequelae, the National Football Head and Neck Injury Registry was established. Initiated in 1975 as an ongoing registry, information was first collected retrospectively to 1971. Criteria for inclusion in the Registry were those head or cervical spine injuries that (1) required hospitalization for more than 72 hours, (2) required surgical intervention, (3) involved a fracture, subluxation, or dislocation, or (4) resulted in permanent paralysis or death.

Information was obtained by several methods. Project descriptions and injury report forms were mailed at the conclusion of each football season to the 40,000 members of the National Association of Secondary School Principals and the 5,000 members of the National Athletic Trainers Association. In addition, a newspaper/media–clipping service was contracted each year to identify those head and neck injuries reported in the press, radio, or television. When an injury was reported, more detailed information was obtained from the athlete, parent, and school officials. Pertinent medical and radiographic data from the physicians and the hospitals responsible for the care of the athlete were also acquired. All the information collected on each athlete was reviewed for (1) the mechanism of injury, (2) the pathologic state of spinal and neural elements, (3) the type of treatment received, and (4) the extent and duration of neurologic deficit resulting from the injury. Injury rates for intracranial hemorrhages, intracranial deaths, cervical spine fractures/dislocations/subluxations, and permanent quadriplegia were calculated for both high school and collegiate participants each year of the study.

When available, game films or videotapes of the injury were studied to determine the mechanism of injury and to calculate the force of impact. Cinematographic records were reviewed for 60 athletes with injuries resulting in neurologic deficits. Stop frame kinetic analysis, a method that allows estimation of the magnitude of injury-producing forces, was performed on 11 films of athletes sustaining injuries that resulted in quadriplegia. The force acting on the athletes' head, cervical spine, and trunk segment was calculated with use of the law of conservation of linear momentum. The orientation of the head, cervical spine, and trunk segment of each athlete was analyzed to determine the mechanism of injury.

A review of the biomechanical literature correlated the clinical observations

documented from the Registry data with the experimental information on cervical spine injury mechanisms.

Analysis of the Registry data revealed definite trends in the incidence of head and cervical spine injuries occurring in both high school and collegiate football. Intracranial hemorrhages demonstrated an apparent increase between the years 1976 and 1982 and then maintained a fairly constant rate for the duration of the study (Fig 8–4). The brief increasing trend was due to the improved diagnostic capabilities in identifying these lesions provided by the advent of computed tomography. Intracranial hemorrhages resulting in death remained relatively constant throughout the study (Fig 8–5).

Fractures, subluxations, and dislocations of the cervical spine demonstrated a progressive decrease between the years 1976 and 1987 (Fig 8–6). The 1976 severe cervical spine injury rates of 7.72/100,000 and 30.66/100,000 occurring in American football at the high school and college levels, respectively, decreased to 2.31/100,000 and 10.66/100,000 during the subsequent 12 years (Table 8–2). These rates represented a 70% reduction in high school injuries and a 65% reduction in college injuries. The largest single year drop occurred between 1977 and 1978, 2 years after the 1976 rule changes. During this year, high school injury rates fell from 7.06/100,000 to 3.72/100,000, a 47% decrease, and college injury rates declined from 20.00/100,000 to 10.66/100,000, also a 47% decrease.

Cervical spine injuries resulting in quadriplegia consistently declined from a total of 34 cases in 1976 to 5 cases in 1984 (Fig 8–7). In 1976 the injury rate was 2.24/100,000 at the high school level and 10.66/100,000 at the college level (see Table 8–2). In 1977, just one year after the rule changes, the rates dropped to 1.30/100,000, a 42% decrease, and 2.66/100,000, a 75% decrease, for high school

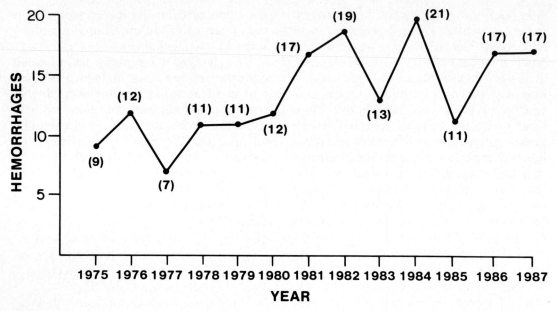

FIG 8–4.
Incidence of intracranial hemorrhages for all levels of participation (1975–1987) demonstrated a gradual increase between 1976 and 1982. Levels remained fairly constant from 1983 to 1987. (From Torg JS, et al: *Am J Sports Med* 1990; 18:50–57. Used by permission.)

and college athletes, respectively. The rates continued to decline at both the high school and college levels until 1984. In 1984 the injury rates had fallen to 0.40/100,000 for high schools, a 82% decrease, and to 0/100,000 for colleges, a 100% decrease. In 1985 the injury rates at both the high school and college levels increased slightly from the low noted in 1984 and remained constant from 1985 to 1987 (see Table 8–2).

Axial compression was identified as the mechanism causing the highest percentage of football cervical fractures/dis-

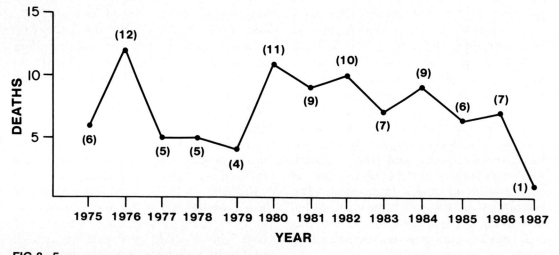

FIG 8–5.
Incidence of craniocerebral deaths for all levels of participation (1975–1987) remained constant for the duration of the study. (From Torg JS, et al: *Am J Sports Med* 1990; 18:50–57. Used by permission.)

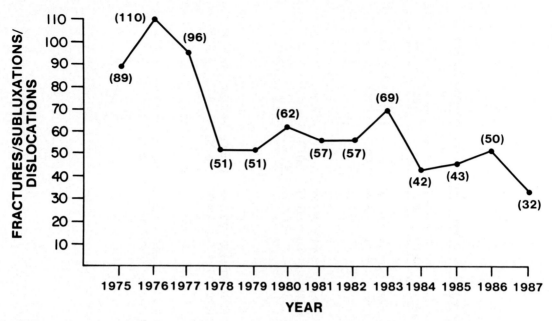

FIG 8–6.
Yearly incidence of cervical spine fractures/dislocations/subluxations for all levels of participation (1975–1987) decreased markedly in 1978 and continued to decline during the remaining 9 years as a direct result of the rule changes instituted in 1976 banning headfirst blocking, tackling, and spearing. (From Torg JS, et al: *Am J Sports Med* 1990; 18:50–57. Used by permission.)

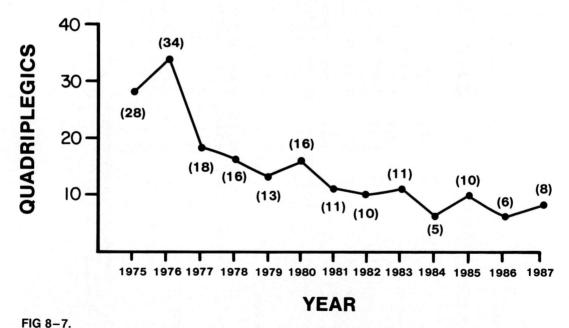

FIG 8–7.
Yearly incidence of permanent cervical quadriplegia for all levels of participation (1975–1987) decreased dramatically in 1977 after initiation of rule changes prohibiting use of headfirst tackling and blocking techniques. The number of injuries continued to decline until 1984, whereupon the dramatically lowered levels were maintained throughout the remainder of the study. (From Torg JS, et al: *Am J Sports Med* 1990; 18:50–57. Used by permission.)

TABLE 8–2.
Twelve-year Data for Severe and Catastrophic Head and Neck Injuries Occurring in American Football at High School, College, and Professional/Recreational Levels*†

Injury	1976	1977	1978	1979	1980	1981	1982	1983	1984	1985	1986	1987
							Year					
Intracranial hemorrhage												
High School	10 (0.89)	6 (0.55)	10 (0.93)	8 (0.85)	8 (0.85)	11 (1.15)	17 (1.88)	12 (1.30)	16 (1.62)	9 (0.96)	15 (1.57)	17 (1.78)
College	1 (1.33)	1 (1.33)	1 (1.33)	1 (1.33)	0	3 (4.00)	1 (1.33)	1 (1.33)	4 (5.33)	2 (2.66)	1 (1.33)	0
Other	1	0	0	2	4	3	1	0	1	0	1	0
Total	12	7	11	11	12	17	19	13	21	11	17	17
Craniocerebral deaths												
High School	11 (0.98)	5 (0.46)	5 (0.46)	1 (0.10)	7 (0.74)	6 (0.63)	8 (0.88)	6 (0.65)	6 (0.60)	3 (0.32)	5 (0.52)	1 (0.10)
College	0	0	0	1 (1.33)	1 (1.33)	2 (2.66)	1 (1.33)	1 (1.33)	1 (1.33)	1 (1.33)	1 (1.33)	0
Other	1	0	0	2	3	1	1	0	2	2	1	0
Total	12	5	5	4	11	9	10	7	9	6	7	1
Cervical spine fixation/dislocation/ subluxation												
High School	86 (7.72)	76 (7.06)	40 (3.72)	42 (4.47)	52 (5.54)	49 (5.16)	46 (5.10)	60 (6.50)	36 (3.65)	32 (3.43)	36 (3.78)	22 (2.31)
College	23 (30.66)	15 (20.00)	8 (10.66)	7 (9.33)	9 (12.00)	8 (10.66)	6 (8.00)	7 (9.33)	5 (6.66)	6 (8.00)	11 (14.66)	8 (10.66)
Other	1	5	3	2	1	0	5	2	1	5	3	2
Total	110	96	51	51	62	57	57	69	42	43	50	32
Permanent quadriplegia												
High School	25 (2.24)	14 (1.30)	14 (1.30)	8 (0.95)	13 (1.38)	7 (0.73)	7 (0.77)	9 (0.97)	4 (0.40)	7 (0.75)	6 (0.63)	7 (0.73)
College	8 (10.66)	2 (2.66)	0	4 (5.33)	2 (2.66)	2 (2.66)	1 (1.33)	1 (1.33)	0	2 (2.66)	0	0
Other	1	2	2	1	1	2	2	1	1	1	0	1
Total	34	18	16	13	16	11	10	11	5	10	6	8

*From Torg JS, et al: Am J Sports Med 1990; 18:50–57. Used by permission.
†Rates in parentheses are per 100,000 participants based on participation numbers from the National Collegiate Athletic Association and the National Federation of State High School Athletic Associations for 11-man football.

locations/subluxations with and without quadriplegia. From 1971 to 1975, 39% of nonquadriplegic cervical spine injuries and 52% of the quadriplegic injuries were attributed to this mechanism. During the years between 1976 and 1987, 52.5% of the quadriplegic injuries and 49% of the nonquadriplegic cervical spine injuries were caused by the same mechanism.

Documentation of axial loading as the responsible mechanism of injury in the production of catastrophic football cervical spine injuries was obtained from the review of game films of actual injuries. Sixty films of injuries resulting in neurologic deficits were available for study. Analysis of these films allowed determination of the mechanism of injury in 85% of the cases. In the 51 films in which it was possible to observe the mechanism of injury, it was determined to be axial loading in every instance. Stop frame analysis performed on 11 of these films determined that 3 distinct types of colli-

sions existed. The first type was a direct collision in which two bodies traveled along the same straight line and in opposite directions before impact. The second type of collision was also direct, but one in which a moving body hit another that was stationary. The third type was an oblique collision in which two moving bodies met at an angle. All 11 of the injuries were determined to be the result of head-first contact, and all resulted in permanent cervical quadriplegia. Four of the injuries were type 1 collisions, three were type 2, and four were type 3. All 11 athletes were injured while tackling an opposing player.

The forces involved with the production of the 11 injuries were calculated based on the law of conservation of linear momentum. By determining the rate of change of the momentum of a body upon collision, the force of that collision can be determined. The impulse of a force (F × Δt) is equal to the change of momentum that it produces ($mv_f - mv_i$). In a

TABLE 8–3.

Presentation of Estimated Force of Impact Values for 11 Axial Loading Injuries Resulting in Quadriplegia Calculated in Stop Frame Analysis*†

Case	Age	M (kg)	V_i (m/sec)	V_f (m/sec)	O_i (degree)	Est. Force (kg f)
Type 1 collisions						
1	19	84	4.90	0	/	700.00
2	19	77	6.63	0	/	368.21
3	17	75	5.08	0	/	667.96
4	15	68	5.83	0	/	674.22
Type 2 collisions						
5	17	80	6.10	0	/	829.89
6	17	75	3.59	0	/	457.91
7	16	75	3.39	0	/	432.40
Type 3 collisions						
8	15	75	4.70	0	10	550.03
9	15	64	3.81	0	90	439.85
10	17	73	6.10	0	30	751.11
11	17	73	5.08	0	90	501.71

*From Torg JS, et al: Am J Sports Med 1990; 18:50–57. Used by permission.
†M = injured player's mass in kilograms; V_i = injured player's velocity measured in meters per second before impact; V_f = injured player's velocity measured in meters per second after collision; O_i = incident angle for those collisions that were oblique; Est. Force = estimated force calculated in stop frame analysis. See Fig 8–8 for a sample calculation of estimated force of impact values.

collision, the respective changes in momentum of the two bodies must be equal and opposite so that the total momentum of the system is unaltered by the impact. A sample calculation (Fig 8–8) and the results for the 11 cases (Table 8–3) are presented. According to the data, the range of axial force that acted on the cervical spine during a direct collision resulting in cervical quadriplegia was approximately 400 to 800 kg f, and the oblique resultant force range was approximately 400 to 700 kg f. This estimated force was similar to the forces calculated by Hodgson and Thomas.[20] They calculated the estimated force of impact in axial loading cervical spine injuries from the work = kinetic energy point of view. The average force involved in each collision they studied was determined from the following formula:

$$\text{Work} = F \times \Delta X = \tfrac{1}{2}\, mv^2$$

where the variables are as follows:

$$x = \text{stopping distance;}$$
$$m = \text{body mass; and}$$
$$v = \text{players' velocity.}$$

Hodgson and Thomas[20] concluded that the average force acting on the neck was between 700 and 1,600 lb f (318.18 kg f to 727.27 kg f), a range nearly identical to

---

Sample calculation, Case 1—type 1 collision:

$$Wt = 84 \text{ kg}$$
$$V_i = 4.9 \text{ m/sec}$$
$$V_f = 0 \text{ m/sec}$$
$$t = 0.06 \text{ sec}$$

According to Newton's second law and the concept of conservation of momentum,

$$F_1 = m_1 a_1 = F_2 = m_2 a_2$$
$$= \frac{(m_1 v_{i1}) - (m_1 v_{f1})}{t} = \frac{(m_2 v_{i2}) - (m_2 v_{f2})}{t}$$
$$\because v_{f1} = 0 = v_{f2}$$
$$\therefore F1 = \frac{m_1 v_{i1}}{t} = F2 = \frac{m_2 v_{i2}}{t}$$

Therefore, $F = \dfrac{(84 \text{ kg}) (4.9 \text{ m/sec})}{0.06 \text{ sec}}$

$$= 6,860 \text{ kg, m/sec}^2$$
$$= 6,860 \text{ newtons}$$

Since 1 kg f = 9.8 newtons,

$$F = \frac{6,860 \text{ N}}{9.8 \text{ N/kg f}} = 700.00 \text{ kg f}$$

700.00 kg f is the estimated axial force acting upon the victim's cervical spine during the injury-producing impact. The same type of calculation is used to estimate the force of impact in type 2 collisions. In type 3 collisions, however the additional variable 0_i (angle of incidence) must be added into the calculation of momentum.

FIG 8–8.
Sample calculation with use of the law of conservation of momentum to estimate force of impact values by stop frame analysis. (From Torg JS, et al: *Am J Sports Med* 1990; 18:50–57. Used by permission.)

that derived from stop frame analysis (see Table 8–3).

Refutation of the "freak accident" concept with the more logical principle of cause and effect has been most rewarding in dealing with the problem of football-induced cervical spine trauma and quadriplegia. Definition of the axial loading mechanism in which a football player, usually a defensive back, makes a tackle by striking his opponent with the top of his helmet has been the key in this process. Implementation of rule changes and coaching techniques eliminating the use of the head as a battering ram have resulted in a dramatic reduction in the incidence of cervical spine injuries, with or without quadriplegia, between 1976 and 1987.

Although these data lead to the conclusion that axial loading is the predominant force involved in the production of athletic cervical spine injuries, classically, these injuries have been attributed either to hyperflexion or to hyperextension mechanisms. Schneider[49] and Schneider and Kahn,[50] the first researchers to catalog head and neck injuries occurring in athletic competition, supported this traditional view. In his series of cervical spine injuries occurring in tackle football, Schneider[49] concluded that the most severe injuries to the cervical spine occur as a result of hyperflexion. Schneider also mentioned that hyperextension may cause cervical lesions, resulting in neurologic damage. He did not list axial loading or vertex impact among the forces associated with football cervical spine neurotrauma.

Other authors have also used these mechanisms to account for a variety of catastrophic athletic cervical spine injuries. Carvell et al.[6] (rugby), Gehweiler et al.[16] (diving), Leidholt[25] (football), Mac-Nab [26] (diving), McCoy et al.[30] (rugby), O'Carroll et al.[33] (rugby), Paley and Gillespie [34] (general sports), Piggot and Gordon[36] (rugby), Scher[41] (rugby),

Williams and McKibbin[67] (rugby), and Wu and Lewis[68] (wrestling) all proposed hyperflexion as the most frequent cause of serious cervical injuries in the activities they reviewed.

Others who, like Schneider, have emphasized both hyperextension and hyperflexion as the two dominant forces producing most types of cervical spine lesions with cord damage, include Dolan et al.[10] (football), Funk and Wells[14] (football), and Silver[51] (rugby). Although some authors, such as Kazarian[22] (general sports), Kewalramani and Taylor[23] (diving), Maroon et al.[28] (football), Mennen[31] (diving), and Rogers[39] (diving), recognized that axial loading is associated with severe cervical spine injuries, they continued to emphasize the dominant role of hyperflexion and hyperextension forces in the production of these lesions.

Traditionally, axial loads have not been mentioned among the major forces contributing to cervical spine fractures, dislocations, or fracture-dislocations occurring in athletes. Allen et al.[4] (diving), Jackson and Lohr[21] (general sports), King[24] (football and diving), and Stauffer and Kaufer[52] (diving) mentioned axial loading as a common mechanism, but they stated that hyperextension, or hyperflexion, or both still accounted for a significant number of the lesions. As a direct result of the National Football Head and Neck Injury Registry data, the axial loading mechanism has been identified as the predominant mechanism of injury for athletic cervical spine injuries. In addition to the studies of Torg et al.,[57–63] Scher[42, 43] in 1980 (diving) and 1981 (rugby), Tator et al.[54–56] in 1981 (diving) and 1984 (ice hockey), and Watkins[64] in 1986 (football) demonstrated vertical impact and axial loading to be the major forces to consider when analyzing cervical spine injuries in athletes.

A review of the literature pertaining to the biomechanics of cervical spine injuries yielded experimental support to the axial loading theory. Mertz et al.,[32] Hodgson and Thomas,[20] and Sances et al.[40] measured stresses and strains within the cervical spine when axial impulses were applied to helmeted cadaver head-spine-trunk specimens. They were able to produce fractures of the lower cervical area of the spine when the impulse was applied to the crown of the helmet. Hodgson and Thomas[20] determined that direct vertex impact imparted a larger force to the cervical vertebra than forces applied further forward on the skull. Gosch et al.[17] investigated three different injury modes, hyperflexion, hyperextension, and axial compression in their experiment involving anesthetized monkeys. They concluded that axial compression produced cervical spine fractures and dislocations. Maiman et al.,[27] Roaf,[38] and White and Punjabi[65] demonstrated vertebral body fractures in the lower cervical spine due to the axial loading of isolated spinal units. Roaf[38] subjected spinal units to forces differing in direction and magnitude, that is, compression, flexion, extension, lateral flexion, rotation, and horizontal shear. He stated unequivocally that he had never succeeded in producing pure hyperflexion injuries in a normal intact spinal unit, and concluded that hyperflexion of the cervical spine was an anatomic impossibility. Roaf was able to produce almost every variety of spinal injury with a combination of compression and rotation.

Bauze and Ardran[5] postulated that axial loads were responsible for cervical spine dislocations as well as fractures. They demonstrated that failure of the facet joints and posterior ligaments occurred when axial loads were applied to cadaveric spines. When the lower portion of the spine was flexed and fixed and the upper part extended and free to move forward, vertical compression produced bilateral dislocation of the facet joints without fracture. If lateral tilt or axial rotation occurred as well, a unilateral dislocation was produced. The forces observed were all less than those required for bony failure, and allowed facet dislocation without associated bony pathology.

This study has delineated the important role axial loading plays in production of football cervical spine injuries. We believe this mechanism is also responsible for similar injuries occurring in other collision sports. Whether it is a football player striking an opponent with the top or crown of his helmet, a poorly executed dive into a shallow body of water where the subject strikes his head on the bottom, or a hockey player checked into the boards headfirst, injury occurs as the fragile cervical area of the spine is compressed between the rapidly decelerated head and the continued momentum of the body. Appropriate rule changes recognizing this mechanism have resulted in a marked reduction of football cervical injuries with and without quadriplegia. The success of the preventive measures advocated by the National Football Head and Neck Injury Registry leads to the suggestion that similar studies, directed toward the prevention of injuries rather than their treatment, would most likely decrease rates for many types of injuries in a wide variety of athletic activities. Continued research, development of clear and concise definitions of the responsible injury mechanisms based on sound biomechanical, epidemiologic, and clinical evidence, education of coaches and players, and enforcement of rules are essential so that the preventive measures may succeed.

REFERENCES

1. Adelstein W, Watson P: Cervical spine injuries. *J Neurosurg Nursing* 1983; 15:65–71.

2. Albrand OW, Corkill G: Broken necks from diving accidents: A summer epidemic in young men. *Am J Sports Med* 1976; 4:107–110.

3. Albrand OW, Walter J: Underwater deceleration curves in relation to injuries from diving. *Surg Neurol* 1975; 4:461–465.

4. Allen BL Jr, Ferguson RL, Lehman TR, et al: A mechanistic classification of closed, indirect fractures and dislocations of the lower cervical spine. *Spine* 1982; 7:1–27.

5. Bauze RJ, Ardran GM: Experimental production of forward dislocation in the human cervical spine. *J Bone Joint Surg* 1978; 60B:239–245.

6. Carvell JE, Fuller DJ, Duthrie RB, et al: Rugby football injuries to the cervical spine. *Br Med J* 1983; 286:49–50.

7. Cloward RB: Acute cervical spine injuries. *Clin Symp* 1980; 32:2–32.

8. Coin CG, Pennink M, Ahmad WD, et al: Diving-type injury of the cervical spine: Contribution of computed tomography to management. *J Comput Assist Tomogr* 1979; 3:362–372.

9. Dall DM: Injuries of the cervical spine. *S Afr Med J* 1972; 46:1048–1056.

10. Dolan KD, Feldick HG, Albright JP, et al: Neck injuries in football players. *Am Fam Physician* 1975; 12:89–91.

11. Dorwart R, LeMasters DL: Application of computed tomographic scanning of the cervical spine. *Orthop Clin North Am* 1985; 16:381–393.

12. Frankel VH, Burstein A: *Orthopaedic Biomechanics.* Philadelphia, Lea & Febiger, 1970.

13. Frykman G, Hilding S: Hop pa studsmatta kan orska allvarliga skador. (Trampoling jumping can cause serious injury.) *Laekartidningen* 1970; 67:5862–5864.

14. Funk FJ Jr, Wells RE: Injuries of the cervical spine in football. *Clin Orthop* 1975; 109:50–58.

15. Garger WN, Fisher RG, Halfmann HW: Vertebrectomy and fusion for "tear drop fracture" o the cervical spine: Case report. *J Trauma* 1969 9:887–893.

16. Gehweiler JH, Clark WM, Schaaf R, et al: Cervical spine trauma: The common combined conditions. *Radiology* 1979; 130:77–86.

17. Gosch HH, Gooding E, Schneider RC: An experimental study of cervical spine and cord injuries. *J Trauma* 1972; 12:570–575.

18. Haines JD: Occult cervical spine fractures. *Postgrad Med* 1986; 80:73–77.

19. Hammer A, Schwartzbach AL, Darre E, et al: Svaere neurologiske skader some folge af trampolinspring. (Severe neurologic damage resulting from trampolining.) *Ugeskr Laeger* 1981; 143:2970–2974.

20. Hodgson VR, Thomas LM: *Mechanisms of Cervical Spine Injury During Impact to the Protected Head.* Twenty-fourth Stapp Car Crash Conference, 1980, pp 15–42.

21. Jackson DW, Lohr FT: Cervical spine injuries. *Clin Sports Med* 1986; 5:373–386.

22. Kazarian L: Injuries to the human spinal column: Biomechanics and injury classification. *Exerc Sport Sci Rev* 1981; 9:297–352.

23. Kewalramani LS, Taylor RG: Injuries to the cervical spine from diving accidents. *J Trauma* 1975; 15:130–142.

24. King DM: Fractures and dislocations of the cervical spine. *Aust NZ J Surg* 1967; 37:57–64.

25. Leidholt JD: Spinal injuries in athletes: Be prepared. *Orthop Clin North Am* 1973; 4:691–707.

26. MacNab I: Acceleration injuries of the cervical spine. *J Bone Joint Surg* 1964; 46A:1797–1799.

27. Maiman DJ, Sances A, Myklebust JB, et al: Compression injuries of the cervical spine: A biomechanical analysis. *Neurosurgery* 1983; 13:254–260.

28. Maroon JC, Steele PB, Berlin R: Football head and neck injuries: An update. *Clin Neurosurg* 1979; 27:414–429.

29. Mawk JR: C7 burst fracture with initial "complete" tetraplegia. *Minn Med* 1983; 66:135–138.

30. McCoy GF, Piggot J, Macafee AL, et al: Injuries of the cervical spine in schoolboy rugby football. *J Bone Joint Surg* 1984; 66B:500–503.

31. Mennen U: Survey of spinal injuries from diving: A study of patients in Pretoria and Cape Town. *South Afr Med J* 1981; 59:788–790.

32. Mertz HJ, Hodgson VR, Murray TL, et al: An assessment of compressive neck loads under injury-producing conditions. *Phys Sportsmed* 1978; 6:95–106.

33. O'Carroll F, Sheenan M, Gregg TM: Cervical spine injuries in rugby football. *Irish Med J* 1981; 74:377–379.

34. Paley D, Gillespie R: Chronic repetitive unrecognized injury of the cervical spine (high jumper's neck). *Am J Sports Med* 1986; 14:92–95.

35. Petrie JG: Flexion injuries of the cervical spine. *J Bone Joint Surg* 1964; 46A:1800–1806.

36. Piggot J, Gordon DS: Rugby injuries to the cervical cord. *Br Med J* 1979; 1:192–193.

37. Richman S, Friedman R: Vertical fracture of cervical vertebral bodies. *Radiology* 1954; 62:536–542.

38. Roaf R: A study of the mechanics of spinal injuries. *J Bone Joint Surg* 1960; 42B:810–823.

39. Rogers WA: Fractures and dislocations of the cervical spine: An end-result study. *J Bone Joint Surg* 1957; 39A:341–376.

40. Sances AJ, Myklebust JB, Maiman DJ, et al: Biomechanics of spinal injuries. *Crit Rev Biomed Eng* 1984; 11:1–76.

41. Scher AT: The high rugby tackle: An avoidable cause of cervical spinal injury? *South Afr Med J* 1978; 53:1015–1018.

42. Scher AT: Diving injuries to the cervical spinal cord. *South Afr Med J* 1981; 59:603–605.

43. Scher AT: Vertex impact and cervical dislocation in rugby players. *South Afr Med J* 1981; 59:227–228.

44. Scher AT: "Crashing" the rugby scrum: An avoidable cause of cervical spinal injury. *South Afr Med J* 1982; 61:919–920.

45. Scher AT: Radiographic indicators of traumatic cervical spine instability. *South Afr Med J* 1982; 62:562–565.

46. Scher AT: "Tear-drop" fractures of the cervical spine: Radiologic features. *South Afr Med J* 1982; 61:355–359.

47. Schneider RC: The syndrome of acute anterior spinal cord injury. *J Neurosurg* 1955; 12:95–123.

48. Schneider RC: Serious and fatal neurosurgical football injuries. *Clin Neurosurg* 1966; 12:226–236.

49. Schneider RC: *Head and Neck Injuries in Football.* Baltimore, Wilkins & Wilkins, 1973.

50. Schneider RC, Kahn EA: Chronic neurologic sequelae of acute trauma to the spine and spinal cord. Part I. The significance of the acute-flexion or "tear-drop" fracture dislocation of the cervical spine. *J Bone Joint Surg* 1956; 38A:985–997.

51. Silver JR: Injuries of the spine sustained in rugby. *Br Med J* 1984; 288:37–43.

52. Stauffer ES, Kaufer H: Fractures and dislocations of the spine, in Rockwood CA Jr, Green DP (eds): *Fractures,* vol 2, chap 12. Philadelphia, JB Lippincott Co, 1975:817–903.

53. Steinbruck J, Paeslack V: Trampolinspringen—ein gefahrlicher Sport? (Is trampolining a dangerous sport?) *Munchen Med Wochenschr* 1978; 120:985–988.

54. Tator CH, Edmonds VE: National survey of spinal injuries to hockey players. *Can Med Assoc J* 1984; 130:875–880.

55. Tator CH, Edmonds VE, New ML: Diving: Frequent and potentially preventable cause of spinal cord injury. *Can Med Assoc J* 1981; 124:1323–1324.

56. Tator CH, Ekong CEU, Rowed DA, et al: Spinal injuries due to hockey. *Can J Neurol Sci* 1984; 11:34–41.

57. Torg JS (ed): Mechanisms and pathomechanics of athletic injuries to the cervical spine, in *Athletic Injuries to the Head, Neck and Face,* chap 11. Philadelphia, Lea & Febiger, 1982.

58. Torg JS, Das M: Trampoline-related quadriplegia: Review of the literature and reflections on the American Academy of Pediatrics' Position Statement. *Pediatrics* 1984; 74:804–812.

59. Torg JS, Quedenfeld TC, Burstein A, et al: National Football Head and Neck Injury Registry: Report on Cervical Quadriplegia 1971 to 1975. *Am J Sports Med* 1979; 7:127–132.

60. Torg JS, Quedenfeld TC, Moyer RA, et al: Severe and catastrophic neck injuries resulting from tackle football. *J Am Coll Heath Assoc* 1977; 25:224–266.

61. Torg JS, Truex R, Quedenfeld TC, et al: The National Football Head and Neck Injury Registry Report and Conclusions. *JAMA* 1979; 241:1477–1479.

62. Torg JS, Vegso JJ, Sennett B, et al: The National Football Head and Neck Injury Registry. 14-Year report on cervical quadriplegia, 1971 through 1984. *JAMA* 1985; 254:3439–3443.

63. Torg JS, Vegso JJ, Yu A, et al: *Cervical Quadriplegia Resulting From Axial Loading Injuries: Cinematographic, Radiographic, Kinetic, and Pathologic Analysis.* Proceedings, Interim Meeting, American Orthopaedic Society for Sports Medicine. Atlanta, Ga, Feb 9, 1984.

64. Watkins RG: Neck injuries in football players. *Clin Sports Med* 1986; 5:215–246.

65. White AA III, Punjabi MM: *Clinical Biome-*

chanics of the Spine. Philadelphia, JB Lippincott Co, 1978.

66. Whitley JE, Forsyth HF: The classification of cervical spine injuries. *AJR* 1960; 83:633–644.

67. Williams JPR, McKibbin B: Cervical spine injuries in rugby union football. *Br Med J* 1978; 2:1747.

68. Wu WQ, Lewis RC: Injuries of the cervical spine in high school wrestling. *Surg Neurol* 1985; 23:143–147.

CHAPTER 9

Fatalities From Intracranial and Cervical Spine Injuries Occurring in Tackle Football: 1945–1988*

Frederick O. Mueller, Ph.D.

Intracranial and cervical spine injuries have been the major cause of football fatalities since the American Football Coaches Association initiated data collection in 1931. The purpose of this chapter is to discuss the cause of tackle football intracranial and cervical spine fatalities from 1945 to 1988. Historical information is presented to demonstrate the evolution of football and its association with fatalities to participants.

Data collected from 1945 to 1988 reveal the frequency of football intracranial and cervical spine fatalities, and also reveal the type of injury, activity at time of injury, level of play, and game or practice injury. Upon establishing the frequency and cause of these fatalities, the data are presented in 10-year spans and concentrate on the variables that have either increased or decreased fatalities. Major preventive measures that have been given credit for the reduction of intracranial and cervical spine fatalities during the

*Material updated from Mueller FO, Blyth CS: Fatalities from head and cervical spine injuries occurring in tackle football: 40 years' experience. *Clin Sports Med* 1987; 6:185–196. Used with permission.

past 12 years are discussed, and recommendations for prevention are given.

HISTORICAL BACKGROUND

The game of football had a rough beginning since that first Princeton versus Rutgers game in 1869. Uniforms were not part of the game, and players actually participated while wearing street clothing.[3] Football helmets were not worn until 1896, and early helmets did not offer much protection. Strategy did not play a role in the outcome of the game in those early years—brute force, physical conditioning, and endurance were the determining factors. The 1905 season ended in protest against the brutality of play, and *The Chicago Tribune*'s compilation of injuries showed 18 football players had died and 159 were seriously injured.[3] In midseason, President Roosevelt met with representatives from Yale, Harvard, and Princeton and told them it was time to save the sport by removing every objectionable feature. The president of the University of California also stated that the game must be made over or abolished. About this same time Columbia University abolished football and did not start again until 1915. In 1906, because of this national concern, rules were initiated to eliminate roughness of play and to reduce the danger of injury to the participants.

REVIEW OF RELATED LITERATURE

In 1961 Schneider et al.[8] published a neurosurgical review of the direct fatalities in the 1959 football season. Three case reports were reviewed, and one of the mechanisms of cervical injury was vascular insufficiency of the vertebral arteries after severe cervical hyperextension resulting in acute central cervical spinal cord injury. On the basis of their research, Schneider et al. suggested revisions of the football helmet to help reduce injury.

Schneider[9] also reviewed data concerning football injuries of a very serious or fatal neurosurgical nature during a 5-year period from 1959 through 1963. From a questionnaire survey of the Harvey Cushing Society and the Congress of Neurological Surgeons, reports of 225 such cases were received and evaluated. There were 11 skull fractures with 4 deaths, 5 extradural hematomas with 4 deaths, 69 subdural hematomas with 28 deaths, 14 intracerebral or intraventricular hemorrhages with 8 deaths, and 17 pontine lesions with 16 deaths. Schneider's report indicated that, besides the skull fractures, other lethal lesions occurred as a result of direct transmission of force to the intracranial contents, intimating strongly that the plastic football helmet did not offer adequate resiliency to dissipate energy. In addition to the craniocerebral injuries, there were 78 spine and spinal cord injuries with 16 deaths. The most tragic group were 30 youths whose fracture-dislocations resulted in immediate, complete, perma-

nent quadriplegia. Eighteen others had partial neurologic deficit and another eight, residual deficit.

In 1969 Snook[10] evaluated field injury reports at the University of Massachusetts during 4 years of football and 2 years of hockey, basketball, and lacrosse. For the first time the head was indicated as the most frequently injured body part among football participants. Knee injuries were next in frequency, followed by neck injuries. Snook also reviewed the common head and neck injuries and presented a classification of them.

Between 1971 and 1975 Torg[11] initiated the National Football Head and Neck Injury Registry. The Registry documented 99 cases of quadriplegia and 58 intracranial football injuries that resulted in death during this time. The Registry has continued to document catastrophic head and neck injuries in football, and based on these data, axial loading of the cervical spine has been established as the mechanism of injury responsible for quadriplegia. Torg has suggested that axial loading of the cervical spine is also responsible for catastrophic injuries in water sports, rugby, ice hockey, and gymnastics.

In 1980 Carter and Frankel[2] published the results of a study designed to examine the guillotine mechanism of injury proposed by Schneider in his early research. Static-free body analyses were undertaken to determine the forces imposed on the cervical spine when the face guard is struck in a manner to create hyperextension of the cervical spine. They concluded, based on the results of their research, that the proposed guillotine mechanism of injury was invalid.

The notion of the posterior rim of the football helmet striking the cervical spine about the C-4 to C-5 level was considered to be without foundation by Virgin[12] in 1980. Virgin studied 16 football players with use of cineradiography to evaluate the possible roles of the posterior rim of the football helmet in causing neck injury. Five different helmets from different companies were used, and no contact existed at any time between the posterior rim of any helmet and the fourth cervical vertebral spinous process.

Maroon et al.[5] published a football head and neck injury update in 1980 in which they discussed the decrease in football deaths and the increase in serious spinal cord injuries. Preconditioning and strengthening of neck musculature were presented as being essential for the prevention of catastrophic head and neck injuries. Proper blocking and tackling techniques were also presented as playing a major role in reducing head and neck injuries.

In a 1982 publication, Bruce et al.[1] stated that accidental injury to the brain and spinal cord in children less than 15 years of age occurs at the rate of 230 per 100,000 children per year. Such injuries requiring hospitalization affect 1 per 100,000 children per year. In children less than 15 years of age, 70% of the head injuries and nearly 100% of the spinal injuries are the result of automobile accidents. Bruce et al. state that, from these figures, it is clear that the frequency of children receiving these types of injuries in sport participation is very low. The rate does increase dramatically in the 15- to 18-year age group.

Hodgson and Thomas[4] stated recently that all the advantage in football rests with those players playing with the head up and that playing with the head up when blocking and tackling will greatly reduce the risk of serious head and neck injury.

INTRACRANIAL AND CERVICAL SPINE FATALITY DATA

In 1931 the American Football Coaches Association initiated the First Annual Survey of Football Fatalities under the direction of Marvin A. Stevens, M.D., of Yale University. In January 1980 I was appointed by the American Football Coaches Association and the National Collegiate Athletic Association (NCAA) to continue this research under the new title, Annual Survey of Football Injury Research.[6] The primary purpose of this Annual Survey of Football Injury Research is to make the game of football a safer and more enjoyable sport. This purpose has been accomplished through rule changes, improved equipment, and improved coaching techniques.

Data Collection

Data are collected on a national level from all organized football programs (public school, college, professional, and youth programs) through personal contact and questionnaires on each football fatality. Information collected includes personal data on the injured player, equipment data, injury type and body part, and pertinent information concerning the exact circumstances of the accident. Football fatalities are classified as direct and indirect.

- Direct: Those fatalities that resulted from participation in the fundamental skills of the game
- Indirect: Those fatalities caused by systemic failure as a result of exertion while participating in football activity or by a complication resulting from a nonfatal injury

For the purpose of this report, only direct fatality information is used in the data.

1945–1988

Each year from 1945 to 1988 a head or cervical spine fatality has occurred in football. During that period there were a total of 670 fatalities in all levels of football. Intracranial injuries accounted for

TABLE 9–1.

Intracranial and Cervical Spine Fatalities (1945–1988)

Body Part	Frequency	Percentage
Intracranial	453	67.6
Cervical spine	115	17.2
Other	102	15.2
Total	670	100.0

TABLE 9–3.

Intracranial and Cervical Spine Fatalities (1945–1988)—Game Versus Practice

	Frequency	Percentage
Intracranial		
Game	281	62.0
Practice	129	28.5
Unknown	43	9.5
Total	453	100.0
Cervical spine		
Game	85	74.0
Practice	21	18.2
Unknown	9	7.8
Total	115	100.0

453 fatalities, or 67.6% of the total, while cervical spine injuries accounted for 115, or 17.2%. Other fatality-producing injuries, not including intracranial or cervical spine injuries, accounted for 102, or 15.2% of the total 670. When intracranial and cervical spine fatalities are combined, they are associated with 568, or 84.8% of the total (Table 9–1).

As illustrated in Table 9–2, a majority of the fatal intracranial and cervical spine fatalities are associated with high school or junior high school football. This would be expected because there are greater numbers of football players at the high school level. As an example, during the 1988 football season there were approximately 1,300,000 high school football players as opposed to 75,000 college players. High school and junior high school football were associated with 74.0% of the intracranial fatalities from 1945 to 1988, sandlot (nonschool football but organized and using full protective equipment), 16.5%, college, 6.6%, and professional, 2.9%. The ranking changes slightly when observing cervical spine fatalities, with high school play associated with 65.2%, college second, associated with 16.5%, professional, 10.4%, and sandlot, 7.9% (Table 9–2).

A majority of the football fatalities, both intracranial and cervical spine, occurred in games, as shown in Table 9–3. Sixty-two percent of the intracranial fatalities and 74.0% of the cervical spine fatalities occurred in games. Most of the unknowns occurred during the early years of the study when data collection was more difficult. One would expect a majority of the fatalities to occur in games, because the competition is much more intense and because there has been a reduction of full-speed contact in practice sessions since the early 1970s (Table 9–3).

Subdural hematomas were related to 77%, or 349, of the intracranial fatalities. Contusions ranked second, with 19, followed by fractures, concussions, and brain stem injuries. Thirty-eight of the fa-

TABLE 9–2.

Intracranial and Cervical Spine Fatalities (1945–1988)—Level of Play

Level of Play	Intracranial		Cervical Spine	
	Frequency	Percentage	Frequency	Percentage
College	30	6.6	19	16.5
High school	335	74.0	75	65.2
Professional	13	2.9	12	10.4
Sandlot	75	16.5	9	7.9
Total	453	100.0	115	100.0

TABLE 9–4.

Intracranial Injuries (1945–1988)—Type of Injury

Type of Injury	Frequency	Percentage
Subdural hematoma	349	77.0
Fracture	18	4.0
Contusion	19	4.2
Concussion	15	3.3
Brain stem	3	0.7
Other	11	2.4
Unknown	38	8.4
Total	453	100.0

TABLE 9–6.

Intracranial Fatalities (1945–1988)—Activity at Time of Injury

Activity	Frequency	Percentage
Tackling	115	25.4
Tackling drill	35	7.7
Tackled	69	15.2
Blocking	24	5.3
Blocked	7	1.5
Collision	60	13.3
Other	22	4.9
Unknown	121	26.7
Total	453	100.0

talities (type of injury) were listed as unknown, and again this is related to problems of data collection during the early years. This is well illustrated by the fact that during the last 14 years there have been only two unknowns (Table 9–4).

Fractures, fracture-dislocations, and dislocations were related to 96.6% of the cervical spine fatalities for the period 1945–1988. Other injuries and unknowns accounted for only 3.4% (Table 9–5).

Tackling was shown to be the major activity related to both intracranial and cervical spine fatalities (Tables 9–6 and 9–7). One third of the intracranial fatalities and almost two thirds (60.9%) of the cervical spine fatalities were related to tackling. The second major activity was being tackled, followed by blocking and being blocked. A majority of these fatal injuries occur in the open field and, as previously stated, a majority involve either tackling or being tackled. It is also well documented that a majority of the cervical spine fatalities involve a defensive back making a tackle in the open field with his head down (contact with the top of the head causing axial loading and injury to the cervical spine).

Intracranial and Cervical Spine Fatalities by Decades

Intracranial and cervical spine fatalities from 1945 to 1984 are depicted in Figure 9–1.

1945–1954

Football fundamentals and the rules of the game play an important role in injury prevention. During this decade the technique used in blocking and tackling involved using the shoulder as the initial point of contact. An important rule change during this period eliminated the requirement that the forward pass be thrown from five yards behind the line of

TABLE 9–5.

Cervical Spine Fatalities (1945–1988)—Type of Injury

Type of Injury	Frequency	Percentage
Fracture	82	71.3
Fracture and dislocation	16	14.0
Dislocation	13	11.3
Other	2	1.7
Unknown	2	1.7
Total	115	100.0

TABLE 9–7.

Cervical Spine Fatalities (1945–1988)—Activity at Time of Injury

Activity	Frequency	Percentage
Tackling	70	60.9
Tackled	12	10.4
Blocking	4	3.5
Blocked	3	2.6
Collision	4	3.5
Other	4	3.5
Unknown	18	15.6
Total	115	100.0

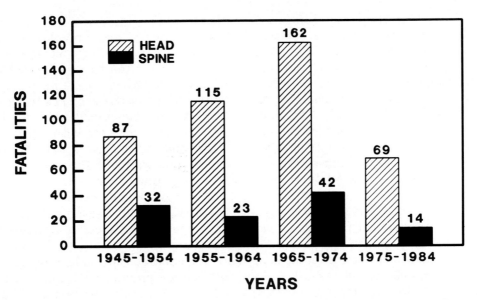

FIG 9–1.
Intracranial and cervical spine fatalities from 1945 to 1984. *(From Mueller FO, Blyth CS: Clin Sports Med 1987; 6:185–196.)*

scrimmage and declared that it could be thrown from anywhere behind the line.[3] Improvement took place in the football helmet during the late 1940s, and the plastic-shelled helmet was introduced. A single-bar face mask was introduced in the early 1950s.

During this decade there were 87 intracranial and 32 cervical spine fatalities in all levels of football. Intracranial and cervical spine injuries were responsible for 77.7% of the fatalities from 1945 to 1954 and 84.8% of the fatalities from 1945 to 1988. A majority of the injured players (57.1%) participated at the high school level, and 67% of the intracranial fatalities and 81% of the cervical spine fatalities took place in games.

Player participation during this decade averaged approximately 700,000 per year. This would give an intracranial fatality incidence rate of 1.24 per 100,000 participants and a cervical spine fatality incidence rate of 0.46 per 100,000 participants for the decade from 1945 to 1954.

Subdural hematomas were related to 80.4% of the intracranial fatalities, and fractures were shown to be the cause of 81.2% of the cervical spine fatalities.

To help prevent serious football injuries and fatalities, it is important to know the exact activity the individual was involved in at the time of the injury. Tackling and being tackled were responsible for 47% of the intracranial and 71.8% of the cervical spine fatalities. When evaluating this area it is important to know exactly how the participant executed the skill (e.g., head down, head-to-head, head-to-knee). These data are difficult to investigate and were not available in some of the earlier surveys.

1955–1964

In the late 1950s the techniques of blocking and tackling used the shoulder as the main area of contact. Players were instructed to keep their heads up, aim their heads at the opponents midsection or chest, and just before contact slide their heads to one side and make contact with their shoulders. Toward the end of this decade there was a move to make initial contact with the head. Improvement of the football helmet continued, and the one-bar face mask was replaced by the two-bar mask; some players had full face masks to protect a fractured nose or other facial injury. From 1955 to 1964 there were 115 intracranial fatalities, 23 cervical spine fatalities, and 37 fatalities related to other causes. Intracranial and cervical spine injuries were responsible for 78.8% of the fatalities during this decade, and 20.6% of the fatalities from 1945 to 1988.

There was an average of approximately 850,000 football participants per year during the decade from 1955 to 1964. The incidence rate for intracranial fatalities from 1955 to 1964 was 1.35 fatalities per 100,000 participants, and 0.27 fatalities per 100,000 participants for cervical spine fatalities.

Fifty-one percent of the intracranial fatalities and 69% of the cervical spine fatalities took place in games, and a majority of the injured players participated at the high school level.

Seventy-seven percent of the intracranial fatalities resulted from subdural hematomas, and 56% of the cervical spine fatalities resulted from fractures.

As was the case in the prior decade, tackling and being tackled were responsible for a major share of the fatalities from 1955 to 1964. Forty-five percent of the intracranial and 60% of the cervical spine fatalities were due to tackling or being tackled. There was a significant increase in the number of tackling drill fatalities in 1955 to 1964 when compared with the 1945–1954 data.

The 1955–1964 data show an increase in the percentage of intracranial fatalities and a slight decrease in the percentage of cervical spine fatalities when compared with data from 1945 to 1954.

1965–1974

The period from 1965 to 1974 in football became well known for terms like "spearing," "butt blocking and tackling,"

"face to the numbers," "face to the chest," "goring," and a number of others. Tackling and blocking techniques involved placing the face of the tackler or blocker into the chest of the individual being tackled or blocked. The initial contact was now being made with the head. All players were now wearing full face masks and felt well protected when striking an opponent with the face or head. It was also a time when cervical spine injuries were causing permanent disability to 25 or 30 football participants per year, and injury data collection systems were being initiated.

The decade starting in 1965 and ending in 1974 produced 162 intracranial fatalities, 42 cervical spine fatalities, and 19 other fatalities. Intracranial and cervical spine fatalities were associated with 91.4% of the fatalities during this decade and 30.5% of the fatalities from 1945 to 1988. The 1965–1974 figures show a dramatic increase over those of the two previous decades.

During the decade from 1965 to 1974, participation figures ranged from a low of 1,100,000 to a high of 1,300,000 per year. The incidence rate for intracranial fatalities ranged from a low of 1.25 to a high of 1.47 fatalities per 100,000 participants. Incidence rates for cervical spine fatalities ranged from a low of 0.32 to a high of 0.38 fatalities per 100,000 participants.

Sixty-seven percent of the intracranial fatalities and 71% of the cervical spine fatalities took place in games, and a majority of the injured players, 77%, participated at the high school level.

Seventy-two percent of the intracranial fatalities resulted from subdural hematomas, and 66% of the cervical spine fatalities resulted from fractures.

Tackling and being tackled have always been associated with a majority of the football intracranial and cervical spine fatalities. Because of incomplete data collection during the early years of this research, type of activity in many fatalities was listed as "unknown." Tackling and being tackled were related to a majority of the fatalities during this decade, and fatalities associated with tackling drills increased again.

The 1965–1974 data reveal a dramatic percentage increase in both intracranial and cervical spine fatalities when compared with the data from the two previous decades. The 1968 football season was also associated with 36 fatalities, the greatest number since the study began in 1931, and all were intracranial and cervical spine fatalities.

1975–1984

Many important changes were made in football during this decade, and they have helped to reduce the number of intracranial and cervical spine fatalities. Data collection indicated a serious problem in head and neck injuries before 1975, and in 1976 a change in the football rules made it illegal to make initial contact with the head or face while tackling or blocking. This rule eliminated using the frontal area or top of the helmet or the face mask, or both to make initial contact with an opponent.[7] The National Operating Committee on Standards for Athletic Equipment (NOCSAE) developed a safety standard for the football helmet that went into effect during the 1978 college football season and the 1980 high school football season. There were many other rules changes made for safety, and, in fact, David Nelson, Chairman of the NCAA Football Rules Committee, has documented that since 1969 there have been 51 injury prevention rules changes involving personal fouls, penalty enforcement, unsportsmanlike conduct, equipment and the field, and officials.

From 1975 to 1984 there were 69 intracranial fatalities, 14 cervical spine fatalities, and 9 other fatalities in football. Intracranial and cervical spine injuries were associated with 90.2% of the fatalities during this decade and 12.4% of the fatalities from 1945 to 1988. The numbers of head and neck fatalities were dramatically fewer than those of the previous decade.

Participation figures for the period from 1975 to 1984 averaged approximately 1,500,000 per year. Incidence rates for intracranial injuries from 1975 to 1984 were 0.46 fatalities per 100,000 participants and 0.09 fatalities per 100,000 participants for cervical spine injuries.

Fifty-eight percent of the intracranial and 71% of the cervical spine fatalities took place in games, and a majority of the injured players, 83%, participated at the high school level.

Eighty-seven percent of the intracranial fatalities resulted from subdural hematomas, and 78% of the cervical spine fatalities, from fractures.

Tackling and being tackled were again involved in a majority of the fatalities. These activities were associated with 52% of the intracranial fatalities and 85% of the cervical spine fatalities.

1985–1988

Data for the decade 1985 to 1994 are, of course, not complete at this time, but the figures for intracranial and cervical spine fatalities are available for the years 1985 to 1988. The data reveal that for this 4-year period there has been a total of 20 intracranial and 4 cervical spine fatalities in football. If these figures continue at the current rate, there should be a decline in intracranial and cervical spine fatalities for the decade 1985–1994.

DISCUSSION

Intracranial and cervical spine injuries accounted for 84.8% of all football fatalities from 1945 to 1988, and the decade with the highest percentage was 1965 to 1974. There was a significant decrease in both numbers and percentages of intracranial and cervical spine fatalities from 1975 to 1984. The following discussion will present preventive measures that were responsible for this reduction and will make recommendations for the next decade.

Data collection plays an important role in the prevention of injuries. The fatality data collected by the American Football Coaches Association since 1931, head and neck surveys that began in the late 1960s and early 1970s, and data collection by the NCAA and the National Federation of State High School Associations have all contributed to the reduction of football fatalities. There is no question that the beneficial changes were the result of reliable data collection and the publication of the results in athletic and medical literature. Persistent surveillance of sports injury data is mandatory if progress is to continue in the prevention of fatalities. Continuous data are needed to observe the development of specific trends, to implement in-depth investigation into areas of concern, and to carry out preventive measures. If continued progress in football injury prevention is to be made, reliable data are a must.

Rules changes that affected the safety of football have played an important role in reducing fatalities. There have been rules changes to help prevent injuries for many years, but the rule change that has played a major role in reducing intracranial and cervical spine fatalities is the 1976 rule that prohibits initial contact with the helmet or face mask when tackling or blocking. This now illegal technique involved driving the face mask, frontal area, or top of the helmet directly into the chest or upper part of the body of the opponent. There is no doubt that this 1976 rule change has made a major contribution to the reduction of intracranial and cervical spine fatalities. The American Football Coaches Association Ethics Committee went on record opposing this type of tackling and blocking, and their report is part of the NCAA football rules book.[7]

To help offset the trend of increasing head and neck injuries and fatalities, the NOCSAE was founded in 1969 to establish safety standards for athletic equipment. The initial effort was directed to head protection for the football player. A safety standard for football helmets was achieved in 1973, and the first helmets were tested on the NOCSAE Standard in 1974. The NOCSAE Standard was accepted by the NCAA for the 1978 season and by the National Federation of State High School Associations for the 1980 season. It is now mandatory for all student athletes in both college and high school to wear a NOCSAE-certified helmet. When helmets are sent to a reconditioner, only those that have passed the NOCSAE test when manufactured may be recertified by the NOCSAE recertification procedures. The development of the NOCSAE research program points out the major role played by everyone interested in athletic injury research.

The education of coaches and the proper techniques of tackling and blocking being taught by coaches have also played an important role in decreasing the number of intracranial and cervical spine fatalities. Research has shown that the safest way to tackle and block is with the head up but with the head not being the initial point of contact. This method of tackling and blocking has proved safer in laboratory research and on the field of play. Both high schools and colleges are making special efforts to coach their players in the correct methods of tackling and blocking, and this has played a role in reducing head and neck fatalities and serious injuries.

Coaches are also doing a better job of getting their players into proper physical condition, and physical conditioning is a major factor in reducing injuries. In addition, coaches are purchasing improved protective equipment and are spending more time in the fitting of their players. Helmet manufacturers have all stressed the importance of proper fit to help reduce injuries.

Improved medical care of football players is also an important area of injury prevention. Physicians and athletic trainers have increased in number on the football fields, and their presence has been a positive factor in injury prevention. Most college programs have a physician and athletic trainer at all games and practices, and some of the smaller programs have athletic trainers on duty. A majority of the states are also setting goals that will have a qualified athletic trainer at each high school. Physicians and athletic trainers have the qualifications to spot possible injuries, and immediate care may prevent an injury from developing into something more serious.

RECOMMENDATIONS

There has been a definite decline in the number of football intracranial and cervical spine fatalities during the past 14 years (1975 to 1988) compared with the number of fatalities in previous decades. Figure 9–2 illustrates the dramatic increase and decline of both intracranial and cervical spine fatalities from 1945 to 1988. An increased effort must be made to continue this trend and to avoid another increase in these types of fatalities. The following are suggestions for reducing intracranial and cervical spine fatalities:

1. Mandatory medical examinations and medical history should be taken before allowing an athlete to participate in football. The NCAA recommends a thorough medical examination when the athlete first enters the college athletic program and an annual health history update with use of referral examinations when warranted. If the physician or coach has any questions about the athlete's readiness to participate, the athlete should not be allowed to play. High school coaches should follow the recommendations set by their state high school athletic associations.

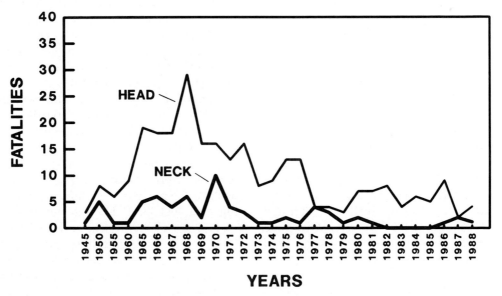

FIG 9–2.
Increase and decline of intracranial and cervical spine fatalities from 1947 to 1988. *(Adapted from Mueller FO, Blyth CS: Clin Sports Med 1987; 6:185–196.)*

2. A physician should be present at all games and practice sessions. If it is impossible for a physician to be present at all practice sessions, emergency measures must be provided.

3. Athletes must be given proper conditioning exercises that will strengthen their necks, enabling them to hold their heads firmly erect when making contact. There are a number of physicians who believe that well-developed neck muscles will help reduce cervical spine fatalities.

4. Coaches should drill the athletes in the proper execution of the fundamental football skills, particularly tackling and blocking. Tackle with the head up and do not make initial contact with the head or face mask.

5. Coaches and officials should discourage the players from using their heads as battering rams when tackling and blocking. The rules prohibiting spearing should be enforced in practice and games. The players should be taught that the helmet is a protective device that should not be used as a weapon.

6. Strict enforcement of the rules of the game by both coaches and officials will help reduce serious injuries.

7. Each institution should strive to have a team trainer who is a regular member of the faculty and is adequately prepared and qualified.

8. Coaches, physicians, and trainers should take special care to see that the players' helmets are properly fitted.

9. When a player has experienced or shown signs of head trauma (loss of consciousness, visual disturbances, headache, inability to walk correctly, obvious disorientation, memory loss), he should receive immediate medical attention and should not be allowed to return to practice or the game without permission from the proper medical authorities.

The following case study demonstrates the importance of proper supervision and medical care:

A 21-year-old college football player received a blow to the head while tackling in the first quarter of a game and lost consciousness. He was allowed to return to the game in the fourth quarter, when he received another blow to the head while making a tackle. He collapsed on the sidelines, went into a coma, and died 10 days later from a subdural hematoma.

SUMMARY

Football intracranial and cervical spine fatalities have been related to 84.8% of all football fatalities from 1945 to 1988. The decade from 1965 to 1974 was related to the greatest number and percentage of intracranial and cervical spine fatalities, and the decade from 1975 to 1984 was associated with the smallest number and percentage (see Fig 1). Data from 1985 to 1988 indicate that the trend in the reduction of these head and neck fatalities will continue.

The data reveal that the majority of intracranial and cervical spine fatalities are related to high school football players either tackling or being tackled in a game. The majority of intracranial fatalities result from subdural hematomas, and a large percentage of the cervical spine fatalities result from fractures, dislocations, or fracture-dislocations.

There has been a dramatic reduction in these types of football fatalities since 1968 (see Fig 2). The preventive measures that have received most of the credit have been the 1976 rule change that prohibits initial contact with the head and face when tackling and blocking, the NOCSAE helmet standard that went into effect at the college level in 1978 and at the high school level in 1980, better coaching in the techniques of blocking and tackling, and improved medical care.

There has been a dramatic reduction in football intracranial and cervical spine fatalities from 1968 to 1984, and the analysis of data from 1985 to 1988 indicates that the trend will continue. Preventive measures that are presently in place must be emphasized, and research efforts that have made this reduction possible must be continued.

REFERENCES

1. Bruce DA, Schutt L, Sutton LN: Brain and cervical spine injuries occurring during organized sports activities in children and adolescents. *Clin Sports Med* 1982; 1:175–194.

2. Carter DR, Frankel VH: Biomechanics of hyperextension injuries to the cervical spine in football. *Am J Sports Med* 1980; 8:302–308.

3. Danzig A: *The History of American Football*. Englewood Cliffs, NJ, Prentice-Hall, 1956.

4. Hodgson VR, Thomas LM: Play head-up football. *Natl Fed News* 1985; 2:24–27.

5. Maroon JC, Steele PB, Berlin R: Football head and neck injuries—an update. *Clin Neurosurg* 1980; 27:414–429.

6. Mueller FO, Schindler RD: *Annual Survey of Football Injury Research 1931–1988*. Orlando, Fla, American Football Coaches Association, 1988.

7. National College Athletic Association: *1988 NCAA Football Rules and Interpretations*. Shawnee Mission, Kan, 1988.

8. Schneider RC, Reifel E, Crisler HO, et al: Serious and fatal injuries involving the head and spinal cord. *JAMA* 1961; 177:362–366.

9. Schneider RC: Serious and fatal neurosurgical football injuries. *Clin Neurosurg* 1965; 12:226–235.

10. Snook GA: Head and neck injuries in contact sports. *Med Sci Sports* 1969; 1:117–123.

11. Torg JS: Athletic injuries to the head, neck, and face. Philadelphia, Lea & Febiger, 1980.

12. Virgin H: Cineradiographic study of football helmets and the cervical spine. *Am J Sports Med* 1980; 8:310–317.

CHAPTER 10

Injuries to the Cervical Spine and Spinal Cord Resulting From Ice Hockey*

Charles H. Tator, M.D., Ph.D., F.R.C.S.(C)

In many countries sports and recreational activities are leading causes of acute spinal cord injury,[13] although the specific types of athletic or recreational activities leading to these catastrophic injuries differ between countries. In Canada diving has always been the leading cause of spinal cord injury in this category,[19, 22, 24, 25] and until recently hockey was a rare cause. Indeed, in my review of 55 acute spinal cord injuries caused by sports-recreational activities that were treated in two Toronto hospitals from 1948 to 1973, not a single one was hockey related.[19, 22] Moreover, there had been no reports in the Canadian literature of spinal cord injury due to hockey before my review of six cases published in 1984.[23] Similarly, no case reports of neck injuries due to hockey were found in the English literature,[†] including the first edition of this book,[26] although Feriencik[6] in 1979 reported the occurrence of lumbar spinal injuries in hockey players in Czechoslovakia.

Beginning in 1977 I began encounter-

ing cases of spinal cord injury in Canadian hockey players. Other Canadian neurosurgeons and orthopaedic surgeons had similar experiences during the late 1970s and early 1980s. Accordingly, in 1981, I organized the Committee on Prevention of Spinal Cord Injuries Due to Hockey, which since then has had the responsibility of performing research into the causes of these injuries and of developing prevention programs. The Committee conducted a Canadian national survey in 1981 to document the extent of the problem, and since then several additional surveys have been made. Questionnaires were sent to all the neurosurgeons, orthopaedic surgeons, and physical medicine and rehabilitation specialists in Canada asking them to report all major injuries. Minor injuries such as strains or whiplash were excluded. In 1985 the Committee on Prevention of Spinal Injuries Due to Hockey became the Committee on Prevention of Spinal and Head Injuries Due to Hockey, a permanent subcommittee of the Canadian Sports Spine and Head Injuries Research Centre, Toronto Western Hospital, University of Toronto. The first detailed report of the Committee's findings was published in 1984,[20] and contained information on 42

*Supported by the Canadian Amateur Hockey Association, Ontario Ministry of Tourism and Recreation, and The National Hockey League Players Association.

†References 4, 6, 9, 10, 12, and 16.

cases of spinal injuries that had been reported to the Committee as a result of its survey conducted in 1982. Since then a permanent reporting system and Registry have been established by the Canadian Sports Spine and Head Injuries Research Centre. By April 1987 there had been 117 spinal injuries due to hockey reported to the Registry. It should be noted that the Registry is strongly supported by the Canadian Amateur Hockey Association, The Ontario Ministry of Tourism and Recreation, The National Hockey League Players Association, The Canadian Paraplegic Association, and Cooper Canada. This report provides demographic details of these 117 injuries, including the possible etiologic mechanisms, and outlines the current prevention programs of the Canadian Sports Spine and Head Injuries Research Centre designed to reduce the incidence of these tragic injuries.

EPIDEMIOLOGY OF SPINAL INJURIES IN HOCKEY

Geographic Location

Except for the six injuries in the United States, all the injuries reported to the Committee occurred in Canada (Table 10–1). Ontario was the site of almost half the injuries (49%), whereas only 12 injuries (10%) occurred in Quebec. This is a major disparity because these two provinces do not differ greatly in total population nor in number of hockey players. The remainder of the Canadian cases were distributed across the country in proportion to population. It is of interest that there have been no recent reports of spinal injuries due to hockey in Western or Eastern Europe, where hockey is played extensively in several northern countries.

Annual Incidence

As shown in Table 10–2, these injuries were rare in the 1960s and 1970s. Beginning in 1980 the annual incidence increased markedly, and from 1982 to 1986 was approximately 15 cases per year.

Sex and Age

Of the 117 injuries, 112 (96%) were in male players, and 5 (4%) of the players were females. Table 10–3 shows that 64% of the players were between the ages of 11 and 20, while only 19% were 21 to 30 years of age. The youngest player with a major spinal injury was 11 years of age;

TABLE 10–1.

Geographic Location of Occurrence of Injuries

	Frequency	Percent
Ontario	57	49
Quebec	12	10
Alberta	9	8
British Columbia	9	8
Nova Scotia	5	4
Saskatchewan	5	4
Manitoba	4	3
Prince Edward Island	3	3
Yukon	3	3
Newfoundland	2	2
New Brunswick	1	0.5
United States	6	5
Unknown	1	0.5
Total	117	100

TABLE 10–2.

Number of Injuries per Year

1966	1
1975	1
1976	2
1977	2
1978	4
1979	2
1980	8
1981	12
1982	15
1983	15
1984	15
1985	12
1986	15
1987 (to April)	6
Missing data	7
Total	117

TABLE 10–3.

Age of Injured Players

Age	Frequency	Percent
11–20	75	64
21–30	22	19
31–40	7	6
41–50	3	3
Missing	10	8
Total	117	100
Range	11–47 years	
Mean	21 years	
Median	18 years	

the oldest was 47. The median and mean ages were 18 and 21 years, respectively.

Level of Injury

Almost 80% of the injuries were to the cervical vertebrae (Table 10–4), with C4–C5, C5, and C-5–C-6 comprising approximately 48% of the injuries. Thoracic, thoracolumbar and lumbosacral injuries were relatively rare. The most common site of injury was C-5–C-6, which comprised 15.6% of the injuries.

Neurologic Deficit

As noted, the Registry excludes minor injuries such as vertebral strains, although fractures or dislocations of the spine were included even if they did not cause neurologic injuries. As shown in

TABLE 10–4.

Vertebral Level of Spinal Injury

	Frequency	Percent
Cervical C-1–C-7/T-1	93	79.5
Thoracic T-1–T-11	3	2.6
Thoracolumbar T-11/12–L-1/2	7	6.0
Lumbosacral L-2–S-5	6	5.1
Missing	8	6.8
Total	117	100

Table 10–5, 52.1% of the injuries were to the spinal cord, while 10.3% caused damage to one or more nerve roots. Of the spinal cord injuries, 29 players sustained complete permanent spinal cord injuries, with no preservation of motor or sensory function below the level of injury, which was cervical in all cases of complete injury. Of the 117 injured players, at the time of preparing this report 5 were known to have died as a result of their injuries. All deaths were due to the complications of spinal cord injury, mostly respiratory failure.

Type of Athletic Event

The largest number of injuries occurred in supervised, scheduled games within an organized hockey league (Table 10–6). Indeed, 85 players (73%) were known to have sustained their injuries in organized games. Only a small number of injuries occurred in practices or in unstructured or unsupervised events (shinny).

Mechanism of Injury

Axial loading was found to be the most common mechanism of cervical spine and spinal cord injury. Axial loading applied to the head when the helmeted head struck another object (especially the boards) and was the most common mechanism, with the most frequent inciting event a push or check from behind (Fig 10–1). In most instances the player was completely unsuspecting of the impact and was hurled horizontally into the boards, with the cervical spinal structure crushed between the abruptly halted, helmeted head and the aftercoming torso.[26] In most instances the axial loading was applied with the head in neutral alignment with the neck and torso, or in slight flexion. Major degrees of flexion or extension were much less

TABLE 10–5.

Neurologic Injuries

	Frequency	Percent
Spinal cord injury		
Complete motor and complete sensory loss	29	24.8
Complete motor and incomplete sensory loss	9	7.7
Incomplete motor loss and incomplete sensory loss	21	17.9
Incomplete sensory loss	2	1.7
Subtotal	61	52.1
Root injury only	12	10.3
No neurologic injury	28	23.9
Missing data/incomplete data	16	13.7
	56	47.9
Overall Total	117	100

common. Impacts with the boards accounted for 76 injuries (65.0%) (Table 10–7). Impacts between players were also a frequent mechanism of injury (10.3%), whereas impacts with the ice or goalpost were less frequent. The mode of injury is shown in Table 10–8, which reveals that the largest number of injuries occurred because the player was pushed or checked from behind (31 injuries; 26.5%); in most of these cases the impact was with the boards. Other frequent causes of injury were from pushes and checks from the front and from sides. In many of these injuries the final impact that injured the spine was with the boards.

tebral injuries. Ruptured disks were less common, although there were examples of ruptured cervical disks causing incomplete spinal cord injury. There were infrequent cases of hockey players with cervical spinal stenosis, with neurapraxia and transient traumatic quadriparesis, as described by Torg et al.[27, 28] in football players. Although spinal stenosis in the hockey players was not accurately documented in this study, there were examples of stenosis due primarily to degenerative rather than developmental causes, associated with transient or permanent spinal cord injury.

Almost all the players in this series were wearing helmets and more than

Other Features of the Injuries

Burst fractures and fracture-dislocations were the most frequent types of ver-

TABLE 10–6.

Type of Athletic Event

	Frequency	Percent
Organized games	85	73
Practices	4	3
Unstructured play (shinny)	1	1
Unknown	27	23
Total	117	100

TABLE 10–7.

Type of Collision

	Frequency	Percent
Boards	70	59.8
Other players	12	10.3
Ice	3	2.6
Goalpost	1	0.9
Boards and players*	5	4.3
Players and ice*	1	0.9
Players and goalpost*	1	0.9
Boards and ice*	1	0.9
Incomplete/missing	23	19.7
Total	117	100

*More than one type of collision.

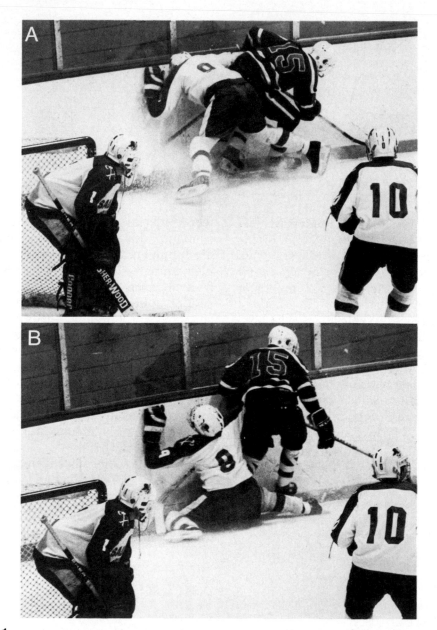

FIG 10–1.
A, the most common mechanism of cervical spinal injury occurring in hockey is axial loading. The helmeted head of the injured player, usually after a push or check from behind, impacts against the boards, as demonstrated in this photograph of an actual injury. **B,** the youngster, having been rendered quadriplegic, slumps to the ice.

TABLE 10–8.

Mode of Injury

	Frequency	Percent
Single mechanisms		
Pushed/checked from behind	26	22.2
Pushed/checked	15	12.8
Slide	6	5.1
Tripped on ice	10	8.5
Trip/fall	3	2.6
Tripped by player	3	2.6
Slide with player	1	0.9
Lost balance	2	1.7
Missed check	2	1.7
Multiple mechanisms		
Tripped on ice + slide	3	2.6
Tripped on ice + slide with player	1	0.9
Trip/fall	1	0.9
Slide + pushed/checked	2	1.7
Slide + pushed/checked from behind	5	4.3
Trip/fall + pushed/checked	1	0.9
Slide + tripped by player	1	0.9
Incomplete/missing	35	29.9
Total	117	100

two-thirds were wearing face masks. Only three cases of serious head injury due to hockey were reported to the Committee during the 1981–1987 period.

ANALYSIS OF ETIOLOGIC FACTORS

The occurrence of spinal injuries in ice hockey is a recent phenomenon, and the Canadian Sports Spine and Head Injuries Research Centre has been able to identify several etiologic factors. Indeed, in our opinion no single factor is responsible for these tragic accidents, but rather they are multifactorial in origin. It should be noted that hockey has also been associated with a high incidence of non–spinal injuries as well. For example, a provincial survey found that in 1986 hockey caused the highest number of major injuries of all types in the province of Ontario. Indeed, in that study hockey caused 79 of the 530 major injuries due to all types of sports and recreational activities during 1986, with the next most frequent causes of injury being water sports and motor sports.[21] It should be noted that an increasing incidence of cervical fractures is beginning to be reported in recent epidemiologic studies of ice hockey injuries in the United States.[8]

The following factors appear to be important in causing the current high incidence of spinal injuries due to ice hockey.[18]

Physical Factors Related to Current Players.—The injured hockey players were taller and heavier, and were skating faster than players in former years. This increased weight and speed increased the force generated by collisions.

Social and Psychologic Factors Among Young Hockey Players.—There was an increased willingness to take risks, and these young players were unaware of the dangers of high-speed impact. Youthful players have attempted to emulate the violence and aggressiveness of professional players in professional leagues, but did not have the physical fitness or conditioning of professionals. There has been a feeling of invincibility among young hockey players, which is most likely related to the large amount of protective equipment worn. Indeed, many of the victims interviewed had been completely unaware of the possibility of spinal cord injury in hockey. The rules were not enforced. Indeed, many of the victims were injured during illegal play, especially illegal pushing or checking from behind.

Coaching.—There was insufficient emphasis on physical conditioning, especially of the neck muscles. The players did not receive sufficient instruction about the risks of hockey and the methods of protecting the spine from injury.

The coaching overemphasized body contact and underemphasized protective maneuvers, especially with respect to avoidance of impact with the boards and strategies for impacting safely. The marked disparity in the incidence of these injuries between Ontario and Quebec, Canada's two most populous and almost equally populated provinces in which there were almost equal numbers of players, suggests that attitude and coaching techniques were extremely important etiologic factors.

Hockey Rinks and Equipment.— Small rinks have been considered a possible factor because collisions are more frequent in smaller rinks. The lack of shock absorption of the boards in most new rinks has been questioned as a possible etiologic factor. The widespread use of helmets occurred in Canadian hockey in the 1970s, and preceded by several years the marked increase in neck injuries. However, biomechanical studies have not supported the notion that the helmet is an important factor.[1] It should be noted that helmets have been extremely effective in reducing the incidence of brain injuries in hockey players. Before their widespread use was approved by the Canadian Standards Association, fatal brain injuries were not uncommon in hockey.[5,7] As noted, our Registry contains only three cases of severe brain injury from 1981 to 1987. Face masks have produced a remarkable reduction of eye and dental injuries in hockey players.[14,15] We have found no evidence that face masks are related to the increase in spinal injuries, a possibility suggested by some hockey observers.[17]

PREVENTION PROGRAMS

The Committee on Prevention of Spinal and Head Injuries Due to Hockey has developed several targeted and specific prevention programs to reduce these tragic injuries.

Player Education and Conditioning.— Canadian hockey leagues and organizations have accepted the responsibility for reducing these injuries by improving player awareness and coaching techniques. Players are being made aware of the risks of certain aspects of play, especially going into the boards "blindly." Several defensive tactics for avoiding spinal injuries are being taught, especially avoiding impact of the helmeted head with the boards, the ice surface, or other players. A videotape entitled "Smart Hockey" was produced in 1989 by the Committee and is being distributed widely to leagues and schools. Coaches and leagues are encouraging players to perform specific neck muscle strengthening exercises, which are detailed in a brochure that has been distributed to all hockey players since 1984.

Rules and Refereeing.— The leagues have taken a leading role in encouraging positive attitudes toward injury reduction and safe hockey. In 1984 the Canadian Amateur Hockey Association introduced specific rules against pushing or checking from behind, and have resolved to reduce violence in the game by rules enforcement. Leagues have adopted other safety measures, including magnetic goalposts, and are promoting the increase in size of rinks to International Ice Hockey Standards.

Equipment Manufacturers and Rink Contractors.— Further research is required to improve the safety of hockey equipment. Helmet shape, friction, and shock absorption require additional research. Research into the shock absorption of the boards should be performed. Placement of concrete backing behind the boards should be discouraged. The leagues have adopted other safety measures, including magnetic goalposts. They are promoting the increase in size of rinks to international standards.

Sports Medicine Experts.—Specialists in sports medicine and other recreation researchers should be encouraged to continue research into these injuries. It is essential to continue the organized reporting system developed by the Canadian Sports Spine and Head Injuries Research Centre. Without that reporting system, it will not be possible to assess the effectiveness of the prevention programs that I have outlined in this chapter. The efforts of these experts in conducting further epidemiologic and equipment research should be strongly encouraged and supported by the hockey associations and by provincial, state, and federal governments.

SUMMARY

Major spinal injuries have been recognized as a common problem in Canadian ice hockey only during the 1980s. The causes of these injuries have been found to be multifactorial.[18] The increased weight, height, speed, and aggressiveness of hockey players are important factors. Lack of awareness of the hazards of small rinks and of certain high-risk maneuvers, such as checking or pushing from behind, is an important factor. There were no specific rules against checking or pushing from behind. Lack of neck muscle strengthening and the feeling of invincibility while outfitted in modern equipment have set the stage for these tragic injuries. After these factors were identified, specific measures were taken to correct them, and a reporting system was established in Canada so that the effects of prevention programs can be monitored. Greater awareness of the risk factors by players, coaches, leagues, refer-

ees, and parents promises to be an effective prophylactic measure. The current, specific prevention programs involve the hockey associations, players, equipment manufacturers, health care professionals and researchers, and governments. Hopefully hockey will follow the excellent example of the reduction of major spinal injuries in U.S. football, which occurred mainly due to the effects of improved awareness and attitude and to rules changes.[2, 3, 11, 29]

REFERENCES

1. Bishop PJ, Norman RW, Wells R, et al: Changes in the centre of mass and moment of inertia of a headform induced by a hockey helmet and face shield. *Can J Appl Sport Sci* 1983; 8:19–25.

2. Clarke KS: An epidemiological view, in Torg JS (ed): *Athletic Injuries to the Head, Neck and Face.* Philadelphia, Lea & Febiger, 1982, chap 2, pp 15–25.

3. Clarke KS, Powell JW: Football helmets and neurotrauma—an epidemiological overview of three seasons. *Med Sci Sports* 1979; 11:138–145.

4. Daffner RH: Injuries in amateur ice hockey: A two-year analysis. *J Fam Pract* 1977; 4:225–227.

5. Fekete JF: Severe brain injury and death following minor hockey accidents: The effectiveness of the "safety helmets" of amateur hockey players. *Can Med Assoc J* 1968; 99:1234–1239.

6. Feriencik K: Trends in ice hockey injuries: 1965–1977. *Phys Sportsmed* 1979; 7:81–84.

7. Feriencik K: Case report: Depressed skull fracture in an ice hockey player wearing a helmet. *Phys Sportsmed* 1979; 7:107.

8. Gerberich SG, Finke R, Madden M, et al: An epidemiological study of high school ice hockey injuries. *Childs Nerv Syst* 1987; 3:59–64.

9. Hastings DE, Cameron J, Parker SM, et al: Study of hockey injuries in Ontario. *Ontario Med Rev* 1974; 41:686–691.

10. Hayes D: Reducing risks in hockey: Analysis of equipment and injuries. *Phys Sportsmed* 1978; 6:67–70.

11. Hodgson VR: Reducing serious injury in sports. *Interschol Athl Ad* 1980; 7:11–14.

12. Kalchman L: *Safe Hockey. How to Survive the Game Intact.* New York, Scribner Book Co, 1981.

13. Kurtzke JF: Epidemiology of spinal cord injury. *Exp Neurol* 1975; 48:163–236.

14. Pashby TJ: Eye injuries in Canadian hockey. Phase III: Older players now at most risk. *Can Med Assoc J* 1979; 121:643–644.

15. Pashby TJ, Pashby RC, Chisholm LJ, et al: Eye injuries in Canadian hockey. *Can Med Assoc J* 1975; 113:663–666.

16. Sim FH, Chao EY: Injury potential in modern ice hockey. *Am J Sports Med* 1978; 6:378–384.

17. Sim FH, Simonet WT, Melton LJ, et al: Ice hockey injuries. *Am J Sports Med* 1987; 15:30–40.

18. Tator CH: Neck injuries in ice hockey: A recent, unsolved problem with many contributing factors. *Clin Sports Med* 1987; 6:101–114.

19. Tator CH, Edmonds VE: Acute spinal cord injury. Analysis of epidemiological factors. *Can J Surg* 1979; 22:575–578.

20. Tator CH, Edmonds VE: National survey of spinal injuries in hockey players. *Can Med Assoc J* 1984; 130:875–880.

21. Tator CH, Edmonds VE, Duncan EG, et al: Danger upstream: Catastrophic sports and recreational injury in Ontario. *Ontario Med Rev* 1988; 55:7–12.

22. Tator CH, Edmonds VE, New ML: Diving: A frequent and potentially preventable cause of spinal cord injury. *Can Med Assoc J* 1981; 124:1323–1324.

23. Tator CH, Ekong CEU, Rowed DW, et al: Spinal injuries due to hockey. *Can J Neurol Sci* 1984; 11:34–41.

24. Tator CH, Palm J: The issue of spinal injuries due to diving and aquatic activities, in Pike B (ed): *Aquatic Spinal Injuries. Proceedings of the Symposium.* The Royal Life Saving Society of Canada, 1980, pp 9–12.

25. Tator CH, Palm J: Spinal injuries in diving: Incidence high and rising. *Ontario Med Rev* 1981; 48:628–631.

26. Torg JS: *Athletic Injuries to the Head, Neck and Face.* Philadelphia, Lea & Febiger, 1982.

27. Torg JS, Pavlov H: Cervical spinal stenosis with neurapraxia and transient quadriplegia. *Clin Sports Med* 1987; 6:115–133.

28. Torg JS, Pavlov H, Genvario SE, et al: Neurapraxia of the cervical spine cord with transient quadriplegia. *J Bone Joint Surg* 1986; 68-A:1354–1370.

29. Torg JS, Vegso JJ, O'Neill MN, et al: The epidemiologic, pathologic, biomechanical and cinematographic analysis of football-induced cervical spine trauma. *Am J Sports Med* 1990; 18:50–57.

CHAPTER 11

Head and Spinal Injuries Associated With Equestrian Sports: Mechanisms and Prevention

William H. Brooks, M.D.
Doris Bixby-Hammett, M.D.

Equestrian sports are uniquely different from any other sporting activity in that the athlete is not fully in control of his own destiny. In no other sport, with the notable exception of dogsledding, are the partners of a team composed of two differing species. Consequently riders must be keenly aware of their "teammate," because an unanticipated decision by the horse is frequently accompanied by accidents and injuries that otherwise might be expected and appropriately avoided. This risk of catastrophic injury is increased further by the kinetic energy involved in equestrian events (Fig 11–1). Horses frequently weigh as much as 2,500 lb and are capable of reaching speeds of 40 mph. Therefore a rider whose head is poised at least nine feet above the ground could be exposed to considerable impact during an unexpected fall. The combination of the unpredictability of the horse and the potential forces generated during falls and impacts is responsible for the significant number of head and cervical spine injuries attributed to equestrian sports. Ac-cordingly, the action of the horse can be incurred during equestrian events.[1]

More than 30 million Americans ride horses; at least half ride on a regular basis.[2,3] Moreover, most horses are kept for recreational purposes and are frequently owned by children and young adults less than 20 years of age; 42,000 of these individuals are treated in the emergency department each year.[4,5] These statistics indicate that despite the potential risks involved in horseback riding, many young people routinely enjoy equestrian sports and seem at the greatest risk of sustaining neurologic injury.[6-8] Although most equestrian-related injuries occur to the upper extremity and shoulder, at least one third involve the head and spine.[9-11] In a study of medical examiner reports from ten states, it was found that as many as 217 deaths per year were attributable to horseback riding.[8] The total number of such fatalities in all states is unknown, yet must certainly be much greater. Because the most common cause of fatality or catastrophic injury in equestrian sports is re-

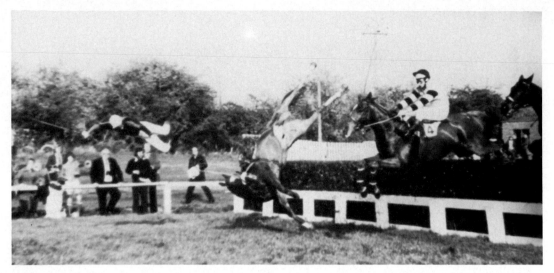

FIG 11–1.
The forces involved in equestrian accidents are capable of exceeding the protective ability of the scalp and skull as well as the musculoligamentous and vertebral components of the spine.

lated to the brain or spinal cord, or both, the purposes of this chapter are to review mechanisms of these injuries and detail specific measures to lessen the risk of serious craniospinal injury.

MECHANISMS OF INJURY

The degree of head-forward position that a participant adopts may be directly linked to the number and severity of craniofacial and cervical injuries. The head-forward position commonly is used to a somewhat exaggerated degree in equestrian sports. When considered in the context of the large potential energies involved in equestrian sports, this stance assures that serious injuries will occur in many riding accidents (Fig 11–2). The velocities and distances obtainable during a fall provide more than enough energy to exceed the limits of the skull and cranium in protecting against intracranial injury. Therefore, the neurologic and facial trauma associated with equestrian activities includes the gamut of injuries seen in other high-speed accidents.

Head injury is the most common neu-rologic injury associated with horseback riding.[11–15] These injuries usually result from falls related to both rider and the horse (Figs 11–3 and 11–4).[1, 8, 16] An inexperienced rider is as likely to be thrown by an experienced horse as an experienced rider is by an inexperienced horse. Experience has not been demonstrated to substitute for carefulness. Unexpected stops or loss of footing of the horse, or both, are most frequently attended by serious craniofacial injuries. Most head injuries (80% to 90%) are limited to concussions or cerebral contusions, and only rarely are associated with skull fracture if proper protective headgear is worn. Skull fracture is commonly seen in those riders refusing to wear protective helmets[12, 14, 17] (Fig 11–5). These individuals often sustain compound and depressed skull fractures as the unprotected head strikes an object or is kicked by an uncontrolled horse.[17, 18] Although most craniospinal injuries occur while mounted, an unexpected kick with an iron-shod foot is capable of delivering sufficient force to cause serious facial and head injury (Fig 11–6).

Injury to the vertebral column or spi-

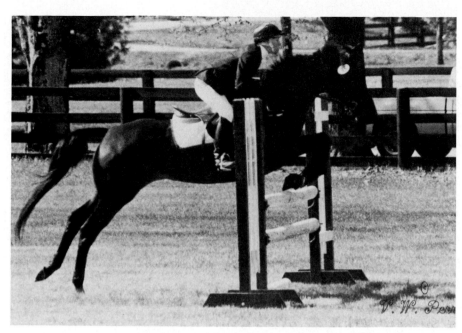

FIG 11–2.
The "classical" poise of jumping increases the risk of craniospinal injury. *(Courtesy of V. W. Perry.)*

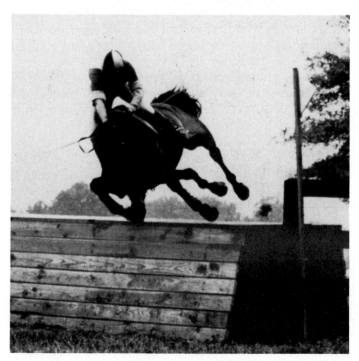

FIG 11–3.
Failure to cross this large obstacle by a well-trained horse resulted in severe concussion.

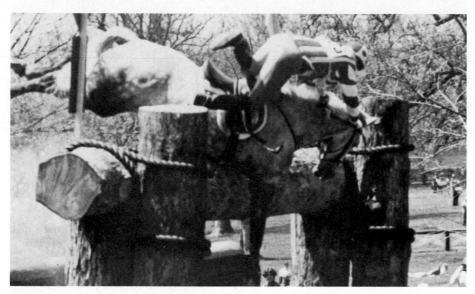

FIG 11–4.
Unexpected stops impart great momentum to riders, contributing to increased potential risk of head and neck injury. *(Courtesy of V. W. Perry.)*

nal cord, or both, occurs less frequently than injuries to the head and face, and comprises approximately 5% to 10% of all neurologic injuries associated with equestrian sports.[17] These injuries frequently involved the spinal cord or the cauda equina. Cervical fractures may occur when the rider is thrown forward over the neck of the horse and strikes the ground. Fractures in this area generally result from exaggerated forced flexion, and hence involve compression of the vertebral bodies and facet dislocation or fracture. These fractures tend to be unstable because both the anterior and posterior elements of the vertebral body have been injured. Cervical fractures rarely are seen in those riders who maintain their head in extension rather than flexion. Moreover, when they do occur they are stable and unassociated with spinal cord injury. Axial loading as seen in football-spearing accidents has not been observed with equestrian activities because riders tend to fall with the upper extremities extended and the neck flexed or extended (Fig 11–7).

The fracture that is unique to equestrian sports is that involving the thoracolumbar spine.[19] These fractures result when a falling rider lands on the buttocks with subsequent rotation and flexion of the spine. The rotation component of this mechanism imparts the high degree of instability and increased likelihood of injury to the cauda equina or the conus medullaris, or both.

Injury to the brachial plexus may occur when a rider fails to release the reins or saddle when thrown (Fig 11–8). These injuries are usually stretch injuries and resolve with conservative treatment. Avulsion of cervical nerve roots has not been reported. Injury to the lumbosacral plexus is preventable with use of heeled boots and "breakaway" stirrups, which prevent the rider from entrapping the leg when falling from a runaway horse.[20]

PREVENTION OF CRANIOSPINAL INJURY

The risk of neurologic injury may be greatly reduced (1) by identification of those individuals who should not ride,

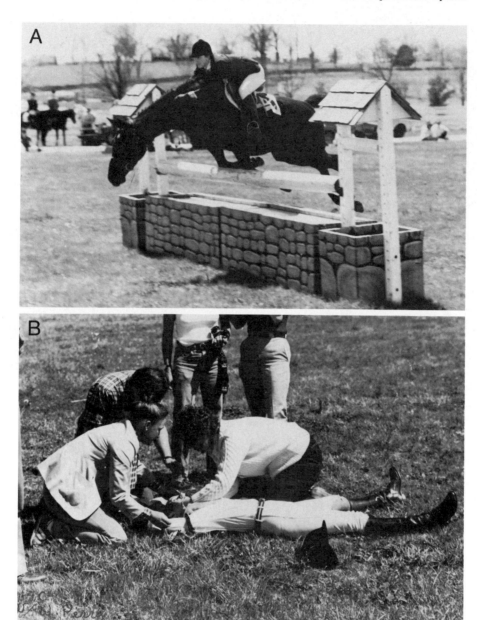

FIG 11–5.
A and **B,** this young rider wears an unsafe helmet without harness. Its loss during this gait resulted in closed-head injury and persistent neurologic deficit.

(2) by development of criteria for determining when riding may be resumed after an accident; and (3) by development of protective equipment as well as mandating its use.

Conditions that absolutely contraindicate equestrian sports include (1) symptomatic (neurologic or pain-producing) abnormalities about the foramen magnum; (2) congenital spinal anomaly with potential instability, which may render the cervical spinal cord vulnerable (significant spinal fracture or dislocation); (3) temporary quadriplegia regard-

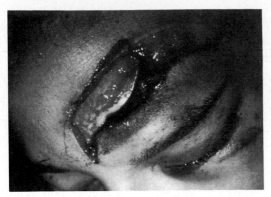

FIG 11–6.
This groom was kicked while attending a mare and foal, sustaining compound depressed skull fracture.

less of the cause; (4) permanent central neurologic sequelae from head injury; (5) spontaneous subarachnoid hemorrhage; and (6) repeated painful injury in the cervical region, particularly in those individuals with radiographic evidence of degenerative osteoarthritis or congenital narrowing of the spinal canal. Well-controlled idiopathic epilepsy is not a contraindication to horseback riding; however, posttraumatic seizures are. These

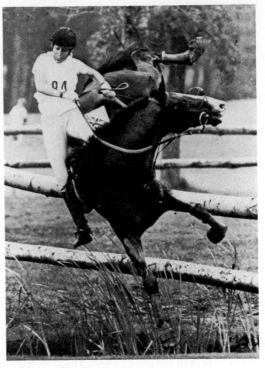

FIG 11–8.
Brachial plexus injuries may result from sudden pull of reins during a fall when the rider attempts to regain balance by holding. Most recover rapidly.

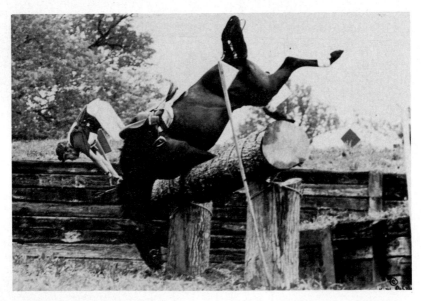

FIG 11–7.
Most riders naturally extend both arms and neck to prevent forced flexion or axial loading of cervical spine.

conditions are to be urged as guidelines for competitive riding; exceptions may be considered for recreational activities. Nevertheless, the risks in both groups are identical; hence the potential risks should be thoroughly discussed with all prospective riders. All riders who sustain head or neck injuries, or both, should be carefully examined before resumption of activities. Brachial plexus injuries producing transient or slight residual loss of function, herniated cervical intervertebral disk with or without surgical treatment, and recurring cervical musculoligamentous injury should be carefully evaluated before the return to regular horseback riding. Repeated concussions are associated with mental deterioration as manifested by loss of attention span, concentration, memory, judgment, and speed of thinking. Thus the repeat occurrence of concussion should be completely investigated to determine the factors involved in the accident (e.g., failure to wear proper protective helmet, attempting feats beyond the skill and scope of the horse and rider, and carelessness). These accidents must not be dealt with passively!

Nothing has done more to improve the safety of horseback riding than the continued research and development of protective headgear. In those riders of the United States Pony Club (USPC) less than 21 years of age, the incidence of head injury has steadily declined since the adoption of helmets with harnesses to prevent loss during a fall. Currently in the United States the standard specifications for helmets to be used in horse sports and horseback riding have been established by the American Society for Testing and Materials (ASTM).[21] The standards set by the ASTM are unique, with particular attention to those objects encountered during horseback riding (e.g., sharp and blunt objects and hoof, relative impact attenuation, retention, fit, and perceived

user acceptability). The minimal performance requirements include: (1) protection from at least 300 Gs at any impact site; (2) presence of a retention system that remains intact during static and dynamic testing without stretch; and (3) peripheral vision clearance of a minimum of 105 degrees horizontally to each side. Those protective headgears that have presently accepted the ASTM standards are individually evaluated by the Safety Equipment Institute (SEI) and must bear this seal inside the helmet (Table 11–1). The American Horse Show Association has made ASTM-SEI–approved helmets mandatory for all junior riders; the USPC requires that all its members wear these helmets when mounted. Although they afford considerable protection against direct blows to the calvaria, protection is lacking at and below the canthomeatal line.[22, 23] This is substantiated by the observation that most fatalities have been the result of head injuries in the squamous portion of the temporal bone or in the suboccipital area below this reference plane in existing helmets.[24]

Although approved helmets are protective to a certain degree, no helmet is fail-safe, and particular features must be considered. The helmet should fit snugly enough to be capable of staying on the head even if unfastened.[25] Damaged helmets should be discarded. Serious head injuries can occur during double impact, when riders fall, strike their heads, and then are kicked. These are among the

TABLE 11–1.

Approved Riding Helmet Manufacturers in First Group of SEI Tests

1. International Riding Helmets, Inc., 1270 36th St., Brooklyn, NY 11218; Frank Plastino.
2. Lexington Safety Products, Inc., 480 Fairman Rd., Lexington, Ky 40511; Bruce Blake.
3. Soyo International Corp., Kobe Port P.O. Box 947, Kobe 651-01 Japan; K. Nishimura. Tel. 078-232-0839; FAX 078 232-0830.

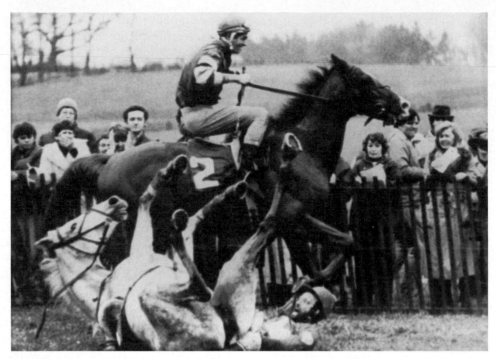

FIG 11–9.
"Double-impact" injuries of ground and hoof are the most lethal of all sport-related injuries.

most lethal of all sports-related accidents (Fig 11–9). The use of body-protective equipment recently has gained considerable popularity among competitive riders. Manufacturers have suggested that the risk of spinal injury is considerably lessened by the routine use of these vests. Detailed investigations are lacking, however, no standards have been developed. Moreover, the existing body protectors are incapable of sufficiently preventing or limiting the rotational and flexion motions involved in the generation of spinal fracture in the thoracolumbar area. Hence their efficiency as "spinal" protectors is nil. Although the ability of these vests to adequately protect against spinal injury is poor, they may afford protection against rib fracture and abdominal injury. Much more detailed research and design are required before these protective vests can be accepted as uniformly indicated in equestrian sports.

As equestrian sports gain popularity, the demand for high-performance horses has sharply increased. Moreover, as younger riders attempt to emulate senior experienced horsemen and horsewomen, the potential for catastrophic injury increases. The coupling of inexperienced riders with aggressive young horses is to be condemned. Additionally, few rules are established to prevent injuries, with the notable exception of the USPC and American Horsemanship Safety Association (AHSA). Many state legislatures and most equestrian organizations lack any safety guidelines. Supervision alone, however, cannot prevent accidents; more than one third of all accidents occur during lessons. Riders often have no means of judging their capabilities or those of their instructors. Unfortunately, instructors are too often selected on the basis of their availability and salesmanship rather than on their knowledge and ability to teach the skills necessary for safe horsemanship. Two organizations that have recognized instructor certification are the American Riding Instructor Certification

Program (P.O. Box 4076, Mount Holly, NJ 08060) and the Horsemanship Safety Association (5304 Reeve St., Mazomanie, WI 53560).

Any equestrian activity is associated with the risk of head and neck injury. The potential for these injuries can be considerably lessened, however, by (1) consideration of those preexisting medical conditions that predispose to neurologic injury, (2) by thoughtful instruction by qualified instructors, and (3) most importantly, by the insistence on the use of approved protective headgear.

REFERENCES

1. Bixby-Hammett DM: Accidents in equestrian sports. *Am Fam Physician* 1987; 36:209–214.

2. Grossman JA, Kulund DN, Miller CW, et al: Equestrian injuries. Results of a prospective study. *JAMA* 1978; 240:1881–1882.

3. *Horse Industry Directory, 1985.* American Horse Council, 1700 K St. NW, Washington, DC 20006.

4. *National Electronic Injury Surveillance System,* US Consumer Product Safety Commission, 5401 Westbard Ave., Washington, DC 20297.

5. Bixby-Hammett DM: Horseback riding in North Carolina. *NC Med J* 1987; 47:530–533.

6. Metropolitan Life Insurance Company: Competitive sports and their hazards. *Stat Bull Metrop Insur Co* 1965; 46:1–3.

7. *MMWR.* Centers for Disease Control, vol 27, no 23, 1978.

8. Bixby-Hammett DM: Youth accidents with horses. *Phys Sports med* 1985; 13:105–117.

9. Gleave JR: *The Impact of Sports on a Neurological Unit.* Read before the Britain Institute of Sports Medicine, Cambridge, England, April 1975.

10. Bernhang AM, Winslett G: Equestrian injuries. *Phys Sportsmed* 1983; 1111:90–97.

11. Barber HM: Horse-play: Survey of accidents with horses. *Br Med J* 1973; B:532–534.

12. Mahaley MS, Seaber AY: *Accident and Safety Considerations of Horseback Riding,* in Proceedings of the 18th Conference on the Medical Aspects of Sports. Dallas, Tex, June 1976.

13. Bliss TF: *Rider Safety—Increase Your Odds.* Read before the Annual Meeting of the US Combined Training Association, South Hampton, Mass, February 1986.

14. Gierup J, Larson M, Lennquist S: Incidence and nature of horse-riding injuries. A one-year prospective study. *Acta Chir Scand* 1976; 142:57–61.

15. Lindsay KW, McLatzhe G, Jennett B: Serious head injury in sport. *Br Med J* 1980; 281:789–791.

16. Williams LP, Remmerg EE, Huff SI, et al: *The Blue-Tail Fly Syndrome: Horse-Associated Accidents.* Presented at the 103rd Annual Meeting of the American Public Health Association, Chicago, Nov 12, 1975.

17. Ilgren EB, Teddy PJ, Va Radis J, et al: Clinical and pathological studies of brain injuries in horse-riding accidents: A description of cases and review with a warning to the unhelmeted. *Clin Neuropathol* 1984; 3:253–259.

18. Muwanga LC, Dove AF: Head protection for horse riders: A cause for concern. *Arch Emerg Med* 1985; 2:85–87.

19. *Justin Sportsmedicine Program, Rodeo Injury Annual Reports.* Mobile Sports Medicine Systems, Inc, Dallas, Tex, 1987.

20. Brooks WH, Bixby-Hammett DM: Prevention of neurologic injuries in equestrian sports. *Phys Sportsmed* 1988; 16:25–30.

21. American Society for Testing and Materials: *Standard Specifications for Head Gear Used in Horse Sports and Horseback Riding.* Annual Book of ASTM Standards 1988; F1163:1–8.

22. Edixhoven P, Sinhask, Dandy DJ: Horse injuries. *Injury* 1981; 12:279–282.

23. D'Arbreu: Brain damage in jockeys, *Lancet* 1976; 1:1241.

24. McGhee CN, Gullan RW, Miller JP: Horse riding and head injury: Admissions to a regional head injury unit. *Br J Neurosurg* 1987; 1:131–136.

25. Pounder DJ: The grave yawns for the horseman: Equestrian Deaths in South Australia 1973–1983: *Med J Aust* 1984; 141:632–635.

CHAPTER 12

Spine Injuries Resulting From Winter Sports

David C. Reid, M.D.

Linda A. Saboe, M.C.P.A., B.P.T.

Many sports have their peak season during the winter months, but traditionally the so-called winter sports include those sports requiring ice or snow as a playing surface. Because of the physical characteristics of this frozen water, most winter sports (with notable exceptions) have evolved into high-speed events. The velocity in sports such as skiing, the hard ice surface and physical contact of hockey, the speed and height of landing in ski jumping, and the bulletlike, but relatively exposed, projectile in bobsledding would lead one to suspect that there would be an unacceptably high incidence of spinal trauma. Nevertheless, considering the large numbers of participants in these pastimes, the relative incidence of spinal fractures is low.[1] The rise in popularity of the snowmobile as a recreational vehicle has added an alarming dimension to the previously unremarkable statistics, however.[2,3] In a series of 1,447 spinal fractures, 202 (14%) were due to sports and recreation[4] (Table 12-1). Of this latter group, nearly half resulted from winter sports, with snowmobile, tobogganing, skiing, and ice hockey being prevalent causes (Table 12-2). The presence of an associated neurologic injury makes even small numbers significant,

and the large amount of associated injuries and the young age of many of the victims give a special cause for concern.

SKIING

Alpine Skiing

Spinal fractures comprise a small, but devastating, percentage of skiing injuries. The incidence in Alpine (downhill) skiing has ranged from 0% to 5.2% in the reported series.[5-10]

The numbers appear to be slowly increasing during the 7 years in Reid's study, but may simply reflect more skiers[1] (Table 12-3). Novice and experienced skiers seem to be injured with equal frequency. The most common mechanisms include attempting a jump and landing poorly and losing control and hitting a tree. The other contributing factors are (1) collisions with other skiers because of their location just over the edge of the slope where they were not seen until the last minute, (2) novice skiers crossing the slopes into the path of fast skiers on the main run, (3) overcrowding of the slopes and the junction of two runs where fast skiers come onto slow skiers, and (4) collisions with the lift support, rocks, and

TABLE 12–1.

Cause and Severity of Spinal Fractures (1980–86)*

Cause of Injury	Total (N)	Injuries (%)	Injuries Neural (N)	With Assoc. Deficit (%)
Motor vehicle accident	768	53	196	26
Occupational	221	15	51	23
Domestic	203	14	13	6
Sporting and recreational	202	14	84	42
Other	54	4	16	4
Total	1448	100	360	25

*Adapted from Reid DC, Saboe LA, Allan DG: Phys Sportsmed 1987; 16:143–152.

TABLE 12–2.

Spine Injuries in Specific Sport*

Sport	Total Injuries	Percent of All Sports	Number With Assoc. Deficit	Percent of Indiv. Sport
Diving	43	21	30	70
Snowmobiles†	20	10	7	35
Parachute/skydiving	20	10	4	20
Equestrian	19	10	6	32
Dirt bikes	18	9	6	33
All-terrain vehicle	15	7	8	53
Toboggan†	11	6	1	9
Alpine skiing†	11	6	4	36
Ice hockey†	6	3	4	67
Rugby	6	3	2	33
Bicycle	5	3	1	20
Football	4	2	1	25
Wrestling	3	1	2	67
Mountaineering	3	1	1	33
Surfing	3	1	1	33
Other	15	7	6	50
Total	202	100	84	42

*Adapted from Reid DC, Saboe LA: Can J Sports Med, in press.
†Wintersports 48 (24%) of injuries.

TABLE 12–3.

Winter Sport Spine Injuries by Year*

Year	Snowmobile	Ice Hockey	Toboggan	Alpine Skiing	Total
1980	2	—	6	1	9
1981	2	—	1	—	3
1982	3	—	2	—	5
1983	4	2	1	—	7
1984	5	1	1	2	9
1985	—	1	—	4	5
1986	4	2	—	4	10
Total	20	6	11	11	48

*Adapted from Reid DC, Saboe LA: Can J Sports Med, in press.

grooming equipment. These etiologic factors are basically of two varieties. The first is essentially related to poor judgment, and this in turn was linked to young age, alcohol, or, in many cases, poorly taught ski etiquette and selfishness. The second big factor is ski slope design, with too many runs converging and overcrowding some parts of the slope. Along with this is inadequate policing of the activity of skiers when dangerous minijumps have been made or when obviously inappropriate behavior is developing on crowded slopes.

These same factors that generate spinal injuries lead to head injury and death. Morrow[11] reported on 22 fatalities among Alpine skiers in Vermont from the 1979–1980 through 1987–1988 ski seasons. However, Alpine skiing fatalities do not usually occur in the typical recreational skier, but in the highly skilled young adult, capable of skiing at very high speeds.[12] There is an estimated rate of one death per 1.6 million skier-days. In addition to the factors cited, Shealy[12] noted that these accidents also resulted from falls on slopes rated above the skier's abilities and from crashes while racing informally with other skiers, as well as while making practice runs for a competitive race. The cause of death is mainly from blunt trauma to the head (82%) and occasionally to the chest and abdomen.

While fractures of the cervical vertebrae occur frequently, burst fractures of L-1, signifying axial loading, with or without a flexion component, predominate in most series. When cervical fractures do occur they are usually midcervical (Table 12–4). The cervical fractures are often associated with head injuries and normally direct impact to the face or forehead. This results in an anteroposterior fore that produces a fracture dislocation in most cases. In the largest series reported, no obvious compressive type fractures were observed.[15] The skiers position at high speed is usually with the head forward and the shoulders raised, and it is suggested that a helmet with an extended posterior rim may afford some protection against cervical spine injury.[13]

In our series the average age was 20.2 years, with the youngest being 13 years; the series included several teenagers and no one more than 26 years of age.[4] Ellison[14] and Margreiter et al.[9] reported 1.8% and 4.7%, respectively, in their series of skiing injuries involving the spine in children and teenagers. Injuries to the spine in young individuals require considerable energy input, but fortunately are frequently usually of lesser severity with little prolonged morbidity[15, 16] (Table 12–5).

Associated injuries are present in about 60% of individuals sustaining a spinal fracture, with approximately one-third having a neurologic deficit (Table 12–6). Long bone fractures, thoracic injury, abdominal injury, and ligament damage to the knee are frequent concom-

TABLE 12–4.

Cervical Injuries From Skiing 1978–1983*

No.	Level	Lesion	Assoc. Concussion	Ages	Male	Female
1	C1–2	Fracture dislocation	Yes	27	1	
3	C2–3	All fracture dislocations	Yes	8, 15, 23	3	
1	C3–4	Fracture dislocation	Yes	10	1	
6	C4–5	All fracture dislocations	Yes	16, 17, 30, 36, 37	5	1
4	C5–6	All fracture dislocations	Yes	15, 3, 5, 4, 1, 57	2	2
3	C6–7	All fracture dislocations	Yes	19, 42, 55	3	

*Adapted from Oh S: Int J Sports Med 1984; 5:268–271.

TABLE 12–5.

Population Characteristics of Individuals Sustaining Spinal Fractures

	Age (Yr)			Sex		Level		
	Mean	(SD)	Range	M	F	C1–C3	C4–C7	Th/L
Snowmobile	28.1	(9.8)	12–57	14	6	1	4	15
Toboggan	19.1	(10.9)	8–35	7	4	1	2	8
Ice hockey	22.0	(7.5)	18–36	6	—	—	3	3
Alpine skiing	20.2	(4.0)	13–26	9	2	—	1	10
All winter sports	24.0	(9.0)	8–57	36	12	2	10	36

itant injuries; these injuries point to the need for careful evaluation before moving the injured individual, as well as skilled management of the transport down and off the ski slopes.[1]

There does not appear to be a specific relationship to the time of day, weather, or (with the exception of head injuries and helmet use) equipment used.

In summary, injuries appear to be specifically related to errors of judgment, and uncontrolled speed is the most prevalent lethal factor. Recommendations for reducing catastrophic injuries include skiing under control. Few serious injuries result from collisions at less than 10 to 15 mph, whereas impacts at more than 20 mph invite disasters. Educating skiers and enforcing speed rules help prevent injuries. Ski patrols should give warning

to individuals who "bomb the slopes" recklessly, and should remove skiers who fail to comply with safety regulations. Altering the design or grooming patterns of specific ski areas or runs might also be effective. Flattening out moguls is a dual-edged sword, since while reducing injuries in general, it promotes faster skiing and may contribute to more severe injuries.

Helmets would reduce the number of catastrophic head injuries, and if appropriately designed may have some effect on cervical spine trauma.

The first most important factor for ski patrollers is to understand that a spinal fracture does not have to be associated with paralysis. Hence a careful assessment is always necessary before moving an individual. The second factor for ski

TABLE 12–6.

Associated Injuries With Spine Fractures*

Degree and Site of Injury	Snowmobiles	Toboggan	Alpine Skiing	Ice Hockey	All Winter Sports
None present	10	7	5	5	27 (56%)
Associated injuries	10	4	6	1	21 (44%)
Another vertebra	—	2	1	—	3
Thoracic trauma	4	—	2	—	6
Head injury	2	2	—	1	5
Long bone fracture	5	1	2	—	8
Abdominal trauma	3	—	1	—	4
Pelvic trauma	2	—	—	—	2
Facial injury	1	—	1	—	2
Brachial plexus	—	—	1	—	1
Urinary tract	—	—	1	—	1
Knee ligaments	—	—	1	—	1
Total injuries	17	5	10	1	33
Multiple trauma	6	1	3	0	10 (21%)

*Adapted from Reid DC, Saboe LA: Can J Sports Med, *in press.*

patrollers to understand is that spinal fractures are often accompanied by one or more other major injuries. These associated injuries are frequently more obvious. A rapid but diligent assessment of the entire skier is necessary in these cases. Otherwise dramatic peripheral injuries may lead to overlooking the spinal fracture with its potentially disastrous results. Ski patrollers must be trained carefully in the difficult task of transporting skiers with spinal fractures with associated multiple trauma.

Freestyle Skiing

The acrobatic nature of freestyle skiing and the temptation for unskilled individuals to mimic the dramatic maneuvers result in the greatest number of spinal injuries in freestyle skiing. As this sport gains in popularity, we can expect the incidence of injuries to rise. Among the more structured events, thoracolumbar fractures alone account for 8% of all time loss injuries in some series.[17] This high figure cited in Dowling's paper is despite the fact that he did not include inverted aerials (flips). These aerials have caused a number of serious spinal fractures and have been banned by the U.S. Skiing Association. Inverted aerials, however, are still included in World Cup Competitions held in Canada and European countries. This event in freestyle skiing is controversial, and careful statistics related to number of exposures should be monitored.[18] The risks from freestyle skiing may be somewhat reduced by good training programs that include adequate dry land gymnastics skills and careful supervision of competitions, with attention to weather conditions, visibility, and takeoff and landing snow conditions.[15, 19]

Ski Jumping

Cross-country and Alpine skiing are enjoyed by millions of people for recreational purposes. Ski jumping, on the other hand, is almost exclusively a competitive sport, with a rather limited number of performers.[20] These jumpers may have on average of about 400 jumps per year. Special facilities are required for Nordic ski jumping. The skier begins at the top of the in run, which is a ramp supported by scaffolding or conformed ground (Fig. 12–1). On the in run, the jumper crouches to minimize wind resistance and hence maximize takeoff speed. At the end of the in run the skier must time the jump perfectly and, almost simultaneously, press the body forward over the skis to mimic an air foil and generate lift. This leaning position is maintained as long as possible. Toward the end of the flight the hips are pushed forward, the shoulders raised, and the trunk extended to a position perpendicular with the slope of the hill. With a crouching movement, one foot is brought slightly ahead of the other as the skis touch the landing hill. The run is completed by skiing through the transition curve and into the long, flat out run, which allows deceleration. Two jumps are completed, and points awarded for style and distance.

The absence of spinal fractures in ski jumping in our series reflects the overall

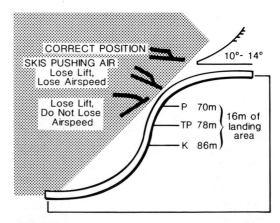

FIG 12–1.
Schematic of a ski jump with influence of correct positioning on lift and speed.

low incidence in this sport.[1] To the casual observer, the ski jump would appear to be a natural setting for catastrophic injuries. Because of the skill level of the ski jumper, proper hill maintenance, and good judgment on the part of the officials, spinal fractures are rare[15] (Table 12–7). Indeed, at the 1980 Lake Placid Winter Olympics, more than 5,000 jumps were made with only two injuries, a mild concussion and a fractured clavicle.

At the Intervale Ski Jump Complex, the largest ski jumping complex in North America, a 5-year record of ski jumping injuries does not include cervical spine fractures or dislocations in its statistics.[21] The most common injuries were contusions (26%), usually involving the shoulder, knee, or elbow, fractures to the extremities (15%), abrasions (14%), and concussions (10%), most of which were mild. Dislocations formed a further 10% of the injuries, and were usually anterior shoulder and acromioclavicular joint separations (Table 12–8). Nevertheless, in a sport in which takeoff speeds of 50 to 56 mph are achieved on 70 m hills and 45 to 55 mph on 50 to 60 m hills, followed by covering up to 70 to 90 m in the air, slightly altered ski placement on the in run because of tracks made by the previous jumpers, loose powder snow dragging on one ski, or poor weight distribu-

TABLE 12–8.

Ski Jumping Injuries*,†

Injury	N	% of Total
Contusion	19	26.4
Fracture	11	15.3
Abrasion	10	13.9
Concussions	7	9.7
Dislocations	7	9.7
Visceral injuries	5	6.9
Sprains	5	6.9
Others	8	12.1

*Adapted from Wright JR, Hixson EG, Rand JJ: Am J Sports Med 1986; 14:393–397.
†At Intervale Ski Jump Complex (1980–85).

tion can lead to a bad takeoff and possibly a fall on the landing hill[23] (Fig 12–2).

In Wester's[20] study of serious ski jumping injuries in Norway, the risk of being seriously injured was approximately 5% in a 5-year period (1977–1981). It was higher in the age groups 15 to 17 years (see Table 12–7). The first jump of the day is particularly dangerous. Most of the serious injuries occur in jumps where the jumper has had previous experience. It is possible that the jumper met unexpected snow conditions on a jump that was believed to be familiar. Other possibilities include the need for a couple of jumps to "remember" or "get the feeling" of the particular jump.[20] When spine fractures do occur, they are usually mid- to low cervical and associated with concussion and paralysis (Table 12–9). High cervical fractures are the most frequent fatal injury in ski jumping.[24] The fatality rate for Nordic ski jumping is estimated at 12 per 100,000 participants annually, which is within the range of other "risky" outdoor sports.[24] Only six fatalities occurred in a 50-year period in the United States; four of these were associated with cervical spine injuries, and at least three were to the C-1–C-2 area.[24]

Despite the fact that many skiers blame personal faults such as rotation at

TABLE 12–7.

Risk of Serious Injury in Ski Jumping*,†

Age	No. of Injuries	Licensed Jumpers	Risk of Injury per Skier per 5 Years (%)
12	1	302	3
13	1	275	4
14	3	211	5
15	3	201	14
16	1	152	7
17	1	125	8
18		83	—
19		79	—
20–34	4	758	5

*Adapted from Shealy JE: Ski Patrol Magazine 1985; 2:21–24.
†Injury causing serious permanent disability (5-year period).

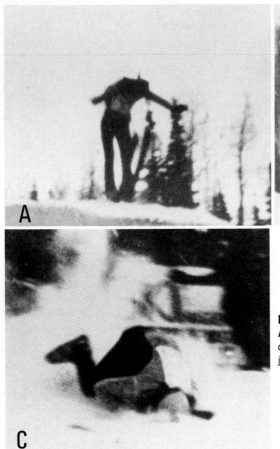

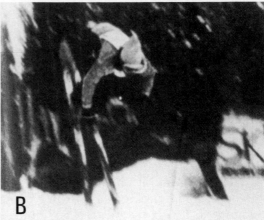

FIG 12–2.
A, incorrect and unbalanced takeoff; **B,** catching tips on landing; **C,** potential for serious head and neck injuries.

the takeoff, too early takeoff, and asymmetric ski placement as the main causes of injury, there are some areas that deserve more detailed discussion in order to formulate a plan for injury prevention.

Injuries are not common in the age group 12 and younger. These youngsters compete on relatively small jumps with lengths up to 30 to 35 m, which are associated with correspondingly lower

TABLE 12–9.

Injuries From Ski Jumping Giving Severe Permanent Disability*

Injury	Medical Disability (%)	Age (Years)	Sex
Cervical fractures with complete cord transection			
C-6	100	17	M
T-6	100	16	M
T-7	100	14	F
Intracerebral hematoma	70	28	M
Amputation, leg			
Poor prosthetic function	25	23	M
Good prosthetic function	45	14	M

*Adapted from Wester K: Am J Sports Med 1985; 13:124–127.

speeds. With flexibility of their spine structures and light body weights, kinetic energy is low. The age 15 to 17 seems to present the greatest risk, with poor judgment and attempts at longer jumps than those for which they are physically or technically qualified being the main contributing factors. The need for careful observation and control by coaches, with progression only when sufficient skill has been obtained, is obvious in reducing injuries.

There may be some bimodal seasonal variation in incidence. Lack of practice may account for the early season problems. Changing snow conditions are more prevalent at both ends of the season. The quality of the in run, the development of ruts, and the uniformity of packing can all alter velocity and balance during the critical moments approaching the takeoff. At the end of the season, or after a heavy snowfall, the landing area can develop knolls or irregularities, or the snow allows sinking in of the ski upon the impact of landing, with sudden deceleration. Only careful inspection and grooming will overcome these difficulties. The increase in confidence and efforts to achieve or surpass personal "bests" may influence the rise in injuries toward the season's end. This, along with more than 50% of the severe injuries occurring on the first jump, indicates the need for the jumper to thoroughly examine all aspects of the jump, including the in run and landing areas, before attempting the course.

Equipment is another key factor, and there has been a remarkable improvement in this area. Skis, bindings, clothing, and, above all, good head protection have added a dimension of protection that, unfortunately, can sometimes lead to recklessness. Previous experimentation with high heel blocks, allowing earlier attainment of the floating position, seemed to increase the incidence of dangerous falls during takeoff, particularly when encountering small decelerations on the in run.[20] Apart from the skiers' equipment, the construction of rails, shields, and fences in all areas of the jump should make it impossible for skis or body parts to get stuck in case of a fall.

Perhaps one of the most significant factors in reducing ski jumping injuries is improvement in technique. The older, less aerodynamically efficient ski jumping techniques required that the jumper be projected high into the air and then "free fall" while flying horizontally. With the modern jump, the jumper mimics an air foil and generates lift. Therefore, it is possible to fly further without needing so much altitude. Hence the vertical component of the flight curve relative to the horizontal component has been decreased. This in turn has allowed the landing hill to be redesigned. The modern ski jump landing hill is not so steep, and as a result the knoll and transition are not as flat. The net effect is an increased margin of safety, since the landing hill more closely resembles the flight curve of a broader range of jumps, including the very long and very short attempts.[24]

In summary, the dangers of Nordic ski jumping have been overestimated because of the remarkable improvement of equipment, hill design, and excellent officiating. Indeed, in Wester's[26] review of catastrophic injuries with permanent disability, he indicated that safety in ski jumping had improved by a factor of 5 in the two time periods studied. The relative safety of both recreational Alpine skiing and ski jumping is illustrated by a comparison of their fatality rates with these or other sporting activities (Table 12–10). Nevertheless, this should not be a cause for complacency in a sport combining the very dangerous elements of speed and height.

TABLE 12–10.

Fatality Rates in Sport (Deaths/100,000/Year)*

Sport	Rate
Recreational Alpine skiing	0.1
Ski jumping	0.12
Use of firearms	1.3
Football	2.0
Alpine ski racing (slalom, giant slalom, downhill)	2.5
Sailing	2.6
Mountain hiking	6.4
Canoeing/kayaking	7.6
Snowmobiling	13.2
Driving an automobile	26.6
Recreational scuba diving	41.7
Professional boxing	45.5
Sail planing	58.5
Motor cycling	90.9
Parachuting	175.4
Hang gliding	178.6
Serious mountain climbing	598.8

Adapted from Reif AE: Risks and gains, in Vinger PF, Hoerrnner EF (eds): Sports Injuries: The Unthwarted Epidemic, ed 2. Littleton, Mass, PSG Publishing Co, 1986.

Snowmobiles

Off-road motor vehicles made their appearance in the late 1960s and early 1970s and have rapidly gained acceptance. With their rise in popularity, the frequency of accidents attributable to them also has risen.[27, 28] There were 3,000 off-road injuries in the United States in 1979, 26,900 in 1983, and 85,900 in 1985.[27] The predominant factor has been the commercial success of the three-wheel all-terrain vehicle (ATV). However, there are more than 2 million snowmobiles in use in the United States, and a larger number per capita in Canada.[2]

Despite the slight decline in popularity of the snowmobile during the last few years, snowmobiles still continue to be a significant source of severe injuries in the winter months (Table 12–11). In Reid's series they formed up to 10% of sport and recreationally induced spinal fractures, and in some publications approximately 35% of them have associated neurologic injury.[1, 2, 29]

Typically, the snowmobiler is injured while driving at night (52%), under the influence of alcohol (53%), and in unfamiliar terrain.[3, 30, 31] Wenzel et al.[29] reported that 11% of injuries occurred in children 10 years of age or younger. Our series also reflected this statistic (see Table 12–5). The incorrect image of the snowmobile as a safe piece of equipment, easy to drive, leads many parents to view it almost as a toy. Ultimately, the key to reducing the number of injuries and fatalities may be setting an age limit and educating drivers[29] (see Table 12–7). Going off embankments, tipping on steep terrain, colliding with another snowmobile, hitting an object (frequently a tree), and becoming airborne are common mechanisms of sustaining spinal fractures (Table 12–12). Occasionally the machine may roll onto the driver. Because of the cold weather conditions, compliance with wearing protective headgear is good, but frequently the impacts are so great

TABLE 12–11.

Frequency of Admission by Vehicle and Year

Vehicle	Admissions—No. (%)					
	1981	1982	1983	1984	1985	Total
ATVs	2 (6)	2 (5)	8 (22)	10 (21)	25 (52)	47 (23)
Snowmobiles	24 (75)	34 (77)	17 (47)	21 (45)	15 (31)	111 (54)
Dirt bikes	2 (6)	3 (7)	7 (19)	9 (19)	1 (2)	22 (11)
Other	2 (6)	4 (9)	2 (6)	3 (6)	2 (4)	13 (6)
Nonrecreational	2 (6)	1 (2)	2 (6)	4 (9)	5 (10)	14 (7)
Total	32 (15)	44 (21)	36 (17)	47 (23)	48 (23)	207 (100)

TABLE 12–12.

Factors Contributing to Spine Trauma in Off-Road Vehicle Accidents*

	ATVs	Dirt Bikes	Snowmobiles	Total
Mechanism				
Collided with object	3	6	8	17
Stayed on machine	—	—	6	6
Crushed by machine	4	3	2	9
Fell off or thrown off	2	12	9	23
Machine tipped over	9	1	—	10
Unknown	2	2	1	5
Terrain				
Hit bump	2	1	4	7
Went over cliff or embankment	1	3	4	8
Flat surface	2	5	3	10
On a hill	6	2	—	8
Ramp or jump	—	1	—	1
Time of day†				
Midnight—7 A.M.	2	—	—	2
7 A.M.—noon	2	2	2	6
Noon—6 PM	6	9	6	21
6 P.M.—midnight	5	6	11	22

*Adapted from Reid DC, Saboe LA, Allan DG: Phys Sportsmed 1987; 16:143–152.
†Fifty-five percent of snowmobile accidents and 47% of ATV accidents occur between 8 P.M. and 4 A.M.; poor lighting and alcohol use are contributing factors.

that these do not eliminate spinal injury or even fatalities.[29, 32] Advertisements showing snowmobilers driving off embankments and doing jumps obviously stimulate sales but do not promote the rational use of these vehicles, nor promote their real capabilities.[33, 34] Spinal fractures in snowmobiling form 3% to 4% of all snowmobile injuries, most involving the thoracolumbar junction.[35–37] Cervical spine injuries account for about a quarter of the overall spinal fractures that occur in snowmobiling.[2] They are also frequently seen as concomitant injuries along with concussion, in series reporting snowmobile deaths[3, 31] (Fig 12–3). Of

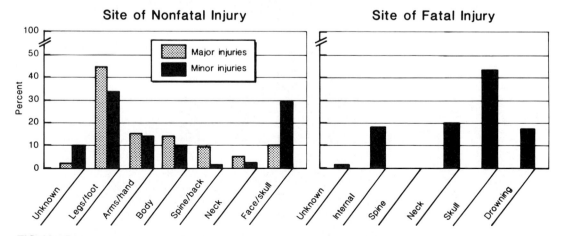

FIG 12–3.
Anatomic sites of nonfatal and fatal injuries suffered by snowmobilers. *(Adapted from Wenzel FJ, Peters RA, Hintz CS, et al: Wis Med J 1973; 72:89.)*

particular concern is the magnitude and number of associated injuries (see Table 12–6).[3] Nearly 50% of individuals have other injuries, and more than 25% have multiple trauma.[1] Long bone fractures, chest trauma, abdominal injury, and head injury make up the bulk of these. Percy[38] reported more than 200 deaths in 1 year in North America, and Wenzel et al.[29] noted that 4% of the fatalities in his series were children 11 years of age and younger.

Both the American and the Canadian pediatric societies, as well as a number of consumer advocacy groups, have expressed their concern about the number of children injured in off-road motor vehicle accidents[31, 34, 39] (Fig 12–4). Their concern extends to the marketing strategies directed at the young rider, the public's misconception of the stability and safety of these vehicles, and the paucity of legislation regulating the vehicles.

Throughout North America generally there is a paucity of legislation relating to the use of off-road motor vehicles.[40] In Canada these vehicles fall under provincial jurisdiction; in Alberta they are included in The Snowmobile Act. They must be registered, licensed, and insured, but drivers need not be licensed providing they are 14 years of age, or 12 and operating under adult supervision. The off-road use of these vehicles, particularly on private property, renders enforcement of the act extremely difficult.

As a result of this and other studies, several recommendations concerning off-road vehicles can be made. Implementation of stricter licensing requirements may reduce the incidence of injury to children.[41–44] Forbidding children younger than 16 years to operate or to be a passenger on off-road vehicles does not seem excessively restrictive when the consequences of accidents in this age group are examined.[27] Since enforcement of legislation is difficult, parents, in particular, and drivers must be made aware of the dangers involved because the majority of accidents are caused by poor driver judgment.

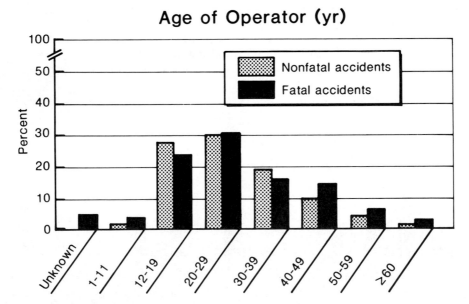

FIG 12–4.
Ages of snowmobile operators, a large percentage of young individuals, involved in nonfatal and fatal accidents. *(Adapted from Wenzel FJ, Peters RA, Hintz CS, et al: Wis Med J 1973; 72:89.)*

Improved headlights have decreased the number of accidents occurring at night, but this is still a significant factor.[36, 37, 45, 46]

In Wenzel et al.'s data,[29] 17% of accidents occurred on public and private trails. They specifically made the point, however, that this figure concealed a shift in accident location (Fig 12–5). With a large number of new trails developed, they supplemented the open fields as the most common accident location by the end of their study. The use of groomed trails was probably responsible for some of the overall decrease in accidents during the 10-year period of study. This contrasts to the toll of accidents involving snowmobiles on highways, which has remained relatively high. Increased enforcement of existing safety laws against snowmobiles on public roads and right-of-ways should be encouraged.

Injury by some part of the snowmobile when it rolls over, or when the rider falls off, along with approximately 8% incidence of injury caused by faulty equipment, suggests that there is still room for improved snowmobile design. Poor judgment, frequently associated with alcohol use, however, is the main contributor to spinal injury in snowmobile and off-road vehicle accidents.[1, 2]

Legislation, better equipment, and public education have made snowmobiling a safer sport during the last few years. The following recommendations should further improve this record:

1. A review of snowmobile legislation to ensure requirements for safety and training programs for all drivers
2. Stricter enforcement and regulation of snowmobiles on public highways
3. Development of designated areas and trails for snowmobiles.
4. Improved safety design of equipment, including helmets as well as the snowmobile.

Tobogganing

As would be anticipated, tobogganing injuries frequently involve very young individuals, and approximately one third

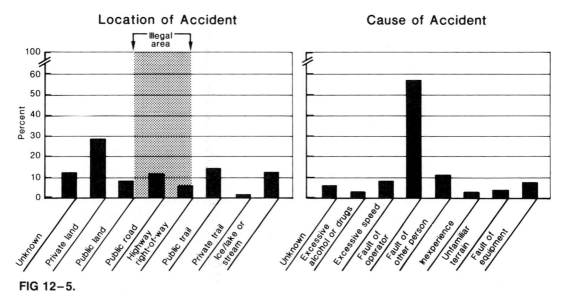

FIG 12–5.
A large percentage of accidents occur in illegal areas, and mainly because of errors of judgment of the operator. *(Adapted from Wenzel FJ, Peters RA, Hintz CS, et al: Wis Med J 1973; 72:89.)*

of the spinal fractures occur in children less than 15 years of age. Poor judgment ranks high in the mechanism of injury, which frequently involves collision with a post, fence, or tree. The other common mechanism was taking off over a bump and becoming airborne. While listed as toboggans in our series, a third of these injuries actually occurred with use of motor vehicle inner tubes. There were no spinal fractures during the last 2 years of our study, and the highest figures were from 1980 (see Table 12–3). This may represent increased parental awareness of the dangers, or more safety features at the popular and frequently used tobogganing slopes.

Axial loading burst type fractures of the thoracolumbar junction occur more frequently than cervical spine fractures.

The key to reduction of these injuries is obviously well prepared and cleared tobogganing areas, safety features to prevent collisions, and adequate education and parental supervision.

Ice Hockey

The typical profile of a spinal fracture in hockey is a young man with a midcervical burst type fracture or fracture dislocation, associated with a significant incomplete or complete spinal cord injury[47] (Table 12–13). The tragedy of these statistics is that there appears to be a rise in incidence during the last few years.[47] In our own series all levels of hockey seemed to be involved, from pickup recreational play to professional, although most injuries come from the more intense levels of competition.[3]

The most frequent event leading to the injury is a push or check usually from behind. An unintentional slide, a trip, and collision with the goalpost or another player may be involved. The fracture is usually the direct result of a blow to the head by contact with the boards, another player, or the goalposts. The

TABLE 12–13.

Spine Injury in Hockey (*N* = 42)*

Injury	No. of Injuries	Percentage
A. Level		
(C1) C1–2	2	4.8
(C2) C2–3	—	—
(C3) C3–4	1	2.4
(C4) C4–5	8	19.0
(C5) C5–6	18	42.9
(C6) C6–7	5	11.9
(C7) (ixC7 T1	5	11.9
T12 L2	3	7.1
B. Type of bony injury		
Fracture-dislocation	27	64.3
Fracture	9	21.4
Dislocation	2	4.8
None	4	9.5
C. Neurologic injury		
Incomplete cord	16	38.1
Complete cord	12	28.6
Nerve root	5	11.9
Nerve	9	21.4
D. Year		
1976	2	4.8
1977	2	4.8
1978	4	9.5
1979	1	2.4
1980	8	19.0
1981	13	31.0
1982 (+Jan. 1983)	12	28.6

*Adapted from Tator CH, Edmonds VE: Phys Sportsmed 1986; 14:157–167.

neck is usually in the slightly flexed position, which has the effect of straightening or slightly flexing the cervical curve. The result is an axial loading type injury. There is a suggestion that the increasing size and speed of hockey players, the feeling of confidence engendered by the protective equipment, and the increasing violence may be factors contributing to an upward swing in numbers of spinal fractures in hockey.[3, 47, 48]

Spinal injuries in hockey are dealt with more fully in the chapter by Dr. Tator. There is, however, one point that needs stressing, and this relates to the immediate management. The ice surface presents special difficulties for inexperienced personnel when it comes to log-rolling a spine-injured player onto a stretcher. It has been our experience that even well-taught and well-rehearsed physicians and therapists do this transfer very poorly unless they have practiced on the ice surface. Failure to take the time to rehearse on the ice will result in a very dangerously executed transfer when attempted for the first time on the slippery surface. Special attention is needed to fix the stretcher. Inasmuch as permanent paralysis is frequently associated with spinal fractures sustained in hockey, the statistics for the sport must be closely observed during the next few years, and each incident must be analyzed carefully for clues as to methods of prevention.

SUMMARY

Considering the large number of participants and the velocities involved in many winter sports, the number of significant spinal injuries is surprisingly small. The notable exception is the snowmobile, where factors leading to poor judgment were obviously important. This includes a young age, alcohol, drugs, poor lighting, and unfamiliar terrain. Misleading advertising of the stability and ease of control of these machines also adds to the danger. We were concerned about the apparent trend toward increasing spinal fractures in ice hockey, and this will have to be monitored carefully. The high skill level of the skiers, excellent grooming of slopes, and good judgment on the part of officials minimize the number of serious accidents in Alpine skiing and ski jumping. A careful analysis of training techniques and aerial maneuvers is necessary if the number of spinal fractures in freestyle skiing is to be contained.

Recreational skiing injuries are difficult to reduce because of the large number of skiers, the young age, and the role that poor judgment plays in the injury.

The frequent association between spinal fractures and other significant musculoskeletal injuries stresses the need for vigilance and excellent training for individuals carrying out first aid on the ski slopes.

REFERENCES

1. Reid DC, Saboe LA: Spine trauma in winter sports. *Sports Med* 1989; 7:393–399.

2. Reid DC, Saboe LA, Allan DG: Spine trauma associated with off road vehicles. *Phys Sportsmed* 1987; 16:143–152.

3. Allan DG, Reid DC, Saboe LA: Off-road recreational motor vehicle accidents: Hospitalization and deaths. *Can J Surg* 1988; 31:233–236.

4. Reid DC, Saboe LA: Spine fractures in sports. *Can J Sports Med*, in press.

5. Frymoyer JW, Pope MH, Kristiansen T: Skiing and spinal trauma. *Clin Sports Med* 1982; 1:309.

6. Davis MW, Litman T, Drill FE, et al: Ski injuries. *J Trauma* 1977; 17:802.

7. Gutman J, Weisbuch J, Wolf M: Ski injuries in 1972-73: A report analysis of a major health program. *JAMA* 1974; 230:1423.

8. Howarth B: Skiing injuries. *Clin Orthop* 1965; 43:171.

9. Margreiter R, Raas E, Luger LJ: The risk of injury in experienced Alpine skiers. *Orthop Clin North Am* 1976; 7:51–54.

10. Tapper EM: Ski injuries from 1939 to 1976: The Sun Valley experience. *Am J Sports Med* 1978; 6:114.

11. Morrow PL: *Downhill Ski Fatalities: The Vermont Experience.* Presented at the National Association of Medical Examiners Annual Meeting, Boston, Nov 5, 1988.

12. Shealy JE: How dangerous is skiing and who's at risk? *Ski Patrol Magazine.* 1985; 2:21–24.

13. Oh S: Cervical injury from skiing. *Int J Sports Med* 1984; 5:268–271.

14. Ellison AE: Skiing injuries. *Clin Symp* 1977; 29:1.

15. Clancy WG, McConkey JP: Nordic and Alpine skiing, Schneider RC, Kennedy JC, Plant ML (eds): *Sports Injuries—Mechanisms, Prevention and Treatment.* Baltimore, Williams & Wilkins, 1985.

16. Garrick JG, Requa RK: Injury patterns in children and adolescent skiers. *Am J Sports Med* 1979; 7:245–248.

17. Dowling PA: Prospective study of injuries in United States Ski Association Freestyle Skiing, 1976-77 to 1979-80. *Am J Sports Med* 1982; 10:268.

18. Keen JS: Thoracolumbar fractures in winter sports. *Clin Orthop* 1987; 216:39–49.

19. Harris JB: Neurological injuries in winter sports. *Phys Sports Med* 1983; 11:111.

20. Wester K: Serious ski-jumping injuries in Norway. *Am J Sports Med* 1985; 13:124–127.

21. Wright JR, Hixson EG, Rand JJ: Injury patterns in Nordic ski-jumpers. A retrospective analysis of injuries occurring at the Intervale Ski Jump Complex from 1980-1985. *Am J Sports Med* 1986; 14:393–397.

22. Reference deleted by author.

23. Eriksson E: Ski injuries in Sweden: A one year survey. *Orthop Clin North Am* 1976; 7:3–9.

24. Write JR: Nordic ski-jumping fatalities in the United States: A 50 year summary. *J Trauma* 1988; 28:848–851.

25. Reif AE: Risks and gains, in Vinger PF, Hoerner EF (eds): *Sports Injuries: The Unthwarted Epidemic*, ed 2. Littleton, Mass, PSG Publishing Co, 1986.

26. Wester K: Improved safety in ski-jumping. *Am J Sports Med* 1988; 16:499–500.

27. Da Sylva NP: Two-, three- and four-wheel unlicensed off-road vehicles (C). *Can Med Assoc J* 1987; 136:233.

28. Trager GW, Grayman G: Accidents and all-terrain vehicles (C). *JAMA* 1986; 225:2160–2161.

29. Wenzel FJ, Peters RA, Hintz CS, et al: Snowmobile accidents in central Wisconsin. *Wis Med J* 1973; 72:89.

30. Hamidy CR, Dhir A, Cameron B, et al: Snowmobile injuries in Northern Newfoundland and Labrador. A 18 year review. *J Trauma* 1988; 28:1232–1237.

31. Two-, three- and four-wheel unlicensed off-road vehicles. Accident Prevention Committee, Canadian Paediatric Society. *Can Med Assoc J* 1987; 136:119–120.

32. Roberts VL, Noyes FR, Hubbard RP, et al: *Biomechanics* 1971; 4:569.

33. Wiley JJ: The dangers of off-road vehicles to young drivers. *Can Med Assoc J* 1986; 135:1345–1346.

34. Haynes CD, Stroud SD, Thompson CE: The three wheeler (adult tricycle): : An unstable, dangerous machine. *J Trauma* 1986; 26:643–648.

35. Chism SE, Soule AB: Snowmobile injuries: Hazards from a popular new winter sport. *JAMA* 1969; 209:1672.

36. Dominici RH, Drake EH: Speed on snow: The motorized sled. *Am J Surg* 1970; 119:483.

37. Damschroder AD, Kleinstiver BS: Homosnomobolilius. *Am J Sports Med* 1976; 4:249.

38. Percy EC: The snowmobile: Friend or foe? *J Trauma* 1972; 12:444.

39. Stevens WS, Rodgers BM, Newman BM: Pediatric trauma associated with all-terrain vehicles. *J Pediatr* 1986; 109:25–29.

40. Smith SM, Middaugh JP: Injuries associated with three-wheeled all-terrain vehicles. Alaska, 1983 and 1984. *JAMA* 1986; 255:2454–2458.

41. Speca JM, Cowell HR: Minibike and motorcycle accidents in adolescents. A new epidemic. *JAMA* 1975; 232:55–56.

42. Golladay ES, Slezak JW, Mollitt DL, et al: The three wheeler—a menace to the preadolescent child. *J Trauma* 1985; 25:232–233.

43. Westman JA, Morrow G III: Moped injuries in children. *Pediatrics* 1984; 74:820–822.

44. Wiley JJ, McIntyre WM, Mercier P: Injuries associated with off-road vehicles among children. *Can Med Assoc J* 1986; 135:1365–1366.

45. Kritter AE, Carnesale PG, Prusinski D: Snowmobile: Fun and/or folly. *Wis Med J* 1972; 71:230–231.

46. Withington RL, Hall LN: Snowmobile accidents: A review of injuries sustained in the use of snowmobiles in northern New England during the 1968-69 season. *J Trauma* 1970; 10:760.

47. Tator CH, Edmonds VE: Sports and recreation are a rising cause of spinal cord injury. *Phys Sportsmed* 1986; 14:157–167.

48. Tator CH, Edmonds VE: National survey of spinal injuries in hockey players. *Can Med Assoc J* 1984; 30:875–880.

CHAPTER 13

Injuries to the Cervical Spine and Cord Resulting From Water Sports

Joseph S. Torg, M.D.

The incidence of cervical spine injuries due to water sports, particularly diving, and the potential dangers of these activities are generally little appreciated.[25, 43] Shields et al.[35] have indicated that the majority of athletic injuries to the cervical cord are a result of water-related activities. Specifically, between June 1, 1964, and Dec 31, 1973, 1,600 patients were admitted to the spinal injury service at Rancho Los Amigos Hospital. Of these, 152, or 9.5%, had been injured in recreational activities. Of these 152 patients, 118, or 78%, were injured while participating in water activities. Of the 118 water-related injuries, 82 were due to diving, 29 to surfing, and 7 to water skiing accidents. Expressed another way, the 82 diving injuries represented 54% of all the sports-related injuries.

A review of the world literature has revealed 13 studies covering the period 1948–1983 that separated the occurrence of cervical spine injuries into specific circumstances that included water sports. Depending on the study, the number of cervical spine injuries reported ranged from 112 to 2,587, and sports-related cervical spine injuries ranged from 12 to 212, with their percentages of the total varying from 5.3% to 39%. Of the sports-related injuries attributed to diving, the number varied from 7 to 131, or a range of 44% to 78% of the sports-related injuries (Table 13–1). The wide variation can be accounted for by the type of institution reporting (i.e., spinal cord injury center, general hospital, children's hospital, orthopaedic hospital) and also to the purpose of the original study. Some dealt with all traumatic spinal injuries, others with sports and recreation injuries, and some specifically with water sports. Of the 8,565 cervical spine injuries reported by this group of 13 authors, 897, or 10.5%, were sports related. And of those identified as sports related, 537, or 60%, were due to diving.

Another group of 20 studies gathered from the world literature covering the period 1948 to 1983 reported cervical spine injuries due to diving in relation to the total number of injuries (Table 13–2). Of these, seven are not included in Table 13–1. In this group of studies, the number of cervical spine injuries reported ranged from 73 to 2,587, and the percentage of those due to diving, from 2% to 42%. Of this group of 20 reports, a cumulative analysis revealed that of the 13,371 cases reported, 1,103, or 8%, were due to diving.

The demographics of a diving injury resulting in spinal cord injury reveals the occurrences evenly divided between pools and natural bodies of water, that is,

TABLE 13–1.

Injuries to Cervical Spine Due to Diving in Relation to Total Number of Cervical Spine Injuries: Report of 13 Studies

Author	Year Published	Years Studied	Location	Total No. of Cervical Spine Injuries	Sports Related Cervical Spine Injuries		Diving Related Cervical Spine Injuries	
					No.	%	No.	%
Cheshire[6]	1967	1959–1966	Victoria	325	41	12.6	27	65.9
Frankel et al.[10]	1969	1951–1968	England	682	71	10.9	42	59.2
Key and Retief[22]	1970	1963–1967	Australia	318	16	5.3	7	43.8
Sutton[38]	1973	1963–1967	Brisbane	207	37	17.9	29	78.4
Gjone[14]	1974	1968–1973	Norway	112	12	10.7	9	75.0
Zrubecky[44]	1974	1957–1965	Austria	725	59	8.2	32*	54.2
Botterell et al.[2]	1975	1969–1970	Canada	224	38	17.0	25	65.8
Kraus et al.[24]	1975	1970–1971	United States	619	43	6.9	33	76.7
Shields et al.[35]	1978	1964–1973	United States	1,600	152	9.5	82	53.9
Minaire et al.[31]	1979	1970–1975	France	351	27	7.8	13	48.1
Steinbruck and Paeslack[37]	1980	1967–1978	Germany	2,587	212	8.2	131	61.8
Hill et al.[19]	1984	1969–1979	USA	122	48	39.3	24	50.0
Tator and Edmonds[42]	1986	1948–1973	Canada	358	55	15.4	38	69.1
Tator and Edmonds[42]	1986	1974–1979	Canada	144	32	22.2	18	56.3
Tator and Edmonds[42]	1986	1980–1983	Canada	191	54	28.3	27	50.0

*Bathing accidents.

TABLE 13–2.

Injuries to Cervical Spine Due to Diving in Relation to Total Number of Cervical Spine Injuries: Report of 20 Studies

Author	Year Published	Years Studied	Location	Total No. Cervical Spine Injuries	Diving Related Cervical Spine Injuries	Diving Related (%)
Cheshire[6]	1967	1959–1966	Victoria	325	27	8.3
Frankel et al.[10]	1969	1951–1968	England	682	42	6.2
Key and Retief[22]	1970	1963–1967	Australia	318	7	2.2
Lougheed et al.[27]	1970	Before 1967	Canada	1,855	128	6.9
Sutton[38]	1973	1963–1967	Brisbane	207	29	14.0
Gjone[14]	1974	1968–1973	Norway	112	9	8.0
Zrubecky[44]	1974	1957–1965	Austria	725	32	4.4
Botterell et al.[2]	1975	1969–1970	Canada	224	25	11.1
Kewalramani and Taylor[20]	1975	1970–1973	United States	126	23	18.3
Kraus et al.[24]	1975	1970–1973	United States	619	33	5.3
Hall and Burke[18]	1978	1955–1977	Australia	917	100	10.9
Shields et al.[35]	1978	1964–1973	United States	1,600	82	5.1
Minaire et al.[31]	1979	1970–1975	France	351	13	3.7
Griffiths[17]	1980	1956–1978	Australia	336	67	19.9
Kiwerski[23]	1980	1965–1978	Poland	924	194	21.0
Steinbruck and Paeslack[37]	1980	1967–1978	Germany	2,587	131	5.1
Mennen[29]	1981	1969–1979	South Africa	575	23	4.0
DePassio et al.[7]	1983	1969–1982	France	73	31	42.5
Hill et al.[19]	1984	1969–1979	United States	122	24	19.7
Tator and Edmonds[39]	1979	1948–1973	Canada	358	38	10.6
Tator and Edmonds[42]	1986	1974–1979	Canada	144	18	12.5
Tator and Edmonds[42]	1986	1980–1983	Canada	191	27	14.1

TABLE 13–3.

Spinal Cord Injuries Occurring in Pools and Natural Bodies of Water

	Diving Into		
Author	Pool	Ocean	Lake/River/Other
Burke[4]	8	16	13
Albrand and Walter[1]	7	—	18
Kewalramani and Taylor[20]	6	—	17
Kewalramani and Kraus[21]	27	7	64
Frankel et al.[11]	44	34	22
Good and Nickel[15]	29	49	31
Green et al.[16]	100	—	—
Steinbruck and Paeslack[37]	—	—	81
Tator and Palm[40]	45%	—	55%
Mennen[29]	10	24	24
Tator et al.[41]	3	5	92
Boyd and Schweigel[3]	54%	17%	29%
Gabrielson[12]	200	←——100——→	
Little[26]	63	←——189——→	

lakes, rivers, and oceans (Table 13–3). With regard to supervision, this varies from none, in most instances, to the presence of a lifeguard, to an organized coaching situation. Gabrielson[13] has estimated that a qualified lifeguard was present at only 12% of the accident sites and an instructor or coach at only 3% of the sites.

The profile of an individual who sustains a spinal cord injury as a result of a diving accident has also been described by Gabrielson.[13]

The injured person is a male between 18 and 31 years of age, none being below the age of 12 years. He is close to 6 feet in height and weighs over 175 lb. He was not intoxicated, but in 40% to 50% of cases had consumed some alcohol, usually beer. He had little or no training in diving. He was visiting the pool for the first time, and the dive he made was the first one in that pool. He was not warned, either verbally or by any signs, that he should not dive where he dived. He had witnessed other people diving before he made his dive. He was removed from the pool by friends who were not aware that he had fractured his neck. No spine board was used. He was not aware that he could break his neck by making a dive where he did. Eighty-eight percent of the accidents resulted in quadriplegia. The most vulnerable vertebra was C5 (29% of injuries); next was C5-C6 (27%).

Noteworthy is that the majority of the victims are males, 13 years of age or older, with little or no formal training; approximately half consumed alcoholic beverages before the accident (Table 13–4).[8]

Important factors regarding the cause of diving injuries to the cervical area of the spine are depth of the water and mechanism of injury.[36] Six investigators who have documented the depth of water into which injured divers have plunged all agree that the danger of diving into shallow water cannot be stressed

TABLE 13–4.

Spinal Cord Injuries in Diving Accidents That Involve Alcohol

Author	Diving Accidents Involving Alcohol (%)
Mennen[29]	50
Gabrielson[13]	40–50
Gabrielson[33]	38–40
Tator and Palm[40]	30
Enis et al.[9]	20
Boyd and Schweigel[3]	30

TABLE 13–5.

Number of Injuries to Cervical Spine in Relation to Depth of Water

Author	No. of Injuries	Depth of Water
Albrand and Walter[1]	13	av = 4 ft (1–7 ft)
Shields et al.[35]	82	av = 5 ft
Gabrielson[13]	NA	>4 ft
McElhaney et al.[28]	NA	≤3½ ft
Frankel et al.[11]	13	>4 ft
Green et al.[16]	52	≤5 ft
Gabrielson[12]	NA	4½–6 ft

NA = not applicable.

enough.[32] Depths recorded vary from as little as one foot to as much as seven feet (Table 13–5). Shields[35] reported the average depth in which his 82 injuries occurred was five feet.

The relationship of depth to injury has been demonstrated by Albrand and Walter,[1] who developed underwater deceleration curves for diving. Specifically, they determined velocity rates of expert divers as they moved through the water after dives from various heights. The subjects were filmed from the point of entry through an underwater window with a Super 8 Bolex camera running at 24 frames per second. Velocity was measured in feet per second, and entrance speeds varied between 15 and 33 ft/sec, depending on the height above the water from which the dive occurred (Fig 13–1).

In no instance was the diver's velocity dissipated before a 12 ft descent.

Injury mechanisms have been proposed by a number or authors. In 1972 Burke[4] reported that "vertical compression or 'burst' fractures were by far the most common injury (45, or 88%)." Albrand and Walter[1] stated that "the hyperflexion-type injury with a wedge fracture of the cervical vertebra was the most common clinical condition noted radiographically, followed by vertical compression or burst fractures and lastly hyperextension injuries." Kiwerski[23] reported that "examining trauma mechanisms, compression fractures were most often found (above 56% of cases). Such fractures occur after striking the head against a hard object under a small layer of water." Steinbruck[37] stated,

In all diving accidents, including high diving, the injuries were located almost exclusively in the cervical vertebrae and were caused by similar accident mechanisms: There were hyperflexion injuries on the one hand and hyperextension injuries on the other. Cases of hyper-rotation or lateral flexion were rare.

Reporting in the South African literature, Mennen[29] stated that the

Radiographs of the cervical spine show that the mechanism of injury in virtually all cases is an axial compression force with vary-

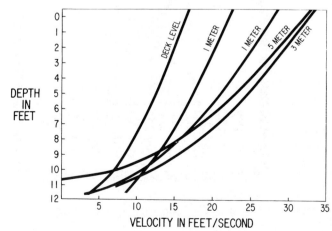

FIG 13–1.
Deceleration rates for dives from deck level, 1, 3, and 5 m. Observe the velocity as it relates to depth and the implications this has for impact to the head and neck.

ing degrees of flexion. . . . An overall picture of the "typical patient" involved in diving accidents was obtained: young male (±24 years), often responding to a challenge at a social gathering where alcohol consumption played an important role; the dive is often not the first attempt and is often into a pool of some sort or at a location that is familiar to the patient; the forehead strikes either the bottom of the pool, a rock, or a sandbank, without any additional injuries, e.g. to the hands; and the radiographs reveal a flexion-axial compression injury to the C4-C6 region of the cervical spine, leaving the majority of patients in a state of permanent and complete tetraplegia.

Scher[34] also reported from South Africa:

The frequency of compression fractures in association with scalp lacerations indicates that most patients sustained injury by direct impact to the vertex when diving into shallow water. Vertical compression injuries can only occur in those parts of the spine which are sufficiently mobile to be straightened, the cervical and lumbar regions. When the neck is slightly flexed, a severe force applied to the top of the head will cause the superior end plate of the vertebral body to fracture; the nucleus of the disc is then forced into the body, which bursts.

Tator et al.[41] observed that "in most cases the cervical spine was fractured and the spinal cord crushed when the top of the head struck the bottom of the lake or pool and not when the head struck the water" (Fig 13–2).

Tator and Edmonds[42] also reported that "shallow-water diving with the head striking the pool or lake bottom was the leading mechanism, with fracture-dislocation the most frequent type of spinal injury" (Fig 13–2). Meyer[30] stated, "When a rock and a hard place—in this case, the bottom of a body of water and one's head—meet, the result is a com-

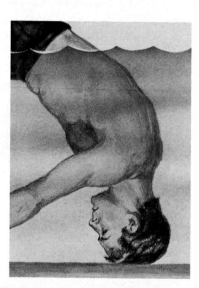

FIG 13–2.
Classic mechanism responsible for cervical spine injuries from diving is that of axial loading. The neck is slightly flexed, straightening the cervical spine. Abrupt deceleration of the head as it strikes the bottom of the lake or pool, associated with continued momentum of the torso, results in compressive deformation and ultimate failure of the cervical spinal structures, causing cord injury and quadriplegia.

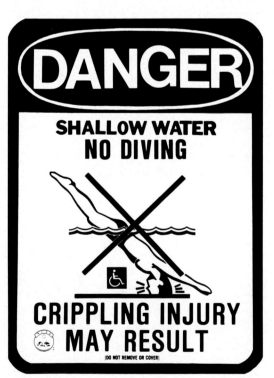

FIG 13–3.
Warning poster. *(Courtesy of the Aquatic Injury Safety Group.)*

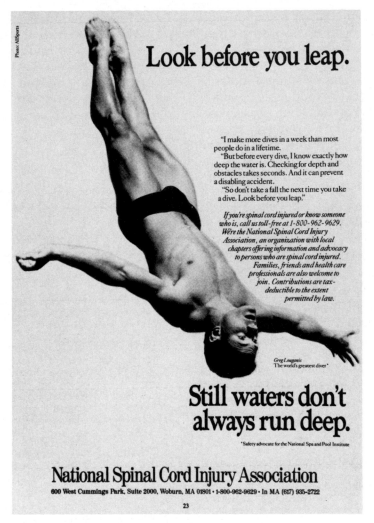

FIG 13–4.
Educational poster. *(Courtesy of the National Spinal Cord Injury Association.)*

pression force sufficient to blow out vertebrae and drive bone fragments into the spinal column."

In the Central Nervous System Trauma Status Report,[5] the following statement was made:

Evidence as to mechanism of injury has been claimed, in almost all reports, to be from contact between the head of the diver and the bottom of the water reservoir. That is, the diver's head strikes the bottom of the reservoir causing depression or burst fractures of the spinal column resulting in neurological damage.

The estimated annual occurrence of cervical spine fractures associated with spinal cord injury in the United States ranges from 600 to 1,800. Clearly, this represents a significant national health problem, a problem that deserves and requires a preventive effort on a national scale. The goal of such an effort should be directed at creating a general awareness of the dangers of diving. In view of the purportedly unblemished record of competitive diving programs, it appears that skill and technique are critical in avoiding these accidents. Consideration of the implementation of a carefully developed program to teach proper diving techniques to those in the at-risk group, that is, male individuals between 13 and 24 years of age, appears appropriate, as does a nationally coordinated educational program conducted on three levels.

Level 1 measures would consist of on-site warning signs and unsupervised educational devices, such as posters, radio and television spots, and newspapers (Figs 13–3 and 13–4).

Level 2 measures involve instruction of all school children in diving safety by professional instructors and teachers. By the age of 13 years, every school child in this country should be well indoctrinated in the danger of diving.

Level 3 instruction would involve teaching proper diving techniques to children and teenagers by qualified instructors.

In view of the potential for disaster associated with unsupervised water activities, it appears that enlightenment of the public with regard to the following guidelines is in order:

1. Do not dive into water that is shallower than twice your height. A 6 ft individual requires 12 ft of depth for safe diving.

2. Do not dive into unfamiliar water. Know the depth and be sure the water is free of submerged objects.

3. Do not assume water is deep enough, Familiar rivers, lakes, bays, and swimming holes change levels. Remember that at low tide there is 6 to 8 ft less depth than at high tide.

4. Do not dive near dredging or construction work. Water levels may change, and dangerous objects may lie beneath the surface.

5. Do not dive until the area is clear of other swimmers.

6. Do not drink and dive. Alcohol distorts judgment.

7. Do not permit or indulge in horseplay while swimming and diving.

8. Do not dive into the ocean surf or lakefront beaches. Diving is best confined to a properly maintained and supervised pool where the depth has been measured and marked.

REFERENCES

1. Albrand ON, Walter J: Underwater deceleration curves in relation to injuries from diving. *Surg Neurol* 1975; 4:461–464.

2. Botterell EH, Jousse AT, Kraus AS, et al: A model for the future care of acute spinal cord injuries. *Ann R Coll Phys Surg Can* 1975; 8:193–218.

3. Boyd MC, Schweigel JF: Diving-related spinal injuries in British Columbia. *BC Med J* 1985; 27:391–394.

4. Burke DC: Spinal cord injuries from water sports. *Med J Aust* 1972; 2:1190–1194.

5. Central Nervous System Trauma Status Report: *Epidemiological Aspects of Acute Spinal Cord Injury*, p 318; correspondence from MJ DeVivo, University of Alabama, Department of Rehabilitation Medicine.

6. Cheshire DJE: *The Complete and Centralized Treatment of Paraplegia: A Report on the Spinal Injuries Centre for Victoria, Australia.* Proceedings of the 16th Annual Clinical Spinal Cord Injury Conference, VA Hospital, Long Beach, Calif, Sept 27–29, 1967, pp 39–49.

7. DePassio J, Toraldo C, Minaire P, et al: Spinal injuries with neurologic signs resulting from the practice of sports. *Sem Hop Paris* 1983; 59:3131–3135.

8. Dietz PE, Baker SP: Drowning: Epidemiology and prevention. *Am J Pub Health* 1974; 64:303–312.

9. Enis JR, Green BA, Hall WJ, et al: Medical analysis of selected swimming pool injuries: Summary report for the US Consumer Product Safety Commission. University of Miami, Fla, 1985.

10. Frankel HL, Hancock DO, Hyslop G, et al: The value of postural reduction in the initial management of closed injuries of the spine with paraplegia and tetraplegia. Part I. *Paraplegia* 1969; 7:179–192.

11. Frankel HL, Montero FA, Penny PT: Spinal cord injuries due to diving. *Paraplegia* 1980; 18:118–122.

12. Gabrielson MA (ed): *Diving Injuries.* Report commissioned by the Council for National Co-operation in Aquatics (U.S.), 1981.

13. Gabrielson MA: *How Injuries Occur.* Presented to National Pool and Spa Safety Association, May 14, 1985.

14. Gjone RN: Personal communication. Sunnaas Sykehus, Nesoodon, Norway, 1974, to JF Kurtzke, Georgetown University School of Medicine, Washington, DC.

15. Good RP, Nickel VL: Cervical spine injuries resulting from water sports. *Spine* 1980; 5:502–506.

16. Green BA, Gabrielson MA, Hall WJ, et al: Analysis of swimming pool accidents resulting in spinal cord injury. *Paraplegia* 1980; 18:94–105.

17. Griffiths ER: Spinal injuries from swimming and diving treated in the Spinal Department of Royal Perth Rehabilitation Hospital: 1956–1978. *Paraplegia* 1980; 18:109–117.

18. Hall JC, Burke DC: Diving injury resulting in tetraplegia. *Med J Aust* 1978; 1:171.

19. Hill SA, Miller CA, Kosnik EJ, et al: Pediatric neck injuries. *J Neurosurg* 1984; 60:700–706.

20. Kewalramani LS, Taylor RG: Injuries to the cervical spine from diving accidents. *J Trauma* 1975; 15:130–142.

21. Kewalramani LS, Kraus JF: Acute spinal-cord lesions from diving—epidemiological and clinical features. *West J Med* 1977; 126:353–361.

22. Key AG, Retief PJ: Spinal cord injuries. Paper read at the International Medical Society of Paraplegia, Annual Scientific Meeting, Tel-Aviv, 1968. *Paraplegia* 1968; 243–249.

23. Kiwerski J: Cervical spine injuries caused by diving into water. *Paraplegia* 1980; 18:101–105.

24. Kraus JF, Franti CE, Riggins RS, et al: Incidence of traumatic spinal cord injuries. *J Chron Dis* 1975; 28:471–492.

25. Kurtzke JF: Epidemiology of spinal cord injury. *Exp Neurol* 1975; 48:163–236.

26. Little AD: *Diving Studies.* Research summary issued by the US National Swimming Pool Foundation (no date).

27. Lougheed WM, Bertrand G, Hay R: Paraplegic care in Canada. *Mod Med* 1969; 25:17–24.

28. McElhaney J, et al: *Biomechanical Analysis of Swimming Pool Neck Injuries.* Society of Automotive Engineers Technical Paper No. 790137, 1980.

29. Mennen U: A survey of spinal injuries from diving. *S Afr Med J* 1981; 59:788–790.

30. Meyer P: *JAMA* 1981; 245:1201–1206.

31. Minaire P, Castanier M, Girard R, et al: Epidemiology of spinal cord injury in the Rhone-Alpes region, France, 1970–75. *Paraplegia* 1978–79; 16:76–87.

32. Raymond CA: Summer's drought reinforces diving's dangers. *JAMA* 1988; 260:119–120.

33. Report of the Data Subcommittee to the National Swimming Pool Safety Commission, Oct 10, 1986.

34. Scher AT: Diving injuries to the cervical spinal cord. *S Afr Med J* 1981; 59:603–605.

35. Shields CL, Fox JM, Stouffer ES: Cervical cord injuries in sports. *Phys Sportsmed* 1978; 6:71–76.

36. Spinal Cord Injury Prevention Program. Position paper, October 1988. Canadian Paraplegic Association, B.C. Division and University Hospital, Shaughnessy site.

37. Steinbruck K, Paeslack V: Analysis of 139 spinal cord injuries due to accidents in water sports. *Paraplegia* 1980; 18:86–93.

38. Sutton NG: *Injuries of the Spinal Cord. The Management of Paraplegia and Tetraplegia,* London, Butterworth, 1973, p 185.

39. Tator CH, Edmonds VE: Acute spinal cord injury: Analysis of epidemiologic factors. *Can J Surg* 1979; 22:575–578.

40. Tator CH, Palm J: *The Issue of Spinal Injuries Due to Diving and Aquatic Activities.* Aquatic Spinal Injuries: Proceedings of the 1980 Symposium, Royal Life Saving Society Canada, pp 9–12.

41. Tator CH, Edmonds VE, New ML: Diving: A frequent and potentially preventable cause of spinal cord injury. *Can Med Assoc J* 1981; 124:1323–1324.

42. Tator CH, Edmonds VE: Sports and recreation are a rising cause of spinal cord injury. *Phys Sportsmed* 1986; 14:157–167.

43. The Report and Recommendations on Safety in

Amateur Sport, Personal Fitness and Physical Recreation in Ontario. The Ontario Sport Medicine and Safety Advisory Board, 1987.

44. Zrubecky G: Personal communication. Rehabilitation Center Tobelbad (Graz), Austria, 1974, to JF Kurtzke, Georgetown University School of Medicine, Washington, DC.

APPENDIX 13–1

Accidents Associated With Pool Use: Report of the Data Subcommittee to the National Swimming Pool Safety Committee,* December 1987

The National Swimming Pool Safety Committee was organized after the 1985 National Safety Conference, cosponsored by the U.S. Consumer Product Safety Commission (CPSC) and the National Spa and Pool Institute (NSPI). The Steering Committee comprises representatives from CPSC, NSPI, the U.S. Department of Education, and the American Academy of Pediatrics. Four subcommittees were formed by the Steering Committee to address issues pertinent to child drownings and diving accidents. The Data Subcommittee was charged with the following tasks: (1) to review research on the incidence of child drownings and diving accidents, making critical comments on this research in both areas; (2) to establish a Clearinghouse of information related to the incidence of child drownings and diving accidents; and (3) to recommend future directions for study and specific research needs. Subcommittee members represent government and municipal groups, the swimming pool industry, and the medical profession. Through their diversity, they have access to a wide range of information on pool use and water-related incidents. Research studies submitted were limited to primary sources published in the last ten years.

*Committee Member: Martha Scotzin, M.S., M.A., Chairman.

The Data Collection Subcommittee first met on Oct 9, 1985, and formulated a plan for commencing its work. It subsequently gathered and reviewed approximately 65 studies; in so doing, the basis for the Clearinghouse was established. A second meeting was held on June 9, 1986, to review an initial draft of this report and to discuss issues relevant to the tasks mentioned. The purposes of this report are (1) to summarize the findings of the research reviewed, (2) to make recommendations that may assist other subcommittees in their work, and (3) to suggest directions in which the CPSC and the NSPI might consider proceeding, based on this review.

Summary of Research Findings

To date, 27 studies on diving injuries and 38 studies on drownings were submitted and reviewed. In addition, ten articles on six state trauma registries (Florida,[4, 29] Maryland,[28, 31] Michigan,[32] New Jersey,[30] Oregon,[23] and Virginia[3]) were reviewed. One study,[39] not directly related to diving or drowning injuries, was reviewed as an example of how data collection and research efforts led to corrective measures in high school and college football programs.

Several problems were found in the diving and drowning research. The first had to do with the Subcommittee's interest in accurate incidence figures vs. the kinds of studies that are being conducted. While the Subcommittee was interested in obtaining a global assessment of the nature and extent of diving and drowning injuries, the studies reviewed were small in scale and focus. Some studies comprised only a few case reports. Large-scale attempts to determine the nationwide incidence of diving-related spinal cord injuries were able only to *estimate* the proportion of all injuries captured in their surveys. Thus there were no national figures for the annual incidence of either diving injuries or nonfatal submersions, and there were no mandatory reporting procedures, except for a few state spinal cord injury (SCI) registries that would either lend credence to, or refute, the incidence studies already conducted. Consequently, there is no mechanism for evaluating changes in incidence over time as a result of prevention efforts or pool technical standards.

The second problem was due to the nature of these accidents, several methodologic issues became apparent that question the validity of published research in this field. For example, none of the outcome studies used control groups and hence provided no basis for describing the extent of impairment or recovery of individuals involved. The difficulty in finding adequate control groups has long been documented in medical research.[38] Retrospective chart review was used extensively to study both diving and drowning. Coroners' records were used to study drownings. The period of time covered by these methods varied and was as long as 12 years. Consequently, little indepth information was available on human or environmental factors that may have led to injuries and drownings. These problems require comprehensive, reliable research about possible precipitating factors, such as the emotional environment at the time of the accident, drug or alcohol use, purpose of pool/spa use, time of day, weather conditions, number of persons present, and whether there was continuous supervision.

Three investigators improved their methodologies by sampling a particular geographic area, several sources of information, or using particularly clear criteria for inclusion in the research project. Gabrielson[12, 13] attempted to increase validity by combining chart review, review of rescue squad reports, newspaper accounts, documents submitted during litigation, and diving victim interviews. His method leads to a convergence of facts, and the resulting reports are remarkable

in breadth and detail. In a 5-year population study of freshwater drownings in Brisbane Australia, Pearn[25a] used loss of consciousness as the criterion for inclusion in the study. Conn et al.[3a, 3b] studied all cases of near drownings at a hospital in Toronto, Ontario, Canada during a 9-year period. Since these three studies have either involved large numbers of injuries or sampled a large proportion of the population at risk, they are helpful to people who are interested in forming tentative conclusions or would like to expand upon existing research.

The third problem is one with respect to definition of terms existing in the child drowning literature. There are differing opinions as to what constitutes a drowning versus a near-drown. Differences in the use of these terms may result in important differences in study design and data analysis. More importantly, since incidence figures are greatly affected by inconsistent terminology, a person may be differentially included or excluded from a treatment condition, based on the label given to his/her condition.

A fourth problem was the lack of control for accident site. It is possible that different types of pools/spas may have been sites of injuries of varying degrees of severity. Concomitantly, the severity of an accident may have been affected by the presence of a safety device. Detailed information regarding pool design and available warnings or protective devices, coupled with accident-specific data, was absent from nearly all of the research we reviewed, and could provide invaluable information to the pool industry and to consumers.

Research on Diving Accidents

Despite the discrepancies noted, there is consistency in the research findings. In most spinal cord injury incidence studies it is reported that approximately 10% of all spinal cord injuries are due to diving incidents.[2, 11, 17, 36] These studies suggest that diving injuries comprise a large proportion of all sports injuries (approximately 50% in the Canadian Paraplegic Association report, 75% in Guttman's[14] report, and 75% in Kurtzke's[17] report).

Similarly, there is agreement as to who is being injured. The prototypic diving accident victim is young, male, and white (see references 1, 2, 11–13, 20, 35, 37; also National Hospital Discharge Survey, 1985); however, blacks have proportionally twice the risk for diving injury than whites.[1, 11, 35] The injuries sustained from diving incidents are more likely to be quadriplegic than paraplegic.[7, 12, 13, 37] Studies of diving accident sites indicate that the majority of injuries occur in private backyard pools (45%[37]; 78%[41]; 54%.)[12, 13]

The New York Regional Spinal Cord Injury System[27] used data from the National Spinal Cord Injury Statistical Center (NSCISC)[22] to compare outcomes of SCI patients injured in diving accidents with SCI patients injured from other causes. The purposes were to (1) determine whether diving victims were different from patients with spinal cord injuries from other causes on a number of dimensions; (2) to document the course of a diving injury, relative to injuries from other causes; and (3) to determine whether patients with diving injuries incurred respiratory complications more frequently than other patients.

Patients injured from diving (N = 924) were first compared with patients of other etiologic categories (N = 9,888, e.g., motor vehicle accidents, gunshot wounds, and other sports injuries) on three demographic variables: age, sex, and race. They were also compared on seven variables related to severity of injury (e.g., functional impairment), course of treatment (e.g., secondary medical complications), and financial costs of SCI (e.g., SCI System hospital charges). Demographic information from the sample

supports the previously documented profiles of people with diving injuries. With use of a large sample of patients, it was demonstrated that patients with injuries from diving are significantly younger than others, are more likely to be white and male, are more severely impaired, and undergo a longer, more costly course of treatment than other patients.

Some reasons for these differences were the level and extent of lesion that was associated with differences on every variable; the cause of diving injuries was associated with age and longer stays in Spinal Cord System hospitals. Thus the severity of a diving injury affects more of the variables under study. The predicted incidence of respiratory complications was no higher than for the rest of the spinal cord–injured population.

Thus the differences found in diving-injured patients in medical status and financial costs were largely due to the type of injury sustained rather than to cause of injury alone. Complete, higher level lesions are associated with more medical complications and surgical procedures in-house, regardless of cause. Diving-injured patients are of serious concern to medical rehabilitation personnel because they comprise the most severely disabled group and require a longer, more costly course of treatment.

From the other research studies reviewed by the Subcommittee, survival rates are difficult to discern because of the differing methodologic designs and reporting techniques. Mesard et al.[20] report differential survival rates by age, time since injury, and level of lesion. The National Hospital Discharge Survey reported 80% of patients to be alive at discharge. Bracken et al.[1] reported an 11% fatality rate during inpatient hospitalization, with death rates increasing with age. In their study, 38% of patients admitted to hospitals in 18 California counties were dead on arrival. Failure Analysis Associates (1985) estimated there were 2,700 diving-related deaths nationwide between 1980 and 1981. Kurtzke[17] estimated that approximately 10% of all diving-injured patients die during hospitalization, and that there is approximately an 18-year life expectancy thereafter.

The possibility of drug or alcohol use as a factor in diving injuries was mentioned in four studies. Tator and Palm,[37] in their long-term (1948–1973) assessment of all acute SCI cases (diving and nondiving) in two Toronto hospitals, found evidence of alcohol intake in 30% of those injured. By comparison, Gabrielson[12, 13] determined in two studies that beer or other alcoholic beverages had been consumed in 40% and 38% of cases, respectively, while drug use was noted in 1% and 3%, respectively. Enis et al.[7] found that some alcohol was consumed by 20% of their sample, while drugs were used by 1%. Although the studies yield similar figures, there is a need for standardized research on the effects of drugs, and difficulties in obtaining accurate data on blood alcohol levels by emergency room personnel lead to the conclusion that drug/alcohol level studies may not be forthcoming.

In general, human factors and environmental conditions at the time of injury should be isolated in follow-up research so that investigators can accurately describe the behavior of victims and the aquatic environment at the injury site. Further, it is likely that many serious injuries not labeled as diving injuries occur at water sites as a result of carelessness or inattention to safety precautions. Working definitions used by researchers affect how an injury is classified. For example, spinal cord injuries may be classified as falls if the victim sustained his/her injury after being pushed into a pool or onto the deck area. In Wiley's[41] sample, 40% of those injured sustained falls near a pool. While these injuries were not classified as diving injuries per se, they may have consequences as serious as diving injuries, and should be sources of concern.

Arthur D. Little, Inc.[33, 34] was commissioned to investigate the mechanisms of diving and the potential for injury in pools of differing designs with different diving surfaces (e.g., springboard, pool deck). The initial study questions (ADL No. I, 1980) were to determine (1) the attainable water entrance velocities for different diver and board combinations, (2) the trajectory of divers, and (3) the velocity of divers in water. Later reports (ADL No. 2–10, 1980–1985) were concerned with suggested NSPI minimum design standards, design configuration changes, their consequences for the "worst case" diver, and diving from different surfaces.[18, 21] Study I argues against pool warning signs, suggesting that they provide a false sense of security and negate an opportunity for training novice divers to dive correctly. Instead, divers are responsible for "steering up" during a dive.

The Arthur D. Little studies make a valuable contribution to the technical literature on diving. The point is made in these reports (ADL 9-B, p 9) that "millions of divers have little or no trouble avoiding bottom contact in residential pools equipped with springboards" and that it is "relatively easy for a springboard diver to maneuver safely to avoid hitting bottom." A letter appended to a later report (ADL No. 10, attachment p 11), however, states, "I do not believe it is reasonable to attempt to design a facility that provides a water envelope . . . to accommodate the dive of one who does not steer up or who projects his dive in the direction of an open and obvious hazard such as a pool wall." The ADL studies advocate placing full responsibility for safe diving on the part of the diver, assuming that, once trained, all persons will dive in the proposed manner. Although no one can design a pool to account for all imprudent behaviors on the part of divers, the ADL report *requires* all divers to steer up on all occasions, making the assumption that human behavior is consistent.

In addition, there is no actual connection made between the presence of warning signs and potentially missed training opportunities. Signs should support training previously given to the diver and should assist in educating the novice. Safety training specialists have not suggested that one method can replace the other, but that multiple training materials and methods be combined. The ADL studies support such a concept (ADL No. IV, p 9) by advising that since engineering cannot possibly account for all human errors, "pools equipped with different types of diving boards be rated and labeled in accordance with the steering effort required to avoid bottom contact. In this way, pool owners and divers can be informed as to what is required to assure safe use." This is an effective suggestion, combining the needs for specific safety information on the product with education of the diver as to the requirements for his/her behavior. The same principle applies to other warning information around pools. It is not a missed training opportunity, but a chance for the swimming pool industry to provide sufficient information for swimmers to dive intelligently. Such labels can be regular reminders to divers of the need to steer up.

Information is available on the efficacy of signs associated with intervention efforts. In Florida, a central SCI registry was established in 1982.[9, 10] In 1980 the Feet First First Time program was established to caution the public about diving into water of unknown depth. Signs, buttons, T-shirts, and a media campaign conveyed their message. Since the Feet First Program commenced, there has been a 40% drop in Florida diving injuries (Campbell T: Personal communication, October 1986).

SUMMARY AND REVIEW—DIVING INJURY RESARCH

To summarize the data reviewed on diving injuries, several points can be made:

1. The diving injury literature presents a consistent profile of the prototypic diving victim as young, white, and male. With this information available, and knowing that diving injuries are preventable, preventive and educational efforts should be particularly geared to *this population* (i.e., young men between the ages of 15 and 30).

2. Though sufficient data do not exist to document the effectiveness of specific warnings and signs around pools, a majority of the Subcommittee agrees that signage is an important factor in all accident prevention, that "no diving" signs should be placed at appropriate locations around pools, and that depth markers should be placed around pools. It is the majority opinion that signs, in general, are effective in guiding and warning the public of potential hazards in all areas of our lives and that it is the obligation of pool owners and/or managers to provide guidance in the safe use of pools. Signs associated with an injury prevention campaign have been effective in dramatically reducing the number of diving injuries in one state. A minority of persons on the Subcommittee is of the opinion that this conlusion is premature without additional substantiating data.

3. Since specific studies of the effectiveness of particular types of pool signs are lacking, investigation should be undertaken to study which are most effective and how swimmers attend to them.

4. Ex post facto investigations of drug and alcohol use before accidents is recommended to explore human factors that may have led to the accident. Two problems inherent in conducting such investigations are recognized: the difficulty

in obtaining blood alcohol levels within a prescribed time period after the accident and the potential invalidity of self-reporting. Despite these difficulties, it is recommended that an independent organization conduct follow-up research on diving accident admissions to emergency rooms.

5. Although accurate yearly figures on the incidence and prevalence of diving injuries are needed, no mechanism currently exists within the federal government to undertake a nationwide investigation of diving injuries, or to establish a national reporting procedure. The Center for Injury Control (CIC) is presently being established in Atlanta, under guidelines from the National Academy of Science Committee on Trauma Research. The CIC is charged with operating a general injury surveillance system. It is recommended that the Steering Committee contact the CIC to determine whether a national injury reporting network is planned, and, if so, whether specific information on diving accidents will be included in the reporting procedures. It is also recommended that the Steering Committee work with as many states as possible in establishing SCI registries. The potential benefits of mandatory reporting are an accurate yearly incidence rate; establishment of a data base that can include information such as etiology and environmental conditions; and use of the data base as a comparison group in future treatment studies.

These five points imply that diving accidents and their prevention are the responsibility of the diver *and* those who build and manage pools. Consumers cannot use pool equipment recklessly, assuming that recreational equipment is foolproof and that they have no responsibility for their behavior. They must know how and where to dive safely through aquatic training programs and reminders. The pool industry is not absolved from providing all information at its disposal to consumers and from taking an active role in consumer education. The most effective approach to safe diving will involve all parties informally and formally, with use of as many methods as possible to create safe recreational activities.

REFERENCES

1. Bracken MB, Freeman DH, Hillenbrand K: Incidence of acute traumatic hospitalized spinal cord injury in the United States, 1970–1977. *Am J Epidemiol* 1981; 113:615–622.

2. Canadian Paraplegic Association: *Spinal Cord Injury Statistics*, 1974–1985.

3a. Conn AW, Edmonds JF, Barker GA: Cerebral resuscitation in near-drowning. *Ped Clinics North Amer* 1979; 26:691—700.

3b. Conn AW, Montes JE, Barker GA, et al: Cerebral salvage in near-drowning following neurological classification by triage. *Can Anaesth Soc J* 1980; 27:201–210.

3. Commonwealth of Virginia Combined Head Injury and Spinal Cord Injury Central Registry, Virginia Department of Rehabilitation Services.

4. Deauville L: *Central Registry for Spinal Cord Injured and Other Severely Disabled Individuals.* Tallahassee, Fla, Department of Health and Rehabilitative Services.

5. DeVivo MJ, Fine PR, Maetz M, et al: Prevalence of spinal cord injury: A reestimation employing life table techniques. *Arch Neurol* 1980; 37:707–708.

6. Dworkin GM: Spinal immobilization in deep water. *J Emerg Med Services* 1983; 35–39.

7. Enis JR, Green BA, Hall WJ, et al: *Medical Analysis of Selected Swimming Pool Injuries: Summary Report for the U.S. Consumer Product Safety Commission.* Miami, Fla, University of Miami, 1985.

8. Ergas Z: Spinal cord injury in the United States: A statistical update. *Cent Nerv Syst Trauma* 1985; 2:19–31.

9. Ferris BC: *Spinal Cord Injury Prevention/ Education Project Fiscal Year 1982–83 Annual Report.* Florida Department of Health and Rehabilitative Services, 1983.

10. Ferris BC: *Spinal Cord Accident Prevention/ Education Project Fiscal Year 1983–84 An-*

nual Report. Florida Department of Health and Rehabilitative Services, 1984.

11. Fine PR, Kuhlemeier KV, DeVivo MJ, et al: Spinal cord injury: An epidemiological perspective. *Paraplegia* 1979; 17:237–250.

12. Gabrielson MA: Preliminary summary: Case studies of spinal cord injury victims who were injured as a result of diving or sliding into swimming pools. Unpublished report, 1985.

13. Gabrielson MA: Regional symposium on spinal cord injuries as a result of diving accidents. Paper presented at the American Alliance for Health, Physical Education, Recreation, and Dance Aquatic Council, Atlanta, Ga, 1985.

14. Guttman L: General Statistics and Legal Aspects. *Spinal Cord Injuries: Comprehensive Management and Research.* Oxford, Blackwell Scientific, 1976.

15. Kalsbeek WD, McLaurin RL, Harris BSH, et al: The national head and spinal cord injury survey: Major findings. *J Neurosurg* 1980; 53:S19–S31.

16. Kraus JF, Franti CE, Riggins RS, et al: Incidence of traumatic spinal cord lesions. *J Chron Dis* 1975; 28:471–492.

17. Kurtzke JF: Epidemiology of spinal cord injury. *Exp Neurol* 1975; 48:163–236.

18. McCarthy GE, Robinson JN: Spa and pool safety: A quantitative risk analysis. Alexandria, Va, National Spa and Pool Institute, 1985.

19. Medical epidemiologist, Department of Health and Human Services: *Report on the National Hospital Discharge Survey.* National Center for Health Statistics, 1985.

20. Mesard L, Carmody A, Mannarino E, et al: Survival after spinal cord trauma. *Arch Neurol* 1978; 35:78–83.

21. National Spa and Pool Institute: 1984 swimming pool and spa industry survey. Alexandria, Va, National Spa and Pool Institute, 1985.

22. National Spinal Cord Injury Statistical Center: *Annual Report No. 3.* University of Alabama in Birmingham, October 1985.

23. Oregon State Health Division Trauma Registry, September 1985.

24. Paralyzed Veterans of America: *SCI Veterans Administration Demographic and Health Care Utilization Data, 1976–1982.*

25. Paralyzed Veterans of America: *Spinal Cord Injury Statistics.* Washington, DC, PVA.

25a. Pearn J: Neurological and psychometric studies in children surviving freshwater immersion accidents. *Lancet* 1977; 1:7–9.

26. Peters GA: Warning signs and safety instructions: Covering all the bases. *Risk Management* 1985; 64–66.

27. Scotzin Shaver M, DeVivo MJ, Rutt RD, et al: A comparison of medical outcomes of diving patients and those of other etiologies. Paper presented at the annual meeting of the American Congress of Rehabilitation Medicine, Kansas City, October 1986.

28. Silverman J: State of Maryland Rehabilitation Information Service, Disabled Individual Reporting System, 1985.

29. Spinal cord injury central registry, 1984–1985, Florida Department of Health and Rehabilitative Services, November 1985.

30. Spinal cord injury early notification system, New Jersey Department of Health.

31. State of Maryland Rehabilitation Information Service, Department of Health and Mental Hygiene. Copy of House Bill proposing a registry of disabled individuals.

32. State of Michigan Amendment to Act No. 368 of Public Acts of 1978, establishing a spinal cord injury registry.

33. Stone RS: Diving safety in swimming pools. A report to the National Swimming Pool Foundation. Arthur D. Little, Inc., 1980.

34. Stone RS: Unpublished reports and correspondence to the National Swimming Pool Foundation. Arthur D. Little, Inc., 1981–1985.

35. Stripling T, Fonsecs JE, Tsou V, et al: A demographic study of spinal cord injured veterans. *J Am Paraglegia Soc* 1983; 6:62–66.

36. Tator CH, Edmonds VE: Acute spinal cord injury: Analysis of epidemiologic factors. *Can J Surg* 1979; 22:575–578.

37. Tator CH, Palm J: The issue of spinal injuries due to diving and aquatic activities in *Aquatic Spinal Injuries.* The Royal Life Saving Society of Canada.

38. Taylor SE, Lichtman RR, Wood JV: Attributions, beliefs about control, and adjustment to breast cancer. *J Pers Soc Psychol* 1985; 46:489–502.

39. Torg J: The National Football Head and Neck Injury Registry, 1971–1984. *JAMA* 1985; 254:3439–3443.

40. Weiner RI: A statistical analysis of quadriplegia and paraplegia from aquatic diving and its implications on effective measures of reduction. Unpublished paper, 1983.

41. Wiley J: Diving injuries: The medical perspective, in *Aquatic Spinal Injuries*. Toronto, The Royal Life Saving Society of Canada.

42. Young JS, Burns PE, Bowen AM, et al: Spinal cord injury statistics: Experience of the regional spinal cord injury systems. Phoenix, Ariz, Rehabilitation Services Administration, 1982.

CHAPTER 14

Spinal Cord Injuries in Football—Rugby Union, Rugby League, and Australian Rules

Thomas K. F. Taylor, M.D.

Myles R. J. Coolican, M.D.

Football in its various forms or codes is a popular game in Australia. As a body contact sport, football carries the inherent risk of injury. This chapter is largely based on information gathered in a retrospective survey of spinal cord injuries sustained by Australian footballers during the period 1960–1985.[14] The study was undertaken because in the early 1980s there were an alarming number of players and notably schoolboys admitted to the Spinal Cord Injuries Unit of The Royal North Shore Hospital, Sydney. It then became apparent that the problem urgently needed definition since there were no accurate data available pertaining to these devastating sporting injuries in this or in any other countries where the games are played.

EARLY HISTORY OF FOOTBALL

The Games—Rugby Union, Rugby League, and Australian Rules*

Most sports played today, including football, have gradually evolved during several centuries. The injuries that may be associated with them are linked in one way or another to the manner in which the games are played, and this, in turn, is the outcome of their evolution. Accordingly, a brief account of the histories of these three codes is in order.

The modern games of football (soccer, Rugby, American football, and Australian Rules) are all derivatives of the melees of ancient and medieval Britain. Rugby League is a derivative of Rugby. In a melee an object, usually an inflated and variously encased animal bladder, was kicked, punched, or carried toward a

*The authors made extensive reference to *Encyclopaedia Britannica* (1971) when researching historical facts pertaining to Rugby Union and Rugby League.

goal. The opponents would, by whatever means possible, attempt to prevent the goal being scored. How medieval Britons came to devise such a game is shrouded in mystery and in myth. The Romans while in Britain probably played a game called harpastum, in which a team of players tried to force a ball beyond a line drawn behind their opponents. The melees may have their origin in this form of contest. Whatever its origins, football grew in popularity and spread across Britain, albeit with many rule variations. History records that a game was played annually on Shrove Tuesday at Chester and that the first ball used was the head of a captured Danish warrior! Football thereby may have its genesis as a form of deterrent to any would-be enemy, as well as being a novel way of celebrating gladiatorial victory.

The popularity of these games increased among the citizens of Britain, and regular matches were arranged between neighboring villages. The ruling classes, however, feared that devotion to such madness would diminish the time young men spent training in archery and in other skills of war. Football was banned by Edward III in 1365, because it was seen as a threat to the ability to defend the country. Further edicts were made by subsequent monarchs, but fortunately these were no more successful than similar Scottish pronouncements against the playing of "Gowffe." In 1602 Richard Carew recorded that goals were set three or four miles apart, and multiple parishes united to play against one another; by the 1800s the games were more like the modern versions. In 1801 Strutt described a match in which an equal number of players from each side took the field and goals were placed 80 to 100 yards apart. The violence of these matches was considerable, and other historians have reported that broken shins and heads were the minor casualties. It

has been said that a Frenchman, after watching a game at Derby, remarked that if the English called this playing, it would be impossible to say what they would call fighting.

The growth of the English public (i.e., private) schools in the 18th century provided the catalyst for modern football. The sons of rich, aristocratic families were confined for long periods in winter without access to their usual sports, particularly horseback riding and fencing. Rowdy games were adopted in one form or another that closely resembled the games long played by the working man. These were regarded by the universities as undignified and unsuited to gentlemen, particularly for those bent on an academic life. Nevertheless, the game flourished at schoolboy level. The type of football played depended on where the school was. For example, Westminster School in London played on cobblestones, and so indulged in a game similar to modern soccer. Rugby School in central England was surrounded by farms. Here the boys had grass to play on, and so a more body contact game was started. Of the original game played at Rugby School, there were two significant rules. First, players were not allowed to pick up the ball—it had to be kicked. Second, if the ball were kicked into the air and caught, all players (including the catcher) stood still. The catcher could either placekick or punch the ball toward his opponents' goal, but he could not run with it, nor could he be tackled. Legend says that in 1823 a 16-year-old lad called William Webb Ellis caught the ball and, instead of standing still in preparation to kicking the ball, ran toward his opponents' goal line. Subsequently this became normal practice. The "pass" was the next step to develop and was allowed, provided the catcher was behind the ball carrier. From these beginnings developed the modern game of Rugby, which was named after the school in central England. Soccer developed in parallel to Rugby, but neither is a derivative of the other.

During subsequent years various rules were developed and distributed, and these allowed matches between schools. Independent clubs were formed, the first being Guy's Hospital Football Club in 1843. Soccer and Rugby finally parted ways in 1863 with the formation of the Football Association and the publication of "Rules of the London Football Association." Rugby formally began in 1871 with the formation of the Rugby Football Union and the drafting of laws.

Rugby Union

Rugby is occasionally referred to as Rugby Union or simply Union to distinguish it from Rugby League. Occasionally the term rugger is used. It is a body contact sport played with an air-filled oval leather ball, slightly larger and less pointed than an American football. Teams of fifteen compete on a grass field of play 100 m long and 69 m wide. Play is divided into two halves, each no longer than 40 minutes plus injury time, with a halftime break of 5 minutes, after which teams change ends. There are no time-outs and no substitutions, except for injury. All players play "offense" and "defense." Coaches are expressly forbidden to send messages onto the field, and the captain of each team makes all on-field decisions.

A Rugby team is divided into eight forwards and seven backs. Each player wears a number on his jersey for identification. Forwards are generally bigger, heavier men who require some of the skills of interior linemen. Forwards participate in scrums, rucks, mauls, and line-outs, while backs assume a positional formation in preparation for either attack or defense, depending on which forward pack wins the contest for the ball. Forwards are divided into the front, second, and back rows (Fig 14–1). The front row consists of two props and a hooker. The left-sided prop is called a loose-head prop, so named because in scrummage his head is free on one side. The tight-head prop and hooker are sandwiched by the opposing front row, which makes them more vulnerable to spinal cord injury in a scrummage collapse. One of the hooker's jobs is to win the ball at scrummage by hooking it back with his feet.

The second row consists of two players, usually big, tall men who may be referred to in New Zealand as locks. These men push in the scrum and jump to catch or deflect the ball in lineouts. The back row consists of two breakaways (flankers) and a lock, who may be known as a number eight (his jersey is always number eight). The back row are usually big, fast men who require the skills and attitudes of the American football linebacker as well as some ball handling skills.

The backs, who tend to be smaller, fast men require good ball handling, agility, and tackling skills. The scrum-half (halfback) is the link between forwards and backs, and needs a good pass to speed the ball to the back line. Scrum-halves are often stockily built men with rapid acceleration from the stationary position. The fly-half, also known as the out-half or five-eighth, is the linchpin of attack and frequently decides which option to use in attack. His abilities should include kicking accurately with both feet and the ability to break a line of defense. The outside backs are referred to as three-quarters and include inside and outside centers and left and right wings. These are players who are frequently fast, with good ball and tackling skills. The full-back is the last line of defense. He is also an attacking player and joins the back line on occasions. He can also relieve pressure with long kicks.

The game is controlled by one referee who is assisted by two touch judges. The touch judges raise a flag if the ball is out

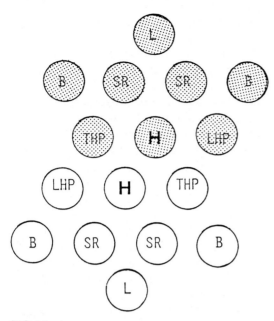

FIG 14–1.
Positions of forwards from opposing teams in a Rugby Union scrum. *L,* lock, *B,* breakaway, *SR,* second row, *THP,* tight-head prop, *H,* hooker, *LHP,* loose-head prop. *(From Taylor TKF, Coolican MRJ: Med J Aust 1987; 147:112–118. Used with permission.)*

of touch (out of bounds), and they are encouraged to report foul play to the referee. The latter has power to overrule the touch judges and has total control, as evidenced by the time-honored phrase of law six: "The referee is the sole judge of fact and law."

The object of the game is (by passing, running with, and kicking the ball) to outscore the opponents and thereby win the match. A try (similar to the touchdown of American football) is worth four points and is scored by a player grounding the ball in his opponents' "in-goal." This is an area beyond the goal line and is equivalent to the end zone of American football. A goal (also known as conversion) is worth two points and is scored when a player either placekicks or dropkicks the ball from opposite the point where the try was scored. The ball must pass above the crossbar and between the uprights, the latter distance being 25% less than in National Football League

(NFL) football. A penalty goal worth three points is a placekick or dropkick passing above the crossbar, from a penalty kick awarded by the referee for an infringement by the opposing team. A field goal, also worth three points, is a dropkick taken at any time in general play where the ball passes above the crossbar.

Play begins with a kickoff, and the team in position may run with, or pass the ball, or kick it upfield or into touch. If the ball or a player carrying it goes into touch (i.e. out of bounds) play is restarted with a lineout. In a lineout both sets of forwards line up parallel to the goal line with their backs in various formations behind them. The nonoffending team throws the ball down the center line where both teams try to gain possession and give the ball to their backs. The backs may run with the ball, kick it, or pass to a teammate provided he is level with, or behind, the ball carrier. When a player is tackled, that is, brought to the ground and held by an opponent, he must release the ball immediately, whereupon other players may gain possession. Frequently a struggle for possession will occur after a tackle, which to the uninformed would appear to be similar to the wild melees of medieval Britain. To the Rugby enthusiast it is a controlled event; it is called a ruck if the ball is on the ground, and a maul if the ball carrier is standing and surrounded by players from both teams. If neither team is able to win the ball quickly, the referee blows a whistle and a scrum is formed.

The scrum, which is by far the most common phase of play that produces cervical spinal cord injuries, is formed by each forward pack forming-up and linking (binding) together in readiness for the ball to be put in down the center line (see Fig 14–1). The ball almost always goes to the team putting the ball (feeding) into the scrum. It is paramount to acknowledge that a scrum is simply a method of restarting play after an infringement and is no more than this. If engagement of the front rows is uncontrolled, or if the players are inexperienced and unsure of which way to put their heads, a clash of heads can occur. The result of major axial loading on the cervical spine on engagement may be one of catastrophic neurologic consequences. While for many years the laws of Rugby expressly forbade a team charging at scrummage, they were observed more in the breach than the concurrence. After engagement and when both sets of forwards push against the other, a "collapse" of the scrum may occur.

The laws of Rugby published by the International Rugby Board include some regulations relating to equipment. Almost all of the standard equipment of American football is illegal. This includes helmets, shoulder harnesses, knee braces, wrestling style ear protectors, and virtually anything containing metal or hard plastic. Most players take the field wearing Rugby shorts and jersey, socks, and Rugby boots. Mouth guards are encouraged but are not essential. Forwards may tape their ears to the sides of their heads to prevent chapping at scrummage, and some players wear a soft leather head and ear protector to help prevent cauliflower ears. Boots and studs (also known as cleats) are inspected at each match, and must conform to regulations.

Rugby League

Rugby League (occasionally known simply as League), which is played predominantly in the north of England, France, and Australia, is a direct descendant of Rugby Union. A split occurred in England during the late 19th century when 22 member clubs formed the Northern Union, later to become the English Rugby Football League. The split was centered on the issue of professionalism. Rugby Union is, and has always been, an amateur game. At the Annual General Meeting of the Rugby Football Union in 1883, a proposal by Yorkshire clubs to permit the payment of compensation for loss of working time due to injury or match commitments during working hours was defeated. A similar split occurred in Australia approximately 10 years later when J. J. Giltinan helped to form what was destined to become the Australian Rugby Football League. The game began in earnest in France in the 1930s after a ban was placed on French Rugby by the British Unions. These Unions were dissatisfied with the control and conduct of the game in France, but quickly restored the French to their former position just before World War II, to halt the spreading popularity of Rugby League in that country.

The Northern Union gradually amended the older Rugby laws to make the game more open and interesting for spectators, and hence to attract larger crowds. The principal differences between Rugby and Rugby League had evolved by the early part of this century. The major variations are that in League:

- The tackled player stands and rolls the ball through his legs with a foot to restart play, rather than releasing the ball.
- When the ball crosses the touch (boundary) line, play is restarted with a scrum and not a lineout.
- Two forwards (breakaways or flankers) have been removed.
- There is a restriction in the time a team may keep possession of the ball. Presently this is for six tackles irrespective of any territory gained or lost.
- There are slight differences in the number of points allocated for the various scoring maneuvers.

Relationships between the two Rugby codes have not always been entirely cordial, but, despite some differences, there have been relatively few major problems.

Most players continue with the code learned at school, but in the adult arena there is some competition for the potential player population. Rugby Union players of exceptional ability are occasionally paid large sums to transfer to Rugby League, and quite a number of men have achieved national representative status in both codes. Professional Rugby League players are automatically banned from Rugby Union for life.

Differences Between Rugby and American Football

There are clearly many differences between American football and Rugby, not the least reason being that neither is a derivative of the other. There are certain fundamental differences between the two games worthy of comment. Both evolved separately from the medieval British melee. American football is territorial; hence one of its names gridiron to describe the transverse lines every 5 yards that are necessary in a game where every inch counts. Defense in such a territorial game therefore attempts to drive a man back, rather than grounding him. Therefore, tackling has become "hitting" that is much harder than in Rugby. Protective pads and helmets are required because of this, or is it that such protection takes away the fear of injury in the defensive player and promotes more violent hitting? Penalties in American football are in yards, rather than in possession of the ball as in Rugby. Substitutes and time-outs are not allowed in Rugby, and players do considerably more running, which promotes a higher level of aerobic fitness. There are few really big men in Rugby (250 pounds or more), perhaps because of the inability of men of this size to achieve the extra level of fitness needed for a continuous, high-athletic performance for 80 minutes. Steroid use in Rugby players is not unknown, but it is extremely rare, probably because it does not confer an advantage to most players.

Australian Rules*

The influx of free settlers from Great Britain and Ireland to this country (then still largely a penal colony) in the early part of the 19th century saw the introduction of football in its nascent forms. While debate continued in England concerning the issue of whether the ball should be carried, this largely centering on class distinctions, the matter was shortly settled in the antipodes. The admixture of English, Irish, and Scottish rules made for confusion. Further, on arrival in Australia the immigrants found themselves in a climate that permitted outdoor games all year round. The catalyst for the needed organization was provided by Thomas Wills, an Australian who had been sent to Rugby School in England for his education. This man, who was a cricketer of exceptional ability, saw football as being a means of keeping cricketers fit during the winter months!

In his now famous letter to Melbourne's sporting journal, "Bell's Life in Victoria," Wills called for the young men of Melbourne to play football during the summer, adding that if the matches were played on existing cricket fields, the grass would be "trampled upon making the turf quite firm and durable." As grass was chosen for the playing surface, both handling the ball and tackling were feasible. Hence the Australian version of football was destined to become a body contact sport. Wills and others were able to draw on the already established cricketing organization, in particular the Melbourne Cricket Club, to promote football. The earlier games were somewhat disorganized as one player recalled:

While a large percentage were Rugby players from England, still not a few hailed from Ireland and Scotland, all eager to refresh

*In writing this section we drew on information contained in Mancini A, Hibbins GM (eds): *Running With the Ball*. Melbourne, Lynedoch Publications, 1987.

their memories with the games of their far-away homes. Englishmen of course played Rugby, Scotchmen a nondescript game, . . . while Irishmen contented themselves by yelling and punting the ball as straight as a die heavenwards. Each man played a lone hand or foot, according to his lights, some guided by their particular code of rules, others by no rules at all.

Rules were needed, and at a historic meeting in May 1859 Wills and several colleagues framed the rules of the Melbourne Football Club. These men were concerned about the violence of the more favored Rugby game and legislated accordingly. The rules were first published in the 1858–1859 edition of *The Australian Cricketers Guide* as "The Rules of the Melbourne Football Club as played in Richmond Paddock." Subsequently, the game rapidly spread to Tasmania and westwards across the country. Today it is the second most popular code of football played in Australia.

Australian Rules is played on an oval, grassed field by 18 players from each side whose object is to kick the ball through the center two of four upright goalposts at their opponents' end of the ground. The field is between 150 and 200 m long and 125 to 140 m wide. A circle, 3 m in diameter, indicates where a field umpire bounces the ball at the beginning of each quarter and after a goal is scored to commence play.

The leather ball is oval shaped and at 725 mm long and 550 mm in maximum circumference is considerably bigger and heavier than an American football.

The game lasts 100 minutes and is divided into 25-minute quarters. In practice most quarters last an average of 30 minutes because the clock is stopped when the ball is not in play. There are no time-outs, but at halftime there is a 20-minute break, and at the end of every other quarter, a five-minute break. The four goalposts are each 6.4 m apart, the center two being slightly taller. The ball kicked

through the center two posts is a goal worth six points; when kicked between the center and outer posts it is called a "behind" and is worth one point.

The match is controlled by six umpires, consisting of two field umpires, two boundary umpires, and two goal umpires. The field umpires working in each half of the ground have full control of play and award penalties in accordance with the laws. Boundary umpires indicate if the ball, or a player carrying it, has crossed the boundary line, and goal umpires indicate scores by the use of flags.

Australian Rules football is built around the kick, which is the only mechanism by which a goal can be scored. The most common type of kick is a drop punt, which results in the ball spinning end over end. It is preferred by most players because of its accuracy. In contrast, the torpedo punt, which some players can kick up to 70 m, is used for distance. Dropkicking is also permitted. When the ball is caught cleanly after a kick, a mark is awarded and the player is entitled to kick the ball from the spot where the mark was taken and without opponent interference. High marking as the ball descends toward a pack of football players is one of the most spectacular features of the game. Players may also run with the ball, but they must bounce it in front of them every 15 yards. The ball may be passed to a teammate in any direction, but this move must be done by tapping it out of the palm of the hand with the fist. Throwing the ball is illegal. A player running with the ball may be tackled in a fashion similar to American football, and the tackler may come from any direction. Hence a ball carrier may be unaware of an imminent tackle. The tackled player must immediately release the ball. If play cannot continue because a tackled player has been unable to release the ball, the umpire restarts play by bouncing the ball between two players, so that each team has an equal chance of gaining possession.

Australian Rules does not have the scrum, ruck, or maul that are so common in Rugby. This means that the combined momentum of several players does not often fall upon a single cervical spine. For this reason alone, catastrophic cervical cord injury in Australian Rules is far less common than in Rugby. The majority of cervical spinal cord injuries occur as a result of "one-on-one" player collisions.

Football in Australia

Rugby Union and Rugby League are played principally in New South Wales and Queensland. Australian Rules is by far and away the major code in Victoria, South Australia, and Western Australia. Soccer is played in all states and is becoming increasingly popular because of the influence of the immigrant population during the last several decades. Not surprisingly, there are no accurate national data on the numbers of games played in each code per season nor on the number of players involved at different levels of the code, including schoolboys.

Estimates of player numbers in 1985 were as follows:

- Soccer   445,856
- Australian Rules   303,100
- Rugby League   162,220
- Rugby Union   83,610

It is relevant to state that there are no data pertaining to player populations, nor are other relevant data back to the early 1960s available.

The Australian Experience in Injuries to the Spinal Cord in Football.— There are six well-organized spinal cord injury centers in Australia, two of which are in New South Wales. These function quite independently of each other. There is no such center in Tasmania nor in the Northern Territory. It has long been accepted by the medical profession that all spinal cord injuries are best managed in these units, and early transfer is both encouraged and strongly supported even though this may involve considerable travel. Despite the popular view of Australia, it is, after Belgium, the second most urbanized country in the world. A great deal of football is played in country areas.

In the period 1960–1985, 107 footballers were admitted to the spinal cord injury centers cited. Inasmuch as hospital records are most often grossly inadequate, as well as incorrect, in describing how the injury was incurred, 92 of these players were personally interviewed, as well as were 7 of the 8 families of those players who had later perished. Seven players, five of whom resided overseas, could not be contacted. It was quite striking, although readily understandable, how players and their families could recall in vivid detail the exact circumstances of their injuries.

Seventeen players were injured in Australian Rules games. There was but a minor increase in the number during the period 1977–1985; 69% of the players sustained their injuries when they collided with other players but were not actually in possession of the ball. Tackles accounted for 19% of the injuries in this code. During the time-span of the study, one patient only was injured at soccer, and he had "headed" a heavy, wet ball. The injury rates for these two codes, given the quoted player populations, speak for themselves in terms of the relative safety of the games compared with the two Rugby codes. The safety factor for these and for other injuries is one reason for the current popularity of soccer, which has recently been introduced in many private schools in Australia, schools that were once the bastions of Rugby Union.

Major axial loading of the cranium

and cervical spine is also capable of producing vascular insufficiency and differential distortion of the brain and the spinal cord.[11] This injury pattern, which may be fatal, has been described in players who used the defensive tactic of "spearing." Schneider et al.[11] suggested that acute vascular insufficiency in the vertebrobasilar system, probably intensified at the C-2 level by a marginal collateral supply, together with disparate distortion between the freely moving brain and the relatively fixed upper cervical cord, were responsible. At autopsy in these patients, petechial hemorrhages at the C2 level were demonstrated. This type of injury was not observed in the Australian survey.

Annual Frequency.—Data are given in Table 14–1 and Fig 14–2. Composite figures for the three codes, excluding soccer, are also depicted. It is to be noted that in Rugby Union no injuries occurred in schoolboys between 1960 and 1976, whereas in the eight subsequent seasons, 11 injuries took place, an alarming figure.

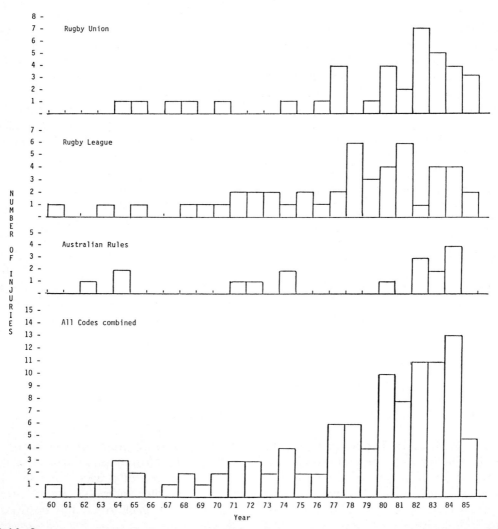

FIG 14–2.
Spinal cord injuries from Rugby Union, Rugby League, Australian Rules, and all codes combined. *(From Taylor TKF, Coolican MRJ: Med J Aust 1987; 147:112–118. Used with permission.)*

TABLE 14–1.

Injuries in Australian Football Players 1960–1985

	No. of Injuries (Average/yr)			
	Adults		Schoolboys	
Code	1960–1976	1977–1985	1960–1976	1977–1985
Rugby Union	7(0.4)	19(2.1)	0	11(1.2)
Rugby League	13(0.8)	29(3.2)	3(0.2)	3(0.3)
Australian Rules	7(0.4)	9(1.0)	0	1(0.1)
Soccer	0	1(0.1)	0	0
Totals	27(1.6)	58(6.4)	3(0.2)	15(1.7)

From Taylor TFK, Coolican MRJ: Med J Aust 1987; 147:112–118. Used with permission.

Age.—The average age for all injured players was 22 years, with a peak incidence at 18 years. The youngest player was 14 years of age, and a total of six players were in the age range of 14–16 years. We were unable to demonstrate that age was a modulating factor either on the mechanism of injury or on the subsequent recovery.

Player Positions.—These are given for both Rugby codes in Table 14–2. Twenty-seven of the players were hookers, but not all were injured in scrummage. In all but one instance, scrum injuries occurred to front row forwards. Approximately one fifth of the injuries occurred when a player was in a position he did not normally play, and two thirds of these injuries were in scrums.

Phase of Play.—These data are given in percentages in Table 14–3. For both codes, where a player was injured in a tackle, in 76% of the cases it was the ball carrier and in the remainder the tackler.

Scrum Injuries.—Thirty-seven players sustained their injuries in scrummage. The mechanisms were analyzed in detail for both adults and schoolboys (Table 14–4). By and large, those injured in scrums, rucks, and mauls were able to recount exactly what had transpired, whereas those injured in tackles often related that the event had happened so quickly that they were uncertain as to what precisely had taken place. For the entire series, forwards accounted for 92% of the injuries in Rugby Union and 41% in Rugby League, an impressive difference. No evidence was detected to suggest that a mismatch of strengths in the opposing front rows was a crucial determinant in neck injuries.

TABLE 14–2.

Player Positions in Rugby Union and Rugby League*

		Schoolboys and Adults, 1960–1985						
Code		Hooker	Loose Head Prop	Tight Head Prop	Other Forward	Backs	Position Unknown	Totals
Rugby Union	Schoolboys	5	2	3	—	1	—	11
	Adults	11	3	6	4	2	—	26
Rugby League	Schoolboys	3	—	1	—	1	1	6
	Adults	8	3	2	10	18	1	42
Totals		27	8	12	14	22	2	85

From Taylor TFK, Coolican MRJ: Med J Aust 1987; 147:112–118. Used with permission.

TABLE 14–3.

Percentages of Total Injuries, 1960–1985*

	Rugby Union	Rugby League
Scrummage	62%	29%
Rucks/mauls	14%	†
Tackles	22%	69%
Open play	2%	†
Unknown	†	2%

From Taylor TFK, Coolican MRJ: Med J Aust 1987; 147:112–118. Used with permission.

Match Standard.—Fifty-one players were injured in club (grade) football, 30 at the lower (subdistrict) level, 14 in schoolboy encounters, and 5 in social games; the exact match standard was not recorded for six players. It is notable that only one player was injured in an international match. Further, none of the injuries were sustained in training sessions.

Stage of Match.—Injuries occurred with comparable frequency throughout the various games, and the stage of game was not related to any other parameter assessed.

Stage of Season.—For Rugby League and Rugby Union the frequency peaked in June and July, respectively, this being in the second half of the football season when an increased competitive edge is in evidence, although the possible significance of this modulating factor cannot be determined.

Long-Term Recovery.—It is correct to say that the long-term prognosis of spinal cord injuries is largely determined at the moment of injury. The least-severe injuries occurred in Australian Rules, where 75% of the players were covered to Frankel grades D and E.[5] The injuries in Rugby Union players were more severe than those in Rugby League players, with 38% and 52% of the players, respectively, reaching the same recovery levels. Eight players died in the immediate postinjury phase. Two later succumbed from complications of their neurologic deficits. Seven of the eight injured loose-head props recovered to Frankel grades D or E, an indication that less severe injuries were sustained by these players.

Neurologic Level on Admission to Hospital.—For the quadriplegic patient the most distal intact spinal cord segment bears strongly on long-term functional prognosis. A C5 quadriplegic is totally

TABLE 14–4.

Scrum Injuries

Mechanism	Rugby Union and Rugby League 1960–1985*			
	Schoolboys		Adults	
	Rugby Union	Rugby League	Rugby Union	Rugby League
Packing	4	2	11	7
Collapse	2	1	2	2
Push after collapse	1	—	2	1
"Popped"	1	—	—	—
Late push after props released bind	—	1	—	—
Totals†	8	4	15	10
	12		25	

From Taylor TFK, Coolican MRJ: Med J Aust 1987; 147:112–118. Used with permission.
†Information not available for an additional 3 schoolboy and 2 adult injuries; 3 for Rugby Union and 2 for Rugby League.

dependent on others for self-care, whereas those with the sixth segment intact can reach a measure of independence. Overall, two thirds of the players had a neurologic deficit at C5 or higher; 76% for Rugby Union players and 58% for those injured in Rugby League (Fig 14–3).

Illegal Play.—Despite some allegations made to the contrary by the injured players, no clear evidence was detected to link spinal cord injuries with illegal play as indexed by the awarding of a penalty or any other action by the referees.

Neck Exercise Programs.—In recent years there has been a particular effort made in this country to encourage players in all codes to undertake exercise pro-

grams to strengthen neck musculature. On careful questioning and evaluation of data, we found no clear evidence of association of compliance with exercise programs to any parameter of either injury or recovery.

Schoolboy Injuries.—A total of 18 injuries were studied (Table 14–5), 11 in Rugby Union and 6 in Rugby League. Three of these players were injured in games against adults, which we consider to be a dangerous practice and one that should be discontinued forthwith. Ten of these Rugby Union injuries occurred after 1980.

Injury Rates Since 1985.—The decrease in injury rate in 1985 (Fig 14–2) was followed by at least six injuries in 1986, of which five were in Rugby Union and one in Rugby League; five of the six injuries occurred in scrums. No attempt has subsequently been made to define the injured players, pending the introduction of an anticipated registry. It is to be noted, however, that only players with a definite spinal cord injury who warranted admission to a specialized spinal cord injury unit have been described in this chapter. Each year all codes of football produce players who sustain minimal or transient spinal cord damage, dislocations with root involvement only, and dislocations without neurologic compromise. This population of injured play-

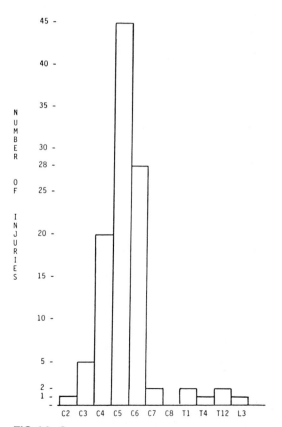

FIG 14–3.
Lowest, normal neurologic level on initial assessment. *(From Taylor TKF, Coolican MRJ: Med J Aust 1987; 147:112–118. Used with permission.)*

TABLE 14–5.

Player Positions for Scrum Injuries*

	Schoolboys, 1960–1985		
	Rugby Union	Rugby League	Totals
Hooker	4	3	7
Loose head prop	2	—	2
Tight head prop	2	1	3
Other forward position	—	—	—
Totals	8	4	12

*From Taylor TFK, Coolican, MRJ: Med J Aust 1987; 147:112–118. Used with permission.

ers has not been delineated. Thus the problem of neck injuries in football is far larger than the reported Australian experience would imply.

Management at the Site of Injury— First Aid and Transport.—First aid is the art of doing the minimum to transfer the patient safely and expeditiously to hospital—no more and no less. The more severe the injury the more applicable is this dictum. Time is often a vital issue in such instances, and delays can be detrimental to the outcome. This basic and sound principle is sometimes forgotten by those involved in first aid, and more so in recent times with the increasing involvement of paramedical personnel in emergency work.

Spinal cord injuries in Rugby are all but exclusively the result of bifacetal or unifacetal dislocations and not the result of fractures. As dislocations, there is an inherent but variable degree of instability, which emphasizes the need for extreme care in lifting and transporting the injured player. While it is well recognized that deterioration of neurologic function in cervical spine injuries can, and does, occur during transport to hospital from the site of the accident, there are no accurate data available.

When, during the course of play, there is reason to suspect the player has incurred a serious neck injury, the referee is obliged to order that the player not be moved in any way until first aid help is present. In particular, the neck should not be rotated to one side or the other by a well-intentioned teammate, attempting to maintain the airway or prevent inhalation of vomit. The absence of a helmet permits ready access to the airway. It is a safe and prudent practice to keep the head in the neutral position at all times, avoiding both flexion and extension. Because of the weight of the head, there is a tendency for the neck and skull to fall back into extension on lifting. If an injured player is lying supine with the head rotated to one side, the neutral position should be gained with gentle longitudinal traction by cupping one hand under the chin and placing the other beneath the occiput. This effective and safe maneuver is strongly advised, and as might be expected, it has been observed on a number of occasions to have reduced the dislocation!

If the player suspected of having a spinal cord injury is lying face down, he should be returned to the supine position. The person in charge, preferably someone with a background in first aid, or a first aid officer, places both forearms on either side of the neck and skull, and another person holds the head and neck against the former's arms. Three other persons should then gently rotate the trunk and lower limbs, pausing at 90 degrees of movement and then completing the arc.

A Jordan frame is ideal for lifting the injured player. This is a rectangular frame with transverse connecting slats, and these are passed under the patient. In the absence of a lifting frame, six persons are required to lift the player with a suspected spinal cord injury safely onto a stretcher. They grasp each other's hands underneath the trunk to ensure good support of the proximal aspect of the torso. One other person holds the neck, either cradling it between both forearms or holding it with one hand under the chin and the other under the occiput. Ideally the person holding the head and neck should give the orders to initiate the moves. The perceived importance of a particular game should in no way influence first aid discipline and procedure.

Assessment of suspected cervical spine injury on a football field is no easy task. The following are symptoms that warrant immediate action: neck pain, temporary paresis, electric sensations in arms and legs and down the back, diffuse paraesthesia in the limbs, and unconsciousness. If any of these are present, it is imperative that the player be handled as if a spinal cord injury has occurred. An unconscious player should be handled with the same protocol, and transient quadriplegia and quadriparesis may be extremely difficult to differentiate from temporary loss of consciousness. If there is any suspicion that a cervical spine injury has occurred, it is imperative that those in charge of the game act on the side of safety. In contrast to the United States, it would be unusual except at representative football matches for a team physician to be present.

It must be acknowledged that there are considerable difficulties in carrying out a detailed neurologic examination at the scene of any accident, let alone one taking place on a football field. Ideally, a simple and quick evaluation of certain joint movements should be done before definitive transport from the site of the game is initiated and this information duly recorded. Only voluntary motor power is of diagnostic value in the immediate post-injury phase. Further, the presence of voluntary movement is much more relevant than the power of such. The following movements should be examined.

	Segmental Value
Upper limb	
Shoulder abduction	C5
Elbow flexion	C5, C6
Wrist extension	C6, C7
Finger flexion/extension	C7, C8
Finger abduction/adductor (interossei function)	T1
Lower limb	
Hip flexion	L2, L3
Knee extension	L3, L4
Ankle dorsiflexion	L4, L5
Ankle plantar flexion	L5, S1

In cervical spinal cord injuries the lowest level of neurologic function in the upper limbs is of extreme practical value in management. This is less relevant in lower limb involvement, which for most injuries tends to be global. An exception to the preceding guidelines is the central cord syndrome, which may occur with dislocations, including those sustained in football.[9] During motor transport to hospital, sandbags on either side of the head are a wise precaution. In those instances in which a long journey to hospital with the inevitable attendant delays is required, a gastric tube should be passed. Rarely, if ever, is catheterization at a small hospital pending transfer to a Spinal Cord Injuries Unit justified. Catheterization is a surgical procedure demanding strict aseptic technique, and a hasty catheterization under less than optimal circumstances may lead to serious long-term urinary tract consequences. It has long been routine practice at our hospital for a medical officer to accompany a patient on a long journey to the unit, and especially so when this is by air. Road transfer is preferable to a helicopter. High cord lesions have occurred with football injuries. When this is so, ventilatory support may be needed during transport.

Treatment of Dislocation of the Cervical Spine.—In the context of this chapter, it is appropriate to encompass briefly the principles of acute surgical management of the injuries under discussion. Fractures of the cervical spine, and particularly burst fractures, are unusual in the codes under consideration unless the injured player was traveling at a high speed. Nearly all the injuries under consideration were dislocations, not fractures.

The early reduction of a dislocation, with loss of spinal cord function, constitutes a true surgical emergency. Prompt restoration of normal canal anatomy offers the best chance for recovery in the compromised neural tissues. The catch phrase in our unit is, "The sun shall neither rise nor set on an unreduced cervical dislocation with spinal cord injury." Time is the essence of the contract, and

20 years' experience has shown this philosophy to be a sound basis for management. In most football injuries, plain radiographs suffice to define the anatomy of the dislocation. Oblique views (angled at 45 degrees) should be taken to delineate foraminal contours. In a unifacetal dislocation the spinous process of the superior vertebra is deviated in an anteroposterior projection toward the side of the subluxation/dislocation. Concomitant fractures of the posterior elements are most unusual in dislocations, but, if suspected, are best documented by computer-assisted tomography. The presence of such fractures may influence surgical technique.

The cervical spine is manipulated under general anesthesia with muscle relaxants as soon as possible after full assessment in hospital. Intubation is required, and not infrequently the gentle extension permitted for this, coupled with the muscle relaxation, will see reduction of a dislocation. In the presence of a suspected complete cord transection, skull calipers are applied. If the cord loss is incomplete, a "Halo" is used. The latter will subsequently be coupled to a plaster jacket for early mobilization. For bifacetal dislocations, unlocking is facilitated by 15 to 20 degrees of flexion before traction is applied; as the articular processes disengage, the proximal spine is extended. The procedure is monitored at all stages by image intensification. With a unifacetal dislocation, the maneuver described by Evans[4] is employed. This entails traction, lateral flexion toward the intact side, and then clockwise rotation to the opposite side followed by extension. It is to be emphasized that the preceding "manipulations" are performed with extreme gentleness. Excessive force is to be avoided. If after two attempts reduction is not achieved, we proceed to posterior open reduction and unisegmental wiring with one-level bone grafting. Wiring technique is dependent on intact spinous processes and laminae. Anterior surgery is reserved for burst fractures and incomplete cord lesions where there is intracanal displacement of a bony fragment. These rare injuries have not been seen in footballers. Manipulation as described is not performed if there is a congenitally narrow spinal canal. In this day and age, we see no place for managing these injuries by continuous skull traction with increasing weights, even though many dislocations will eventually reduce in this way. Time is the essence of the contract, and provided due care is exercised, manipulation and open reduction carry no risk of further loss of root or cord function, or both. While we have not experienced these complications, we have seen patients in whom overvigorous manipulation under anesthesia has led to increased neurologic deficit.

DISCUSSION

As early as 1977 reports began to appear in the literature suggesting that spinal cord injury in football (Rugby Union) was on the increase. It was concerned doctors in Rugby Union—playing countries (not the governing authorities and their medical advisors) who focused attention on the problem and brought the matter to public attention (see references 2, 6, 8, 10, 12, 13, 17). Indeed, the public still has good reason to question the lack of prompt action by administrators of the game. Hence one has cause to wonder what might have happened, or not happened, if the authors cited had not reported their concerns. There is as yet no official registry in Australia of spinal cord injury from sports, although some tentative steps have been taken in this direction. Neither is there one in the United Kingdom.[7] The action taken by our American colleagues in introducing a National Football Head and Neck Injury Registry is an excellent example of what can be achieved. Torg et al.[16] were able to present a 14-year experience of the Registry and, moreover, to speak with authority on crucial issues such as frequency of occurrence of the injuries and so on. A Registry is the only way by which spinal cord injury from sports can be monitored. Then appropriate safety measures can be instituted. Even then, several seasons have to elapse before the effectiveness or lack of effectiveness of such measures can be gauged. In this matter, time is on no one's side, and least of all for the players at risk.

As Rugby Union officials became more aware of the problem, steps were taken to stabilize the scrum, on the premise that "collapse" was the principal cause of the injuries. As we have shown, this was an inappropriate approach. In simple terms, the relevant research had not been done. Alterations to scrummage laws must be directed toward " "depowering" the scrum in every possible way, and to making it more stable. There have been some alterations to the laws in this regard. Improvements in binding techniques should be constantly reappraised, and scientifically so. Such experiments are now eminently feasible.

In 1988 changes to the laws for scrummage as they apply to Rugby Union players less than 19 years of age were belatedly introduced to lessen the impact of engagement in the front rows; the same rules applied to all other levels of play in 1989 (interstate and international matches excepted). This is viewed as a positive step of merit, but it is still up to the referees, and indeed to all concerned, to see that legislated scrum discipline is rigidly followed. As yet, existing laws are so often observed more in the breach rather than in concurrence.

One obvious way to remove the problem of the "crashing" engagement, and one that we have suggested, is for the two front rows to engage first, with the second and back rows then packing down

sequentially.[15] This proposal was supported in principle by Burry and Calcinai.[3] They also reported that the New Zealand Rugby Football Union had obtained dispensation from the International Rugby Football Board to introduce modified laws, in an attempt to make scrummage safer. These included alteration in binding methods, minimizing the duration of a scrum, prohibiting the scrum to move more then 1.5. m, and "wheeling" of a set scrum. These modifications were employed in New Zealand for all domestic matches below senior level in the 1985–1986–1987 seasons. Burry and Calcinai[3] came to the conclusion, on the basis of existing data, that nine spinal cord injuries could have been anticipated for these three seasons, yet only one occurred.

The role of neck exercise programs in the prevention of spinal cord injuries warrants some comment. In our review no evidence was found to indicate that compliance with an exercise program had an effect either on the occurrence of, or on the recovery from, a spinal cord injury. Axial loading to the spine in American football has been shown to be the critical factor in the pathomechanics of dislocation.[16] The anatomy of the cervical spine, and particularly the obliquity of the facet joints, predisposes it to dislocation when it is experimentally axially loaded with forces far less than the load that can be generated in a scrum.[1] The latter may be in the order of 1.5 tons at impact of the front rows. These data account for the occurrence of luxation from what is apparently relatively minor trauma. The explanation we have put forward for the infrequent occurrence of these injuries in boys less than 16 years of age is that until they reach the later teens they do not have the muscular power and development for power scrummage and its potential consequences. There was but one representative player with a spinal injury in our study. At this level of competition the forwards, particularly the front row forwards, are highly skilled, extraordinarily fit, and very well versed in scrummage, just as are their opponents. In these circumstances, cervical spine injury is unlikely to occur. The immunity of the cervical spine to injury in football in boys less than 14 years of age is likely to be closely associated with the high degree of normal spinal mobility in the very young, and with the ability of the immature cervical spine to deform without dislocation. Mobility protects against injury. In birth paraplegia and severe cervical spine injuries in childhood, spinal cord disruption may take place without any demonstrable damage to the bony and soft tissue elements of the spinal column. On the other hand, a rigid cervical spine, such as in ankylosing spondylitis, is much at risk from fracture with even minor trauma. Children less than 10 years of age constitute less then 5% of all published series of spinal cord injuries, and these are most often the result of violent trauma in motor vehicle accidents.

In recent years there have been some public pronouncements (unsubstantiated by sound evidence) in Australia that boys with "long, thin necks" should not play in the front row of the scrum. This premise was the basis of a successful lawsuit in 1987, with the award of 2.2 million dollars to an injured schoolboy. In handing down his decision, the judge indicated that the Education Department had been negligent in not making the player and the coach aware of the vulnerability of this loosely described body habitus to scrum injury. In our view, time will place the sagacity and the correctness of this judgment in a different perspective. The opinions concerning scrum injuries and the role of neck exercise, as well as body habitus, in their occurrence should be viewed against what is known about dislocations in general and the experimental evidence for cervical luxations.[1] Dislocations occur when a force is applied to a joint in a particular way. A joint may simply dislocate or a fracture-dislocation may be sustained. For example, at one end of the spectrum of the injuries that may be sustained from a fall on the outstretched arm is a fractured scaphoid bone, and at the other end is a dislocated shoulder. The latter is a joint with low inherent stability, as is the cervical spine. The outcome of a fall on the outstretched upper limb depends on the magnitude of the force applied, the position of the limb at impact, and the manner in which the force is applied. Irrespective of the strength of the shoulder musculature, the joint dislocates when the protective muscles are not "on guard." The analogy to scrum injuries is put forward as equally tenable. Emphasis on neck exercise programs and body habitus, as part of preventive programs, tends to distract from the central issues. Strong neck muscles in fact encourage the type of play that characterizes power scrum. Powerful neck musculature may help prevent injury, however, when a scrummage collapses and the back rows keep pushing. This tactic is now prohibited. A hidden benefit of neck exercise programs is to make players more aware of the possibility of neck injury. In contrast to thoracic and lumbar spine fractures and fracture-dislocations, in the common cervical dislocation it is quite noticeable at open reduction how little, if any, disruption of the posterior musculature has taken place.

The increase of injuries in the seventies cannot be precisely ascribed to any one factor alone. As Silver[13] has pointed out, the changes to Rugby Union tackle laws, and subsequently more rucks and mauls, are likely responsible, at least in part, for what has transpired. These phases in play are handled somewhat differently in the various Rugby-playing countries. They present certain difficulties to a referee, for he can see only one side of a ruck or maul at any one time. Rucks and mauls do constitute what can reasonably be called "controlled violence," and in the heat of the moment this easily becomes uncontrolled, as our Sunday papers so frequently attest. Only too often does a "football game" become all but instantly transformed into a "free-for-all-brawl." It is notable that the changes introduced in New Zealand for rucks and mauls also led to a significant reduction in the number of spinal injuries sustained.[3]

"Power scrummage," popularized by the British Lions in the early seventies, became a feature of Rugby Union in that decade. This, together with increase in rucks and mauls, changed a running and passing game into something quite different. While spectators are always enthralled by a fast, open match with scintillating back line play, it is curious that the power aspects of the game today also evoke an enthusiastic response in some quarters of our communities.

Aggression is one aspect of football that is also far more in evidence (also found in other sports) than it once was, and not so long ago either, although the temporal sequence of change in the ethos of the games is hard to define. All sports are becoming more competitive. In body contact sports increased competitiveness kindles aggressive behavior in the contestants. Men, not unexpectedly, meet aggression with aggression; violence breeds counterviolence. We all live in a more violent society, and our people now mutely sanction such behavior in sports, behavior that once would have been intolerable. To win at all costs has become a driving force in most forms of athletic endeavor, and an extreme of this attitude is the taking of anabolic steroids and other drugs. This is a far cry from the Olympic ideal of true sportsmanship. These days, however, sports have become a major component of the entertainment industry, and there are rich, even huge prizes for those young men and women who reach the top of their chosen sport. Hence sport is no longer "sport" in the literal sense of the word, and, more importantly, has ceased to be what the world once understood it to be. Now, it would be both foolish and quixotic to attempt to change all this, but societies need to come to terms with these events that have gradually become part of their mores.

"Psyching up" of players by coaches before games, media involvement, spectator enthusiasm, and peer pressure among the players themselves summate to have a catalytic effect so often culminating as violence on the field of play. The glory of the school may be another factor at schoolboy games. Those interested in this aspect of the topic should read the incisive letter from an injured schoolboy published by Silver.[13] In these terms there is a clear case for schools to make a concerted attempt to teach, foster, and reward sportsmanship (old meaning). The value of leading by example at school cannot be emphasized enough. Therein lies the hope for the future.

The increase of spinal cord injuries in schoolboys playing football in the 1980s was a matter for grave concern, and this was echoed around the Rugby-playing countries. In sports, schoolboys tend to style their play and behavior generally on that of their heroes. It is understandable that tacitly approved violence and aggression in football at senior and representative levels will have an effect on young, impressionable footballers. There is a wide compass of responsibility in this regard. As the figures clearly show, Rugby Union has been a far more dangerous game for schoolboys than has Rugby League.

CONCLUSION

The Australian experience in spinal cord injuries from football has been reviewed. The need for a registry of these injuries in Australia remains urgent and unmet, as it is in some other countries. Continued surveillance is the sole way by which the problems can be monitored and corrective measures taken to alter laws accordingly. The administration of Rugby Union and other codes has correctly been put on notice by Burry and Calcinai[3] when they stated, "Failure to alter the procedures of a game despite the knowledge that existing practises were hazardous and safe alternative existed could well be held by a court to constitute culpable negligence." There is no question whatsoever that both codes of Rugby must be made safer than they have been in the past decade or so. The medical profession, through its influence and writings, must do all possible to help put the matter right.

Acknowledgments

The authors gratefully acknowledge the assistance of Mrs J. Mitchell and Miss J. Lord in the preparation of the manuscript.

REFERENCES

1. Bauze RJ, Ardran GM: Experimental production of forward dislocations in the human spine. *J Bone Joint Surg (Br)* 1978; 60–B:239–245.

2. Burry HA, Gowland H: Cervical injury in Rugby football: A New Zealand survey. *Br J Sports Med* 1981; 15:15–19.

3. Burry HC, Calcinai CJ: The need to make Rugby safer. *Br Med J* 1988; 296;149–150.

4. Evans DK: Reduction of cervical dislocations. *J Bone Joint Surg (Br)* 1961: 43–B:552–555.

5. Frankel HL, Hancock DO, Hyslop G, et al: The value of postural reduction in the initial management of closed injuries of the spine with paraplegia and tetraplegia. Part 1. *Paraplegia* 1969; 7:178–192.

6. Horan FT: Injuries to the cervical spine in schoolboys playing Rugby football. *J Bone Joint Surg (Br)* 1984; 66–B:470–471.

7. Hoskins TW: Prevention of neck injuries playing Rugby. *Public Health* 1987; 101:351–356.

8. McMoy GF, Piggot J, Macafee AL, et al: Injuries of the cervical spine in schoolboy Rugby football. *J Bone Joint Surg (Br)* 1984; 66–B:500–503.

9. Merriam WF, Taylor TKF, Ruff SJ, et al: A reappraisal of acute tramatic central cord syndrome. *J Bone Joint Surg (Br)* 1986; 68–B:708–713.

10. Scher AT: Rugby injuries to the cervical spinal cord. *S Afr Med J* 1977; 51:473–475. Rugby injuries to the cervical cord (editorial). *Br Med J* 1977; 1556–1557.

11. Schneider RC, Gosch HH, Norell J, et al: Vascular insufficiency and differential distortion of brain and cord caused by cervicomedullary football injuries. *J Neurosurg* 1970; 33:363–375.

12. Silver J, Davies JE, Walkden L, et al: *Report: Annual General Meeting of the Medical Officers of Schools Association.* London, Medical Officers of Schools Associations, 1979.

13. Silver JR: Injuries of the spine sustained by Rugby. *Br Med J* 1984; 288:37–43.

14. Taylor TKF, Coolican MRJ: Spinal-cord injuries in Australia footballer, 1960–1985. *Med J Aust* 1987; 147:112–118.

15. Taylor TKF, Coolican MRJ: Rugby must be safer: Preventive programmes and rule changes (letter). *Med J Aust* 1988; 148:224.

16. Torg JS, Vegso JJ, Sennett B: The National Football Head and Neck Injury Registry: 14 year report of cervical quadriplegia (1971–1984). *Clin Sports Med* 1987; 6:61–72.

17. Williams JPR, McKibbin B: Cervical spine injuries in Rugby Union football. *Br Med J* 1978; 2:1747.

EDITOR'S NOTE

Joseph S. Torg, M.D.

Rugby football, a game indigenous to the United Kingdom, Wales, South Africa, New Zealand, and Australia, is played in the United States on a quasi-organized club basis. Although there is no indication that injuries to the head and neck are a significant problem in this country, recently there has been great concern in the Commonwealth nations.

Silver[1] initially reported on 63 patients who had sustained serious injuries to the cervical spine in England between 1952 and 1982. More recently he has added another 19 who had sustained their injuries between 1983 and 1987. Of these, 13 were paralyzed, 3 had transient quadriplegia, 1 died, and 2 had dislocation without neurologic involvement. Silver did not present the data in terms of injury rates, and whether there has been a real increase cannot be determined. He described the injuries as resulting from "blows to the head or the head being driven into the ground." Seven injuries occurred in scrums, five players were injured while tackling, and six in a ruck and maul situation when they were pushed to the ground while stooping to pick up the ball.

Silver[1] points out that it has been suggested that Rugby League code results in a safer game because the ruck and maul has been abolished. The incidence of four cervical spinal injuries for 26,000 players in Rugby League as opposed to five injuries out of 500,000 for Rugby Union does not support this claim, however.

After the report of the 63 injuries to the administrators of the Rugby Union at a joint meeting of doctors, Rugby players, and administrators in 1983, a committee was set up to make recommendations on an experimental basis for schoolboys in the United Kingdom, in an attempt to make the game safer. The suggestions were supported by other unions, particularly by the New Zealand Rugby Football Union, and subsequently adopted by the International board. The rule changes concentrated on keeping players on their feet, both at the set scrum and in the ruck and maul; shoulders were not to dip below waist height in the scrummage. With the emphasis on the safety of players, recommendations were made (1) to reduce irresponsible modes of play; (2) to match players in terms of strength and skill; (3) to instill correct attitudes; and

(4) to provide training for specific positions. Subsequently, a survey of all spinal units in the United Kingdom revealed a reduction in the number of injuries from ten in 1983 to five in 1986–1987.

Silver[1] is of the opinion that, as mentioned, the injury mechanism results from a blow to the head or by the head, or by the head being driven into the ground, or results from a poorly executed tackle, and that the current rules are adequate, but must be enforced.

Williams and McKibbin[2] have reported 18 spinal cord injuries occurring in Welsh Rugby Union Players during the 19-year period from 1964 through 1984. One injury was reported to have occurred in 1964, the next was 10 years later in 1974, and since they have continued at a steady rate of two per year.

The total number is small but the victims are derived from a well-defined group of players, and therefore in accord with the findings in all the other studies in the United Kingdom, indicating that there is sufficient evidence of a trend to cause concern.

An attempt was made to go back earlier than 1962, but the records were too unreliable. Nevertheless, the fact that only two patients with injury to the spinal cord can be identified during the entire 20 years before the present study is surely noteworthy.

During the period of study when records were available there was only one injury in the first decade. A sudden increase appears to have occurred in 1974, and once established the number has not risen. During the period 1974–1978 inclusive, there were six complete tetraplegias, including one death, in a Rugby-playing population of 33,000, whereas in the series from New Zealand during the same 5-year period there were 16 complete tetraplegias, again including one death, from a playing population of 200,000; when corrected to the same population of players, there are in New Zealand only half the number of tetraplegias found in Wales.[3]

It might have been anticipated that, because the increase in these injuries occurred in 1974 and has remained fairly constant since, some single factor might explain this. Despite a detailed analysis, however, none has emerged. If there had been some change in laws or technique of play, one might have expected this to affect a particular phase of the game, whereas, in fact, all phases appear to be equally affected.

Certain types of play became more popular in the midseventies, including deliberately collapsing the scrum and placing emphasis on the ruck, which, if incorrectly set up, resulted in multiple pileups. Changes in the laws have since been introduced to avoid this, and it remains to be seen whether this will reduce the incidence of serious injuries to the neck. The limited evidence to date (see Table 14–2) suggests that while the incidence is not increasing it has not reverted to the pre-1974 level.

Injuries in scrums call for a separate comment because these appear to follow a more set pattern than in other phases of the game. The proportion of these among the total injuries is remarkably constant, being 35% in the New Zealand series,[3] while in South Africa Scher[4] reported 40% and Silver[5] 38% in Britain. The incidence in the present series was 44%. The injury involves predominantly players in the front row, and the characteristic injury of flexion accompanied by restraint of the vertex described by Williams and McKibbin[6] in 1978 has been demonstrated. This injury is particularly serious because it frequently leads to dislocations of both facets, which are usually associated with transection of the cord.[4] Nine of the 12 injured in scrums in this series suffered severe injury of the spinal cord.

Most of the injuries in scrums occurred early in the season, with only one occurring after the New Year. This, coupled with the finding that many injuries were sustained during the first quarter of the game or in training, suggests that injury is more likely to occur if packs are not used to each other and are uncertain of their combined course of action in the event of a collapsed scrum.

Injuries sustained during tackles and in the ruck/maul are inevitably more varied in their mechanism, but, even so, the effect of violent flexion predominates. In these instances the element of restraint of the vertex is often absent, and the amount of damage to the spinal cord therefore may be less severe. There was no instance of extension injury.

The most comprehensive study of spinal cord injuries resulting from Rugby was recently reported by Taylor and Coolican.[7] They reviewed 107 injuries that occurred between 1960 and 1985 from participants in the four major codes: Australian Rules, Rugby League, Rugby Union, and soccer. The study was prompted by concern at the number of schoolboys who were admitted to the Spinal Cord Injuries Unit at the Royal North Hospital of Sydney in 1982 and 1983 and attempted to determine the exact incidence of the injuries as well as any feature of play in which preventive measures might be applied.

With the cooperation of the six Australian spinal cord injury units, 103 cases were identified and reviewed, including 92 patients who were interviewed personally. In each of the four major codes there has been a marked increase in spinal cord injuries since 1977, from an average of 1.8 injuries per year between 1960 and 1976, to 8.2 injuries per year between 1977 and 1985; 81% of the injuries in Rugby Union have occurred since 1977, as have 67% of the injuries in Rugby League and 59% of the injuries in Australian Rules (see Table 14–1). An even sharper increase has taken place in the number of injuries to schoolboys: all schoolboys who were injured in Rugby Union and Australian Rules have been injured since 1977, and 50% of schoolboys who were injured in Rugby League were injured in this period. There has been only one injury in soccer in the time span of the study.

The average age of all the injured payers was 22 years; the average age of an injured player in Rugby Union and Australian Rules was 24 years; in Rugby League the average age was 20 years. The peak frequency of injury for the combined codes occurred at 18 years. The youngest player was 14 years of age at the time of injury, and the oldest was 56. The latter had cervical spondylosis, which probably contributed to his vulnerability to injury. Age was shown not to have a bearing on either the mechanism of injury nor on the degree of subsequent recovery. The average age of players in the different team positions for all codes did not vary significantly.

It is not possible to estimate accurately the relative probabilities of injury in a given football season for the four major codes. There are approximately at least twice as many players in Rugby League as in Rugby Union, however. Irrespective of how the data are viewed, the risk of injury in both schoolboy and adult Rugby Union would appear to be much higher than that in Rugby League. Compared with Australian Rules, this risk is amplified further. It should be noted that the number of players on the team for each code is different: soccer, 11 players; Rugby League, 13 players; Rugby Union, 15 players; and Australian Rules, 18 players.

The player at maximal risk in Rugby Union is the hooker, who is at the center of the scrum. Of the 85 injured players in both Rugby codes, 27 players were hookers, but not all of them sustained their spinal cord injuries at scrummage. Spinal cord injuries in scrums occur almost exclusively in the front row; only one injured forward had not played in one of the three front row positions: tight-head prop, hooker, and loose-head prop (see Fig 14–2).

For both Rugby Union and Rugby League, 22% of the injured players were not playing in their usual positions, and two thirds of these players were injured in a scrum.

Apart from the eight loose-head props (seven of whom recovered to Frankel grades D or E), the chance of recovery was not influenced by the team position. Unlike the hooker and tight-head prop, the loose-head prop is free on one side, which gives a measure of immunity from neck injury in scrums (see Fig 14–2).

No particular team position could be pinpointed for the 17 injured Australian players.

In Rugby Union, 62% of the players were injured in scrums, 22% in tackles, 14% in rucks and mauls, and 2% in open play. Conversely, in Rugby League, tackles accounted for 69% of the injuries, scrums for 29%, and 2% of players were injured in an unknown manner; the ball carrier was injured in 76% of the tackles, and the tackler was injured in the remainder.

In Australian Rules, 69% of the players were injured in a collision when neither player had the ball, and 19% were injured in tackles. One other player was kicked in the head and died subsequently as a result of his neck injury, and another was injured when hit by a ball in flight (12% of injuries).

MECHANISM OF SCRUM INJURIES

The high frequency of injuries in scrums led Taylor and Coolican[7] to pay particular attention to this facet of play. Thirty-seven players were injured in scrums, but collapse was not, as is stated so frequently, the most relevant factor.

Rather, it was the force of impact at the engagement of the two sets of forwards. As already mentioned, the players' recall for what had transpired remained extraordinarily clear even many years after the injury. When interviewed, a near-identical history was so often given: "We formed our pack and just as we engaged my head hit something hard and twisted—I felt my neck crack and my whole body went numb. I couldn't strike for the ball and when my props ran off, I fell and couldn't get up."

Direct questioning of players indicated that 24 (65%) of the 37 scrum injuries occurred at engagement; 19% of injuries at the collapse of the scrum; 11% of injuries by pushing after the collapse of the scrum; 3% of injuries when "popped" (which refers to a maneuver whereby a front rower uses his neck and shoulders to so lift an opponent that his feet leave the ground and he cannot push); and 3% of injuries occurred by a push from the opposition after the props had released their bind (see Table 14–3). Whereas all those who were injured in scrums, rucks, and mauls were able to give a clear description of what happened, those who had been hurt in tackles generally believed that the incident had taken place so quickly that they could not be sure of the manner in which it occurred. The exceptions were the victims of "spear-tackles."

Over all, 92% of Rugby Union injuries, compared with 59% of injuries for Rugby League, occurred to forwards. Apart from the hooker in Rugby League, the injury rates for other positions varied little. A discrepancy in strength between opposing front rows may contribute to scrum instability. In the players' judgment of the relative strength of front rows, however, injuries occurred with almost equal frequency to players in both the adjudged stronger or weaker front rows.

No precise explanation could be offered for the increase in injuries since 1977. It could, in part, be due to increases in the number of players who were involved, as well as to increases in the number of games that were played each season; we have no accurate information on these trends. The concept of power scrummaging, which was introduced to New Zealand in 1971 and subsequently to Australia, certainly changed the role of the rugby scrum in that country, but the increase in the frequency of injuries includes all phases of play, and is mirrored in all codes except soccer. It seems likely that increased aggression is a major factor, although this is difficult to discuss, or to attempt to analyze, in even quasiscientific terms. It is true to say that all sports have become more competitive, and in body contact sports, increased competitiveness is the inevitable corollary of more aggressive play.

In football, the competitive atmosphere is encouraged by the coaches, the players, the media, the spectators, and, in some instances, for junior players, by the schools. In this context, the fact that no injuries occurred in training is considered highly relevant. Most players spend at least twice the time training as they do playing matches, but in training, the competitive edge is usually not there to kindle aggression. Further supportive evidence for the role of aggression is the finding that the frequency of these injuries peaks toward the latter part of the season when the competitive spirit is more in evidence. At this time the prospect of a team reaching the finals, or, conversely, of being relegated to a lower division, looms large in the minds of all concerned. In the higher grades of Rugby Union and Rugby League, the players are more fit, more experienced, more committed to the game, and, most importantly, more expert. Further, in these standards of play it is much less likely that there will be a wide discrepancy in the talent and strength of the opposing teams.

It is to be noted that there were no schoolboy injuries to players less than 14 years of age. A simple but plausible explanation for this is that younger players do not have the strength to create the forces that are necessary to produce injuries either in scrummage or in other phases of play for both Rugby codes.

In 1985 the Australian Rugby Football Union, in an effort to prevent serious neck injuries, introduced a new set of rules for players less than 19 years of age and altered the laws for adults, particularly in relation to scrummage. Most of the changes that were made to the scrum rules were to prevent collapse—Taylor and Coolican's[7] study has shown clearly that this is of much less importance than are the impact forces generated by the engagement of the two sets of forwards. These rule changes to "depower" and to control the engagement of the scrum cannot be regarded as adequate. The present study has identified 24 spinal cord injuries that were probably preventable, given the data that are presented here. Theoretically at least, scrum injuries could largely be eliminated from Rugby Union and Rugby League if the two front rows were to pack separately and then to add, in succession, the second and the back rows.

Far more emphasis is attached to scrummage in Rugby Union than in Rugby League, although this is of relatively recent origin. In Rugby Union, a strong scrum and a forward pack that advances in rucks and mauls have become high priorities, particularly at the representative level. Players in lower grades, especially schoolboys, inevitably style their game on the example that is set by representative football in all codes. No doubt the additional two players in the Rugby Union scrum add to the impact force that can be generated at the engagement of the two sets of forwards. There is every good reason for immediate changes in the rules to "depower" Rugby scrums. The stabilization of a scrum, although important, is less relevant in the prevention of these tragic injuries. After all, in simple terms, a scrum is a method by which to bring the ball back into play after a rule infringement; in 95% of cases, possession goes to the nonoffending team. The falloff in the numbers of injuries in 1985 (see Fig 14–1), when no schoolboys were injured, is encouraging at first glance. One would like to think that the decrease was the result of appropriate corrective measures, but this cannot be substantiated. In the 1986 season, for which full details are not yet available, six Australian footballers sustained a spinal cord injury (five in Rugby Union and one in Rugby League). Four of these injuries took place in scrums. One of the players was a schoolboy Rugby Union hooker who went on the field as a replacement hooker in his school's first team shortly after having just completed a match in the lower grade.

A national register for spinal cord injuries as a result of playing football is needed urgently, so that close scrutiny of the problem can be maintained. A register is the only way by which the frequency of such injuries can be monitored, the public kept informed, and the effectiveness, or otherwise, of rule changes evaluated.[7]

REFERENCES

1. Silver JR, Gill G: Injuries of the spine sustained during Rugby. *Sports Medicine* 1988; 5:328–334.

2. Williams P, McKibbin B: Unstable cervical spine injuries in Rugby—a 20-Year Review. *Injury* 1987; 18:329–332.

3. Burry HA, Gowland H: Cervical injury in Rugby football: A New Zealand survey. *Br J Sports Med* 1981; 15:5–9.

4. Scher AT: Rugby injuries to the cervical spinal cord. *S Afr Med J* 1977; 51:473–475.

5. Silver JR: Injuries of the spine sustained by Rugby. *Br Med J* 1984; 288:37–43.

6. Williams JPR, McKibbin B: Cervical spine injuries in Rugby Union football. *Br Med J* 1978; 2:1747.

7. Taylor TKF, Coolican MRJ: Spinal-cord injuries in Australia footballer, 1960–1985. *Med J Aust* 1987; 147:112–118.

CHAPTER 15

Legal Aspects of Athletic Injuries to the Head and Cervical Spine

Daniel Patterson, J.D.

Athletes who sustain permanent injuries to the head and cervical spine suffer devastating emotional shock, unfathomable physical pain, potential financial ruin, and undirectable rage. The excitement and pride of participation and competition are extinguished the instant a catastrophic injury irrevocably reduces a young life to a footnote of human potential. To spectators, this particular tragedy is an unfortunate accident, part of the inherent risk of sports. To the family and athlete, it is much more.

After a catastrophic injury has occurred, neither the family nor the injured athlete is willing to accept retrospective responsibility for having assumed the risk of such a catastrophic injury in exchange for the fellowship, teamwork, self-discipline, and personal satisfaction that athletic participation offered. Those affected often feel a desperate need to shift responsibility outside the family, to find fault in order to explain the tragedy. The legal system offers those who suffer such an injury the potential for economic compensation and what amounts to moral absolution.

ATHLETIC INJURY LAWSUITS

Once litigation is instituted, coaches, administrators, trainers, medical practitioners, and equipment manufacturers are accused of neglect and incompetence. Products that have protected millions of athletes in hundreds of millions of similar situations through decades are labeled defective. All potential defendants must justify their actions and products in a courtroom atmosphere steeped in sympathy and pathos and with emotions inflamed by attorneys motivated by large contingent fee contracts.

Regardless of the evidence presented, jurors viewing a youngster who will never rise on his own from a wheelchair because of quadriplegia, or the photographs of one interminably comatose from a head injury, are often disposed to ignore rules of law and substitute an understandable compassion for the plight of the catastrophically injured athlete and his emotionally stricken loved ones. Although the process compensates a few injured athletes and certainly enriches lawyers, it also extracts each year unconscionable millions of dollars from the "deep pockets" of school districts, equipment manufacturers, doctors, and others who are dragged into athletic litigation.

HISTORY

The imposition of litigation upon athletics is a relatively recent phenomenon. Twenty-five years ago, this subject had little relevance to individuals or corporations involved with athletics. Before the mid-1960s, millions of young people enthusiastically participated and competed in many forms of athletics that involved some risk of serious injury or death. When the occasional catastrophic injury occurred, no one was accused of negligence. Athletic injuries were viewed as unfortunate but infrequent, and the slight risk of injury was considered acceptable when weighed against the benefits of athletic participation.

In 1905, with a fraction of the present number of participants, there were 18 deaths and 149 serious injuries in intercollegiate football alone. President Theodore Roosevelt considered seeking a ban of football and convened a conference of representatives from Harvard, Yale, and Princeton to consider these problems and suggest solutions. There is no record, however, to suggest that any litigation resulted from any of these incidents.

In 1984, with 75,000 college football players and more than one million high school football players, there were 9 deaths and 5 cases of permanent quadriplegia. Of these 14 incidents, we can anticipate at least 7 will result in litigation, and 3 or 4 will result in awards to the plaintiff of tens of millions of dollars. Times and attitudes have changed; so has the law.

Although lawsuits involving athletic injuries to the head and cervical spine can be found in appellate reports across the country before the mid-1960s, they are relatively infrequent. The liability theories used also were different from those used today. Defenses were then available that have since been eroded or extinguished. Recovery in extracurricular athletic activities was virtually impossible. Suits were not brought against equipment manufacturers, trainers, or doctors.

Early cases made clear distinctions between required athletic activities, such as physical education classes, and those in which students voluntarily participated. Where students were required to participate and injury occurred, courts generally allowed the player to sue and recover when there was evidence of negligent supervision. A young man, for example, required to box without instruction or warnings, an inexperienced wrestler required to allow his more experienced opponent to use a risky maneuver, a young woman required to attempt a back flip she was afraid to attempt, a girl required to tumble with a physical disability that made it difficult for her to execute the maneuver, and a young man required to race toward a ball from a 75 ft circle of students and get the ball before an opponent all successfully sued when they suffered head or neck injuries and obtained verdicts that were upheld on appeal.

A 1942[9] appeals court stated a principle of law that is still the law in most jurisdictions today:

We entrust the safety of our children to public school authorities during school hours. They are bound to exercise an amount of care for their safety during school hours. They are bound to exercise an amount of care for their safety during that period commensurate with the immaturity of their charges and the importance of their trust.

Another court[6] was equally articulate, but more succinct 7 years later: "Parents do not send their children to school to be returned to them maimed because of the absence of proper supervision or the abandonment of supervision."

Courts today continue to follow these holdings.

ASSUMPTION OF RISK AND CONTRIBUTORY NEGLIGENCE

The change that has gradually occurred during the past two decades is the approach toward extracurricular athletic activities. The law that once was generally applied to these activities was as follows: "Voluntary participation in lawful games, sports and even roughhouse, assumes the risk of injury at the hands of their fellow participants (and, of course, of "hurting themselves") so long as the game is played in good faith and without negligence."[3]

Assumption of risk simply meant that the plaintiff, in advance, had agreed to relieve the defendant of any obligation toward him and to take his chances of injury from a known risk. It did not matter if the athlete specifically said or read anything. His or her voluntary participation in an athletic activity was viewed as an implied waiver of the right to later claim negligence in the event of an injury.

Assumption of risk was the rule of law that completely barred a plaintiff's recovery. This defense was applied in many extracurricular athletic injury cases. When a 16-year-old high school baseball player, for example, became paralyzed after using his head as a battering ram to jar the ball loose from the catcher while attempting to score at home plate, an appellate court[7] reversed a plaintiff's verdict, saying:

It is important to realize that unlike physical education courses in school, participation in interscholastic activity is a purely voluntary act. The great majority of accident cases involving schools deal with situations in a gymnasium during school hours. The incident event dealt with an extracurricular activity. The plaintiff assumed the risk of injury when

he tried out for and played on the high school varsity team.

The same reasoning was applied to a football injury that occurred when a ninth grader used his head as a battering ram when being tackled. In response to claims that he was an inexperienced player, not physically coordinated, was tackled hard, and had not received proper instruction or equipment, the court concluded he had voluntarily assumed the risk of his injury: "No one expects a football coach to extract from the game the body clashes that cause bruises, jolts and hard falls. To remove them would end the sport."[11]

Another line of defense available in early cases was contributory negligence, which is defined as "conduct on the part of the plaintiff, contributing as a legal cause to the harm he has suffered, which falls below the standard to which he is required to conform for his own protection."[8] This doctrine of defense placed the responsibility for reasonable care on the athlete himself[7]:

The coaches had the right to assume that he possessed the intelligence and stock of information of a normal young man. Thus, they had the right to assume that he knew of the possibility of injury that comes to an individual who uses his head as a battering ram.

Assumption of risk and contributory negligence were powerful deterrents to the instigation and successful conclusion of many athletic injury lawsuits. Exceptions, however, were carved out when injuries resulted from reckless or deliberate acts or when injuries were exacerbated by negligent actions in dealing with an already injured player. In these cases, neither assumption of risk nor contributory negligence would bar recovery. Two examples illustrate this. A goalie in a soccer game was kicked in the head as he was in a crouched position holding the ball in the penalty area. The opponent-defendant had time to avoid contact with the plaintiff. In this case, *Nabozny vs. Barnhell*,[5] the appellate court reversed a defense verdict, holding that a reckless disregard for safety of other players cannot be excused in the name of athletics:

This court believes that the law should not place unreasonable burdens on the free and vigorous participation in sports by our youth. However, we also believe that organized, athletic competition does not exist in a vacuum. Rather, some of the restraints of civilization must accompany every athlete onto the playing field. One of the educational benefits of organized athletic competition to our youth is the development of discipline and self-control. . . . Individual sports are advanced and competition enhanced by comprehensive sets of rules. Some rules secure the better playing of the game as a test of skill. Other rules are primarily designed to protect participants from serious injury.

The *Nabozny* case is similar to the celebrated lawsuit in which Rudy Tomjanovich won a multimillion dollar verdict against Kermit Washington and the Los Angeles Lakers. Washington had deliberately hit Tomjanovich in the jaw with his fist during a game. Courts have consistently held athletes do not assume the risk of deliberate or totally reckless actions by opponents during competition.

A tragic second example of an exception to the assumption of risk rule was the case, in 1958, in which a California appellate court affirmed a $325,000 award for a high school football player. The young athlete was unable to get up after being tackled as he attempted a quarterback sneak. The coach checked the players' condition and then had the young man carried off the field without a stretcher by eight teammates. The boy became permanently quadriplegic. The appellate court had no trouble agreeing with the jury's determination that removing the plaintiff from the field without a stretcher was improper. Medical experts testified that additional injury occurred because of the move. This athlete was not held to have assumed the risk of improper medical care; nor was he held to have been contributorily negligent himself.[12] No one would expect these cases to be viewed differently in 1990 than they were when they were tried.

COMPARATIVE NEGLIGENCE

Comparing early cases and the laws by which each party's conduct was measured with the changes in the law in the past 25 years, we can see why both the numbers of lawsuits and their scope have literally exploded. Contrary to the pronouncements of the press and propaganda of the insurance industry, our society did not become "sue happy" overnight. Three alterations in the constantly evolving legal system have combined to make personal injury cases attractive and incredibly profitable for the plaintiff's bar. They are as follows: (1) the wholesale abolition, by the late 1970s, of contributory negligence and the adoption of comparative negligence in its place; (2) additionally, the abolition or dilution of assumption of risk, the traditional barrier to extracurricular athletic injury lawsuits; and (3) the creation of "strict products" liability in 1963.

These three changes, when combined with the traditional damage doctrine of "joint and several" liability, have created a nightmare for everyone involved with athletics. In the early cases, a finding that the plaintiff was 1% negligent or that he assumed the risk of his injury completely barred his recovery. To eliminate what was viewed as a fundamental unfairness of this rule of law, many states dropped contributory negligence and adopted comparative negligence. By 1978, 37 states had made this change. The concept is simple. Rather than deny the injured plaintiff any recovery if he negligently contributed to his own injury, his award would simply be reduced by the percentage of his own negligence. If a jury found that the plaintiff's total damages were $100,000 and determined that the plaintiff was 25% negligent, he was entitled to recover $75,000 from the defendants who also contributed to the injury.

Individual states approach comparative negligence differently, but there are two basic plans: pure and modified. Under the pure comparative approach, a plaintiff theoretically could recover 1% of his damage even if the jury found he was 99% responsible for causing his own injury. The modified approach is a compromise between contributory and comparative negligence. Under this approach, a plaintiff can recover if his fault is equal to or less than that of the defendants, but his damages are still reduced by the percentage of his own fault just as they are in states with pure comparative negligence. Some states require that the plaintiff be less negligent than the defendants; other states require that he be no more negligent than they. Regardless of which approach is applied, the result has been a dramatic increase in litigation.

State legislatures and courts opened the way for the negligent injured person to obtain a favorable verdict that would previously have been denied. Even people who seemingly caused their own injuries were allowed to sue and collect on the ground that someone else was at least partially responsible for their accident. The rule of comparative negligence allowed the family of a man who killed himself by throwing himself in front of a subway train to collect $650,000 from the New York Transit Authority. The family claimed the train operator should have stopped sooner. Comparative negligence also allowed the family of a man in California to collect $500,000 from Ventura County after the man committed suicide in his jail cell. The family claimed the sheriff's officers should have discovered the attempt and prevented him from taking his own life. Fault was apportioned 10% to the man who committed suicide; 90% to the Sheriff's Department for not stopping him.

Comparative negligence has also opened the courthouse doors to lawsuits over athletic injuries to the plaintiffs who under the principles of contributory negligence would probably have been unable even to find lawyers to take their cases. In California, a gymnastics instructor sued the manufacturer of a mat designed for pole vaulters for injuries he received when he underrotated while attempting a somersault off a trampoline. He had done the same trick 300 to 400 times. When he hit the mat headfirst, he broke his neck and injured his spinal cord. His theory against the mat manufacturer was that the mat had not been tested for gymnastic use and the manufacturer had failed to warn him of the dangers of using the mat for gymnastics. Absurd? To everyone perhaps, except the jury. The gymnasium instructor was awarded $14.7 million.

ABOLITION OF ASSUMPTION OF RISK

Comparative negligence largely abolished the defense of assumption of risk. It was subsumed into comparative negligence. This prior bar to recovery evaporated. Participants in extracurricular athletics were no longer considered to have assumed the risk of anything. If they could establish fault on the part of anyone else for their injury, whether coach, athletic administrator, trainer, team physician, state athletic association, or equipment manufacturer, they could obtain a verdict and collect; the only question was how much. With the abolition of traditional defenses, a proliferation of litigation became inevitable.

STRICT PRODUCTS LIABILITY

The creation of strict products liability further fueled the explosion of litigation in general and of athletic litigation in particular. In 1963, in the case of *Greenman vs. Yuba Power Products, Inc,*[2] the California Supreme Court declared: "A manufacturer is strictly liable in tort when an article he places on the market, knowing that it is to be used without inspection for defects, proves to have a defect that causes injury to human beings." The reasoning of *Greenman* was that losses due to defective products should be borne by the manufacturer because he is in the best position to insure against the liability and to distribute that liability to the public by factoring its costs into the price of the product.

This judicial legislation effectively mandated verdicts against the manufacturing community, and plaintiffs' lawyers wasted no time in exploiting the invitation. Fault was suddenly irrelevant. An injured person need only have an "expert" testify a product was defective and a jury would then be allowed to decide whether the injured person would collect and, if so, how much. Neither contributory negligence, assumption of risk, nor plain stupidity was allowed as defenses.

Since *Greenman,* the California Supreme Court has even eliminated the plaintiff's burden of proving a defect. An injured player's sole liability burden is to prove he was injured while using the product. The burden of proof then shifts to the defendant, who must prove that the benefits of the product's design outweigh the risks inherent in the product. If the defendant is unable to convince a jury, the plaintiff wins.

This economic spreading-the-cost process has been a circuitous but overwhelming success from the injured person's standpoint. Krepps[4] accurately described the mechanics in this way: "Juries hand down large judgments seemingly regardless of blame. Insurance companies pay the judgements, then raise the premiums on the insured. Finally, the insureds pass along the premiums to the rest of us in the price of their products and service." A football helmet that cost $23.95 in 1960 retailed for $100 in 1985. Of that $100, $35 to $40 is for product liability exposure. The premise of *Greenman* seemed to be that there would always be a sufficient number of manufacturers and insurance carriers willing to participate in a no-fault giveaway. This is simply not true.

Between 1975 and 1982, eight football helmet manufacturers left the marketplace. Of the six major manufacturers remaining at the beginning of 1982, Medalist Gladiator dropped out of the industry as of Oct 1, 1982; MaxPro and Bill Kelley, who had merged in the hope of being able to collectively afford product liability insurance, closed their doors as of Feb 1, 1983. There now remain three major helmet manufacturers, who are facing at least 60 catastrophic head and neck injury cases yet to be tried. Profits for the entire football helmet industry are estimated to be between $2 million and $3 million on sales between $30 and $35 million. In 1983, when coverage was still available, the total liability premiums were estimated to be about $2.5 million. Today, the three remaining manufacturers are self-insured or have coverage through parent corporations and are probably hopelessly underinsured. The manufacturer with the smallest market share pays approximately $1 million for coverage. The remaining two, with a combined market share of 85% to 90%, are setting aside or paying similar amounts for their liability exposure. Assuming none of these manufacturers ever have to pay a multimillion dollar verdict, simply the minimum amounts they are setting aside for liability exposure meet or exceed the profits for the entire industry. There is no business incentive for anyone to stay in the football helmet business.

Similar situations can be found with trampolines, wrestling mats, hockey helmets, and baseball helmets. In lacrosse, one of the two manufacturers of helmets has been forced to market their product without insurance. Their $8,000 premium paid in 1984 for $25 million of coverage was increased to $200,000 for $1 million worth of liability coverage for 1986. The president of the company[1] was quoted in *Time* magazine as saying, "If we have a large judgement against us, it could be the end of lacrosse." The same is true of football.

JOINT AND SEVERAL LIABILITY AND DEEP POCKET LITIGATION

Whereas the adoption of comparative negligence, strict product liability, and the abrogation of assumption of risk has dramatically increased the number of athletic lawsuits in the past 20 years, the application of joint and several liability has increased the number of potential defendants in litigation. Joint and several liability has fostered what is commonly referred to as deep pocket litigation.

Joint and several liability is a rule of law dealing with damages. Where multiple defendants are each found to have contributed to a plaintiff's injury, each is responsible, individually, for the entire verdict. The reasoning behind this rule is that the injured person is entitled to the full amount of his verdict and should not be deprived of his damages because one or more of the defendants are unable to pay their proportionate share of an award. A plaintiff, thus, may collect his judgment from any defendant regardless of the percentage of fault of that party. A defendant 1% at fault can be required to pay 100% of a verdict.

When this doctrine is combined with comparative negligence, it virtually guarantees that everyone even remotely related to an accident will be named in a lawsuit. It allows the attorneys to shop for the "deepest pocket," the defendant or defendants with enough assets to pay

an award even if their involvement is peripheral. Additionally, the more defendants named, the larger the potential settlement pot becomes.

MORE LAWSUITS, HIGHER AWARDS

In the world of athletic litigation, an event which would otherwise be accepted as an unfortunate accident or a deliberate act of malice by a fellow player becomes a very serious and complicated circus orchestrated by an attorney with a large financial stake in convincing 12 jurors to find that someone other than, or in addition to, the injured player caused or contributed to a particular injury. A finding of any fault, however slight, can have devastating financial consequences for school districts, coaches, trainers, officials, team and treating physicians, and equipment manufacturers.

During the period 1970–1985, in football alone, 25 cases involving head and neck injuries have been tried to verdict. Of these 25 verdicts, 11 have been in favor of injured athletes. These 11 verdicts total $45.8 million. They were rendered against football helmet manufacturers, school districts, coaches, athletic associations, and doctors. Of this $45.8 million, $38.7 million was awarded between 1980 and 1985. These were verdicts only; settlements during the same period of time would increase the payout at least another $5 million.

Verdicts in the same 5-year period for noncatastrophic football injuries and against defendants involved in gymnastics, wrestling, track, baseball, basketball, hockey, lacrosse, and even cross-country track would easily quadruple the $38 million awarded for football injuries during that same period. A $14.7 million verdict for a gymnastic instructor in November 1985 was described earlier in this chapter. A former football player was awarded $1.5 million against the District of Columbia Public School system because he injured his arm while making a tackle. He claimed his coach had played him despite the fact he had injured the same area in practice the week before. A Portland, Ore, football player was awarded $80,975 against his coach and school district because he suffered a spinal column stress fracture as a result of his participation in a drill that required him to carry another player on his back. A high school pole vaulter settled his $32 million suit against the school district and mat manufacturer for $5 million after 7 days of trial. While competing, he landed only partially on the mat, which he claimed was not properly placed. The mat manufacturer contributed to the settlement.

In Colorado, a young man suffered a spinal cord injury while using a privately owned trampoline at a fraternity house. He sued the university, the fraternity house, the trampoline manufacturer, and others, claiming the trampoline was in poor condition and unsupervised. All defendants except the university settled with the plaintiff before trial. The result: a $7.2 million verdict against the university that was reduced to $5.25 million because the jury found the plaintiff to have been 28% contributorily negligent. To many, it is incomprehensible that someone who gets on a trampoline knowing it is in poor condition and unsupervised is allowed to sue, much less collect. He can.

RISKS OF ATHLETIC PARTICIPATION

In many athletic injury cases, plaintiff's counsel argue that the sport or activity itself is unnecessarily dangerous. Sometimes they are correct. The spring-loaded tackling dummy is an example of a device that was much too dangerous for the benefit it offered. It is no longer used. Trampolines may be another good exam-

ple. Torg and Das[10] reviewed 23 years of literature on trampoline-related spinal injuries. They found 114 catastrophic spine injuries with quadriplegia. They also found that more experience with trampolines did not reduce the chance of serious injury. They concluded: "It is our opinion that both the trampoline and the minitrampoline are dangerous devices when used in the best of circumstances, and their use has no place in recreation, educational or competitive gymnastics."

This same argument is made about football. Attorneys argue that the game is not worth the statistically inevitable few catastrophic head and neck injuries that will occur each year. Plaintiffs' attorneys call on the jury to "send a message across America" that the game must be made "safer" by awarding an enormous verdict in their particular case. This well-rehearsed tactical invocation often has an irresistible emotional appeal; however, it is plain and pure sophistry and cannot be rationally supported. A look at the injury statistics for neurotrauma, cervical injuries, and deaths should illustrate that the "message" plaintiffs' attorneys are still imploring juries to send was received and collectively heeded a decade ago.

It may be impossible to make football any safer without fundamentally altering the structure of the game to reduce or eliminate physical contact between players. Society cannot continue to cheer and support an activity such as football without accepting the inevitable fact that some catastrophic injuries and deaths are certain when large, well-conditioned young men are constantly running into one another at incredible velocities as an integral part of the game. If society is unwilling to accept the risks inherent in football, it must diminish contact and dramatically alter the game. Neither football equipment manufacturers, national associations, school districts, athletic directors, nor coaches can make that decision.

Statistically, the fact remains that on a time-risk basis, football is one of the safest activities in which a young person can be involved, except for those other sports that are associated with even fewer catastrophic injuries. The irony is that litigation in athletics in general and football in particular is inversely proportional to injury statistics; during the period in which both neurologic and cervical injuries decreased, litigation increased. Although there were fewer and fewer potential plaintiffs, those who were injured were more inclined to sue, and juries were more disposed to find fault and award enormous damages.

Statistics are obviously meaningless to the 10 or 15 high school and college athletes and their parents who will suffer each year when a catastrophic athletic injury occurs. Litigation is going to continue, and school districts, coaches, state and national associations, and sports medicine practitioners will have to make the same decision that manufacturers have been forced to face: Can we afford to continue our involvement in athletics?

CONSEQUENCES OF ATHLETIC INJURY LAWSUITS

Several school districts and leagues are considering dropping those athletic activities that generate litigation, while others already have. The controversy over football may be the loudest, but football is not the only sport under attack. The Riverside, New York, Little League settled a lawsuit in 1985 brought by a young man whose parents sued his coaches because he misplayed a fly ball during practice and was hit in the eye. The coach, who was also the president of the youth athletic association that sponsored the town's Little League, said he was disappointed that he was denied his day in court. He reported that his organization was considering cancelling the rest of the schedule, including participation in the Little League World Series Tournament, and he doubted that the association could obtain adequate insurance in the future.

For those individuals who administer athletic programs or who teach, treat, or supply athletes, the implications of the increase in the number and scope of athletic injury lawsuits are obvious. Such an individual stands a much better chance today than he did a decade ago of being named as a defendant, regardless of how the injury occurred or his involvement in it. Once he is named, his insurance carrier will pay large sums of money to defend, settle, or try his case. Defense costs alone in a catastrophic injury case, not including any verdict that might be awarded, can run in the hundreds of thousands of dollars. Plaintiffs' lawyers know and exploit this fact.

Once a case is filed, a judge who is more concerned with the administration of justice than justice itself may practice what lawyers refer to as "judicial blackmail." Every available ounce of judicial influence will be mustered against defense counsel to settle the case, no matter what the merits and regardless of the defendant's wishes. Judges want cases off already crowded calendars. The insurance carrier will be caught between two undesirable options: pay now and stop the costs of defense from increasing or continue with the risk that there will be defense costs. To insurance carriers, economics, not right or wrong, determine which cases settle and which are tried.

Regardless of the outcome of a particular case, once an individual or group is sued, the costs of insurance will increase dramatically or insurance will simply become unavailable. This fact has been a reality for the manufacturing community and medical profession for some time. It has recently hit hard against school districts, private leagues, and organizations. Today the insurance industry is reluctant to write any kind of liability insurance. The industry's representatives cite statistics that show 13 million civil suits filed last year, one for every 15 citizens of the United States. From 1977 to 1981, the number of civil lawsuits filed in state courts increased four times as fast as the population. Between 1974 and 1984, the number of products liability lawsuits increased 680% in federal courts. There was one multimillion dollar verdict in 1962. There were 401 in 1984. No one wants to write liability coverage when the number of lawsuits filed continue to proliferate and verdicts continue to increase. In California, many public entities, including school districts, have no liability coverage at all. Even the U.S. Olympic Committee has been told that its liability coverage will not be renewed when the policies expire.

The fundamental fallacy of the *Greenman* philosophy is now exposed; for those being sued for athletic injuries there is no way to pass on the costs of litigation to the general public. Even if coverage remains available, the cost of increased insurance premiums cannot be paid, much less passed on. Quoting premiums of $875,000 for $1 million worth of coverage is not an offer of coverage. A manufacturer can add $30 or $40 to the price of a football helmet in an attempt to cover its liability exposure, but how many schools can afford to purchase football helmets at $100 apiece? Even those schools that can afford the increased price in equipment still have their own independent liability exposure. To whom can they pass on that exposure when insurance is unavailable? Without liability coverage, coaches will be reluctant to participate in athletics, and school districts will find it necessary to cut back or eliminate programs. This will be unfortunate for those youngsters who appreciate the benefits of athletics.

EDUCATION AND PRECAUTIONS

Those involved with athletics are unfortunately unable to insulate themselves from being named in lawsuits. Assuming they choose to continue to participate, however, they can take steps to minimize the chances of being found at fault. Every school district should institute a program of education for athletes and their parents that would include a candid discussion of the risks as well as the benefits of their particular sport. Coaches who are reluctant to discuss the dangers of athletic competition for fear of losing good players or dulling their desire to win are not only kidding themselves but also failing to fulfill an obligation they owe athletes. They are also guaranteeing themselves judicial damnation and possible bankruptcy if an injury does occur and they are sued. Athletes who are injured and their parents invariably claim that they never appreciated the risks because no one told them. The realization and acceptance of those risks can only come from the coaching staff and schools.

Through this educational process, every school district should obtain a written waiver of liability from each athlete (or in the case of a minor, his parents). The waiver should repeat the risks of participation clearly and candidly. Signing such a waiver should be a condition of participation in athletics. The Seattle School District faced a $6.4 million verdict in 1982 when a jury accepted a football player's testimony that he was not taught not to run with his head down. The case was later settled for $3.2 million. The school district then instituted a policy requiring parents to waive their right to sue the school district in the event of an athletic injury as a condition of a student's participation. In February, the King County Superior Court upheld the school district's right to institute such a policy. Every school district in the county should attempt to utilize some sort of a waiver that would protect the school district, all its employees, and any outside personnel who act as part-time trainers or team doctors.

With or without a waiver, there are many precautionary actions schools can take to reduce the number of serious athletic injuries. A medical examination and a full medical history should be required before an athlete is allowed to participate in sports. Yearly follow-up examinations also should be required. If any questions are raised in routine examination, referrals should be made to appropriate medical specialists before an athlete continues in a program.

Excellent safety films and written material are available from the National Federation of State High School Associations in Kansas City, the Athletic Institute in North Palm Beach, Fla, and the American Academy of Orthopaedic Surgeons. At least one safety film should be shown to athletes at the start of each season. Their parents should be invited. Coaches should advise players that head injuries that can be fatal are often traceable to persisting minor symptoms such as recurring headaches and blurred vision. They should emphasize that any athlete with recurring episodes of these symptoms should inform the coaching staff immediately. The staff should then make certain that any such complaint is referred to a doctor immediately, and only when the doctor releases the athlete should he be allowed to resume participation. Coaches should document the attendance at all risk education classes by a roll record or sign-in sheet, and the particular subject matter of the discussion should be outlined, whether a lecture, a film, or a combination of both is used.

Ideally, every school should have a team doctor present at all games and practice sessions. In today's world, however, that usually is not economically possible. If a school cannot afford a team physician, it should attempt to employ a trainer who is a regular member of the faculty and who is adequately prepared and qualified. If neither team doctor nor trainer is a realistic possibility, each team must have someone who serves as a team first aid person. Whoever takes on the responsibility for this position should be trained by a qualified physician so that he can recognize symptoms of head injury and signs that identify potential problems and can use accepted measures to ensure that there are no symptoms of concussion before an athlete is allowed to continue participation.

Coaches must teach safe techniques in athletics. They should ensure that each athlete is properly conditioned; they should not encourage athletes to attempt risky maneuvers prematurely; and they should never force an athlete to proceed with any activity for which he or she is not ready either physically or psychologically. In football, coaches should explain helmet safety. Equipment people should make certain that each helmet is individually fitted to each player. All contact drills, especially blocking and tackling, should be explained thoroughly and then practiced at quarter speed initially until players become familiar with the purpose and execution. Only then should full-speed practice be allowed. In gymnastics, qualified spotters should always be available and used during practice sessions. Wrestling coaches should use care to ensure that only athletes of comparable size and skill are allowed to participate. Finally, safety equipment for all sports should be inspected regularly to make certain it is still capable of providing the protection for which it was designed. All equipment should be reconditioned or replaced when appropriate.

Basically, everyone responsible for athletics should be aware of the mechanics of cervical spine injuries and the danger signs that often precede permanent cerebral injuries. Athletes should be warned that lowering their heads and driving them into an opponent or falling headfirst onto a mat can cause a fracture dislocation resulting in quadriplegia. Although most athletes have little choice as to head positions during participation, knowledge, training, and practice may prevent cases of quadriplegia when the athlete knows what he or she should attempt to avoid. Be well informed yourself, teach safe practices, be sensitive to the possibility of serious injuries, and have a prepared plan for dealing with an injury if one does occur.

Defense counsel cannot prevent athletic lawsuits from being filed. They can, however, successfully defend them if those responsible conform to the standards of their professions by providing the instruction and care each athlete deserves and has the right to expect.

REFERENCES

1. Church GJ: Sorry, your policy is cancelled. *Time,* March 24, 1986.

2. *Greenman v Yuba Power Products, Inc,* 59 Cal 2d 57, California Supreme Court, 1963.

3. Harper and James: *The Law of Torts,* 21.5, p 1181.

4. Krepps W: Review of recent tort trends. *28 Defense Law Journal* 1979; I:65.

5. *Nabozny v Barnhell,* 334 NE 2d 74, Illinois Court of Appeals, 1975.

6. *Ohman v Board of Education,* 90 NE 2d 474,476, New York Court of Appeals, 1949.

7. *Passantino v Board of Education of City of New York,* 395 NYS 2d 628, New York Court of Appeals, 1976.

8. Prosser WL: *Handbook of the Law of Torts,* ed 4, 1971, pp 416–417.

9. *Satriano v Sleight,* 54/Cal App 2d 278,284, California Court of Appeals, 1942.

10. Torg JS, Das M: Trampoline-related quadriplegia: A review of the literature and reflections on the American Academy of Pediatrics' position statement. *Pediatrics* 1984; 74:804–811.

11. *Vedrell v School District 26C, Malheur County,* 376, p 2d 406, 413, Oregon Supreme Court, 1962.

12. *Welch v Dunsmuir Union High School District,* 326 p 2d 633, California Court of Appeals, 1958.

PART TWO

Intracranial Injuries

CHAPTER 16

Anatomy of the Brain and Its Coverings

Robert J. Johnson, M.D.

THE SCALP

The scalp is the first tissue that receives the trauma of blows or impacts to the head. It may be described as consisting of five layers. The first is the skin, which consists of epidermis and corium. We may include the hair, which under certain circumstances may have some protective value. Second, we have the superficial fascia, or subcutaneous layer, which consists of dense fatty areolar tissue tightly bound to both the skin above and to the next layer below, the galea aponeurotica. Because the subcutaneous layer is well vascularized, blows are prone to rupture its small vessels and lead to sharply localized hemorrhages trapped within this layer (Fig 16–1).

The third layer is a muscular one consisting of the epicranial muscle, with its two bellies at the front and two at the rear of the scalp, and the expansive galea aponeurotica between them. The galea is, in reality, a flat intermediate tendon between the bellies of this anteroposteriorly oriented digastric muscle. The right and left occipital muscles originate from the superior nuchal lines of the skull, and the right and left frontal muscles insert anteriorly into the skin at the two eyebrows. Because the fibrofatty subcutaneous layer is densely bound to the galea, blood or fluid within the former cannot disperse readily from its site of origin.

The fourth layer is loose areolar tissue that intervenes everywhere between the galea aponeurotica, or epicranius, and the underlying periosteum of the skull. This loose aerolar layer permits the scalp to move freely upon the skull and also allows blood or pus to spread easily within its substance. These may pass forward and into the tissues of the upper eyelid and deep to the orbicular muscle of the eye. Scalping injuries involve the separation of the scalp from the skull along this weak connective tissue plane. Last, the fifth layer of the scalp is the pericranium or periosteum of the skull bones.

THE CRANIUM

The primary duty of the cranial portion of the skull is to support and protect the brain. To this end the cranium and the contained dural folds are configured so as to offer internal compartments that provide several weight-supporting surfaces. These private loges for the several parts of the brain can prevent it from becoming displaced, and can prevent the

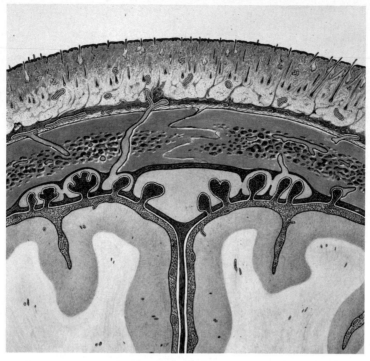

FIG 16–1.
Frontal section through scalp, cranium, meninges, and upper part of brain. *(From Clemente CC:* Anatomy, a Regional Atlas of the Human Body, *ed 3. Baltimore-Munich, Urban & Schwarzenberg, 1987. Used with permission.)*

tendency to roll and rotate that the brain would otherwise suffer if it were contained inside a single sphere.

The cranium is somewhat spheroid, and this allows it, like a true sphere, to provide maximum protection against the indentations produced by external impacts with the minimum of structural mass or substance; however, because of variations in the shapes of skulls, some are more spheroid than others. The short brachycephalic skull more closely approximates a sphere, while the elongated dolichocephalic skull is not as spherical. If a brachycephalic skull is compressed from any direction, its volume decreases, thereby compressing the brain inside. However, if a dolichocephalic skull is compressed along its anteroposterior axis, its internal volume increases slightly.[5] Thus, the shape of the cranium, as well as the thickness of the cranial bones, modifies the effects of blows.

Because of the foramen magnum and the tentorial incisure, any compressive force applied to the brain has a component of elongation distortion downward through these two apertures. Thus longitudinal tensions may be set up within the diencephalon and the brain stem.

At certain sites, the bones of the cranial vault are reinforced to receive the forces delivered upward from the facial skeleton via the heavier buttresses of bone present. Thus the forces of mastication, as well as the forces of blows to the face, are ultimately transferred to the cranium via the facial buttresses of bone that are prolonged into the cranium. These strengthened lines of bone in the cranium modify or determine lines of stress, and, therefore, lines of fracture.

Foramina or other apertures of the skull may modify fracture lines, because they offer zones of weakness. However, some of the margins of these apertures may be so thickened that they actually become zones of strength. Fractures that pass through foramina may involve the contents of those foramina. Nerves and vessels in foramina may tear, and the hemorrhage, in turn, may damage the nerves, piercing the foramen.

THE CRANIAL CAVITY

The floor of the cranial cavity is arranged in three fossae: anterior, middle, and posterior. The floors of these fossae resemble three steps, each with tread and riser, which descend anteriorly to posteriorly. The lateral floor of the anterior cranial fossa is the orbital plate of the frontal bone, which also serves as the roof of the orbital cavity. Frequently this plate of bone is pneumatized by the horizontal extension of the frontal sinus. If a fracture occurs here, the risk of meningitis is increased. More medially, the floor is formed by the cribriform plate of the ethmoid, which may communicate with the nasal cavity in case of fracture. The orbital surfaces of the frontal lobes of the brain rest on the floor of the anterior cranial fossa.

The middle cranial fossa is divided into right and left depressions by the higher-standing body of the sphenoid bone, which is indented by the fossa hypophyseos for the pituitary gland. Thus the middle cranial fossa is shaped somewhat like a butterfly with wings spread. The fossa for the hypophysis represents the body of the butterfly, and the lateral parts of the fossa, upon which the temporal lobes of the brain rest, are positioned like the spread wings. The riser between the right and left wings of this fossa and the anterior fossa is that part of the or-

bital plate of the great wing of the sphenoid bone that separates the middle fossa from the orbital cavity. On its other side, this orbital plate serves as the posterior half of the lateral wall of the orbit. Because this orbital plate fails to meet the lesser wing of the sphenoid bone, a space between them (the superior orbital fissure) permits communication between the middle cranial fossa and the orbital cavity.

The posterior cranial fossa supports the cerebellum and houses the pons and the medulla in its anteromedian region. Its floor is formed by the occipital bone, with the foramen magnum in its center anteriorly. The riser between it and the middle fossa is formed laterally by the posterior (or cerebellar) surfaces of the petrous portions of the right and left temporal bones. In the median area, the riser or anterior wall of this fossa is formed by the basilar portion of the occipital bone and the posterior surface of the body of the sphenoid bone, including the dorsum sellae.

The posterior cranial fossa is roofed in by the tentorium cerebelli (Figs 16–2 and 16–3). Since the tentorium has a U-shaped central defect anteriorly (the tentorial incisure), the mesencephalon or upper part of the brain stem ascends through this defect or space, and is continuous with the right and left diencephalons of their respective cerebral hemispheres. As it passes through the tentorial incisure, the mesencephalon has about 1 to 4 mm of free space between it and the edge of the tentorium cerebelli on either side. This limited tolerance should be remembered, because lateral shifts of the brain stem, due to supratentorial hematoma or other expanding lesions, force the cerebral peduncle of the opposite side to impinge against the firm, unyielding edge of the tentorium. This produces a Kernohan's notch or groove in the peduncle, with consequent hemiple-

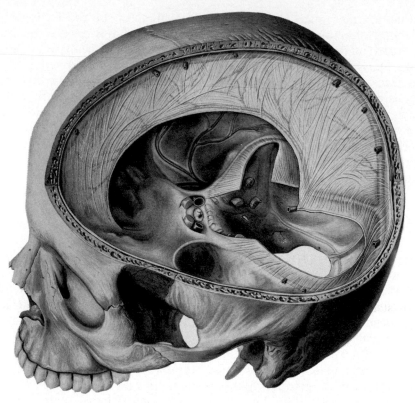

FIG 16–2.
The intracranial dura mater and the dural venous sinuses. *(From Clemente CC:* Anatomy, a Regional Atlas of the Human Body, *ed 3. Baltimore-Munich, Urban & Schwarzenberg, 1987. Used with permission.)*

gia, which is contralateral to the notch. Thus, hemiplegia develops on the same side as the original lesion (the hematoma). If supratentorial pressure increases, the uncus of the parahippocampal gyrus may herniate downward through this same available space between the cerebral peduncle and the margin of the tentorium cerebelli. The herniating uncus may produce a force that causes a lateral shift of the mesencephalon, with a Kernohan's groove as a possible result.

The downward-herniating uncus can also impinge on the oculomotor nerve below it, and damage it by stretching or compressing it against the dural fold known as the clivus ridge. When the mesencephalon shifts laterally, the oculomotor nerves may be damaged by yet another mechanism. Since the oculomotor

nerves not only descend at a 45-degree angle but also diverge at a 45-degree angle, it is apparent that a shift to one side or the other soon stretches the nerves on the side opposite to the direction of mesencephalon displacement.

Another possible mode of damage to the oculomotor nerve occurs with descent of the brain stem. Such descent carries the basilar artery downward, along with its terminal branches, the posterior cerebral arteries. The posterior cerebral artery on either side lies directly above the oculomotor nerve and crosses it at approximately a right angle. Descent of the posterior cerebral artery may drag downward on the oculomotor nerve, and either stretch it or compress it against the clivus ridge (see Fig 16–3). The adjacent trochlear nerve escapes comparable injuries because it is shielded by its position lat-

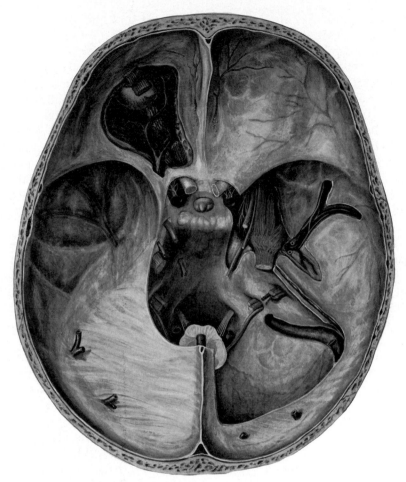

FIG 16–3.
The base of the cranial cavity showing dura mater and vessels and nerves. *(From Clemente CC:* Anatomy, a Regional Atlas of the Human Body, *ed 3. Baltimore-Munich, Urban & Schwarzenberg, 1987. Used with permission.)*

erally under the protection of the free edge of the tentorium cerebelli. Any downward displacement of the brain stem immediately stretches the abducens nerve, causing a lateral rectus muscle paresis.

THE MENINGES

The cranial cavity is lined everywhere with the dura mater. The dura mater consists of two layers. Where it is apposed to the skull, the two layers are the meningeal and the periosteal (or en-

dosteal) layers. The latter lies directly against the bone. Although their fibers run in different directions in any given area, and thus maintain some individual identity, the two layers cannot be separated by dissection. However, at the sites of the superior sagittal sinus and the lateral dural venous sinuses, these two layers are fully separated by the presence of these sinuses. The endothelial walls of the sinuses fit against the separated surfaces of the two dural layers. It thus appears that the dural venous sinuses run within the dura mater. There are three major sites where the meningeal layer alone is drawn inward as a double-layered fold, thereby creating the falx cerebri, the tentorium cerebelli, and the inconspicuous falx cerebelli.

In the midsagittal plane of the cranial cavity, the meningeal layer is drawn downward in a double-layered fold, in the lower-free margin of which is the inferior sagittal sinus (see Fig 16–2). This median sagittal fold is the falx cerebri, and it stands as a firm plate between the cerebral hemispheres. Its lower border falls short of reaching the corpus callosum, a massive commissural bundle, which links the two hemispheres. In unilateral expanding masses a portion of the hemisphere on the involved side may be forced under the lower margin of the falx cerebri to herniate toward the opposite side, with consequent local damage to brain tissue.

The tentorium cerebelli is a fold of dura mater that forms a roof over the posterior cranial fossa below, and at the same time serves as the floor for supporting the posterior part of the supratentorial brain. It is chiefly the occipital lobes of the brain, which rest upon the upper aspect of the tentorium cerebelli, and which are thus separated from the cerebellum. The tentorium cerebelli is not horizontal, but peaks upward centrally to somewhat resemble a conical tent. And, like an Indian teepee, it has an anterior opening through which the mesencephalon ascends. This opening, the tentorial notch or incisure, has already been discussed. The tentorium cerebelli has, therefore, an attached margin, like the base of the tent, and a free margin, which forms the edges of the tentorial incisure (see Fig 16–3). The attached margin is anchored to the cranium along a nearly horizontal curved line where it houses the right and left lateral dural venous sinuses. This attached margin extends forward and medially on either side along the petrosal crest and finally bridges the short gap between the apex of the petrosal crest and the posterior clinoid process. These last few millimeters of the attached margin create the clivus ridge, mentioned previously in connection with compression of the oculomotor nerve.

In the midline, the extensive falx cerebri separates the two cerebral hemispheres, while posteriorly the tentorium cerebelli separates the cerebellum from the inferior aspect of the occipital lobes and serves as a support for the latter. The smaller falx cerebelli projects along the midline in the floor and posterior part of the posterior cranial fossa. It forms a small partition separating the right and left posteriormost portions (arciform lobes) of the cerebellum. These three dural folds thus extend into the interior of the cranial cavity like baffle plates and create separate lobes for the several parts of the brain. As previously mentioned, these separate compartments have a protective value since they prevent a tendency for the brain to roll and rotate (or twist) with the various motions of the head.

The dural folds also house the dural venous sinuses, which receive all of the venous drainage from the brain. The superior sagittal sinus, running in the attached margin, and the inferior sagittal sinus, in the lower-free margin of the falx cerebri, both receive superficial cerebral veins from the hemispheres. The lateral dural venous sinuses (right and left) run in the attached margin of the tentorium cerebelli and receive the veins draining the cerebellum below, as well as superficial cerebral veins from the occipital lobes. All of these veins coming from brain tissue must pass through the subarachnoid space, pierce the arachnoid, and enter the dural sinuses. As they pass from the arachnoid to the dura mater they cross the potential subdural space. If displacements of the brain stretch these bridging veins and the veins tear while in this interval, they bleed into the subdural space. Several bridging veins leave the sylvian fissure (superficial middle cerebral veins) to pass to the small sphenoparietal venous sinus that runs along the posterior free border of the lesser wing of the sphenoid bone. Posterior displacements of the brain put these bridging veins in jeopardy, and may cause subdural hematomas.

THE MENINGEAL ARTERIES

On the external surface of the dura mater, and intimately and firmly attached to it, are a number of so-called meningeal arteries with their accompanying venae comitantes. These vessels lie between dura mater and bone and branch to both the dura mater subjacent to them and to the overlying bone. As stated, they are firmly attached to the dura mater when it is stripped away from the bone. What is not usually obvious is that their many small osseous branches, which supply the overlying bone, are broken by such dural stripping, even though the main trunk of the artery remains intact. By far the greater part of the blood flowing in these meningeal vessels is actually destined for the overlying bone of the skull. Not only does bone itself have a higher metabolic demand than dura mater, but the diploë between the inner and outer tables of cranial bone is filled throughout life with hematopoietic tissue for the production of red blood cells.

Breaking the osseous branches of the meningeal arteries is the primary source of bleeding in epidural or extradural hematomas. Note that this bleeding occurs at arterial pressure. Obviously the venae comitantes, as well as the occasionally torn dural venous sinus, can also be sources of bleeding. The mere stripping of dura mater from the overlying bone, which has been indented by impact and has snapped back to a normal configuration without fracturing, is sufficient to rupture the osseous branches. At certain places the main trunks of the meningeal arteries may lie in bony canals, or be so deeply embedded in bone that they are likely to be torn in any fracture that occurs here. This is clearly not the only mechanism that causes bleeding, however.

The middle meningeal artery, which runs across the floor of the middle cranial fossa and spreads its branches widely up the side of the skull, is by far the largest of the meningeal arteries. Smaller meningeal arteries, derived from the ophthalmic artery, supply the dura mater and bone of the floor and walls of the anterior cranial fossa. Several equally small meningeal arteries, derived from the external carotid system, supply the dura mater and bone of the floor and walls of the posterior cranial fossa. Thus epidural hematomas are more common in the middle cranial fossa and over the dorsolateral aspect of the brain, but they can also occur in the anterior and posterior cranial fossae.

The leptomeninges consist of the arachnoid and the pia mater. Between these two membranes lies the subarachnoid space, which is filled with about 150 mL of cerebrospinal fluid. The arachnoid is applied to the inner aspect of the dura mater but does not adhere to it except at certain sites, such as at arachnoid granulations and the places where veins pierce it to enter the dural venous sinuses. The pia mater is a thin layer of connective tissue intimately adherent to the surface of the brain and spinal cord. It must be penetrated by all the branches of the cerebral arteries and veins that enter the neural substance. A forest of trabeculae, composed of arachnoid cells, extends from the inner aspect of the arachnoid membrane across the subarachnoid space to spread upon and fuse with the pia mater. Thus the subarachnoid space is actually an extensive cleft in the meshwork of arachnoid cells. Arteries and veins on the surface of the brain, if ruptured or torn, bleed into the subarachnoid space.

ARTERIES OF THE BRAIN

The blood supply to the brain is derived from four arteries, the right and left internal carotid arteries and the right and left vertebral arteries (Fig 16–4). Each of these can be damaged by cervical as well as intracranial trauma. Such trauma may result in laceration, contusion with thrombosis, and vasospasm.

In the neck the internal carotid artery, together with the internal jugular vein and vagus nerve, is embedded in the carotid sheath. This artery enters the carotid canal in the petrous part of the temporal bone and makes its way into the cranial cavity via the upper aspect of the foramen lacerum. It is immediately contained within the cavernous sinus on the lateral aspect of the body of the sphenoid bone. In the event of fractures here, small branches of the internal carotid artery may establish arteriovenous aneurysmal connections with the venous network within the cavernous sinus. Passing through the roof of the cavernous sinus, each internal carotid artery establishes communications with the other and with the right and left posterior cerebral arteries, which are derived from the vertebrobasilar system. Thus the circle of Willis forms in which the four arteries that supply the brain communicate with one another by means of anastomoses. However, this anastomotic system varies in effectiveness or completeness from one person to another.

The three cerebral arteries are the anterior, the middle, and the posterior. The anterior and middle cerebral arteries are derived from the internal carotid artery, while the posterior cerebral artery is derived from the vertebrobasilar system. However, occasionally one or the other posterior cerebral artery arises, as they do in the embryo, from the internal carotid artery.

The right and left vertebral arteries ascend in the neck through the foramina transversaria of the cervical vertebrae (see Fig 16–4). Typically, each artery skips the foramen of the seventh cervical vertebra and enters that of the sixth. Thereafter it passes successively through each of the foramina, finally to exit from the transverse foramen of the first cervical vertebra or atlas. The artery then turns sharply posteriorly to pass around the lateral and posterior aspects of the lateral mass of the atlas. Next it crosses the posterior arch of the atlas, pierces the atlanto-occipital membrane, and enters the neural or vertebral canal. It then penetrates the dura mater and the arachnoid, ascends in the subarachnoid space through the foramen magnum, and enters the posterior cranial fossa. The right and left vertebral arteries now incline toward one another as they ascend in front of the medulla. They meet and fuse to form the basilar artery at the level of the junction of the pons and medulla (inferior pontine sulcus). The basilar artery continues to ascend within the subarachnoid space, remaining in the midline between the pons and the clivus. At the junction of the pons and the mesencephalon (superior pontine sulcus), the basilar artery divides into the right and left posterior cerebral arteries. These leave the posterior cranial fossa by passing onto the superior aspect of the tentorium, and thereafter supply the right and left occipital lobes (see Fig 16–4).

Several sites of the vertebrobasilar system are in particular jeopardy from athletic trauma. As the vertebral artery ascends through the foramina transversaria, it may be damaged by fractures or dislocations. Osteophytic protrusions at the uncovertebral joints, a late sequel of degenerative disk disease and past trauma, may compress the vertebral artery and lead to vertebrobasilar insufficiency. Because of stiffening of the arte-

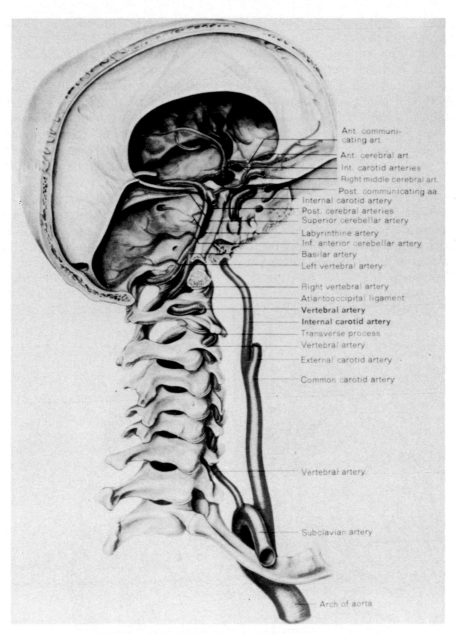

FIG 16–4.
The vertebral and internal carotid arteries shown in the neck and in the cranial cavity. In this specimen ossification in the atlanto-occipital membrane immediately adjacent to the aperture for the vertebral artery has created the posticulus posterior. This, with the posterior arch of the atlas, creates a bony foramen for the vertebral artery, which is a variation occasionally found. *(From Clemente CC:* Anatomy, A Regional Atlas of the Human Body, *ed 3. Baltimore-Munich, Urban & Schwarzenberg, 1987. Used with permission.)*

rial wall and a reduction in the caliber of the lumen, there is increased likelihood of even minor cervical spine trauma, causing critical vascular impairment in the older individual, with atherosclerotic changes in the vertebral artery. This is particularly true at the atlantoaxial joint level. Turning the head to one side or the other while looking upward may stretch and angulate the artery so much that these motions result in abrupt reductions of arterial flow to the brain stem and occipital lobes (transient ischemic attacks). As the right and left vertebral arteries cross the posterior arch of the first cervical vertebra and pierce the atlanto-occipital membrane, they may be subject to hazardous compression between the arch of the atlas and the occipital bone, in severe and forcible hyperextension of the head and cervical spine.[4] Such traumatic compression may be more than a mere momentary occlusion, for it may cause intimal contusion, laceration, and thrombosis, with consequent prolonged occlusion. Arterial wall trauma may also precipitate vasospasm in the arterial distribution beyond the site of trauma. At a higher level, the basilar artery may be involved in fractures through the clivus.

During their ascent in relation to the brain stem, the vertebral and basilar arteries give off a series of innumerable branches to the medulla, the pons, and the mesencephalon. These branches penetrate the brain stem as paramedian and short and long circumferential branches. In general, all such branches pass into and irrigate brain stem tissue in the horizontal plane. Since the brain stem is essentially vertical when the head is erect, we can compare the penetrating branches to the teeth of a comb when the comb is held vertically. Not to be forgotten is the

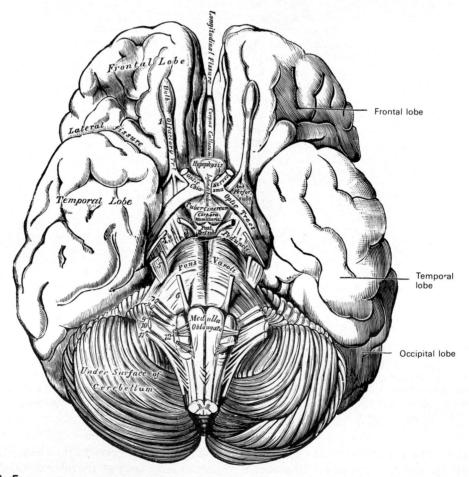

FIG 16–5.
Inferior surface of the brain. *(From Williams (ed):* Gray's Anatomy of the Human Body, *ed 37. New York, Churchill-Livingstone, 1989. Used with permission.)*

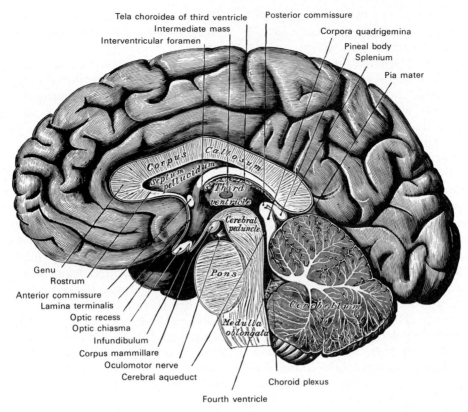

Tela choroidea of third ventricle
Intermediate mass
Interventricular foramen
Posterior commissure
Corpora quadrigemina
Pineal body
Splenium
Pia mater

Corpus Callosum
Septum pellucidum
Third ventricle
Cerebral peduncle

Genu
Rostrum
Anterior commissure
Lamina terminalis
Optic recess
Optic chiasma
Infundibulum
Corpus mammillare
Oculomotor nerve
Cerebral aqueduct

Pons
Cerebellum
Medulla oblongata

Choroid plexus
Fourth ventricle

FIG 16–6.
Medial surface of the brain demonstrating the major divisions visible in the sagittal section. *(From Williams   (ed): Gray's Anatomy of the Human Body, ed 37. New York, Churchill-Livingstone, 1989. Used with permission.)*

origin of the uppermost part of the anterior spinal artery, which supplies central branches to the cervical cord as well as to the medulla. This anterior spinal artery originates by the fusion of two short trunks from the right and the left vertebral arteries. Therefore, the upper cervical cord may also be endangered in trauma to the vertebral arteries.

A series of branches arise from the proximal parts of the anterior, middle, and posterior cerebral arteries and penetrate into the basal surface of the brain to supply the basal ganglia (basal or ganglionic arteries) and the thalamus (thalamogeniculate arteries). Lateral shifts of the cerebral tissue caused by hematomas may angulate these small, but often long, basal arteries and thus impede their blood flow. Cerebral contusions and lacerations may damage the branches of the three great cerebral arteries (anterior, middle, and posterior), which spread over the surface of the hemispheres. Their many penetrating branches irrigate the cortex and the subjacent white matter, and extend to the walls of the ventricular cavities.

THE BRAIN

The cerebral hemispheres (Figs 16–5 and 16–6) reside within the right and left sides of the supratentorial portion of the cranial cavity. The hemispheres are partially separated from each other in the midline by the falx cerebri. On the other hand, they are connected to each other by the tethering band of commissural fibers known as the corpus callosum. Displacement of the hemispheres may contuse their medial surface (particularly at the cingulate gyrus) against the resistant falx cerebri. This displacement may produce internal stress and strain within the corpus callosum and cause focal lesions of some length anteroposteriorly.

Although the cerebrum is protected and buffered everywhere by cerebrospinal fluid within the subarachnoid space, this space allows a certain amount of cerebral displacement before impact against the cranial wall or the dural folds. This displacement, plus further deformity from indentation of the skull or from inertial loading of the brain, can lead to contusions against not only the dural folds (falx cerebelli and tentorium cerebelli) but also the basal and polar areas of bony contact. Thus contusions are prone to develop at the frontal pole of the brain; in the adjacent surfaces of the frontal and temporal lobes, from impingement against the sphenoidal ridges (free margins of the lesser wings of the sphenoid bone); on the orbital surface of the frontal lobe; and on the inferolateral surface of the occipital lobes. The uncus of the parahippocampal gyrus may be contused against the margin of the tentorium, as well as herniated downward through the tentorial incisure by forces of long duration, such as cerebral swelling and intracerebral hematoma. The inferior surface of the cerebellum may be contused against the floor of the posterior cranial fossa. As previously mentioned, the cerebral peduncles may impinge against the free margins of the tentorium cerebelli during lateral displacements. Since the brain stem may also be displaced downward and even undergo slight torsion, it is apparent that it can be subjected to internal stresses as well as those that may occur in the cerebral hemispheres. Such internal stress may produce minute and diffuse neuronal and microglial damage, as well as vascular damage at the capillary level.

Internal shear stress, as well as cortical and surface vascular damage, may lead to degeneration and atrophy of long-fiber tracts in the cerebrum and in the brain stem. Thus there may be diffuse atrophy of cerebral white matter, which leads to enlargement of the various parts of the ventricular system that it surrounds. Areas of long-tract degeneration likely seen in the brain stem include the brachium conjunctivum cerebelli (the major outflow tract from the cerebellum), the corticospinal tracts, the medial lemnisci, and the central tegmental fasciculus (a multipurpose bundle best seen in the tegmentum of the pons).[1] Loss of cells in the hippocampus (Ammon's horn) and the presubiculum, as well as reduction of Purkinje cells in the inferior part of the cerebellum, has been noted, particularly in boxers.

REFERENCES

1. Adams JH: The neuropathology of head injuries, in Vinken PJ, Bruyn GW (eds): *Handbook of Clinical Neurology*, vol 23, part 1. New York, Elsevier Science Publishing Co, 1975.

2. Clemente CC: *Anatomy, a Regional Atlas of the Human Body*, ed 3. Baltimore-Munich, Urban & Schwarzenberg, 1987.

3. Netter F: *Atlas of Human Anatomy*, ed 1. Summerville, NJ, Ciba-Geigy Corp, 1989.

4. Schneider RC: Vascular insufficiency and differential distortion of brain and cord caused by cervicomedullary football injuries. *J Neurosurg* 1970; 33:363.

5. Unterharnscheidt F, Sellier K: Mechanics and pathomorphology of closed brain injuries, in Caveness WF, Walker AE (eds): *Head Injury*. Philadelphia, JB Lippincott Co, 1966.

6. Williams (ed): Gray's Anatomy of the Human Body, ed 37. New York, Churchill Livingstone, 1989.

Color Plates

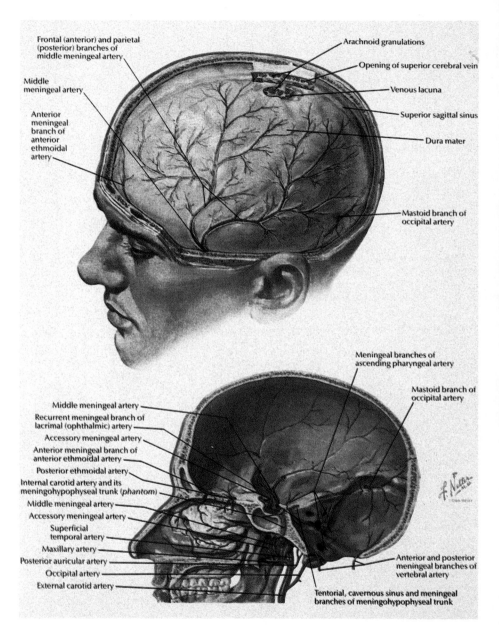

Frontal (anterior) and parietal (posterior) branches of middle meningeal artery

Middle meningeal artery

Anterior meningeal branch of anterior ethmoidal artery

Arachnoid granulations

Opening of superior cerebral vein

Venous lacuna

Superior sagittal sinus

Dura mater

Mastoid branch of occipital artery

Meningeal branches of ascending pharyngeal artery

Mastoid branch of occipital artery

Middle meningeal artery

Recurrent meningeal branch of lacrimal (ophthalmic) artery

Accessory meningeal artery

Anterior meningeal branch of anterior ethmoidal artery

Posterior ethmoidal artery

Internal carotid artery and its meningohypophyseal trunk (*phantom*)

Middle meningeal artery

Accessory meningeal artery

Superficial temporal artery

Maxillary artery

Posterior auricular artery

Occipital artery

External carotid artery

Anterior and posterior meningeal branches of vertebral artery

Tentorial, cavernous sinus and meningeal branches of meningohypophyseal trunk

PLATE 1.
Meningeal arteries.

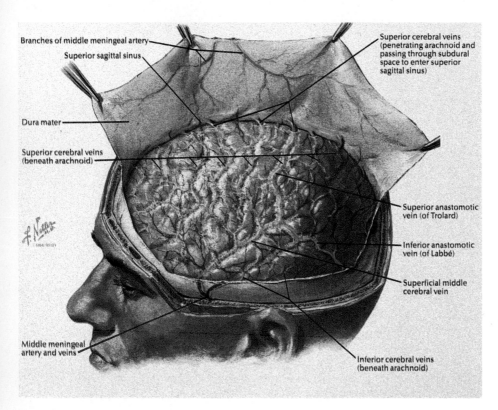

Branches of middle meningeal artery

Superior sagittal sinus

Dura mater

Superior cerebral veins (beneath arachnoid)

Middle meningeal artery and veins

Superior cerebral veins (penetrating arachnoid and passing through subdural space to enter superior sagittal sinus)

Superior anastomotic vein (of Trolard)

Inferior anastomotic vein (of Labbé)

Superficial middle cerebral vein

Inferior cerebral veins (beneath arachnoid)

PLATE 2.
Meninges and superficial cerebral veins.

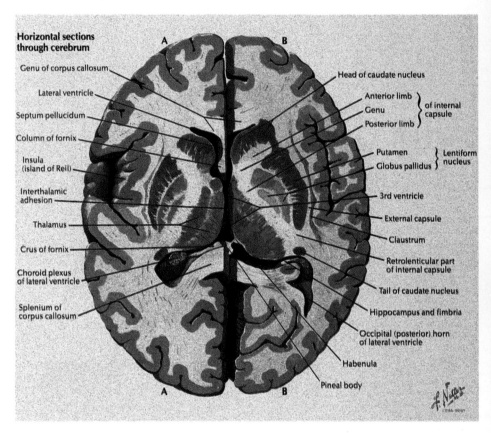

Horizontal sections through cerebrum

A B

Genu of corpus callosum

Lateral ventricle

Septum pellucidum

Column of fornix

Insula (island of Reil)

Interthalamic adhesion

Thalamus

Crus of fornix

Choroid plexus of lateral ventricle

Splenium of corpus callosum

Head of caudate nucleus

Anterior limb ⎫
Genu   ⎬ of internal capsule
Posterior limb ⎭

Putamen   ⎫ Lentiform
Globus pallidus ⎭ nucleus

3rd ventricle

External capsule

Claustrum

Retrolenticular part of internal capsule

Tail of caudate nucleus

Hippocampus and fimbria

Occipital (posterior) horn of lateral ventricle

Habenula

Pineal body

A B

PLATE 3.
Basal ganglia.

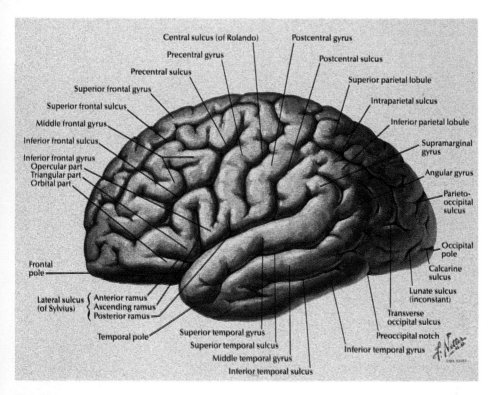

PLATE 4.
Cerebrum: Lateral view.

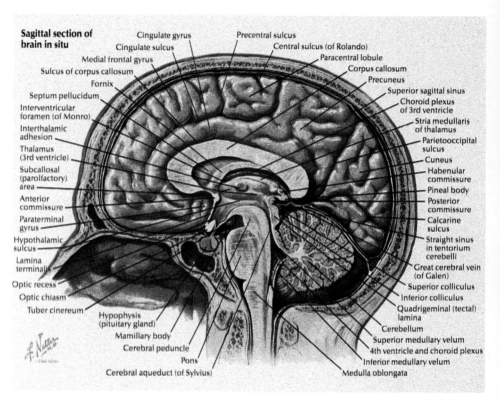

Sagittal section of brain in situ

Cingulate gyrus
Cingulate sulcus
Medial frontal gyrus
Sulcus of corpus callosum
Fornix
Septum pellucidum
Interventricular foramen (of Monro)
Interthalamic adhesion
Thalamus (3rd ventricle)
Subcallosal (parolfactory) area
Anterior commissure
Paraterminal gyrus
Hypothalamic sulcus
Lamina terminalis
Optic recess
Optic chiasm
Tuber cinereum
Hypophysis (pituitary gland)
Mamillary body
Cerebral peduncle
Pons
Cerebral aqueduct (of Sylvius)

Precentral sulcus
Central sulcus (of Rolando)
Paracentral lobule
Corpus callosum
Precuneus
Superior sagittal sinus
Choroid plexus of 3rd ventricle
Stria medullaris of thalamus
Parietooccipital sulcus
Cuneus
Habenular commissure
Pineal body
Posterior commissure
Calcarine sulcus
Straight sinus in tentorium cerebelli
Great cerebral vein (of Galen)
Superior colliculus
Inferior colliculus
Quadrigeminal (tectal) lamina
Cerebellum
Superior medullary velum
4th ventricle and choroid plexus
Inferior medullary velum
Medulla oblongata

PLATE 5.
Cerebrum: Medial view.

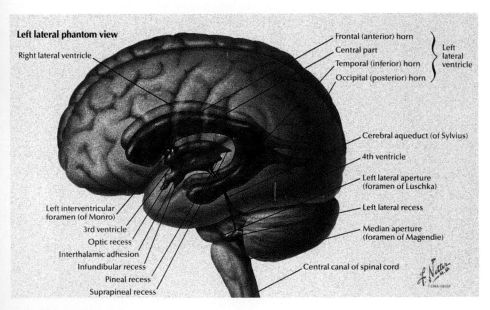

Left lateral phantom view

Right lateral ventricle

Frontal (anterior) horn
Central part
Temporal (inferior) horn
Occipital (posterior) horn

Left lateral ventricle

Cerebral aqueduct (of Sylvius)

4th ventricle

Left lateral aperture (foramen of Luschka)

Left lateral recess

Median aperture (foramen of Magendie)

Central canal of spinal cord

Left interventricular foramen (of Monro)
3rd ventricle
Optic recess
Interthalamic adhesion
Infundibular recess
Pineal recess
Suprapineal recess

PLATE 6.
Ventricles of brain.

CHAPTER 17

Field Evaluation and Management of Intracranial Injuries

Joseph J. Vegso, M.S.
Joseph S. Torg, M.D.

The purpose of this chapter is to present clear, concise guidelines for classification, evaluation, and emergency management of injuries that occur to the head as a result of participation in competitive and recreational activities.

Although all athletic injuries require careful attention, the evaluation and management of injuries to the head should receive special consideration. The clinical picture is not always representative of the seriousness of the injury. An intracranial hemorrhage may manifest only minimal symptoms, yet follow a precipitous downhill course, whereas a less severe injury, such as neurapraxia of the brachial plexus, which is associated with alarming paresthesias and paralysis, will resolve swiftly and allow for a quick return to activity. Although the more severe injuries are rather infrequent, this low incidence results in little, if any, management experience for the on-site medical staff.

There are several principles that should be considered by individuals responsible for the care of athletes who may sustain injuries to the head and neck.[4] They are as follows:

1. The team physician or athletic trainer should be designated as the person responsible for supervising on-the-field management of the potentially serious injury. This person is designated as the "captain" of the medical team.

2. Prior planning must ensure the availability of all necessary emergency equipment at a site of potential injury. At a minimum, this should include a spine board, stretcher, and equipment necessary for the initiation and maintenance of cardiopulmonary resuscitation (CPR).

3. Prior planning must ensure the availability of a properly equipped ambulance and a hospital equipped and staffed to handle emergency neurologic problems.

4. Prior planning must ensure immediate availability of a telephone for communicating with the hospital emergency room, ambulance, and other responsible individuals in case of an emergency.

INTRACRANIAL INJURIES

Injuries to the brain that occur as a result of sports may be either focal or diffuse lesions. The athlete who sustains such an injury may be conscious and ambulatory, conscious and nonambulatory, or unconscious. The initial state of the patient is not necessarily a reliable indicator of either the pathologic diagnosis or the severity of the injury. Rather, specific parameters must be used to determine the nature and severity of the insult, and to determine how the injured athlete should be managed.

The athlete who receives a blow to his head or a sudden jolt to his body that results in a sudden acceleration-deceleration force to the head should be carefully evaluated. In those instances in which the individual is ambulatory and conscious, the entire spectrum of intracranial pathology must be considered, ranging from a grade I concussion to a more severe intracranial condition. Initial on-the-field examination should include the following: (1) evaluate facial expression; (2) determine orientation of time, place, and person; (3) test for posttraumatic amnesia; (4) test for retrograde amnesia; and (5) evaluate gait.

An individual with a grade I concussion (Fig 17–1) will be confused and have a dazed look on his face. There may also be mild unsteadiness of gait. Posttraumatic and retrograde amnesia are not prominent features, however.[2] This clinical picture is best described by the athletes themselves who say, "I had my bell rung." Usually the state of confusion is short lived, and the athlete is completely lucid in 5 to 15 minutes. When his mind is clear, he may return to the activity under the watchful supervision of the team physician or the trainer. Associated symptoms such as vertigo, headaches, nausea, photophobia, and labile emotions should preclude returning to the game, however.

A grade II concussion is characterized by confusion associated with posttraumatic amnesia. The signs and symptoms described for grade I concussion also may be present. Individuals manifesting posttraumatic amnesia, the inability to recall events that have occurred from the moment of injury, should not be permitted to return to play that day. These athletes require postinjury evaluation. They may develop the "postconcussion syndrome," which is characterized by persistent headaches, difficulty with vision, inability to concentrate, and irritability. In some instances, these symptoms may last for several weeks postinjury, and participation in sports is precluded as long as symptoms are present.

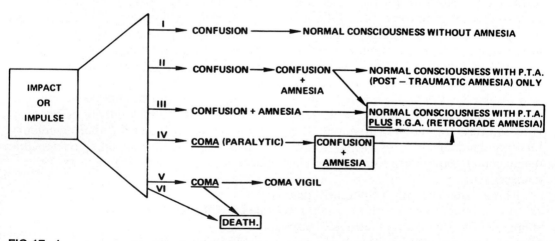

FIG 17–1.
Diagram of the six grades of cerebral concussion.

In addition to the symptoms mentioned, grade III concussions are characterized by retrograde amnesia,[2] which is the inability of the individual to recall events before the injury. These athletes should not be permitted to return to the game, and the general rules for observation and follow-up care as given should be followed. When there is a traumatic intracranial lesion that produces a gradual increase in intracranial pressure, as in epidural and subdural hemorrhages, the individual may be conscious and ambulatory to the point of appearing capable of fulfilling his usual activity and then suddenly collapse.

Frequently a more severe grade II or grade III concussion may result in the injured player being disoriented and unable to ambulate because of vertigo or an ataxic gait. The all-too-common practice of having such an individual literally dragged off the playing area by two of his teammates leaves much to be desired. Because the player may have a serious intracranial injury, or, in some instances, an associated cervical spine injury, an injured player who cannot walk unaided from the playing field after a reasonable period of time should be transported on a rigid stretcher or spine board.

A grade IV concussion involves the "knocked-out" player. This individual is at first in a paralytic coma, usually recovers after a few seconds or minutes, and then passes through states of stupor, confusion with or without delirium, and finally an almost lucid state with automatism before becoming fully alert.[2] Most certainly retrograde and posttraumatic amnesia will be present. If the loss of consciousness lasts more than several minutes or if there are other signs of a deteriorating neurologic state, the patient should be immediately transported to a hospital (Fig 17–2).

Immediate, initial examination of the athlete who has been rendered unconscious should involve making certain that he is breathing and that he has a pulse and then evaluating his level of consciousness. If unobstructed respirations and an adequate pulse are present, there is no immediate need to do anything. It is important to keep in mind, however, that head and neck injuries are frequently associated. Therefore, the player should be protected from injudicious manipulation or movement.

Such patients frequently remain semistuporous for more than several minutes. It should be emphasized that these individuals should be carried off the field on a spine board or stretcher. An athlete who has been rendered unconscious for any period of time should not be allowed to return to contact activity, even if he is mentally clear. Overnight observation in a hospital should be seriously considered for these athletes.

Grade V concussions are those in which injury produces paralytic coma that may be associated with secondary cardiorespiratory collapse.[2] In those instances in which associated cardiorespiratory failure develops, CPR should be implemented immediately.

Signs and symptoms that demand emergency action in an athlete who has sustained a blow to the head are increasing headache, nausea and vomiting, inequality of pupils, disorientation, progressive or sudden impairment of consciousness, a gradual rise in blood pressure, and, finally, a diminution of pulse rate. The development of any one or a combination of these may be indicative of increasing intracranial pressure. In this case, immediate evacuation to a medical facility is necessary.

An epidural hematoma may occur in the athlete who receives a severe blow to the head, for example, a baseball player who had been struck by the ball. If a fracture occurs across the middle meningeal groove, severing the middle meningeal artery with subsequent formation of a "high-pressure" hematoma, the player

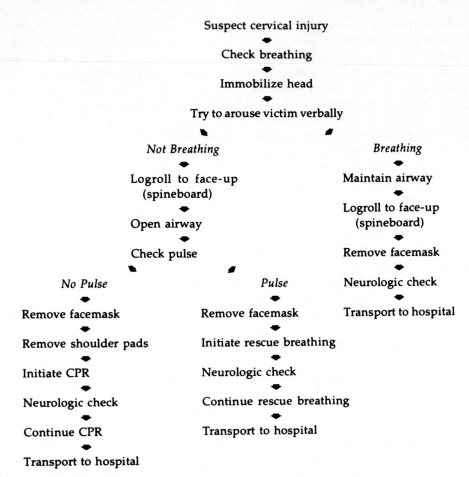

FIG 17-2.
Field decision making: head and neck injuries (unconscious athlete).

may do well for a short time; however, 10 to 20 minutes later he will develop one or more of the aforementioned danger signs. Such an individual should be transported immediately to a hospital.

A subdural hemorrhage occurs when the bridging veins between the brain and the cavernous sinus are torn as a result of contrecoup or rotational acceleration-deceleration injury. Low-pressure venous bleeding occurs, hematoma formation is slow, and the signs and symptoms of increasing intracranial pressure may not be evident for hours, days, or even weeks after the injury. In Schneider's[3] series of 69 patients with acute subdural hematoma, 24 had surgery or died within 6 hours of injury. Thus the physician and the trainer should be suspicious of a blow to the head and should watch the patient carefully. If an athlete develops any of the aforementioned danger signs and symptoms, he should be transported immediately to a hospital for neurologic evaluation and treatment.

In cases of collapsed or unconscious persons, the adequacy or absence of breathing and circulation must be determined immediately. If breathing alone is inadequate or absent, rescue breathing may be all that is necessary. If circulation is also absent, artificial circulation must be started in combination with rescue breathing. The methods of recognizing adequacy or absence of breathing or circulation and the recommended techniques for performing artificial ventilation and artificial circulation are presented below.

If the victim is breathing, simply remove the mouth guard, if present, and maintain the airway. It is necessary to remove the face mask only if the respiratory situation is threatened or unstable, or if the athlete remains unconscious for a prolonged period. Leave the chin strap on.[5]

Once it is established that the athlete is breathing and has a pulse, evaluate the neurologic status. The level of consciousness, response to pain, pupillary response, and unusual posturing, flaccidity, rigidity, or weakness should be noted.

At this point, simply maintain the situation until transportation is available, or until the athlete regains consciousness. If the athlete is face down when the ambulance arrives, change his position to face up by logrolling him onto a spine board. Make no attempt to move him except to transport him or to perform CPR if it becomes necessary.

If the athlete is not breathing or stops breathing, the airway must be established. If he is face down, he must be brought to a face-up position. The safest and easiest way to accomplish this is to logroll the athlete into a face-up position. In an ideal situation your medical-support team is made up of five members: the leader, who controls the head and gives commands only; three members to roll; and a fourth to help lift and carry when it becomes necessary.[5] If time permits and the spine board is on the scene, the athlete should be rolled directly onto it. Breathing and circulation are much more important at this point, however.

With all medical-support team members in position, the athlete is rolled toward the assistants: one at the shoulders, one at the hips, and one at the knees. The assistants must maintain the body in line with the head and spine during the roll. The leader maintains immobilization of the head by applying slight traction and by using the crossed-arm technique. This technique allows the arms to unwind during the roll (see Figs 30–3 and 30–4).

The face mask must be removed from the helmet before rescue breathing can be initiated. The type of mask that is attached to the helmet determines the method of removal. Bolt cutters are used with the older single- and double-bar masks. The newer masks that are attached with plastic loops should be removed by cutting the loops with a sharp knife or scalpel. Cut the loops on the side away from the face. Remove the entire mask so that it does not interfere with further rescue efforts (see Figs 30–5 and 30–7).

Once the mask has been removed, initiate rescue breathing following the current standards of the American Heart Association.[1]

Once the athlete has been moved to a face-up position, quickly evaluate breathing and pulse. If there is still no breathing, or if breathing has stopped, the airway must be established.

Opening the airway and restoring breathing are the basic steps of artificial ventilation. The steps can be performed quickly under almost any circumstances and without adjunctive equipment or help from another person. They constitute emergency first aid for airway obstruction and respiratory inadequacy or arrest. Respiratory inadequacy may result from an obstruction of the airway or from respiratory failure. An obstructed airway is sometimes difficult to recognize until the airway is opened. At other times, a partially obstructed airway is recognized by labored breathing or excessive respiratory efforts, often involving accessory muscles of respiration, and by soft tissue retractions of the intercostal, supraclavicular, and suprasternal spaces. Respiratory failure is characterized by minimal or absent respiratory effort, failure of the chest or upper part of the abdomen to move, and inability to detect air movement through the nose or mouth.

Opening of the Airway

Material in this and the following two sections is from *Healthcare Provider's Manual for Basic Life Support.*[1] The most important action for successful resuscitation is immediate opening of the airway. In the absence of sufficient muscle tone, the tongue and/or epiglottis will obstruct the pharynx and/or the larynx, respectively. The tongue is the most common cause of obstruction in the unconscious victim. Since the tongue is attached to the lower jaw, moving the jaw forward will lift the tongue and the epiglottis away from the back of the throat and open the airway. Also, either the tongue or the epiglottis, or both, may produce obstruction when negative pressure is created in the airway by inspiratory effort, causing a valve-type mechanism to occlude the entrance to the trachea. Opening the airway may be all that is needed to relieve the obstruction and allow the victim to breathe.

Head-Tilt/Chin-Lift

Head-tilt/chin-lift is recommended for opening the airway. Head-tilt is accomplished by placing one hand on the victim's forehead and applying firm, backward pressure with the palm to tilt the head back (Fig 17–3). To complete the head-tilt/chin-lift maneuver, place the fingers of the other hand under the bony part of the lower jaw near the chin and lift to bring the chin forward and the teeth almost to occlusion, thus supporting the jaw and helping to tilt the head back. The fingers must not press deeply into the soft tissue under the chin, which might obstruct the airway. The thumb

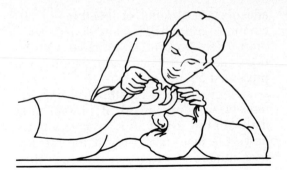

FIG 17–3.
Head-tilt/chin-lift maneuver for opening the airway. Used if jaw thrust is inadequate or if a helmet is being worn. *(Reprinted with permission of the American Heart Association.)*

should not be used for lifting the chin. The mouth should not be completely closed (unless mouth-to-nose breathing is the technique of choice for that particular victim). When mouth-to-nose ventilation is indicated, the hand that is already on the chin can close the mouth by applying increased force and, in this way, provide effective mouth-to-nose ventilation. If the victim has loose dentures, head-tilt/chin-lift maintains their position and makes a mouth-to-mouth seal easier. Dentures should be removed if they cannot be managed in place.

Jaw-Thrust

Additional forward displacement of the jaw by use of the jaw-thrust maneuver may be required. This can be accomplished by grasping the angles of the victim's lower jaw and lifting with both hands, one on each side, displacing the mandible forward while tilting the head backward (Fig 17–4). The rescuer's elbows should rest on the surface on which the victim is lying. If the lips close, the lower lip can be retracted with the thumb. If mouth-to-mouth breathing is necessary, the nostrils may be closed by placing the rescuer's cheek tightly against them.

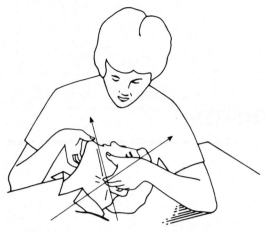

FIG 17–4.
Jaw-thrust maneuver for opening the airway of a victim with a suspected cervical spine injury. *(Reprinted with permission of the American Heart Association.)*

Jaw-thrust (or chin-lift), without head-tilt, is the safest first approach to opening the airway of the victim with a suspected neck injury because it usually can be accomplished without extending the neck. The head should be carefully supported without tilting it backward or turning it from side to side. If this maneuver is unsuccessful, the head should be tilted backward very slightly.

REFERENCES

1. *Healthcare Provider's Manual for Basic Life Support.* American Heart Association, Dallas, Tex, 1988.

2. Ommaya AK, Gennarelli TA: Cerebral concussion and traumatic unconsciousness. Correlation of experimental and clinical observations on blunt head injuries. *Brain* 1974; 97:638.

3. Schneider RC: *Head and Neck Injuries in Football. Mechanisms, Treatment, and Prevention.* Baltimore, Williams & Wilkins, 1972.

4. Schneider RC, Kriss FC: Decisions concerning cerebral concussions in football players. *Med Sci Sports* 1969; 1:115.

5. Torg JS, Quedenfeld TC, Newell W: When the athlete's life is threatened. *Phys Sportsmed* 1975; 3:54.

CHAPTER 18

Head Injury Mechanisms

Thomas A. Gennarelli, M.D.

Considerations of determining how a particular mechanical input to the head results in a particular outcome require an analysis of multiple factors. First the nature, the severity, and the site and direction of the input to the head are of importance. The primary mechanical damage which that input causes may then affect either the scalp, the skull, or the brain. Finally, the overall result of mechanical input is determined by a complex interaction of pathophysiologic events that result in temporary or permanent neurologic disability.

In general terms, head injuries can be viewed as comprising three distinct varieties: skull fracture, focal injuries, and diffuse injuries. Skull fracture can occur with or without damage to the brain, but is itself not an important cause of neurologic death nor disability. The injuries to the neural substance of the brain are rather the causes of neurologic dysfunction and can readily be divided into two categories. Focal injuries cause local damage and comprise entities such as cortical contusion, subdural hematoma, epidural hematoma, and intracerebral hematoma. These injuries comprise approximately 50% of all head injury patients admitted to the hospital and are responsible for two thirds of head injury deaths.

Diffuse injuries are not associated with localized damage but rather with widespread disruption of either the structure or the function of the brain. These diffuse injuries account for approximatly 40% of head injury patients admitted to hospital, and, although they comprise only one fourth of the deaths, they are the most serious cause of persisting neurologic disability in the survivors.

BIOMECHANICAL MECHANISMS OF INJURY

The types of mechanical input to the head are numerous and complex. Fig 18–1 provides a flow chart analysis of the known and proposed mechanisms of injury. Mechanical input to the head can either be slow (static loading) or, as more commonly occurs, rapid (dynamic loading). Static loading of the head implies that forces are applied in a gradual manner, usually exceeding 200 to 500 msec or longer. This is comparable to a slow squeezing effect on the skull and results in serious fracturing of the skull. Only after multiple comminuted skull fractures occur is consciousness lost and the brain itself injured. Static loading is not a commonplace situation, particularly in sports

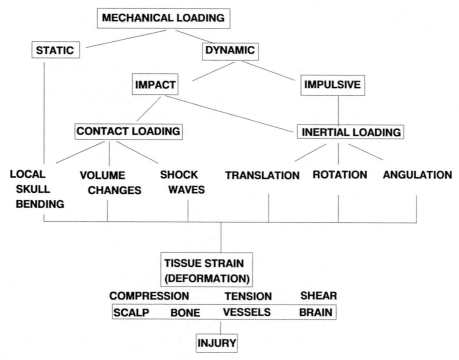

FIG 18–1.
Flow chart of the biomechanical mechanisms of head injury. *(From Abel J, Gennarelli TA, Segawa H: Incidence and severity of cerebral concussion in the rhesus monkey following sagittal plane angular acceleration, in* 22nd Stapp Carr Crash Conference Proceedings. *New York, Society of Automotive Engineers, 1978.)*

injuries. The more common dynamic loading occurs during time periods less than 200 msec, and usually involves two components, impact and impulsive loading. Impact to the head is the most common event of dynamic loading, but impulsive loading of the head can also occur. Impulsive loading occurs in situations in which the head is not directly struck, but is set into motion, and either is accelerated or is decelerated. Such loading results from impact to the thorax where the head is freely movable. Impact produces the most frequent mechanical input to the head, and usually does cause acceleration of the head (inertial loading) as well as many regionalized effects known as contact phenomena.

The contact phenomena are a complex group of mechanical phenomena that occur both locally and distant from the point of impact. The magnitude and importance of these contact phenomena vary with the size of the impacting device and with the magnitude of force of the impact. Immediately beneath the point of impact there is localized skull deformation with in-bending of the skull, surrounded by a periphery of out-bending. If the degree of local skull deformation is significant, penetration of the skull, perforation, or fracture occurs. Additionally, shock waves that travel with the speed of sound propagate throughout the skull from the point of impact as well as directly through the brain substance. The role of shock waves in causing local changes in brain tissue pressure and, consequently, brain injury has been a matter of debate. Because of the extremely rapid transmission of these waves through the brain, however, shock waves are probably not the most important injury mechanism for the brain.

CONTACT PHENOMENA AND SKULL FRACTURE

Local contact phenomena that result from impact are, however, the most important mechanism for skull fracture. The occurrence of skull fracture is dependent on the material properties of the skull, the magnitude and direction of impact, the size of the impact area, and the thickness of the skull in various areas. The material properties of the skull are similar to those of other bony structurees in the body. In general, mechanical failure of the skull occurs in tensile stress more readily than in compression. Thus when a patient falls and strikes his head on an object, or when an object strikes the patient's head at the point of in-bending of the skull beneath the impact point, the inner table of the skull is placed under a tensile strain, whereas the outer table is put into compression. If the impact is of sufficient magnitude and the skull is sufficiently thin at the point of impact, a skull fracture will begin in the area of tensile loading on the inner table of the skull. Alternately, if the region of impact is over a thick portion of the skull, the local in-bending will have no effect. There is an area of out-bending of the skull peripherally around the impact zone, however, which puts the outer table under tension and the inner table under compression. If this area of out-bending is in a thin area of the skull, a fracture may be in some distance from the point of impact in the outer table. Propagation of a skull fracture from its origin will then occur along lines of least resistance. It is therefore not surprising that not all skull fractures occur immediately beneath the impact area.

The common locations of skull fractures will, to some degree, reflect the direction of impact forces. Low frontal impacts, those on the forehead or supraorbital area, propagate fractures up the vault along the frontal bone as well as down along the base of the skull into the anterior cranial fossa. Most of the fracture line may be along the thin cribiform plate at the base of the skull or along the orbital roofs rather than on the surface of the skull. If the impact point is higher in the frontal area, vault fractures are more common than basilar fractures. An impact site that is frontolateral propagates a fracture line through the very thin inferolateral aspect of the skull rather than over the thicker frontal bone. Thus fractures occur into the squamous portion of the temporal bone and orbital roofs. Higher lateral impacts, above and behind the ear, similarly tend to propagate fractures at a distance from the impact, again because of the thinness of the inferior portion of the temporal bone. These fractures will progagate along the floor of the middle cranial fossa and upward toward the site of impact. Posterior impacts involving the occipital or posterior parietal areas cause fracture lines that travel downward through the occipital bone and aim for the foramen magnum.

Skull fractures can be viewed in the same light as fractures elsewhere in the body. Healing is anticipated within several weeks after fracture, and therefore the fracture itself is of no clinical importance. The exceptions to this rule include fractures of the skull base, fractures that cross meningeal vessels, and fractures that are compound or open. The terminology of the latter is slightly different than for fractures elsewhere in the body. Compound fractures are associated with skin lacerations above them, whereas open fractures mean that the dura mater has been lacerated. These fractures run a greater risk of infection within the brain substance and are more severe than closed fractures. Fractures that cross meningeal blood vessels may lacerate these vessels and cause extradural hemorrhage that can be life threatening. Basilar skull fractures are important because of dural, arachnoid, or cranial nerve lacerations that are associated with the fracture. The fractures of the base of the skull anteriorly may cause anosmia by transection of the olfactory nerve, or blindness because of transection of the optic nerve. Frequently a fracture through the cribiform plate beneath the olfactory nerve causes cerebrospinal fluid to leak into the nose and can cause a potential input for bacteria into the head, with resulting meningitis. Fractures of the middle and posterior cranial fossa base usually involve the petrous ridge that houses the facial, auditory, and vestibular nerves. Involvement of these nerves can cause a facial palsy, deafness, or vertigo, and additionally can cause cerebrospinal fluid to leak out through the external ear. With the exceptions of basilar skull fractures, fractures across the meningeal vessels, and open skull fractures, skull fractures in and of themselves are of little clinical importance.

Depressed skull fractures may be of clinical importance if they result in brain contusion, laceration, or compression. These fractures are the consequence of impacts from an object small in diameter that causes skull perforation. Because the skull fails in tension before compression, fracturing of the inner table is always more serious than that of the outer table. In-driven bone fragments can then perforate or lacerate the dura mater or brain and cause local brain damage. This cortical injury is associated with a serious risk of infection and seizures. Thus while linear skull fractures, with the exceptions noted, are usually of limited clinical significance, depressed skull fractures can be the cause of long-standing neurologic problems.

INERTIAL (ACCELERATION) EFFECTS

The effects of inertial loading of the head, whether caused by an impact or by impulsive loading, result in acceleration or deceleration of the head. From the mechanical point of view, acceleration and deceleration are the same physical input, differing only in direction. Acceleration of the head may result in a straight movement (translational acceleration; Fig 18–2, *A*) or in rotation of the head and neck (angular acceleration; Fig 18–2, *B*). There is mounting evidence that the effects of translational and angular acceleration on the brain differ markedly. This was tested directly in a series of primate experimental head injuries. In these tests the effects of impact were eliminated by encasing the head in a special helmet that diffused the head loading over the entire skull rather than provide focal impact loading. Two groups of animals were then subjected to pure acceleration loads. In the first group pure translational acceleration was provided in a posteroanterior direction, with the axis of acceleration along the sagittal plane. The second group of animals was subjected to angular acceleration by rotating the head and neck through a 45- to 60-degree arc with the center of rotation being in the cervical spine (see Fig 18–2). The physiologic and pathologic results in these two groups differed markedly. At the maximum accelerations used, it was impossible to induce a cerebral concussion in monkeys undergoing translational acceleration. On the other hand, it was very easy to induce concussion from rotational acceleration. It is therefore evident that the type of acceleration delivered to the head has a profound influence on the type of resulting neurologic dysfunction. Furthermore, it was apparent from this group of experiments that focal structural lesions such as contusions were much more common after translational acceleration, and diffuse injuries of the brain, such as concussion, were principally the results of rotational acceleration.

The initial experiments were followed by a series of 100 primate head injuries with use of a nonimpact angular

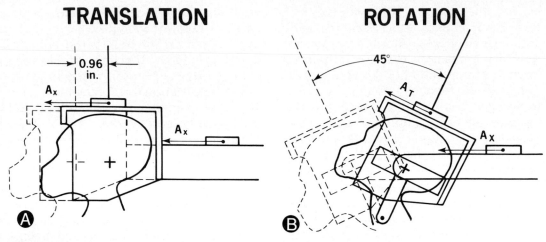

FIG 18–2.
Types of inertial loading of the head. Acceleration can be either translational **(A),** where the center of gravity (+) moves in a straight line, or angular **(B),** where the center of gravity travels in an arc. Pure acceleration loads are delivered into experimental animals by placing their heads within helmets so that no impact occurs during head movement. *(From Gennarelli TA, Thibault LE, Ommaya AK: Pathophysiologic responses to rotational and translational acceleration of the head, in* 16th Stapp Carr Crash Conference Proceedings. *New York Society of Automotive Engineers, 1978.)*

acceleration mechanism. In this series the animals' heads were once again placed within a helmet so that the input forces were diffused widely over the head to avoid contact forces associated with impact. As angular acceleration was increased, changes in heart rate and blood pressure occurred before there was any evidence of loss of consciousness. Brief periods of apnea, followed by respiratory irregularities, occurred if angular acceleration was increased further. Only at substantial acceleration levels did concussion appear. Thus a continuum of events was defined and was related to the level of acceleration input into the head.

It is evident from these experiments that considerable physiologic dysfunction can occur with subconcussive injuries and that impact is not necessary for cerebral concussion. Furthermore, at very high levels of acceleration the subdural bridging veins were torn and large acute subdural hematomas of sufficient size to cause death occurred. In fact, detailed neuropathologic examination of the animal brains disclosed virtually every type of head injury pathology that is seen in human head injuries.

Therefore, many of the physiologic and pathologic consequences of head injury can be produced by a single injury mechanism, namely, angular acceleration. This is an important conceptual point because of the not infrequent occurrence of subdural hematoma in sports, particularly football and boxing. It must be understood that the mechanism of production of these is not related to the contact forces of impact but rather is a consequence of the angular acceleration of the head. This must be taken into account when designing safety equipment for sports. In a contact sports environment it is almost impossible to protect against the effects of head acceleration. Protective headgear, however, can decrease the local contact effects of the impact phenomena. Thus sports helmets could be expected to decrease skull fracture but not to substantially influence the production of acceleration-related injuries such as concussion and acute subdural hematoma.

In summary, the biomechanical events that occur as a result of mechanical input to the head are extremely complex. They can be viewed more simply as occurring from either acceleration or from contact phenomena. Contact phenomena from an impact produce principally focal effects, and result in skull fracture and cerebral contusion. In sports activities these can be mitigated to a considerable degree by adequate head protective devices. Acceleration affects the brain principally, but not exclusively, by angular (rotational) acceleration and causes more diffuse injuries to the brain. The mechanical properties of the brain are such that it is most susceptible to shear strains, and these strains are maximized by angular acceleration. Therefore, concussion, diffuse brain injury, and the production of acute subdural hematoma by tearing of bridging veins occur, not because of impact but because of head acceleration. These injuries, as well as others due to acceleration, are less likely to be minimized by protective headgear since these safety devices do not substantially change the direction and magnitude of head acceleration.

PATHOPHYSIOLOGIC MECHANISMS OF HEAD INJURY

The response of the brain to mechanical input is itself a complex series of events. Although the specific result of the brain's response varies with the magnitude of mechanical input, as well as with the direction and type of input, the pathophysiologic mechanisms that occur in the brain can be viewed as primary or secondary events. The primary brain injury mechanisms are entirely dependent on the mechanical damage to the brain caused by the mechanical input. Fortunately, in most instances the mechanical damage to the brain substance is not overwhelming. Usually secondary injury

mechanisms, such as ischemia-hypoxia, hemorrhage, edema, and the liberation of neurotoxic substances, comprise the mechanisms that cause more injury to the brain than the primary mechanical damage. Primary mechanical damage can affect either the brain fibers themselves, as is seen in cerebral contusions or in shearing damage to white matter axons, or can effect cerebral, dural, or meningeal blood vessels. The latter causes disruptions of arteries or veins within or around the brain and can lead to subsequent hemorrhaging. Often it is the degree of hemorrhaging rather than the disruption of the arterial and venous structures that causes the brain damage. Hemorrhage into the extradural, subdural, or intracerebral areas is therefore a secondary event that, if treated appropriately, can result in a favorable outcome. If the amount of hemorrhage is massive or if treatment is unable to reverse the effects of hemorrhaging, however, the outcome will not be favorable.

Another secondary event that occurs after the primary mechanical damage is cerebral ischemia or hypoxia. These events can be caused by inadequate ventilation, resulting in systemic, whole body hypoxia. The cerebral vascular reaction to injury may be such that the cerebral blood flow is insufficient to meet the metabolic demands of the brain. This then results not in whole body hypoxia but rather in ischemia localized to the brain or to part of the brain. If inadequate blood flow or inadequate oxygen delivery to the brain persists long enough, death of tissue or cerebral infarction will occur. This is a secondary complication of head injury that should be preventable. If it is not, permanent damage to the brain will be additive to that primary mechanical damage caused by the mechanical input. The role of cerebral edema, that is, increased tissue water, is still debated, but recent evidence suggests that cerebral edema itself is important only as a cause of cerebral dysfunction if it is sufficient to cause increased intracranial pressure.

Even less is known about the secondary effects of toxic substances released at the time of mechanical input. In areas of cerebral ischemia, increased tissue acidosis and lactic acid accumulation occur and further embarrass cerebral function. If synaptic or axonal damage has occurred, intracellular contents, such as neuroactive peptides or neurotransmitter substances, are released. The action of these neurotransmitter substances can further embarrass cerebral function. This postulate remains to be proved, however.

Therefore the final biologic result of the mechanical input is dependent not only on the primary mechanical damage that occurs at the time of injury but also on the ischemic-hypoxic event, on the amount and location of cerebral hemorrhage, on the amount of cerebral edema and its effect on intracranial pressure, and on the amount of toxic agents that further embarrass cerebral function. The final result of a head injury in any particular patient therefore depends on the location and amount of the influence of these interacting factors.

The combination of these injury factors causes one of two series of events to predominate, focal injuries and diffuse injuries. Focal injuries result from primary mechanical damage in a localized area of the brain. Local hemorrhaging, edema, or ischemia causes localized swelling around primary mechanical damage and results in a local mass effect. The local mass effect causes an increase in local tissue pressure and pressure gradients within the brain. These rapidly result in shifts of the brain and herniations of brain tissue beneath the falx cerebri, to the tentorial incisura, or through the foramen magnum. These herniations, if of sufficient magnitude, cause compression of the brain stem, and if they act long enough will cause secondary hemorrhaging into the brain stem. At this point vital

centers controlling awakeness and respiratory and cardiac function are permanently damaged. Thus a cascade of events can occur from focal injuries that cause localized damage to affect remote areas in the brain stem. It is therefore not the primary mechanical event nor the primary mechanical brain damage that is most injurious, but rather the consequences of this damage. Therapy for focal injuries is therefore aimed at stopping the potential progression of this series of events.

Diffuse injuries to the brain have a different pathophysiologic mechanism. In these injuries there is no localized damage, but rather widespread damage throughout the cerebral hemispheres. This damage can be physiologic and therefore only temporarily cause neurologic dysfunction. In this instance there is very little actual mechanical damage to the brain; therefore, if the secondary factors of ischemia, hemorrhage, and edema are controlled, the patient should have a good-quality survival. If the injury is more severe, the anatomic disruption of axons in the white matter of both hemispheres can occur and is irreversible. The widespread cerebral dysfunction is usually associated with diffuse swelling of the brain that at first is a vascular event. Diffuse swelling can result from massive vasodilatation and an increase in intravascular cerebral blood. This condition, if it exists, then causes true edema or increased tissue water, with a consequent rise in intracranial pressure. Even if these factors are controlled with therapy, the end result will be dependent on the amount of primary disruptive damage that occurred at the moment of injury.

The principal difference between focal and diffuse injuries is that in the former localized areas of primary damage occur, whereas in the latter there is often widespread damage throughout the brain. These conditions can be viewed in that focal injuries cause a lot of damage in a small area, while diffuse injuries cause less pronounced damage but occur over a much wider area of the brain. The end result of these injuries depends on the severity of secondary factors and how adequately these secondary factors are controllable. When these factors are adequately controlled, the final result then relates to the amount of primary mechanical damage. In focal injuries the final result will depend on the location and size of the focal damage. If this damage, such as from a contusion, is in a "silent" area of the brain, no abnormality may be detectable. If, however, the focal damage is in the speech, sensory, motor, or visual areas of the brain, a focal neurologic deficit will result. In diffuse injuries the final result will depend on the number of axons physically disrupted. If these are small in number, the outcome will be good; however, if the number of axons disrupted is large, global injury to the brain will result. This often is reflected as personality changes, memory disorders, cognitive deficiencies, or intellectual dysfunction.

SUMMARY

The most common type of sports injury to the head results in a rapidly applied mechanical input to the head. Most often this is a direct blow or an impact. An impact causes two phenomena to be set in motion. First, local factors beneath the site of impact (contact phenomena) cause deformation of the skull and shock wave propagation through the skull and brain. The magnitude, direction of impact, and size of impacting device are the factors that affect resulting mechanical damage. Damage is maximized by high-magnitude forces, forces that are applied to thin areas of the skull and impact with small objects. Resulting skull deformation can cause skull fracture and underlying cerebral contusion. The events result-

ing from contact phenomena of impact can be minimized by decreasing the magnitude of impact forces and by diffusing the size of the impact over the head. Protective headgear should be aimed at achieving these goals.

Head injury is also caused by acceleration or deceleration of the head. In this regard it does not matter whether an impact to the head has occurred or whether the head is set in motion by impacts elsewhere on the body. Acceleration forces cause shear, tensile, and compression strains to be created within the brain substance, with shear being the most injurious. The injuries that result from acceleration are principally due to rotational components and tend to cause contusions at a distance from the site of impact, diffuse injuries to the brain, and subdural hematoma. Head injury protective devices are less able to keep the head from accelerating or decelerating, and are thus less likely to minimize the type of injuries caused by acceleration forces.

The response of the brain to mechanical input and the ultimate biologic result of the input relate to several pathophysiologic mechanisms. The primary mechanical damage occurs at the time of head injury, is irreversible, and is maximal at the time of injury. If other factors are controlled, this primary mechanical damage is the sole determinant of the outcome. Secondary factors such as ischemia, hypoxia, hemorrhaging around or within the brain, cerebral swelling, and the possible effects of toxic substances can all complicate the primary mechanical damage, however. Potentially, these events should be controllable to a greater or lesser degree. If these mechanisms of injury cannot be controlled, they will add more dysfunction to the primary mechanical damage. If control of these problems is successful, no further damage will occur, and the ultimate outcome will then be dependent on the primary mechanical damage.

BIBLIOGRAPHY

1. Abel J, Gennarelli TA, Segawa H: Incidence and severity of cerebral concussion in the rhesus monkey following sagittal plane angular acceleration, in *22nd Stapp Car Crash Conference Proceedings*. New York, Society of Automotive Engineers, 1978.

2. Gennarelli TA, Thibault LE, Ommaya AK: Pathophysiologic responses to rotational and translational acceleration of the head, in *16th Stapp Car Crash Conference Proceedings*. New York, Society of Automotive Engineers, 1972.

3. Gennarelli TA: Head injury in man and experimental animals: Clinical aspects. *Acta Neurochirurg* 1983; (suppl 32):1–13.

4. Gennarelli TA, Thibault LE: Biomechanics of head injury, in Wilkins RH, Rengachary S (eds): *Neurosurgery*. New York, McGraw-Hill, 1985, pp 1531–1536.

5. Gennarelli TA: The state of the art of head injury biomechanics, in *29th Proceedings American Association of Automotive Medicine*, 1985, pp 447–463.

6. Gennarelli TA: Mechanisms and pathophysiology of cerebral concussion. *J Head Trauma Rehabil* 1986; 1:23–29.

7. Gennarelli TA: Mechanisms of cerebral concussion, contusion and other effects of head injury, in Youmans J (ed): *Neurological Surgery*. Philadelphia, WB Saunders Co, 1990, pp 1953–1964.

8. Goldsmith W: Physical processes producing head injuries, in Caveness W, Walker AE (eds): *Head Injuries*. Philadelphia, JB Lippincott Co, 1966.

9. Goldsmith W, Ommaya AK: Head and neck injury criteria and tolerance levels, in Aldman B, Chapon A (eds): *The Biomechanics of Impact Trauma*. New York, Elsevier Science Publishing Co, 1984, pp 149–187.

10. Gross AG: A new theory on the dynamics of brain concussion and brain injury. *J Neurosurg* 1958; 15:552.

11. Gurdjian ES, Webster JE, Lissner HR: Observations on the mechanisms of brain concussion, contusion, and laceration. *Surg Gynecol Obstet* 1955; 101:684.

12. Gurdjian ES; *Impact Injury and Crash Protection*. Springfield, Ill, Charles C Thomas, Publisher, 1970.

13. Gurdjian ES; *Impact Head Injury*. Springfield, Ill, Charles C Thomas, Publisher, 1975.

14. Hirsch AE, Ommaya AO, Mahone RH: Tolerance of subhuman primate brain to cerebral concussion, in Gurgjian ES (Ed): *Impact Injury and Crash Protection*. Springfield, Ill, Charles C Thomas, Publisher, 1970.

15. Holbourn AHS: Mechanics of head injuries. *Lancet* 1943; 2:440.

16. Ommaya AK, Gennarelli TA: Cerebral concussion and traumatic unconsciousness. Correlation of experimental and clinical observations on blunt head injuries. *Brain* 1974; 97:633.

17. Ommaya AK, Hirsch AE: Tolerance for cerebral concussion from head impact and whiplash in primates. *J Biomech* 1971; 4:13.

18. Sances A, Yoganandan N: Human head injury tolerance, in Sances A, Thomas DJ, Ewing CL, et al (Eds): *Mechanisms of Head and Spine Trauma*, Goshen, NY, Aloray, 1986, pp 189–218.

19. Thibault LE, Gennarelli TA: Biomechanics and craniocerebral trauma, in Povlishock J, Becker D (Eds): *Central Nervous System Trauma Status Report*. NINCDS 1985; 370–390.

CHAPTER 19

Radiographic Evaluation of the Skull and Facial Bones

Helene Pavlov, M.D.

RADIOGRAPHIC TECHNIQUES AND ANATOMY

Radiographic examination of the skull and facial bones and the central nervous system is difficult to obtain and interpret, especially in the acutely injured patient who is confused, semiconscious, or in pain. Diagnosis of injuries to the head and cervical spine injuries in the acutely traumatized patient requires trained technicians and the cooperative effort of the orthopaedic and radiologic personnel in order that the correct radiographic examinations are obtained and additional injury to the patient is avoided.

Skull and Facial Bones

Because of the spatial relationship of the skull and facial bones, there is always superimposition of these structures on plain radiographs. The number of projections in a skull series differs in every radiographic department, but includes at least four films—one anteroposterior (AP) view, both lateral views, and one posteroanterior (PA) view. In addition, there are special views performed or monitored by a radiologist that enhance the detail of a specific area.

Plain Films

The most utilized plain films for a trauma series are the AP and lateral views to evaluate the skull and the Waters' view to evaluate the facial bones.

The *straight AP view* is obtained with the person's head lying on a grid cassette and the central ray perpendicular to the cassette. This view is essential in the unconscious patient with possible cervical spine fractures because it can be obtained while the patient is still on the litter. The orbitomeatal line (OM), that is, the line between the outer canthus of the eye and the external auditory meatus, is perpendicular to the cassette.[11, 13, 14, 18] This view demonstrates the orbits, ethmoid sinuses, frontal and maxillary sinuses, nasopharynx, internal auditory canal, and a calcified pineal gland.[12]

The *inclined AP view* is obtained with the same patient position, but the central ray is angled 15 degrees cephalad to the OM line. This view demonstrates the frontal, maxillary, and ethmoid sinuses, the nasopharynx, mandible, and orbits (Fig 19–1, A).

The *AP (half-axial) Towne view* uses the same patient position, but the central ray is angled 30 degrees caudad to the OM line. This view demonstrates the occipital bone, including the foramen mag-

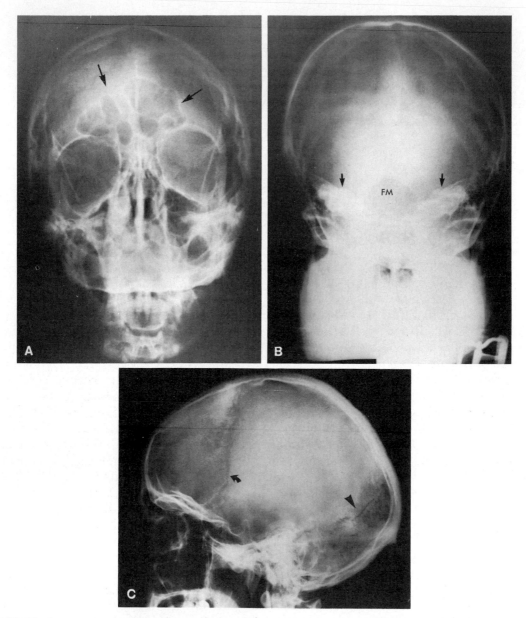

FIG 19–1.
A, inclined AP view demonstrating the orbits, frontal sinuses *(arrows),* nasopharynx, and mandible. **B,** towne view demonstrating occipital bone, foramen magnum *(FM),* and petrous ridges *(arrows).* **C,** lateral view of skull demonstrating nasopharynx, multiple sinusoidal vascular channels *(arrow),* and interdigitating cranial sutures *(arrowhead).*

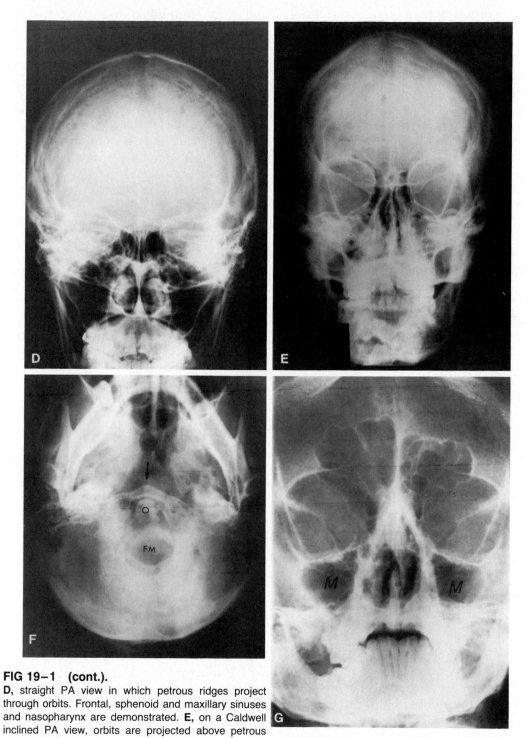

FIG 19–1 (cont.).
D, straight PA view in which petrous ridges project through orbits. Frontal, sphenoid and maxillary sinuses and nasopharynx are demonstrated. **E,** on a Caldwell inclined PA view, orbits are projected above petrous ridges. **F,** submentovertical or axial view demonstrating mandible, foramen magnum *(FM)*, odontoid *(O),* and anterior arch of C-1 *(arrow)*. **G,** Waters' view is specific for facial bones, including the orbits, and frontal and maxillary sinuses *(M)*.

num, petrous pyramids, and mastoid air cells (Fig 19–1, *B*).

For the *lateral views*, the side closest to the cassette distinguishes right or left. Both lateral views should be obtained. Initially this view can be obtained with the patient supine on the litter with use of a horizontal central ray. Lateral views demonstrate the nasopharynx, the maxillary, ethmoid, sphenoid, and frontal sinuses, the mastoid air cells, external auditory canal, and temporal and parietal bones (Fig 19–1, *C*).

The *straight PA view* is obtained with the patient's face against the cassette and the OM line and the central ray perpendicular to the cassette. In this view the petrous ridge projects through the orbits. The ethmoid, frontal, and maxillary sinuses, nasopharynx, and mandible are also demonstrated (Fig 19–1, *D*).

The *inclined PA-Caldwell view* is obtained with the same patient position but the central ray angled 15 degrees caudad to the OM line. This view demonstrates the orbits unobstructed by the petrous ridges, the superior orbital fissure, and frontal and ethmoid sinuses (Fig 19–1, *E*).

The *submentovertical* view, axial, or base view is obtained only when it is certain that the neck can safely be hyperextended. The cassette is placed under the vertex of the head. The central ray is perpendicular to the cassette and the OM line is parallel to the cassette. This view demonstrates the base of the skull, mandible, foramen magnum, and nasal cavity, and may identify a basilar skull fracture in a patient with pneumocephalus and normal routine skull radiographs (Fig 19–1, *F*).

The *Waters' view* is specific for examination of the sinuses and facial bones. It is obtained with the patient's nose and chin positioned against the cassette and the central ray angled approximately 37 degrees caudad to the OM line. This view demonstrates the orbits, maxillary, fron-tal, and ethmoid sinuses, and the nasopharynx (Fig 19–1, *G*).

Additional facial bone views are the specific AP, lateral, and oblique views that best delineate the individual facial bones, such as the orbits, sinuses, nose, zygomatic arches, or mandible. Simply ordering a "facial bone" examination is improper. The request should be specific, that is, nose, mandible, orbits, or sinuses (Fig 19–2).

Special Views

Coned down, oblique, stereoscopic, and tomographic views are performed or monitored by a radiologist, and should be obtained when a specific area is not clearly seen on the routine views and computed tomography (CT) is not available.

Coned-down views center the central ray on the specific area of interest, and narrow the area exposed in order to increase detail. This technique is particularly useful in examining the orbit and sinuses.

Oblique views are obtained by rotating the skull so that the abnormal area is in tangent to the radiographic beam. This is especially useful in evaluating a depressed skull fracture to determine the depth of the fracture fragments.

Stereoscopic views are obtained by taking two exposures, each with a slight change in the tube angle while the patient remains stationary. These two radiographs provide evaluation of the special relationships. They are useful to locate intracranial fracture fragments and radiopaque debris and to identify facial bone fractures.

Tomographic views blur the structures outside the plane of interest in order to increase detail in the plane of interest. Tomography is useful in examining the orbit, maxillary sinuses, and internal ear, and should be used when a facial bone fracture is suggested on the initial plain films, but is not definite.

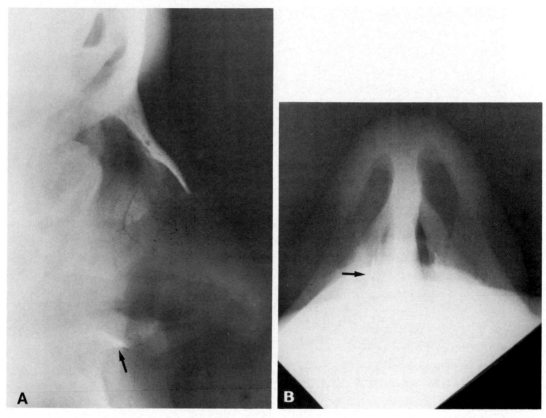

FIG 19–2.
A, lateral view of nose demonstrating nasal bone, soft tissues, and maxillary spines *(arrow).* **B,** occlusal view is specific for showing maxillary spines. Right maxillary spine is medially displaced and fractured *(arrow).*

Brain

When a brain injury is suspected either because of the trauma sustained or the change in the patient's neurologic status, computed tomography (CT) or magnetic resonance imaging (MRI), or both are the most diagnostic studies. In most emergency room situations, however, the radiographic examination of the brain starts with routine skull films. Additional diagnostic modalities include an arteriogram, and a radionuclide brain scan.

Plain Films

The plain films of the skull suggest brain injury when there is a fracture, especially if there are depressed fracture fragments or radiopaque debris within the cranial vault. The demonstration of intracranial air indicates communication with a sinus or a fracture through the base of the skull, even though the fracture may not be documented on the routine films.

A displaced pineal gland on the plain film confirms intracranial and possible brain injury. The pineal gland is small; it can calcify by the age of 6 years, and is calcified in 60% of adults.[12] It is normally midline (Fig 19–3).

Computed Tomography and Magnetic Resonance Imaging

The CT and MRI examinations evaluate the cranial vault, brain, ventricles, and osseous structures. Both examinations display multiple cross-sectional

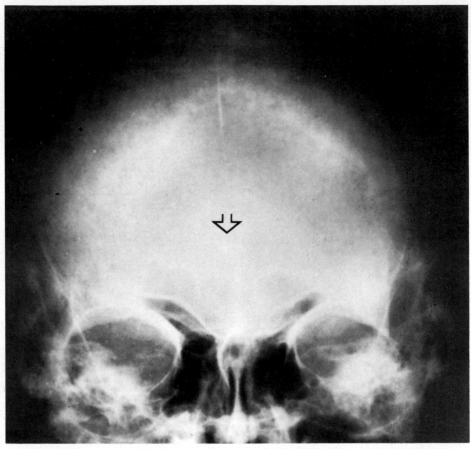

FIG 19–3.
Calcified pineal gland *(arrow)* should be midline on the frontal views. Displacement of more than 2 mm from midline results from increased intracerebral pressure in one hemisphere, displacing the pineal gland toward the opposite side.

slices of the skull and brain at different levels and document the location and size of an intracranial injury. Coronal, sagittal, and oblique reconstructions can be performed. Both examinations are noninvasive; however, intravenous contrast is usually to enhance an abnormality. The CT and MRI examinations of brain trauma are discussed in a separate chapter.

Cerebral Arteriography

Cerebral arteriography is the intraarterial injection of contrast to delineate the arterial, capillary, and venous blood flow of the brain.[9, 15] Although the CT head scan has replaced arteriography as an emergency procedure, an arteriogram is still often necessary to demonstrate a subdural hematoma, a posttraumatic aneurysm, an arteriovenous shunt, or the site of a bleeding vessel.

Nuclear Medicine

Radionuclide studies involve injecting an isotope and then scanning the patient with a gamma camera to detect the radiation. The intravenous injection of sodium pertechnetate ^{99m}Tc can be traced by dynamic and static brain scanning. Dynamic scanning, obtaining multiple scans at 2-second intervals, demonstrates the gross vascular flow to the brain (Fig 19–4, *A*). The static scan, ob-

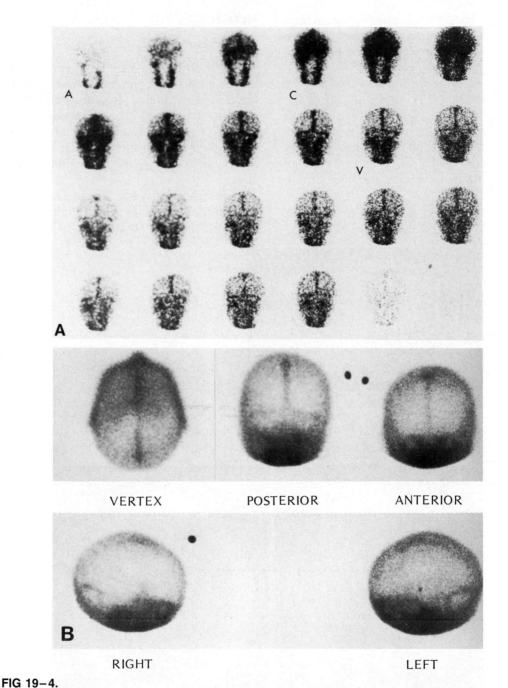

VERTEX   POSTERIOR   ANTERIOR

RIGHT   LEFT

FIG 19–4.
Radionuclide brain scan as seen on the gamma camera after intravenous isotope injection. **A,** Dynamic brain scan in sequential 2-second displays. Each row is read from left to right. Blood flow can be followed by isotope augmentation. Arterial *(A),* capillary *(C)* in which entire brain is perfused, and venous *(V)* phases are demonstrated. **B,** Normal static brain scan includes anterior, posterior, and both lateral and submentovertical vertex views. These views are obtained by placing that portion of the head against the gamma camera for radiation detection and display. Normal isotope uptake should be uniform and symmetric. *(Courtesy of Jay W. MacMoran, M.D., Director, Department of Radiology, Germantown Hospital, Philadelphia, Penn.)*

tained minutes after the injection, and the dynamic scan demonstrate the integrity of the skull and the blood-brain barrier (Fig 19–4, *B*).

The intrathecal injection of sodium pertechnetate ^{99m}Tc or ^{111}In DTPA (diethylenetriamine pentaacetic acid) is used to evaluate the ventricular system in cases of posttraumatic hydrocephalus, and is most useful in cases of persistent posttraumatic cerebro-spinal fluid rhinorrhea or otorrhea.

FRACTURES

Skull Fractures

Skull fractures can be linear or depressed, and both can be associated with brain injury. Linear fractures are occasionally complicated by extension into a sinus or across a blood vessel. Depressed fractures are often complicated by brain injury and subsequent infection or abscess.

Identification of a linear skull fracture on plain films, especially when bilateral, can be difficult because of the nor-

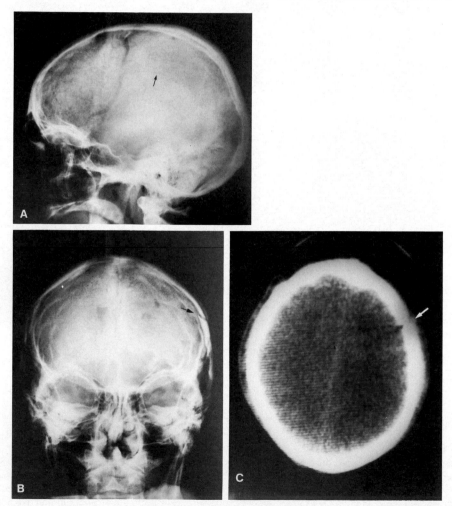

FIG 19–5.
A, linear fracture *(arrow)* is straight with sharp margins as opposed to the sinusoidal vascular grooves or interdigitating suture lines. **B,** AP view of **A** that is tangential to the fracture *(arrow)*. **C,** CT scan of skull can also document a cranial vault fracture *(arrow)*. At this window setting, adjacent brain tissue can also be examined.

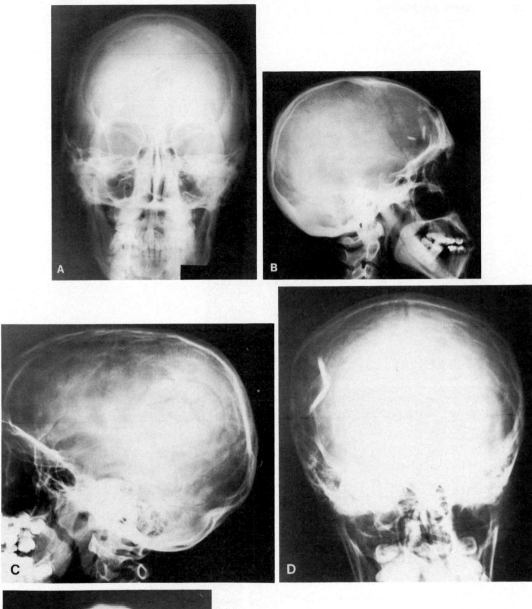

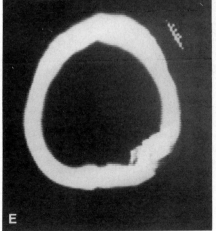

FIG 19–6.
A, on PA view of skull multiple osseous fragments are seen in the midline. **B,** lateral view of **A** confirming frontal location of a comminuted depressed skull fracture. **C,** lateral view of a different patient demonstrating a confluence of linear lucencies in the posteroparietal area. **D,** frontal view of **C,** demonstrating a depressed fracture. **E,** CT scan at bone-window setting demonstrating a depressed skull fracture. Scan performed at window for brain tissue revealed no injury.

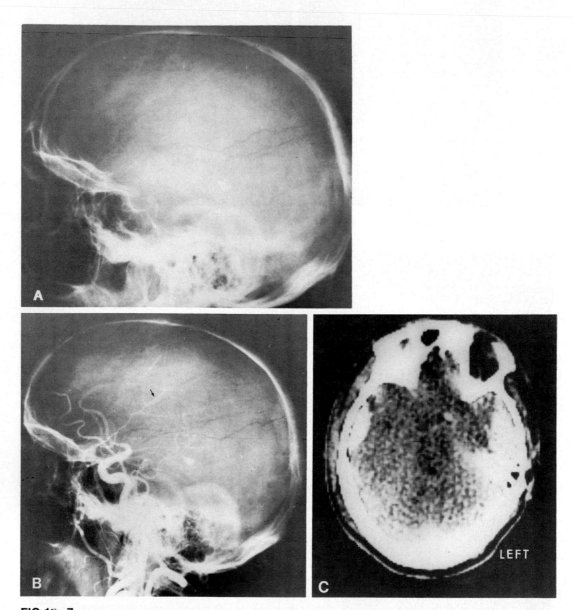

FIG 19–7.
A, bilateral linear fractures through temporoparietal bones. Pineal gland is calcified. **B,** retrograde brachial arteriogram demonstrating the "tram track" sign *(arrow),* indicating arteriovenous communication and confirming that the temporoparietal fracture extends through the middle meningeal artery. **C,** cerebral contusion and hematoma in left temporo-occipital area. There are bilateral asymmetric epidural hematomas in midtemporal to anterotemporal areas, and a localized area of edema medial to the left epidural hematoma.

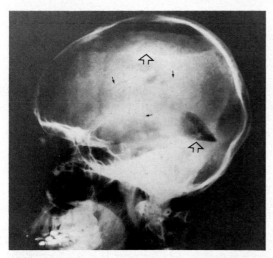

FIG 19–8.
Lateral view of this patient reveals a comminuted linear fracture *(small arrows),* but, more importantly, a large pneumocephalus. There are air fluid levels *(open arrows)* because the patient was sitting and a horizontal radiographic beam was used. *(Courtesy of Jay W. MacMoran, M.D., Director, Department of Radiology, Germantown Hospital, Philadelphia, Penn.)*

mal vascular grooves and sutures. In addition, scalp lacerations, dirt, foreign bodies, and hair produce multiple artifacts that can simulate fractures.[1, 17] A linear skull fracture is a straight linear lucency with sharp edges. Because of the occasionally confusing shadows, demonstration on more than one view, or on a CT scan, may be necessary (Fig 19–5). Linear fractures are not always associated with brain damage, but a CT head scan is indicated whenever there is clinical suspicion of neurologic impairment.

A depressed skull fracture is evaluated best on a CT head scan in which the depth and location of the bony fragments can be determined (Fig 19–6).

A fracture in the temporoparietal region is frequently associated with rupture of the middle meningeal artery and an epidural hematoma. An arteriogram will document an arterial injury. CT or MRI examination is also usually necessary to determine the size of the hematoma and its involvement of the ventricles and midline structures (Fig 19–7).

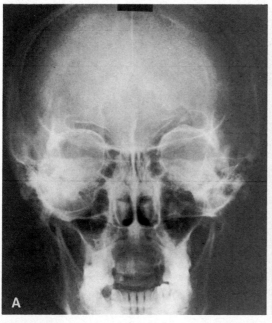
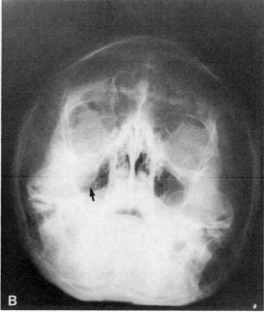

FIG 19–9.
A, PA view demonstrating asymmetry in infraorbital areas. **B,** Waters' view demonstrating a depressed fracture of floor of right orbit, showing orbital contents *(arrow)* extending into superior portion of maxillary sinus.

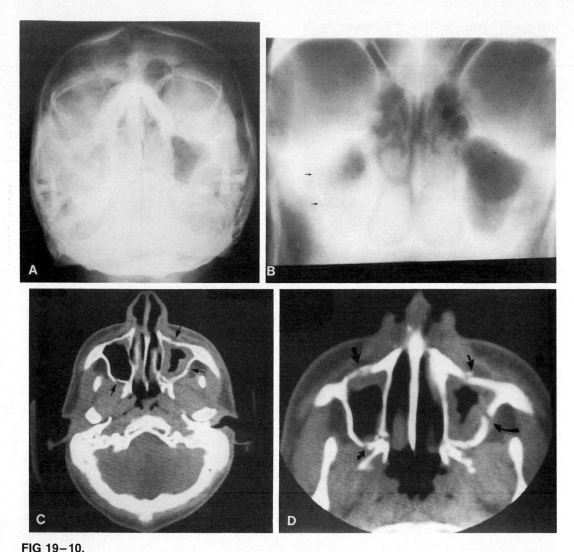

FIG 19–10.
A, Waters' view demonstrating asymmetry. Right side of face is more dense than left. A definite fracture is not seen. **B,** tomogram of both maxillary sinuses, demonstrating fractures of lateral wall of right maxillary sinus *(arrows)*. Increased density in inferior portion of sinus represents blood. **C,** CT scan of a different patient, demonstrating comminuted bilateral maxillary sinus fractures *(arrows)*. **D,** close-up CT view clearly delineating maxillary sinus fractures and location of fragments *(arrows)*. Edematous lining of maxillary sinuses is also evident. **(C** and **D,** *courtesy of James C. Hirschy, M.D., New York, NY.)*

A pneumocephalus is air around the brain and is associated with a fracture through a sinus or base of the skull (Fig 19–8).[4, 7] Occasionally the fracture may be demonstrated only with tomography or on the submentovertical view.

Persistent bloody or clear discharge from the nose (rhinorrhea) or the ear (otorrhea) after trauma is associated with fracture through a sinus or the temporal bone, respectively. Because the actual fracture cannot always be demonstrated, the origin of the fluid may not be obvious, and a nuclear medicine examination may be helpful. The intrathecal isotope is injected, and a cotton plug is placed in the nose or ear; this is measured for isotope collection 6 to 24 hours later.[3] The

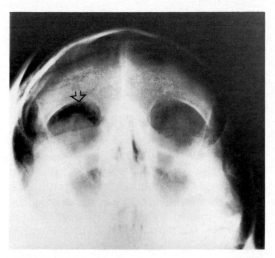

FIG 19–11.
Waters' view demonstrating asymmetry. The right orbit is too lucent due to periorbital air *(arrow)*, which usually indicates an ethmoid sinus fracture.

presence of the isotope on the cotton confirms that the discharge is cerebrospinal fluid.

Facial Bone Fractures

Facial bone fractures are easy to overlook radiographically, and the best way to examine the radiographs for possible fractures is to note asymmetry.

Orbital fractures may involve the floor, rim, roof, or walls of the orbit. Specific orbital views and a Waters' view should be obtained whenever an orbital fracture is suspected. A fracture of the orbital floor is a blowout fracture, and the eye may descend into the maxillary sinus (Fig 19–9).[4, 6] A blowout fracture is best demonstrated on the Waters' view; however, tomography and a CT scan always should be employed when the diagnosis is uncertain.

Comparison of one side of the face with the other is also useful in identifying maxillary sinus fractures (Fig 19–10,A). Tomography, both routine and CT, is important and further delineates the number and position of the fractures, as well as the associated soft tissue swelling and hematoma (Fig 19–10,B–D).

Subcutaneous air, especially intraorbital air, is an indication of an ethmoid or paranasal sinus fracture, even without demonstrating the fracture (Fig 19–11).

Fractures of the zygomatic arch are suspected by asymmetry on the Waters' view, but are best demonstrated on an

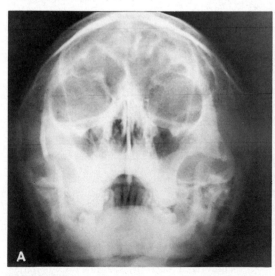
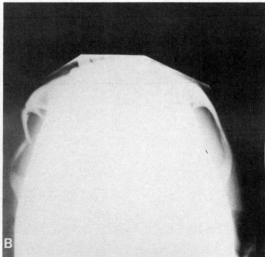

FIG 19–12.
A, asymmetry of face is noted, with increased density on right, and irregularity of right zygoma. **B,** underpenetrated submentovertical view demonstrating a comminuted fracture of right zygomatic arch.

underpenetrated submentovertical view in which the arch is projected in tangent (Fig 19–12). The position of the fracture fragments of a mandibular fracture is demonstrated on oblique views or on a submentovertical view of the skull (Fig 19–13,A and B). Fracture through the condyles of the mandible is best seen in the Caldwell view (Fig 19–13,C). Faciomaxillary fractures, as described by Le-Fort,[4, 16] are best demonstrated in the Caldwell and Waters' views.

INTRACRANIAL INJURY

Intracranial injury should be expected whenever plain films of the skull reveal a skull fracture, intracranial osseous fragments, radiopaque foreign debris, a pneumocephalus, or a shift of a calcified pineal gland more than 2 mm to one side of midline. Unfortunately a midline pineal gland does not exclude bilateral brain injury or generalized cerebral edema.

Brain injury after acute trauma includes cerebral edema, contusion, and hematoma. Subsequent brain damage includes hydrocephalus and atrophy. The CT and MRI examinations are the most useful radiographic modality for evaluating brain injury.[2, 5, 8, 10] They analyze the displayed structures by their relative densities. The density of a vascular lesion can be increased by the intravenous injection of various contrast materials. The CT and MRI examinations of the brain are discussed in separate chapters.

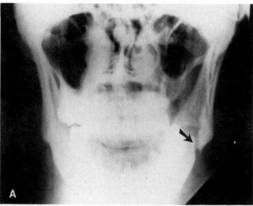

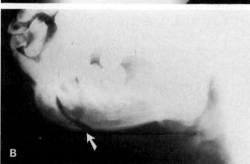

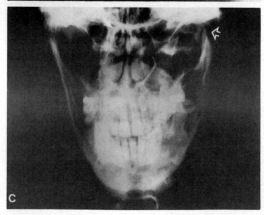

FIG 19–13.
A, mandibular fracture on PA view *(arrow),* demonstrated clearly on oblique view **(B). C,** fracture through mandibular condyle seen on Caldwell view *(arrow).*

REFERENCES

1. Allen WE, Knir EL, Rothman SLG: Pitfalls in evaluation of skull trauma—a review. *Radiol Clin North Am* 1973; 11:479.

2. Davis KR, et al: Computed tomography in head trauma. *Semin Roentgenol* 1977; 12:53.

3. DiChiro G, Reames PM: Isotopic localizations of cranionasal cerebrospinal fluid leaks. *J Nucl Med* 1964; 5:376.

4. Dolan KD, Jacoby CG: Facial fractures. *Semin Roentgenol* 1978; 13:37.

5. Dublin AB, French BN, Rennick JM: Computed tomography in head trauma. *Radiology* 1977; 122:365.

6. Fueger GF, Milauskas AT, Britton W: The

roentgenologic evaluation of orbital blow-out injuries. *AJR* 1966; 97:614.

7. Greenfield JG, Russell DS: Traumatic lesions of the central and peripheral nervous system, in Greenfield M (ed): *Neuropathology*. Baltimore, Williams & Wilkins, 1963.

8. Koo AH, LaRoque RL: Evaluation of head trauma by computed tomography. *Radiology* 1977; 123:345.

9. Lee TP: Techniques of cerebral angiography. *Radiol Clin North Am* 1974; 12:223.

10. Merino-de Villasante J, Taveras JM: Computerized tomography (CT) in acute head trauma. *AJR* 1976; 126:765.

11. Merrill V: *Atlas of Roentgenographic Positions*. St Louis, Mosby–Year Book, 1967.

12. Ozonoff MB, Burrows EH: Intracranial calcification, in Newton TH, Potts DG (eds): *Radiology of the Skull and Brain*, vol I. St Louis, Mosby–Year Book, 1971.

13. Potts DG: A system of skull radiology. *Radiology* 1970; 94:25.

14. Rumbaugh CL, Davis DO: The normal skull: Techniques and indications. *Semin Roentgenol* 1974; 9:91.

15. Taveras JM, Wood JH: Diagnostic neuroradiology, in Robins LL. (ed): *Golden's Diagnostic Radiology*, vol II, ed 2. Baltimore, Williams & Wilkins, 1976.

16. Tilson HB, McFee AS, Soudah HP: The *Maxillofacial Works of Rene LeFort*. Houston, University of Texas Press, 1972.

17. Tomsick TA, Chambers AA, Lukin RR: Skull fractures. *Semin Roentgenol* 1978; 13:27.

18. Weathers RM, Lee A: Radiologic examination of the skull. *Radiol Clin North Am* 1974; 12:215.

CHAPTER 20

Computed Tomography and Magnetic Resonance Imaging for Evaluation of Head Trauma

Caren Jahre, M.D.

Helene Pavlov, M.D.

Michael D. F. Deck, M.D.

While the introduction of computed to- mography (CT) in the early 1970s revolu- tionized the evaluation of head trauma, the more recent development of magnetic resonance imaging (MRI) has even sur- passed CT in its ability to define the ex- tent of cerebral and extracerebral trau- matic injury. Before the existence of CT and MRI, only limited information could be obtained from plain x-ray films of the skull. On these x-ray films fractures and indirect signs, such as a shift of a calci- fied pineal gland, could be identified; however, little else about the much more important intracranial injuries could be detected. Angiography provided more in- formation about mass effects resulting in displacement of normal vascular struc- tures; however, it was relatively nonspe- cific, and, being an invasive procedure, was associated with small but finite risks to the patient. CT and MRI are noninva- sive procedures that provide specific de- lineation of pathologic processes. This chapter reviews the principles of CT and MRI, the indications for these techniques, and the appearances of head trauma se- quelae on both CT and MRI evaluation.

PRINCIPLES

Computed Tomography

CT involves the use of a series of finely collimated x-ray beams and detec- tors covering a span of 360 degrees sur- rounding the specific body part of the pa- tient. The data obtained are relayed to a computer that rapidly constructs axial images with use of a gray scale. Radio- dense structures, such as bone or blood, appear white, whereas less radiodense substances, such as fat and fluids, are black. Blood is considered a radiodense substance because it contains iron and appears white on the scan. Soft tissues, including muscle and brain tissue, are in- termediate, and are represented by vary- ing shades of gray. The gray scale can be manipulated on the CT console screen to produce brain or bone "windows" in or- der to optimize evaluation of the corre- sponding underlying structure (Fig 20–1).

With modern equipment, each axial image can be obtained in approximately 2 seconds; thus images are obtainable in all but the most uncooperative patients.

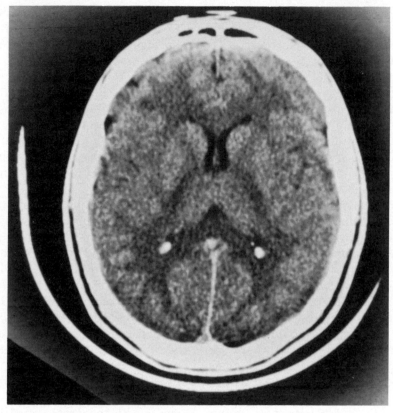

FIG 20–1.
Axial CT image through the brain at the level of the frontal horns of the ventricles showing typical symmetry and normal differentiation between gray matter and white matter. The image is displayed at a brain "window" to emphasize the normal brain parenchymal anatomy.

A complete head scan, consisting of approximately 13 10 mm axial images, can be performed and reconstructed in approximately 5 minutes. In cases of suspected fractures of the base of the skull, thin sections of 1.5 mm and direct coronal images may be useful. Intravenous iodinated contrast is generally unnecessary in trauma cases.

Magnetic Resonance Imaging

MRI is a noninvasive technique that does not involve the use of ionizing radiation but, instead, magnetic forces and the hydrogen ions present within the body's water; water is the major component of the body's weight.[1] The patient is supinely positioned within the center of a large magnet housed in the MRI unit. The hydrogen nuclei throughout the body are naturally spinning, but become aligned when within the magnet field. Coils are placed around the body part; these produce pulses of radiofrequency waves, providing energy to deviate the spinning hydrogen nuclei away from the direction of the main magnetic field. When the radiofrequency pulse from the coils is stopped, the hydrogen nuclei realign themselves with the magnetic fields and emit the radiofrequency waves that were just applied. The radiofrequency coils measure these signals, and computers convert them into images.

Normal structures and pathologic processes, such as edema and blood, can be exquisitely differentiated secondary to differences in the amount and state of the hydrogen nuclei (protons) they contain. The overall magnetic resonance signal is dependent on proton density, proton velocity, and the T1 and T2 relaxation times. Proton density refers to the concentration of hydrogen ions. Velocity refers to the movement of the protons, such as those in flowing blood, which appear as a signal void (black) on the images because they do not remain in the imaging plane long enough to emit a signal. The T1 and T2 relaxation times are time constants measuring the radiofrequency signals from the hydrogen ions as they relate to different geometric planes. It is the uniqueness of the T1 and T2 relaxation times of the various types of tissues that allows them to be differentiated.

Standard magnetic resonance images are referred to as "spin echo images" (Fig 20–2). Substances with a short T1 or long T2 have a high intensity on magnetic resonance images and appear white. Substances with a long T1 or short T2 have a low signal intensity and appear black. Intermediate values appear at various levels on gray scale. The differences in T1 and T2 among various substances can be accentuated by varying machine parameters used in obtaining the images. These machine-imaging parameters are the repetition time, TR, which is the time between applications of the radiofrequency pulse, and TE, the echo time, at which time the signal emitted by the hydrogen nuclei ("the echo") is collected.

Images obtained with a short TR of approximately 500 msec emphasize the differences in the T1 among various tissue types and are often referred to as "short TR (STR)" or "T1-weighted images" (see Fig 20–2,A and D). Proton density images emphasize neither T1 nor T2 and have a TR of approximately 2,000 msec and a TE of 20 to 40 msec (see Fig 20–2,B). Long TR (LTR) images, with TRs of approximately 2,000 msec and TEs of 50 to 80 msec, emphasize differences in T2 and are often referred to as "T2-weighted images" (see Fig 20–2,C). The signal intensities on short TR and long TR images allow one to characterize tissues as normal soft tissue, cerebrospinal fluid (CSF), blood, tumor, fat, or increased protein. The short TR images provide superior anatomic resolution compared with the proton density and long TR images, which are generally more sensitive to areas of abnormal signal intensity.

MRI can provide images in sagittal and coronal planes by changing the directions in which the signals are applied and collected, so that the patient does not have to be moved (see Fig 20–2,D). A routine head study generally involves short TR axial and sagittal images and long TR axial images. In trauma cases, a gradient echo sequence may be added to the routine. A gradient echo sequence is another method of varying the way in which the radiofrequency pulses are applied. Gradient echo images are more sensitive to the presence of hemorrhage and can be obtained more quickly than routine long TR spin echo images, although their resolution is inferior.

INDICATIONS FOR IMAGING

The clinical indications for CT and MRI scanning in the setting of head trauma have been a matter of some debate.[5] It is generally agreed that depressed or decreasing levels of consciousness, focal neurologic signs, depressed skull fracture, and penetrating skull injury are strong indications for scanning. Less definite indications include transient loss of consciousness, seizures, vomiting, and amnesia; however, in clinical practice scanning is frequently done in many patients with such symptoms. A group with low risk for intracranial injury includes those with simple headache, dizziness, and scalp injury.

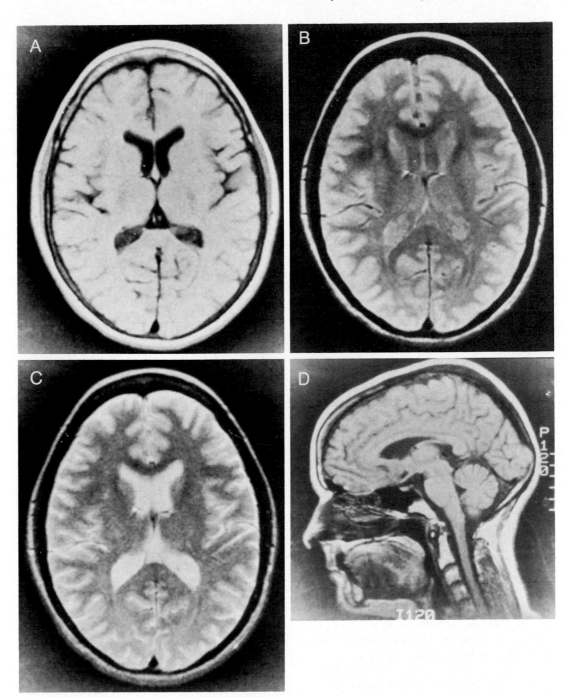

FIG 20-2.
A-D, normal anatomy seen with magnetic resonance imaging. **A,** short TR axial image through the level of the frontal horns demonstrates the excellent visualization of normal anatomic structures such as the cerebral sulci. Note that the outer and inner tables of the skull are seen as two thin black lines surrounding the marrow space, which has a higher signal intensity. **B,** example of a proton density image, with a long TR, at the same level as **A.** This type of image is very sensitive to subtle alterations in normal tissue water content. **C,** example of a long TR image through the same level as *A* and *B*. The normal CSF signal is very bright on these images. **D,** midline sagittal short TR image showing normal midline structures of the brain and the cervical-medullary junction.

Since the advent of MRI, once the decision for imaging has been made, one must choose between CT and MRI. MRI, in our opinion, is the procedure of choice for imaging after head trauma, except in fracture cases (such as depressed skull fractures and petrous temporal bone fractures), in which CT is needed to visualize osseous structures. Although the number of MRI units available continues to increase, CT is still the more readily available modality. Also, although studies have demonstrated the superiority of MRI over CT in detecting subdural hematomas and parenchymal injuries, this advantage is primarily in the diagnosis of small subdural hematomas (SDHs) that generally do not require surgery. Therefore, if MRI cannot be utilized, CT scanning remains a highly accurate method for diagnosis of subdural and epidural hematomas of larger size that may require prompt surgical intervention. Medical management and prognostic evaluation are optimized with the use of MRI.

There are several types of patients in whom MRI cannot be used, such as those on respirators and monitors, uncooperative patients, and those with contraindications to MRI. Each MRI sequence is obtained in approximately 5 to 10 minutes, requiring approximately 30 minutes for a complete examination. Thus the patient must be able to cooperate and lie still during the 5 to 10 minutes of imaging time per sequence or significant motion degradation will occur. Approximately 5% of patients cannot tolerate the examination because of claustrophobia. Sedation may be helpful in some cases.

Monitoring of critically ill patients within the magnetic resonance unit is a problem because the magnetic field disrupts the function of ventilators, cardiac monitors, and intravenous infusion pumps. MRI can be used for evaluation of patients on respirators if special long tubing is available to connect the patient to a ventilator that is placed outside the influence of the magnetic field. Ventilators and other monitoring equipment are being developed that will be functional within the magnetic field area. There are also several important contraindications to MRI because of the strong magnetic field. Patients in whom MRI is contraindicated are those with ferromagnetic cerebral aneurysm clips, programmable pacemakers, cochlear implants, and intraorbital metallic foreign bodies.

TRAUMATIC LESIONS

Skull Fracture

The diagnosis of an uncomplicated linear skull fracture is of little clinical importance because most require no therapeutic intervention. These fractures are often better seen on plain radiographs than with CT, especially when the plane of the fracture corresponds to that of the axial CT. MRI is not useful for evaluation of fractures because of the absent signal from cortical bone.

CT is helpful for delineating the amount of displacement of the depressed skull fractures, which may require surgical elevation (Fig 20–3). Fractures through the paranasal sinuses that may result in CSF leaks or compromise of the dura mater, such as in fractures of the posterior wall of the frontal sinus, are well evaluated by CT. Thin-section high-resolution CT, with 1.5 mm axial and direct coronal images, is indicated in possible fractures of the petrous temporal bones, which may result in ossicular dislocation and facial and eighth nerve injuries.

Subdural Hematoma

SDHs may result from laceration of the dura mater, venous sinuses, bridging veins between the cortex and the dural sinuses, and parenchymal injury.[6] Blood

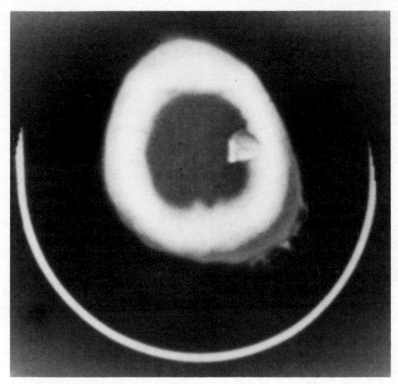

FIG 20–3.
Axial CT image performed with bone "window" to demonstrate wedge-shaped displaced left parietal skull fracture.

in the subdural space spreads over the hemisphere, resulting in the typical crescentic configuration conforming to the calvarium and brain (Fig 20–4 and 20–5). Both CT and MRI are valuable in detecting this lesion. On CT, the SDH usually has a high radiodensity (white) in the acute stage (see Fig 20–4). The density diminishes with time, and may become isodense to the underlying brain in 1 to 3 weeks. The chronic SDH is typically of low density. Occasionally, an acute SDH may also be hypodense. The mass effect resulting from SDH is usually appreciated on the ipsilateral lateral ventricle, which is compressed, and, in severe cases, with evidence of midline shift. A small SDH may not be seen readily when its density merges with that of the adjacent calvarium, but its presence may be suspected because of unexplained mass effect on the ventricular system. Widening the window width of

the images on the CT console is helpful in this regard (see Fig 20–4,B).

SDHs are usually not associated with fractures, and are bilateral in approximately 25% of cases. They often are associated with multiple episodes of re-bleeding, resulting in mixed density patterns.

On MRI the signal intensities of SDH are variable, depending on the age of the hematoma (see Fig 20–5). The mechanisms responsible for the signal intensity of hemorrhage on MRI are extremely complex and are dependent on numerous factors that are also time dependent. These factors include hemoglobin and its breakdown products, oxygenation, clot retraction, intactness of the red blood cells, and magnetic field strength.[7] In general, hematomas in the first 24 hours are mildly hyperintense (brighter) compared with normal brain on short TR images and minimally hyperintense or isointense on long TR images. They be-

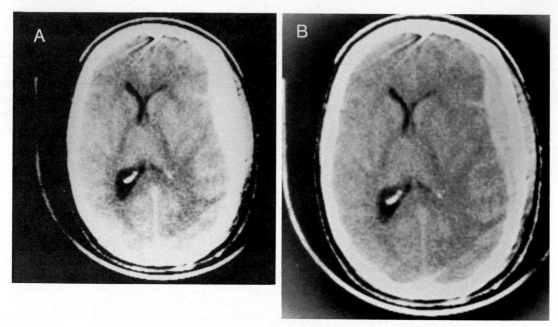

FIG 20–4.
CT of left frontal SDH. **A,** moderately large, dense left frontal SDH with marked mass effect and midline shift of the ventricles to the right. **B,** by changing the window levels on the CT console, the left frontal SDH is better differentiated from the adjacent dense calvarium.

come hypointense (darker) to brain on long TR images and isointense on short TR images during the next 1 to 2 days. On approximately day 4, hematomas increase in signal on both sequences, but faster on the short TR compared with the long TR images. By day 6, hematomas have reached maximal signal intensity and are bright on both sequences. After weeks to months, if the hematoma is not reabsorbed, the chronic SDH has low signal intensity on short TR images and remains bright on long TR images.

MRI is superior to CT in detection of SDH for several reasons.[2–4] Because there are no mobile hydrogen nuclei in cortical bone, the inner table of the skull cannot produce a signal on MRI and appears dark, as an area of signal void. Thus even a small SDH can be visualized on MRI because the calvarium does not obscure it, in contrast to CT where a small SDH can merge and be radiographically inseparable from the calvarium. Another advantage of MRI is superior soft

tissue discriminating ability compared with CT—an abnormal mass such as an SDH can be more readily appreciated. Signal abnormalities on MRI are more dramatically different from the underlying brain compared with CT, and persist for weeks to months. On CT, SDH in its isodense stage may be indistinguishable from normal brain.

Epidural Hematoma

Epidural hematoma (EDH) results from bleeding between the calvarium and the dura mater and is often associated with skull fracture.[6] The dura mater is firmly attached to the inner table of the skull, but it can be separated by bleeding under sufficient pressure. The edges of the dura mater remain adherent and are sharply defined on CT; the medial border bulges into the brain parenchyma, producing the classic lentiform configuration of EDH (Fig 20–6). Most commonly, the middle meningeal artery is lacerated, re-

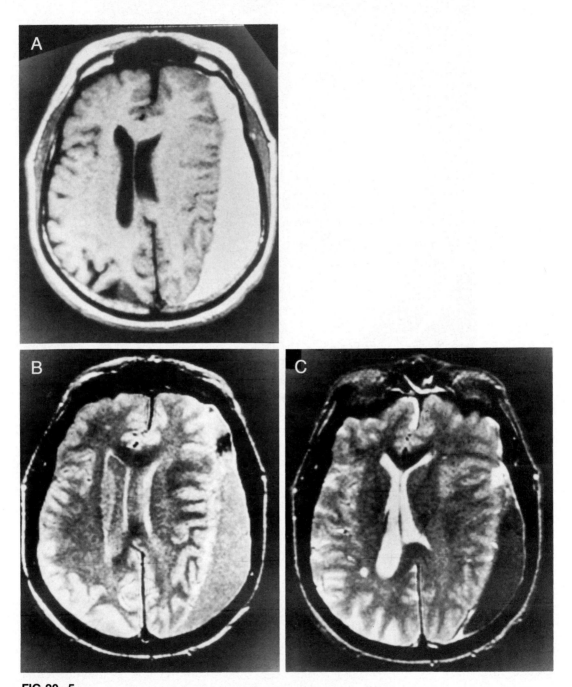

FIG 20–5.
MRI of large subacute left-convexity SDH, with a typical crescentic configuration and large associated mass effect with shift of the ventricles to the contralateral side and compression of the underlying sulci. The different signal intensities on the short TR image **(A),** proton density image **(B),** and long TR image **(C)** are typical for evolving hemorrhage.

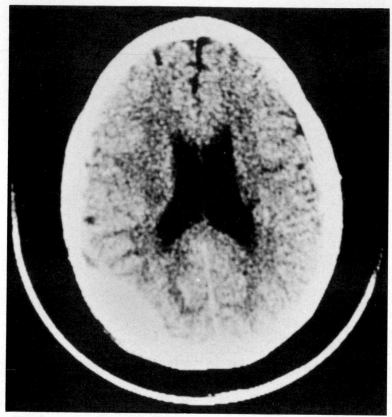

FIG 20–6.
Axial CT image demonstrating acute right parietooccipital EDH with classical lentiform configuration and mild associated mass effect.

sulting in a temporal EDH. Other frequent sites are the frontal and occipital regions. EDH can also result from venous bleeding, particularly after rupture of venous sinuses.

As in SDH, an acute EDH is usually hyperdense on CT. An associated skull fracture may be visualized on the bone "windows." Since EDH is usually a surgical emergency and most are promptly evacuated, the chronic phases are rarely seen. With time, EDH will decrease in density and size.

Most EDHs are relatively large and detectable on CT; however, MRI is superior to CT in delineating their full extent and anatomic distribution (Fig 20–7).[2–4] Again, signal intensity varies with the age of the hematoma, and are similar to those described for SDH. On MRI, the dura mater may be seen as a thin, hypointense curvilinear structure medially displaced by the hematoma, thus confirming its epidural location. MRI may not visualize associated fractures, since the cortical bone does not produce a signal.

Subarachnoid and Intraventricular Hemorrhages

Subarachnoid and intraventricular hemorrhages are sometimes seen in the setting of trauma, and almost always in association with extra-axial hemorrhage or other injuries. These entities are well seen on CT as areas of increased density in the subarachnoid space, basilar cis-

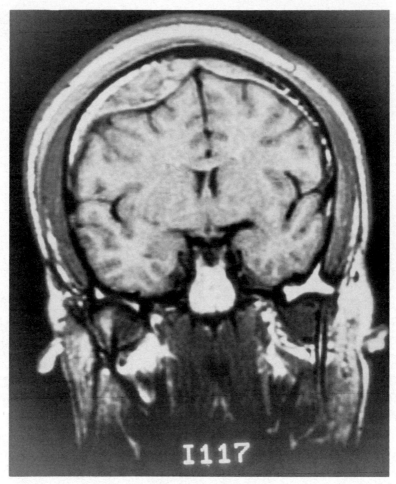

FIG 20–7.
MRI of acute EDH. Short TR coronal image demonstrates bifrontal EDH, greater on the right side compared with the left. Note the classic lentiform configuration and compression of the underlying brain. *(Courtesy of Dr. Thomas P. Naidich, Miami, Fla.)*

terns, sulci, sylvian fissures, or in the ventricles. MRI is notoriously poor in detecting these lesions, because blood mixed with CSF diffuses and remains relatively well oxygenated, thus not producing the typical signal alterations by which MRI readily detects blood in the parenchymal and extra-axial spaces. Subarachnoid and intraventricular hemorrhages themselves, however, do not require treatment unless they result in hydrocephalus—thus their direct detection is not of great therapeutic importance. Hydrocephalus, if it develops, is easily detected on both CT and MRI.

Parenchymal Injury

Although brain parenchymal injury does not require surgery in the vast majority of cases, its accurate diagnosis remains an important goal for several reasons. Medical management may be altered according to the severity of parenchymal abnormality. The presence or absence of extensive parenchymal injury, particularly in the unconscious patient, has important prognostic implications.

MRI is significantly superior to CT in its ability to detect parenchymal injury, especially with regard to nonhemorrhagic

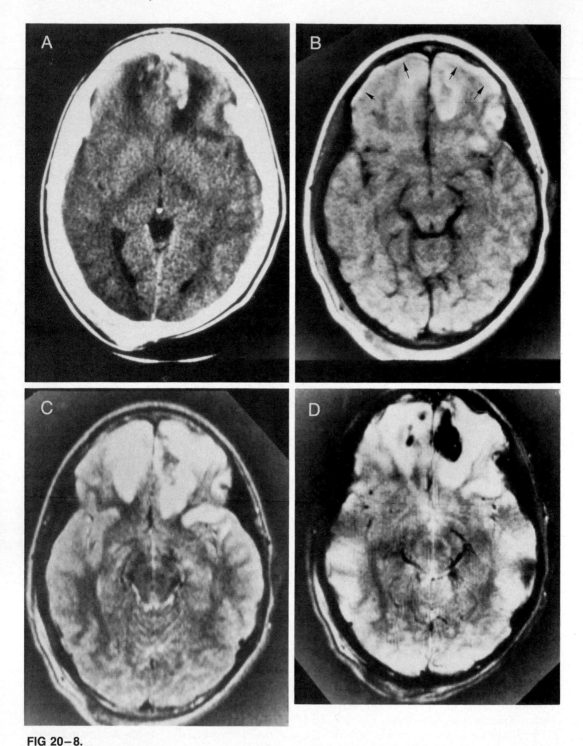

FIG 20–8.
Bifrontal hemorrhagic contusions. **A,** axial CT image demonstrates bilateral low density in the frontal lobes interspersed with areas of high density representing hemorrhage. These findings are consistent with hemorrhagic contusion. **B,** short TR axial MR image at the same level demonstrates parenchymal hemorrhage as areas of high signal intensity. Note the small bifrontal acute SDHs *(arrows),* which were not visualized on the CT study. Their ready visibility on the magnetic resonance image is possible because the adjacent calvarium is black and

lesions.[2-4] The advantage of MRI is not as pronounced for the diagnosis of hemorrhagic lesions. MRI is better than CT because it is more sensitive to subtle alteration in tissue water content, and it is free of the artifacts that obscure some CT images, particularly in the anterotemporal and inferior frontal lobes, which are frequent sites of parenchymal contusions (Fig 20–8). In patients with profound neurologic deficits unexplained by CT, MRI may reveal extensive shear injuries that unfortunately have a poor prognosis. Injury to the brain parenchyma may take several forms, including contusions and shear lesions.

Contusions primarily involve the cortex adjacent to bony surfaces. They are most commonly located in the temporal, frontal, and parieto-occipital regions. Contusions are often multiple and may be nonhemorrhagic or hemorrhagic; the hemorrhage may also be delayed. On CT, contusions appear as areas of low density, with areas of irregular increased density if hemorrhage is present (see Fig 20–8,A). On MRI, long TR images are the most sensitive, showing areas of high signal intensity in the cortex and subcortical regions; the short TR images may show areas of low signal intensity (see Fig 20–8,B and C). Both sequences will show areas of increased and decreased signal intensity if hemorrhage is present. Mass effect with swelling of gyri, obliteration of sulci, and distortion of the ventricles is also well depicted on MRI. Gradient echo images are more sensitive for the presence of hemorrhage, which will appear as areas of low signal intensity (see Fig 20–8,D).

Another important parenchymal injury is diffuse axonal injury or shear lesions. These are small lesions, often less than 1 cm, located in the white matter or at the gray–white matter junction. They are usually multiple, and the majority are not hemorrhagic (Fig 20–9). Common locations include the frontal and temporal lobes, subcortical white matter, corpus callosum, and corona radiata. These lesions appear as small areas of hypodensity on CT, along with higher density if hemorrhagic. MRI reveals these white matter lesions as high signal lesions on long TR images, and areas of hypointensity may be seen on short TR images. As with cortical contusions, associated hemorrhage may be seen on the routine spin echo images, but gradient echo images increase sensitivity.

Long-Term Sequelae

Focal atrophy is often seen to develop in previous areas of contusion, appearing as enlargement of the sulci and adjacent ventricle. When an area of encephalomalacia ("softened brain") communicates with the ventricular system or subarachnoid space and forms a cystic cavity containing CSF, this is referred to as porencephaly. After severe head trauma, diffuse cerebral atrophy may sometimes result, with enlargement of the ventricles and sulci.

All of these abnormalities are readily detected with both CT and MRI examination. MRI, with its superior anatomic resolution and multiplanar imaging capability, offers better delineation of the anatomic relationships of these lesions,

does not obscure the high signal of the hematoma, as it does on the CT images. The edema of the contusion is not well seen on the short TR image. **C,** long TR magnetic resonance image through the same area as *A* and *B* demonstrates extensive abnormal high signal representing contusion that is more extensive on the MRI compared with CT examination. The hemorrhagic component on this image is seen as irregular low signal within the area of high signal intensity. **D,** gradient echo magnetic resonance image at the same level demonstrates hemorrhage as areas of markedly decreased signal intensity (black). The small hemorrhages in the right frontal lobe are best seen on the gradient echo images. The gradient echo images also demonstrate the high signal edematous component of the contusion.

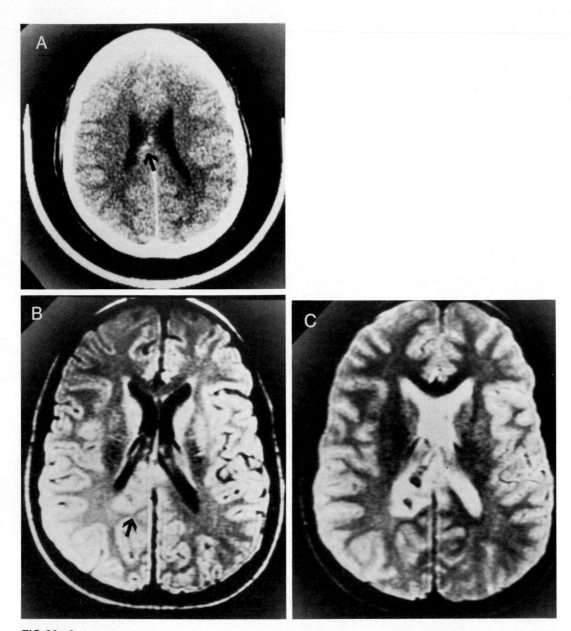

FIG 20–9.
Corpus callosum hemorrhagic shear injury. **A,** CT image shows small foci of hemorrhage in the corpus callosum *(arrow).* **B,** proton density magnetic resonance image through the same level shows more marked abnormality with hyperintensity in the corpus callosum *(arrow).* **C,** long TR image at the same level as *A* and *B* again demonstrates more extensive hyperintensity in the corpus callosum compared with the CT image. The areas of low signal intensity represent hemorrhage. Note that the hyperintensity of the shearing injury merges with the hyperintensity of the CSF. This problem is avoided on the proton density images where the CSF is dark and the abnormal parenchyma is bright.

such as the communication of a poren-cephalic cyst with a ventricle. MRI can also detect the presence of small areas of hemosiderin and gliosis consistent with previous trauma, which is not visible with CT examination. Hemosiderin appears as hypointense areas on gradient echo images and gliosis as areas of hyperintensity in long TR images surrounding focal areas of atrophy or porencephaly.

Communicating hydrocephalus may result after head trauma when subarachnoid hemorrhage blocks reabsorption of CSF at the arachnoid villi. On both CT and MRI, enlargement of the entire ventricular system is seen without corresponding sulcal enlargement such as that seen in cerebral atrophy.

REFERENCES

1. Brant-Zawadski, M: Magnetic resonance imaging principles: The bare necessities in magnetic resonance imaging of the central nervous system, in Brant-Zawadski M, Norman D (eds): New York, Raven Press, 1987, pp 1–12.

2. Gentry LR, Godersky JC, Thompson B, et al: Prospective comparative study of intermediate-field MR and CT in the evaluation of closed head trauma. *AJNR* 1988; 9:91–100.

3. Gentry LR, Godersky JC, Thompson B: MR imaging of head trauma: Review of the distribution and radiopathologic features of traumatic lesions. *AJNR* 1988; 9:101–110.

4. Kelly AB, Zimmerman RD, Snow RB, et al: Head trauma. Comparison of MR and CT experience in 100 patients. *AJNR* 1988; 9:699–708.

5. Masters SJ, McClean PM, Arcarese JS, et al: Skull x-ray examinations after head trauma. Recommendations by a multidisciplinary panel and validation study. *N Engl J Med* 1987; 316:84–91.

6. Zimmerman RD, Danziger A: Extracerebral trauma. *Radiol Clin North Am* 1982; 20:105–121.

7. Zimmerman RD, Heier LA, Snow RB, et al: Acute intracranial hemorrhage: Intensity changes on sequential MR scans at 0.5 T. *AJNR* 1988; 9:47–57.

CHAPTER 21

Cerebral Concussion and Diffuse Brain Injuries

Thomas A. Gennarelli, M.D.

Traumatic injuries to the brain can be classified into focal brain injuries and diffuse brain injuries. Focal brain injuries are those in which a lesion large enough to be visualized with the naked eye has occurred; they comprise cortical contusions, subdural hematoma, epidural hematoma, and intracerebral hematoma. These lesions cause neurologic problems not only by virtue of the local brain damage but also by causing masses within the cranium that lead to brain shift, herniation, and, ultimately, brain stem compression. Diffuse brain injuries, on the other hand, are associated with more widespread or global disruption of neurologic function and are not usually associated with macroscopically visible brain lesions. Diffuse brain injuries are the consequence of the shaking effect of the brain within the skull and are thus lesions caused by the inertial or acceleration effects of the mechanical input to the head. Both theoretic and experimental evidence points to rotational acceleration as the primary injury mechanism for diffuse brain injuries.[6, 7]

Since diffuse brain injuries, for the most part, are not associated with visible macroscopic lesions, they have historically been lumped together to mean all injuries not associated with focal lesions.

Recently, however, diagnostic information has been gained from computed tomographic (CT) scanning as well as from neurophysiologic studies, which enables us to better define several categories within this broad group of diffuse brain injuries.[21] These injuries are discussed in detail. Three categories are now recognized:

1. Mild concussion: Several specific concussion syndromes exist that involve temporary disturbance of neurologic function without loss of consciousness.
2. Classical cerebral concussion: Classical cerebral concussion is a temporary, reversible neurologic deficiency caused by trauma that results in temporary loss of consciousness.
3. Diffuse axonal injury: Diffuse axonal injury (DAI) is a traumatic brain injury with prolonged loss of consciousness (more than 24 hours). Often residual neurologic, psychologic, or personality deficits result.

Diffuse axonal injury can be classified into three classes of severity[8, 9, 11]:

1. Mild DAI: Coma from 6 to 24 hours.
2. Moderate DAI: Coma lasting more

than 24 hours without concomitant brain stem signs, that is, decerebration or decortication.

3. Severe DAI: Coma lasting more than 24 hours, with prominent motor signs of brain stem dysfunction.

MECHANISMS OF CONSCIOUSNESS

Since most diffuse brain injuries involve a disturbance of consciousness, a brief review of the mechanisms that subserve the consciousness state is in order.[18] Consciousness, although difficult to define, is that easily recognized state in which a person can meaningfully interact with his environment. The neuroanatomic substrate of the awake state is a complex interaction involving the cerebral cortex, subcortical structures including the hypothalamus, and numerous brain stem centers. The disconnection of one of these functions from the other two results in an altered state of consciousness. In general terms, the awake state requires the neural activity of the ascending reticular activating system of the brain stem to be projected to the cerebral cortex of both cerebral hemispheres. This projection may be either direct or indirect via hypothalamic-diencephalic centers. Similarly, feedback from the cerebral cortex of both hemispheres onto both the diencephalon and the reticular activating system of the brain stem is necessary for awakeness.

In more general terms, unconsciousness can be produced either by dysfunction of the diencephalon—brain stem or, on the other hand, by dysfunction of both cerebral hemispheres. Head injuries cause loss of consciousness in the former instance by compression or by hemorrhage into the brain stem from supratentorial mass lesions produced by focal injuries. Diffuse cerebral injuries, on the other hand, cause widespread dysfunction of both cerebral hemispheres, and thereby alter consciousness by disconnecting the diencephalon or brain stem activation centers from hemispheric activity. Extremely severe diffuse brain injuries, such as seen in the shearing injury, can cause not only bilateral cerebral hemisphere dysfunction but also direct anatomic damage within the brain stem itself.

THE SPECTRUM OF DIFFUSE BRAIN INJURY

Diffuse brain injuries form a continuum of progressively severe brain dysfunction that is caused by increasing amounts of acceleration damage to the brain (Table 21–1). Since normal brain function is a delicately balanced electrochemical series of events occurring in billions of cells at any one moment, it is easy to understand how mechanical forces can alter brain function. At low levels of input, this function can be disrupted, at least temporarily, without causing any structural disruption of the tissue. Thus *physiologic dysfunction can occur in the absence of structural or anatomic disruption.* This concept is the basis for our understanding of the concussion syndromes that, by their definition, are transient, reversible events. It is also easy to imagine that if more profound mechanical input is delivered to the brain, structures within the brain can become physically, anatomically disrupted. In this instance, permanent sequelae would occur in those structures that are anatomically disrupted. Therefore, as the magnitude of mechanical input increases function is first interrupted, and later when anatomic disruption occurs, both function and structure are disrupted. *The degree of functional disruption, since it precedes anatomic disruption, is always greater than the degree of anatomic disruption.*

TABLE 21–1.

Diffuse Brain Injuries

	Mild Concussion	Cerebral Concussion	Diffuse Axonal Injury		
			Mild	Moderate	Severe
Loss of consciousness	None	Immediate	Immediate	Immediate	Immediate
Duration of coma	None	<6 hr	6–24 hr	Days	Days-weeks
Decerebrate posturing	None	None	None	Rare	Common
Posttraumatic amnesia	Min	Min/hr	Hr	Days	Weeks
Memory deficit	None	Min	Mild	Moderate	Severe
Motor deficits	None	None	None-mild	Mild-moderate	Moderate-severe
Outcome at 3 mo			%		
Good recovery	100	95	63	38	15
Moderate deficit	0	2	15	21	13
Severely disabled	0	2	2	12	14
Vegetative	0	0	1	5	7
Dead	0	0	15	24	51

To illustrate this concept, one can envision a set of ten axons each of which participates to an equal degree in a particular neurologic function. Each of the ten axons is, for purpose of illustration, stronger and more resistant to mechanical strain than the one that precedes it. If a very mild mechanical stress is applied to the ten axons, none will be disrupted, but the first axon (the most sensitive one) will have a temporary loss of function. The overall result may not be noticeable because the other nine axons are still functioning perfectly normally. A more severe mechanical stress may cause dysfunction of the first five axons, and by this point a decrease in the overall neurologic function would be apparent. Since none of the axons is structurally damaged, the function will soon return, however. A still larger mechanical input now causes physical disruption of the first three axons and physiologic dysfunction of the remaining seven axons. Now all ten axons have had an anatomic or physical disruption, so that the neurologic function is totally abolished. However, seven of the axons will recover their function so that little if any neurologic deficit will be identified. This example should clarify the concept of physiologic disruption being more sensitive to mechanical input than is anatomic disruption.[13]

MILD CEREBRAL CONCUSSION SYNDROMES

The syndromes of mild cerebral concussion are included in the continuum of diffuse brain injuries because they represent the mildest form of injury in this spectrum. Mild concussion syndromes are those in which consciousness is preserved but there is some degree of noticeable temporary neurologic dysfunction. These injuries are exceedingly common, and, because of their mild degree, they are often not brought to medical attention. They are the most common group of injuries to the brain that will be encountered in sports medicine.

The mildest form of head injury is that resulting in confusion and disorientation unaccompanied by amnesia. This temporary confusion without loss of consciousness lasts only momentarily after the injury, and is so commonplace that it needs no further description. This concussion syndrome is completely reversible and is associated with no sequelae.

Slightly more severe head injury causes confusion, with amnesia that develops after 5 or 10 minutes. Again, this is an extremely frequent event, particularly in sports medicine. Football players may experience such a "ding" and, although confused, continue coordinated sensorimotor activities after the accident. If examined immediately after the accident, these players possess intact recall of the events immediately before impact. Posttraumatic amnesia then develops 5 or 10 minutes later, however, and thereafter the player does not remember the impact or events immediately after impact. The amnesia usually extends for only several minutes before the injury, and although it may shrink somewhat, the player will always have some degree of permanent, although short, retrograde amnesia despite resumption of a completely normal consciousness.[20] The confusion and disorientation completely resolve in a matter of moments.

As the mechanical stresses to the brain increase, confusion and amnesia are present from the time of impact. Football players commonly can continue to play while having no recollection of prior events. By this stage some degree of retrograde amnesia (forgetting of events before the injury) also occurs in addition to posttraumatic amnesia (forgetting of events after the injury). The patient's length of confusion may last many minutes, but then his level of consciousness returns to normal usually with some permanent degree of both retrograde and posttraumatic amnesia.[5]

These three syndromes of mild cerebral concussion have been witnessed frequently and described in detail.

Although consciousness is preserved, it is clear that some degree of cerebral dysfunction has occurred. The fact that memory mechanisms seem to be the most sensitive to trauma suggests that the cerebral hemispheres (rather than the brain stem) are the location of mild injury forces. The degree of cerebral cortical dysfunction, however, is not sufficient to disconnect the influence of the cerebral hemispheres from the brain stem activating system, and therefore consciousness is preserved. No other cortical functions except memory seem at jeopardy, and the only residual deficits that patients with mild concussion syndromes have is the brief retrograde or posttraumatic amnesia.

CLASSIC CEREBRAL CONCUSSION

Classic cerebral concussion is the posttraumatic state that results in loss of consciousness. This state is always accompanied by some degree of retrograde and posttraumatic amnesia. In fact, the length of posttraumatic amnesia is a good measure of the severity of cerebral concussion. Inherent in the usual concept of classic cerebral concussion is the fact that the disturbance of consciousness is transient and reversible. In clinical terms this means that full consciousness has returned within 6 hours. It has also been frequently stated that classic cerebral concussion is not associated with pathologic damage to the brain. Because of its transient and reversible state, however, patients with cerebral concussion do not have neuropathologic examinations. Evidence from experimental cerebral concussion does suggest some mild degree of microscopic neuronal abnormalities. In practical terms, however, classic cerebral concussion can be viewed as a phenomenon of physiologic neurologic dysfunction with no anatomic disruption.

There is unconsciousness or coma from the moment of head impact in patients with classic cerebral concussion. Although systemic changes, such as bradycardia, hypertension, and brief apnea, or neurologic signs, such as decerebrate posturing, pupillary dilatation, or flaccidity, may occur, they do so only fleetingly and disappear within several seconds. The patient then awakens and is temporarily confused before regaining full alertness and orientation. As in the mild concussion syndromes, classic cerebral concussion is always associated with both retrograde and posttraumatic amnesia. Although these states vary in length, they tend to be longer in cerebral concussion than in the mild concussion syndromes.

Insufficient attention has been placed on the precise events of recovery from classic cerebral concussion. Although, by definition, the loss of consciousness is transient and reversible, sequelae of concussion are commonplace.[14] Certainly, some sequelae such as headache or tinnitus may reflect injuries to the inner ear or other noncerebral structures. Subtle changes in personality, however, or subtle changes in psychologic or memory functioning have been documented and must be of cerebrocortical origin. Thus, although the great majority of patients with classic cerebral concussion have no sequelae other than amnesia for the events of impact, some patients may in fact have more long-lasting, although subtle, neurologic deficiencies that must be investigated further.

The mechanisms that underlie classic cerebral concussion are but an extension of those of the mild concussion syndromes. With classic cerebral concussion, not only have the mechanical stresses and strains on the brain caused dysfunction of those cortical functions involving memory, but also in this instance have caused sufficient physiologic disturbance to temporarily result in diffuse cerebral hemispheric disconnection from the brain stem reticular activating system. Since this dysfunction is physiologic and not structural, when the electrochemical milieu of the brain returns to normal, the usual interaction between the cerebral hemispheres and the brain stem is reestablished and consciousness is resumed.

DIFFUSE AXONAL INJURY

Diffuse axonal injury is the term given to a more serious type of diffuse brain injury. It is evidenced by loss of consciousness from the time of injury and continuing beyond 6 hours. It is common for patients with DAI to be unconscious for days or weeks before beginning a recovery period. In its severe form, there are signs of decerebrate posturing and no increased sympathetic activity (hypertension, hyperhidrosis). Patients with DAI are comatose, with either purposeful movements to pain or with withdrawal movements to pain; only occasionally they have brain stem reflexive decorticate or decerebrate posturing. These patients often appear to be restless and may have an increased amount of random motor movements.

The longer duration of consciousness in DAI suggests a more profound disturbance of cerebral function than occurs in classic cerebral concussion. Since unconsciousness may last for weeks, it is likely that DAI represents that transition between pure physiologic dysfunction and anatomic disruption. Therefore, it is not surprising that if some degree of anatomic disruption occurs, recovery is incomplete. This indeed is the case with DAI. As patients awake from coma, they are confused and have long periods of posttraumatic and retrograde amnesia. Deficits of intellectual, cognitive, memory, and personality functions may be mild to severe. Some patients, however, do make an adequate recovery and are capable of resuming all normal activities; thus the degree of anatomic injury may be little or marked.

DAI results from the same types of mechanical strains on the brain that cause the mild concussion syndromes and classic cerebral concussion. Physiologic function is impaired in a widespread area throughout the cerebral cortex and diencephalon, and actual tearing (anatomic disruption) occurs in some weaker fibers in both hemispheres. The degree of recovery is then dependent on the amount and location of anatomic damage. Since the cerebral hemispheres are disconnected from the brain stem reticular activating system for a prolonged period, the resulting prolonged coma makes these patients prone to the numerous complications of the comatose state. Therefore the recovery process can be curtailed by secondary complications that can result in death.

SEVERE DIFFUSE AXONAL INJURY

Severe diffuse axonal injury, also called diffuse white matter shearing injury or diffuse impact injury, is the most severe form of all the diffuse brain injuries. It is the next step in severity from DAI and is associated with severe mechanical disruption of many axons in both cerebral hemispheres. Additionally, axonal disruption extends into the diencephalon and brain stem to a greater or lesser degree.

Patients with shearing injury are immediately deeply unconscious and remain so for a prolonged period of time. They are differentiated from patients with diffuse injury by the presence of abnormal brain stem signs such as decorticate or decerebrate posturing. In addition, they usually exhibit evidence of immediate autonomic dysfunction, such as hypertension, hyperhidrosis, and hyperpyrexia. Although these patients were formally diagnosed as having "primary brain stem injury" or brain stem contusion, there is now ample evidence that such injuries are exceedingly rare, and that shearing injury is present in most patients with this clinical picture.[16, 17]

The abnormal brain stem signs of decortication or decerebration, or both, are often asymmetric, and, if the patient survives, will decrease after several weeks and eventually disappear. The same is true of the autonomic dysfunc-

tion. These events are suggestive that recovery of the physiologic dysfunction of brain stem function is occurring; residual deficiencies are profound, however.

Three types of recovery suggest that there is indeed a continuum of injury within this category of shearing injury. Patients with least anatomic damage, that is, with fewest axons torn, can recover to a greater or lesser degree. Recovery rarely is good, however, but rather severe intellectual or bilateral sensorimotor deficits occur. A second pattern of shearing injury occurs in which the patient survives but does not recover. These patients remain in a vegetative state, and although their eyes are open they have no cognitive connection or response to their environment. However, the most common pattern with the shearing injury is death. This indeed is the far end of the spectrum of all diffuse cerebral injuries, and is associated with so much anatomic disruption that it is incompatible with life.

Pathologic evaluation of patients who die after shearing injury shows very little macroscopic change. Careful examination does disclose two lesions that are regularly associated with shearing injury. Hemorrhagic lesions in the superior cerebellar peduncle and corpus callosum are virtually always present. These may be the only visible findings, but disruption of the fornix or hemorrhages in the periventricular regions may also be seen.

The principal pathologic findings in shearing injury are seen only on microscopic examination of the brain. The lack of such examinations has caused an inadequate appreciation for the frequency of this severe lesion in the past. Careful microscopic examination, however, discloses evidence of axons that have been torn throughout the white matter of both cerebral hemispheres. Depending on the time from injury to death, this is reflected by axonal retraction balls or microglial clusters. Degeneration of the long white matter tracts extends into the brain stem if the patient has survived for many weeks.

Thus pathologic information verifies the concept that at this end of the spectrum anatomic disruption of innumerable axons has occurred. It is postulated that the survivors have slightly lesser amounts of anatomic damage.*

THE SPECTRUM OF DIFFUSE CEREBRAL INJURIES

Diffuse cerebral injuries form a spectrum of severity, beginning with the mild concussion syndromes and ending with severe diffuse axonal injury (Fig 21–1). It is postulated that as mechanical input increases, brain acceleration causes progressively more shear, tensile, and compression strains to the brain substance.

*The occurrence of diffuse axonal injury in nonvehicular sports is unusual. These injuries require such a large amount of angular head acceleration that they are most commonly seen in motorcyclists, vehicle occupants, and pedestrians. Consequently, DAI will usually be seen only in sporting events related to these activities.

At first these strains are insufficient to cause any injury. As they increase, mild physiologic disruption of cortical processing causes the mild concussion syndromes. More severe input increases the strains in the brain. These are insufficient to cause disruption of axons, but are sufficient to cause temporary global dysfunction of cortical activity. This results in a temporary disconnection of the cerebral cortex from the reticular activating system necessary for consciousness, and classic cerebral concussion results. As mechanical strains increase further, the structurally weakest axons fail, and anatomic disruption begins. Physiologic dysfunction is still more prominent than mechanical disruption however. As more and more axons break, the severe DAI is seen. Here, sufficient physiologic dysfunction of brain stem activity occurs, prolonged unconsciousness is produced, and, depending on the amount of anatomic damage to axons, either partial recovery, nonrecovery, or death occurs. Thus a fatal DAI is a situation in which the mechanical input forces cause such

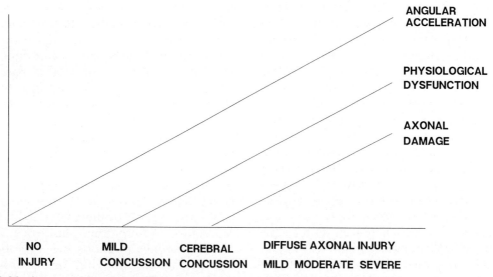

FIG 21–1.
The continuum of diffuse brain injuries is illustrated. As mechanical strains increase, the mild concussion syndromes (three) occur, followed by classical cerebral concussion, diffuse axonal injury, and shearing injury. Functional activity of the brain is always more disturbed than anatomic disruption.

large strains that an overwhelming number of nerve fibers are destroyed.

PHENOMENA RELATED TO DIFFUSE BRAIN INJURIES

Several events are related to diffuse brain injuries that, because of different mechanisms of causation or because of different pathophysiologic effects, must be differentiated from diffuse brain injuries. These events include vasovagal phenomena and brain swelling.

Vasovagal syncope must be distinguished from the mild concussion syndromes and from classic cerebral concussion. This event is a fainting spell caused by intense, brief stimulation of the vagal parasympathetic nervous system. Activation of vagal centers occurs commonly from impacts or punches to the abdomen (the solar plexus punch of boxers), but may also be caused by head movements that stimulate the vagus nerve in or around the head. Blows to the face can cause sufficient head movements to activate the vagus. That this commonly occurs before the input forces are sufficient to cause classic cerebral concussion is well evidenced in experimental head injury.[1]

Whatever the cause, vagal hyperactivity results in profound bradycardia and hypotension. If mild, it may lead to light-headed or swooning sensations. If severe, the bradycardia and hypotension can decrease cerebral blood flow sufficiently to result in loss of consciousness. Thus a mild vasovagal episode may mimic one of the mild concussion syndromes, while a more severe event can cause fainting and loss of consciousness, resembling a classic cerebral concussion. The true brain injury syndromes can usually be differentiated from vagal events by the lack of retrograde or posttraumatic amnesia and the presence of a slow, bounding pulse in the latter situation. Additionally,

a momentary delay often occurs before the vasovagal syncope results in loss of consciousness, and thus the patient may stagger for a few seconds before collapsing. Classic cerebral concussion, on the other hand, occurs exactly at the time of impact and is always caused by head, rather than body, impact.

Brain swelling is a poorly understood phenomenon that can accompany any type of head injury. Swelling is not synonymous with cerebral edema, which refers to a specific problem in which there is an increase in extravascular brain water. Such an increase in water content may not occur in brain swelling, and current evidence favors the concept that brain swelling is due, at least in part, to increased intravascular blood within the brain. This is caused by a vascular reaction to head injury that disturbs the normal actions of the cerebral blood vessels and leads to vasodilatation and increased cerebral blood volume. If this condition of increased cerebral blood volume continues for a long period of time, vascular permeability may be increased and true edema may result.

Although brain swelling may occur in any type of head injury, the magnitude of the swelling does not correlate well with the severity of the injury. Thus both severe and less severe injuries may be complicated by the presence of brain swelling. The effects of brain swelling are thus additive to those of the primary brain injury, and may, in certain instances, be more severe than the primary injury itself.

Despite a lack of knowledge of the precise mechanism of causation of brain swelling, it can be conceptualized in two general forms (see Table 21–2). It should be remembered that many different types of brain swelling may exist and that the following represents a phenomenologic, rather than a mechanistic, approach to brain swelling.

Acute brain swelling occurs in sev-

TABLE 21–2.

Brain Swelling

I. Acute swelling
   A. Associated with focal lesions
      1. Acute SDH—hemispheric
      2. Contusions—focal
   B. Associated with DAI—generalized
II. Delayed swelling
   A. Associated with lethargy
   B. Associated with light coma
   C. Associated with deep coma

eral circumstances. Swelling that accompanies focal brain lesions tends to be localized, whereas diffuse brain injuries are associated with generalized swelling. Focal swelling is usually present beneath contusions, but does not often contribute additional deleterious effects. On the other hand, the swelling that occurs with acute subdural hematomas, although principally hemispheric in distribution, may cause more mass effect than does the hematoma itself. In such circumstances, the small amount of blood in the subdural space may not be the only reason for the patient's neurologic state. If the hematoma is removed, the acute brain swelling may progress so rapidly that the brain protrudes through the crainiotomy opening. Every neurosurgeon is all too familiar with this condition of external herniation of the brain that is most difficult to treat.

In an experimental model of acute subdural hematoma, this type of "malignant brain swelling" occurs regularly.[2, 19] Shortly after the subdural blood is removed, the brain swells so massively that it protrudes well above the outer table of the skull (Fig 21–2). Measurement of tissue water content, studies with labeled sucrose, and electron microscopic observations have failed to find signs of cerebral edema in the swollen brain. This is indirect evidence that this variety of acute brain swelling is not due to cerebral edema, but rather is due to increased cerebral blood volume.

The more serious types of diffuse brain injuries are associated with generalized, rather than focal, acute brain swelling. Although not all patients with DAI or shearing injury have brain swelling, the incidence of swelling is higher than in patients with either classic cerebral concussion or one of the mild concussion syndromes. Because of the serious nature of the underlying injury, it is difficult to determine the importance of swelling in these patients. The swelling, although widespread throughout the brain, may not cause a rise in the intracranial pressure for several days. This late rise in pressure probably reflects the formation of true cerebral edema, and diffuse swelling associated with the severe diffuse brain injuries may be deleterious because it produces edema. In any event, this type of swelling is very different from the type of swelling associated with acute subdural hematomas.

Delayed brain swelling may occur minutes to hours after head injury. It is usually diffuse and is often associated with the less severe forms of diffuse brain injuries. Whether delayed swelling is the same or a different phenomenon than the acute swelling of the more serious diffuse injuries is unknown. However, in less severe diffuse injuries there is a distinct time interval that exists before delayed swelling becomes manifest, thus confirming that the primary insult to the brain was not serious. Considering the high frequency of the mild concussion syndromes and of classic cerebral concussion, the incidence of delayed swelling must be very low. When it occurs, however, delayed swelling can cause profound neurologic changes or even death.

In its most severe form, severe delayed swelling can cause deep coma. The usual history is that of an injury associated with a mild concussion or a classic cerebral concussion from which the patient recovers. Minutes to hours later, the patient then becomes lethargic, then stu-

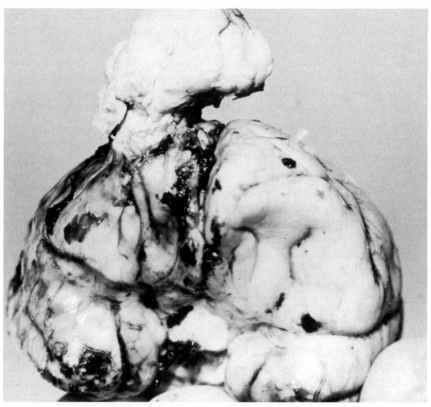

FIG 21–2.
This frontal view of a monkey brain demonstrates the massive amount of acute brain swelling that can occur after the removal of an acute subdural hematoma. The "mushroom" over the frontal lobe (viewers' left) is swollen brain that protruded through the craniotomy defect moments after a subdural hematoma was evacuated.

porous, and then lapses into a coma. The coma may either be a light coma, with appropriate motor responses to painful stimuli, or a deep coma associated with decorticate or decerebrate posturing.

The key difference between these patients and those with DAI is that in the latter the coma and abnormal motor signs are present from the moment of injury, whereas with delayed cerebral swelling there is a time interval without these signs. This distinction is of major significance, however, since with DAI a certain amount of primary structural damage has occurred from the moment of impact that is not present in delayed swelling. Therefore, the deleterious effects of delayed swelling should be potentially reversible, and, if these effects are controlled, the

outcome should be good. Control of the effects of brain swelling may be difficult, however. Vigorous monitoring of, and attention to, intracranial pressure is necessary and prompt, and vigorous treatment of raised intracranial pressure is required to control brain swelling. If this is successfully accomplished, the mortality rate from the increased intracranial pressure associated with diffuse brain swelling should be low.[14]

The severe form of delayed brain swelling often appears in a stereotyped fashion principally involving children between 4 and 10 years of age.[4] It may result from any variety of head injuries and is usually characterized by a more or less completely lucid interval immediately after injury. The children then become lethargic and lapse into coma, often in association with an early posttraumatic seizure. A dynamic sequence of events occurs during the next several months. First brain swelling is manifest on CT scanning by the absence of cerebral ventricles and subarachnoid spaces. If intracranial pressure is adequately controlled, a week or more after the injury brain swelling begins to diminish, often to the point that extracerebral collections occur. By 1 month after injury these collections disappear spontaneously, and the brain, which had been swollen, begins to shrink. Thus the ventricular system becomes enlarged. This is often associated with enlargement of the sulci around the brain, giving an appearance of cerebral atrophy with CT examination. By this time some degree of neurologic recovery from the deep coma has occurred. Still later (approximately 6 to 9 months after injury), the appearance of cerebral atrophy disappears on CT examination, and the brain resumes its normal configuration. The exact mechanisms that cause this prolonged series of events to occur is unknown, but the final outcome in these patients, if their intracranial pressure is controlled, is a good result with no residual neurologic deficit.

Less severe amounts of delayed cerebral swelling may also occur with the mild concussion syndromes and with classic cerebral concussion. These are not often diagnosed because they are associated only with early posttraumatic lethargy that soon disappears. However, these patients undergo the same type of early clinical course as those patients with more severe delayed cerebral swelling. Again, after a mild concussion or classic cerebral concussion, the patient awakens and is normal for some moments to hours. Thereafter, a degree of lethargy occurs that lasts for hours to days. This state is reasonably common and probably represents a mild degree of delayed brain swelling.

Whether mild or severe, delayed brain swelling is an epiphenomenon of diffuse brain injuries that is poorly understood. Since it does not occur in all patients with diffuse brain injuries, it can be viewed as a reaction to injury rather than as a primary injury itself. As with the immediate types of brain swelling, it is likely that delayed brain swelling initially represents a vascular reaction to injury in which the cerebral blood vessels lose their normal vascular control mechanisms and widely vasodilate. This results in increased cerebral blood flow and increased cerebral blood volume.[15] True edema formation may subsequently occur and result in increased intracranial pressure. Thus the effects of brain swelling, whether immediate or delayed, are added to the effects of the primary brain injury, and, in the case of the milder forms of diffuse brain injury, may represent the most serious threat to survival.

SUMMARY

Diffuse brain injuries are consequences of shaking of the brain and the violent head motions caused by head impacts. They result from acceleration effects of head trauma and have little if anything to do with localized phenomena of the impact. Acceleration causes shear, tensile, and compression strains to be generated throughout the brain, and these strains are the primary injurious factors. Since the brain is weakest in the shearing mode, rotational acceleration is more injurious than other types of acceleration because of the high shear strains it induces. The primary injuries to the brain caused by acceleration form a continuum of injury severity that increases as acceleration of the brain increases. Very low strains, caused by low levels of acceleration, may cause no injury whatsoever. As acceleration increases, the mild concussion syndromes result, but these are not associated with loss of consciousness. Classic cerebral concussion is caused by a further increase in acceleration and is associated with transient reversible loss of consciousness. If still further strains are induced in the brain by higher levels of acceleration, anatomic damage begins to occur and is associated with more severe functional changes of the brain. DAI is a primary injury associated with prolonged loss of consciousness and variable amounts of diffuse anatomic damage. Shearing injury is the most severe form of diffuse brain injury, and is accompanied by deep coma, signs of decerebrate posturing, and autonomic dysfunction. It is associated with widespread disruption of axons throughout the white matter of both cerebral hemispheres. Although patients may recover with mild forms of DAI, most patients with severe DAI either die or remain in a vegetative or severely impaired state.

The continuum of the diffuse brain injuries is associated with both physiologic dysfunction and, at the most severe end of the spectrum, anatomic disruption. Although the individual primary diffuse brain injuries are distinct, they are a continuum, and one syndrome may merge indistinguishably into the next. This can provide difficulty in making a precise diagnosis in certain cases. However, the end result of the primary injury is dependent on the amount of anatomic disruption that occurs at the moment of injury, since the functional changes, in themselves, are reversible.

Brain swelling may be superimposed on the primary diffuse brain injuries. Although brain swelling does not occur in every case of diffuse brain injuries, it can add deleterious effects to the primary injury by causing increased intracranial pressure. Rapidly occurring brain swelling is associated with severe diffuse brain injuries, whereas delayed brain swelling appears in conjunction with the less severe varieties of diffuse brain injuries.

Diffuse brain injuries and brain swelling form a distinct group of head injuries that have different mechanisms of causation, different pathophysiologic influences on the brain, and different outcomes than do focal brain injuries.

REFERENCES

1. Abel J, Gennarelli TA, Segawa H: Incidence and severity of cerebral concussion in the rhesus monkey following sagittal plane angular acceleration. In *22nd Stapp Car Crash Conference Proceedings.* New York, Society of Automotive Engineers, 1978.

2. Adams JH: The neuropathology of head injuries, in Vinken PJ, Bruyn GW (eds): *Handbook of Clinical Neurology,* vol 23. Amsterdam, North Holland Publishing, 1975.

3. Adams JH, et al: Diffuse brain damage of immediate impact type. *Brain* 1977, 100:489.

4. Bruce DA, et al: Outcome following severe head injuries in children. *J Neurosurg* 1978, 48:679.

5. Fischer CM: Concussion amnesia. *Neurology* 1966; 16:826.

6. Gennarelli TA, Thibault LE, Ommaya AK: Pathophysiologic responses to rotational and translational acceleration of the head, in *16th Stapp Car Crash Conference Proceedings.* New York, Society of Automotive Engineers, 1972, pp 296–308.

7. Gennarelli TA, Ommaya AK, Thibault LE: Comparison of linear and rotational acceleration in experimental cerebral concussion, in *15th Stapp Car Crash Conference Proceedings.* New York, Society of Automotive Engineers, 1971, pp 797–803.

8. Gennarelli TA, Spielman G, Langfitt TW, et al: The influence of the type of intracranial lesion on outcome from severe head injury: A multicenter study using a new classification system. *J Neurosurg* 1982; 56:26–32.

9. Gennarelli TA, Thibault LE, Adams JH, et al: Diffuse axonal injury and traumatic coma in the primate. *Ann Neurol* 1982; 12:564–574.

10. Gennarelli TA: Emergency Department management of head injuries. *Emerg Med Clin North Am* 1984; 2:749–760.

11. Gennarelli TA, Adams JH, Graham DI: Diffuse axonal injury—a new conceptual approach to

an old problem, in Baethmann A, Go KG, Unterberg A (eds): *Mechanisms of Secondary Brain Damage.* New York, Plenum Publishing Corp, 1986, pp 15–28.

12. Groat RA, Windle WF, Magoun HW: Functional and structural changes in the monkey's brain during and after concussion. *J Neurosurg* 1945; 2:26.

13. Holbourn AH: Mechanics of head injury. *Lancet* 1943; 2:438.

14. Jane JA, Rimel R, Poberstein L, et al: Outcome and pathology of minor head injury. In Grossman R (ed): *Seminars in Neurological Surgery,* New York, Raven Press, 1982, pp 229–238.

15. Jane JA, Steward D, Gennarelli TA: Axonal degeneration induced by experimental noninvasive minor head injury. *J Neurosurg* 1985; 62:96–100.

16. Mitchell DE, Adams JH: Primary focal impact damage to the brain stem in blunt head injuries: Does it exist? *Lancet* 1973; 1:215.

17. Obrist WD, et al: Relation of cerebral blood flow to neurological status and outcome in head-injured patients. *J Neurosurg* 1979; 51:292.

18. Ommaya AK, Gennarelli TA: Cerebral concussion and traumatic unconsciousness. Correlation of experimental and clinical observations on blunt head injuries. *Brain* 1974; 97:633.

19. Strich SJ: The pathology of brain damage due to blunt head injuries. In Walker AE, Caveness WF, Critchley M (eds): *The Late Effects of Head Injury.* Springfield, Ill, Charles C Thomas, Publisher, 1969.

20. Yarnell PR, Lynch S: The "ding": Amnestic states in football trauma. *Neurology* 1973; 23:186.

21. Zimmerman RA, Bilaniuk L, Gennarelli TA: Computed tomography of shearing injuries of the cerebral white matter. *Radiology* 1978; 127:393.

CHAPTER 22

Football-Induced Mild Head Injury*

Wayne M. Alves, Ph.D.

OBJECTIVES OF PROSPECTIVE STUDY

We have completed a prospective study of football-induced mild head injuries sustained by players from ten university teams. The importance of mild head injuries is now clear,[1, 2, 5, 8] but our knowledge of the *frequency of occurrence, how often intellectual functioning is impaired, how long impairment lasts,* and *whether multiple injuries have cumulative effects* is not complete. Our study was designed to address these questions. The major objectives were the following:

1. To *estimate* the incidence of football-induced head injuries and to determine the extent and nature of neuropsychologic and psychosocial deficits of injured players.

2. To *determine* the recovery curve for players with minor head injuries and to develop guidelines for when players can resume normal activities, including football.
3. To *identify* the personal and football-related factors predisposing players to risk of head injury.
4. To *evaluate* the longer-term neuropsychologic and psychosocial consequences of sustaining more than one minor head injury during the player's college career.

In this chapter we give an overview of the design and conduct of the study and present major descriptive findings.

By design, football is a contact sport that naturally places participants at risk for a variety of injuries, especially neural trauma. The occurrence of severe head and spinal cord trauma in football has been well documented and fortunately is low, but there are a much larger unmeasured number of mild head injuries often referred to as "dings." Based on our previous studies of mild head injury patients admitted to the hospital,[5, 14, 15] we would expect that many football players would have uneventful recoveries after mild head injury. We also would anticipate that a heretofore unmeasured number of

*Supported by a grant from the Pew Charitable Trusts (Philadelphia, Pa.) entitled "A Prospective Study of Minor Head Injuries in Football." The principal investigators were Wayne M. Alves, Ph.D. (Division of Neurosurgery, University of Pennsylvania School of Medicine) and Rebecca W. Rimel, B.S.N., M.B.A. (Executive Director, The Pew Charitable Trusts, Philadelphia). Other investigators were John A. Jane, M.D., Ph.D. (Professor and Chairman, Department of Neurological Surgery, University of Virginia), Jeffrey T. Barth, Ph.D. (Director of the Neuropsychological Assessment Laboratory, University of Virginia), Thomas J. O'Leary, Ph.D. (Coordinator, University of Virginia Cancer Center), and William E. Nelson, M.D.

injured players would experience significant neurophysical, psychologic, and psychosocial sequelae. There is little detailed information available as to the mechanisms of sports-induced head injuries and the deficits that arise from these injuries. We believed that we could achieve the study aims by monitoring college football players during several seasons, and evaluating the neurobehavioral deficits and psychosocial problems of those players sustaining mild head injuries.

University of Virginia Pilot Study

In Fall 1981 we conducted a pilot study at the University of Virginia.[3] During the usual preseason medical examinations, we administered a brief battery of neuropsychologic tests, and players completed a questionnaire that described their previous organized sports experience, any history of head injuries, including documented loss of consciousness and hospitalization, and a series of psychosocial measurement scales to tap dimensions such as anxiety, sleep problems, confused thinking, sadness, and enervation (all described in more detail later herein). The entire 1981 University of Virginia football team was tested (N = 116), and during the season players meeting the inclusion criteria were identified by participating trainers present at every practice and game. Twenty players were identified during the season, and all were retested after the completion of the season. In addition, five players were tested within 24 hours of their injury. Sixty-seven uninjured players were also tested at the season's end. In sum, 75% of all players were retested.

Data from the pilot study conducted in 1981–1982 were sufficient to convince us that players sustaining mild head injuries experienced disruption of cognitive functioning, exhibiting problems of attention, concentration, and memory.[3] Further, it appeared that these deficits would diminish quickly. This led us to wonder what factors might explain differences in recovery rates. The data collected in this pilot effort were not adequate for determining how long deficits remained or whether repeated injuries had cumulative effects. Accordingly, we organized the main study with ten university football teams to study players on these teams during a period of nearly 5 years. The participating schools were the eight Ivy League universities and colleges, the University of Pittsburgh, and the University of Virginia. Table 22–1 lists the team physicians and trainers who assisted with the study. We monitored players during a four-season period and evaluated neurobehavioral impairments and psychosocial problems of players sustaining mild head injuries. *A total of 2,300 players were monitored up to 4 years during the study period.*

Why Be Concerned About Mild Head Injuries?

Why should we be concerned about mild head injuries? After all, they may be considered as just part of the game. Concern for football-induced mild head injuries is well founded. First, a high incidence, combined with the potential for complications and persisting impairments, make it imperative that concerted efforts be made to prevent and treat these injuries. Second, the morbidity of the less severe forms of brain injury appears to have been underestimated by a considerable margin. Of course, since factors of life-style and the life cycle play important roles in both the incidence and the outcomes of mild brain injury, we cannot attribute all posttraumatic difficulties to brain injury per se.[2, 5] Third, there is no singular recovery pattern after mild brain injury. For example, Gronwall and Wrightson[9] have estimated that even in the case of uncomplicated mild head in-

TABLE 22–1.

Participants in the Prospective Study of Football-Induced Head Injuries

Institution	Physician	Trainer(s)
Brown	Kenneth Knowles, M.D.	Frank George
Columbia	Charles Schetlin, M.D.	James Gosset
		Michael Cappeto
Cornell	Russell Zelko, M.D.	Bernie DePalma
		Scott Withers
Dartmouth	John Turco, M.D.	Fred Kelly
Harvard	Arthur Boland, M.D.	William Coughlin
Pennsylvania	Joseph Torg, M.D.	Donald Frey
		Mitch Biuno
Pittsburgh	Richard Ray, M.D.	Francis Feld
		Kip Smith
Princeton	Louis Pyle, M.D.	Richard Malacrea
Virginia	Frank McCue, M.D.	William Nelson
		Anthony Decker
Yale	Daniel Larson, M.D.	Daphne Benas
		Molly Meyer

jury recovery may take 35 days or longer. The exact time of recovery is less important than the fact that significant brain damage may have occurred.[7, 9–13, 16, 17] Finally, milder forms of injury may serve as a model for selected aspects of more severe forms of traumatic brain damage.[2, 5]

METHODS OF STUDY

Inclusion Criteria

The study design called for any player who sustained a documented loss of consciousness or a "ding" to be tested at 24 hours, 5 days, and 10 days post-injury. A "ding" was defined, for this study, as (1) a period of disorientation to name, time, and place, (2) an inability to remember the previous play(s) the player was active in, or (3) the sudden expression of posttraumatic complaints, such as headaches, dizziness, tinnitus, or confused thinking. Each injured player was then retested again 12 weeks post-season, along with a player not injured during that season who was randomly selected from the roster of uninjured players. Players had been tested before enrollment in the study according to the proto-col described later; 2,300 players were enrolled in the study. In addition, 50 student controls and 56 selected players with orthopaedic injuries were also studied. *There were 196 injuries involving 183 players identified by trainers or physicians during the study. There were 12 second injuries and 1 third injury among the 196 injuries identified.* Table 22–2 describes the number of players enrolled and injuries studied, and Table 22–3 presents the number of players recruited and injured by school.

Undetected Injuries

Although it is difficult to give an accurate estimate from the data we collected, we believe it is likely that many

TABLE 22–2.

Players Enrolled in Study

Total players enrolled	2,350	
Players	2,300	
Student controls	50	
Head injuries identified	196	100.0%
1st injury	183	93.4%
2nd injury	12	6.1%
3rd injury	1	0.5%
Orthopaedic injuries studied	58	56 players

TABLE 22−3.

Players Recruited and Number Injured by School

School	Total Players	%	Number Injured	%	Total Injuries
Brown	244	10.61	26	14.21	26
Columbia	171	7.43	9	4.92	12
Cornell	249	10.83	29	15.85	30
Dartmouth	228	9.91	5	2.73	5
Harvard	205	8.91	17	9.29	18
Pennsylvania	286	12.43	17	9.29	17
Pittsburgh	242	10.52	20	10.93	21
Princeton	253	11.00	20	10.93	21
Virginia	214	9.30	28	15.30	33
Yale	208	9.04	12	6.56	13
Total	2,300	100.0	183	100.0	196

players (possibly a number equal to or greater than those identified by trainers and physicians as having experienced a mild head injury) were "dinged" or otherwise injured but *either* failed to report such injuries or they went unnoticed. We do not address this question further in this chapter, but plan to do so in later reports.

An Overview of the Study Design

The study design was a longitudinal or panel design in which injured players were tested up to five times before, during, and after the football season (including bowl game appearances). Any player who sustained either a concussion (documented loss of consciousness) or a "ding" was to be included in the study. A "ding" was defined for this study as (1) a period of disorientation to name, time, and place; (2) a failure to remember the previous play(s) the athlete was active in; or (3) the player reported posttraumatic complaints such as headaches, dizziness, tinnitus, or confused thinking.

Before the start of the 1982−1983 season, a team of investigators from the University of Virginia traveled to each participating institution and administered a brief neuropsychologic test battery and a questionnaire documenting the player's year in school, years of organized sports activities, position on the team, and previous history of head injury. We completed the pre-season evaluations with the assistance of graduate and medical students recruited from the psychology department and the medical school at their respective institutions. The test battery and questionnaire items have been described in detail elsewhere, and are briefly described in Tables 22−4 and 22−5.[4, 6] The study Protocol provided to the team physicians and trainers is reproduced in the Appendix to this chapter. The entire test administration took approximately 15 to 20 minutes per player. Players completed the questionnaire portion of the assessment protocol while they waited for their testing session. In subsequent years of the study, only new players, or players not tested in the previous year (for example, late walk-on players), were tested at the beginning of each season. All players in later study years were asked to complete the pre-season questionnaire at the beginning of each season. Nearly 1,800 of the players completed the pre-season neurobehavioral test protocol (Table 22−6).

Players injured during practice sessions or games were retested within 24 hours of their injury by the *team trainer*. A training session on test administration for the trainers was held before the start of each season by the project investigators from the University of Virginia. At

TABLE 22-4.

Neurobehavioral Test Protocol*

Reitan's Trailmaking Tests A and B
  A highly reliable and well-validated test that assesses attention, concentration, complex new problem solving, and perceptual motor integration. Trails A and B have proved sensitive to impairments associated with head injuries.
Smith's Symbol Digit Test
  This well-validated test measures complex visuomotor processing, fine motor coordination, and speed.
Gronwall's Paced Auditory Serial Addition Task (PASAT)
  The PASAT measures sustained auditory attention and concentration as well as rapid mental manipulation of simple configural information. A shortened version of this test was used.
Ammon's Quick Test
  This test is a widely used and reliable measure that provides a brief way of assessing verbal intelligence. It was administered only at the pre-season test session.

*In the University of Virginia Pilot Study, additional tests were used: Buschke's Selective Reminding Task (verbal learning) and Benton's Controlled Word Association (verbal fluency).

TABLE 22-5.

Psychosocial Assessment Protocol

Psychiatric Research Epidemiology Interview (PERI)*
  Anxiety scale A six-item scale that assesses conscious fears, worries, and mild anxiety.
  Sadness scale A four-item scale that measures mild depressive mood.
  Enervation scale A six-item scale measuring lack of energy or general listlessness.
  Insomnia scale A three-item scale that measures difficulty in falling asleep and problems with early morning wakefulness.
  Confused thinking A four-item scale measuring perceived difficulty in concentration, memory, and thought processes.
Other Questionnaire Items
  Symptoms and complaints
  Previous athletic experience
  Medical history of head injury
  Injury event and details
  Problems with school, family, and other life domains

*The PERI is a set of psychometric scales developed by Dr. Bruce Dohrenwend and his colleagues at the Social Psychiatry Research Unit at Columbia University.

TABLE 22-6.

Count of Data Records by Time of Study

Time of Study	Data Record	Players	Student Controls	Count
Pre-season	Psychosocial (PS) questionnaire	3,514	49	3,563
	Neurobehavioral (NB) tests	1,745	49	1,794
In-season	Injury data	265	48	313
	Post-injury NB tests	263	48	311
	Post-injury PS questionnaire	262	48	310
	Injury description (card)	260	48	308
Post-season	Injured NB tests	366	46	412
	Injured PS questionnaire	249	46	295
	Post-season questionnaire	2,134	0	2,134
Total		9,058	382	9,440

this training session the team trainers received intensive practice experience with the test battery and its administration, and we reviewed the problems experienced during the previous season. At 24 hours after injury, the trainer also recorded information regarding the injury event, including activity of the player and the time and location of the injury, as well as player symptoms and complaints. Injured players were then retested at 5 days and 10 days after injury. At the 5-day and 10-day test sessions, the injured players also completed a questionnaire describing their symptoms or complaints and completed the psychosocial assessment scales.

We also tested 56 players who sustained 58 orthopaedic injuries, and we recruited 50 nonathlete student controls from the University of Virginia to be tested according to the same test protocol. At the beginning of a fall semester the student controls were recruited from introductory psychology courses and tested during a 1-week period. Throughout the semester these students were randomly recalled, and a series of three tests was administered to simulate the 24-hour, 5-day, and 10-day post-injury tests. Finally, at the end of the semester the entire group of students was retested. Forty-eight students completed the protocol.

At the end of each season a questionnaire containing the same items for symptoms and complaints and psychosocial assessment scales were given to all players. Twelve weeks after the last game (including bowl games), players who were injured during the season were retested with the neuropsychologic tests, and they filled out a questionnaire describing symptoms and complaints they were still experiencing. In addition, a random sample of players who were not injured during the season were retested. The study protocol called for the sample of uninjured players to be approximately one-half the number of head-injured players.

The data base provided by this study is extensive and provides important pre-injury measurement of some simple parameters of neurobehavioral and social functioning. We have described the data base in more detail in another publication,[4] and Table 22–6 describes the data records from the study available for analysis.

Pre-season Testing

A brief neuropsychologic test battery and a questionnaire documenting their year in school, years of organized sports activities, position on the team, previous history of head injury, and psychosocial assessment scales were filled out by the players (see Tables 22–4 and Table 22–5). Table 22–7 presents the number of players completing neurobehavioral tests and questionnaires; *1,730 players completed pre-season test batteries, and 2,229 players completed pre-season questionnaires during the four study seasons.* For 1,926 players both pre- and post-season questionnaires are available, and pre- and post-season tests are available for 224 players.

In-season Testing

At 24 hours after injury the trainer recorded information regarding the injury event, including activity of the player and time and location of injury as well as player symptoms and complaints. At the 5-day and 10-day test sessions, the player completed a questionnaire describing his symptoms or complaints and completing the psychosocial assessment scales mentioned in the pre-season testing described. The numbers of players and student controls completing the in-season testing protocol are presented in Table 22–8.

TABLE 22–7.

Study Wave Player Completion Counts

Pre-season Test/Quex	Uninjured	Injured	Orthopaedic Controls	Others*	Total
Both same season	1,465	142	38	4	1,649
Questionnaire (Quex) only	480	31	16	3	530
Tests only	29	2	0	0	31
Tests before Quex	33	0	1	0	34
Quex before tests	12	3	1	0	16
Neither done	32	5	0	3	40
Total	2,051	183	56	10	2,300
Pre- and Post-Season Quex†	1,773	116	31	6	1,926
Pre- and Post-Season Tests†	90	77	9	2	224

*Uninjured players who were tested with the in-season protocol.
†Both tests or questionnaires within the same season.

TABLE 22–8.

Completeness of In-Season Testing Protocol

Pattern		Total	Complete	Incomplete	Excluded
24 hr–5 days–10 days					
Total	Tests	313	249	50	14
	Quexs	313	231	67	15
Injuries	Tests	196	149	33	14
	Quexs	196	145	38	13
Controls	Tests	50	42	6	2
	Quexs	50	42	6	2
Orthopaedics	Tests	58	50	6	2
	Quexs	58	42	14	2
Pre–24 hr–5 days–10 days					
Total	Tests	313	207	92	14
	Quexs	313	225	73	15
Injuries	Tests	196	124	58	14
	Quexs	196	141	42	13
Controls	Tests	50	42	6	2
	Quexs	50	42	6	2
Orthopaedics	Tests	58	36	20	2
	Quexs	58	40	16	2
Pre–24 hr–5 days–10 days–post					
Total	Tests	313	174	125	14
	Quexs	313	143	155	15
Injuries	Tests	196	111	71	14
	Quexs	196	82	101	13
Controls	Tests	50	42	6	2
	Quexs	50	42	6	2
Orthopaedics	Tests	58	17	39	2
	Quexs	58	17	39	2

Quexs = questionnaires.

Post-season Testing

A questionnaire containing the same items for symptoms and complaints and psychosocial assessment scales was given to all players 12 weeks after the last game (including bowl game appearances). Players who were injured during the season were retested and filled out a questionnaire detailing symptoms and complaints they still experienced. In addition, a random sample of players who were not injured during the season were retested; *418 post-season tests were administered during the study, approximately 50% to injured players and 50% to uninjured control players; 2,180 post-season questionnaires (given to all players) were also completed.*

Student Control Series

Forty-eight student controls completed all questionnaires and, with a few exceptions, all test sessions. These data provide us with estimates of the learning effects of repeated testing; that is, the normal testing behavior of healthy young men for the selected tests used in this study.

Orthopaedic Control Series

Fifty-six players with 58 orthopaedic injuries were tested with use of the head injury protocol. This "injury control" series enables us to look at the possible consequences of injury per se on the neurobehavioral tests and other assessment measures used in this study. It should be noted that participation in this series was by invitation; thus, through self-selection, this group may be (and probably is) an unrepresentative series. Team trainers were asked to invite all players sustaining orthopaedic injuries that were expected to keep the player away from activity for a duration comparable to players with mild head injuries.

Symptom Incidence Study

Interpretation of the incidence of posttraumatic symptoms in players sustaining football-induced mild head injuries is difficult. While to some extent the reporting of symptoms may simply reflect the pre-morbid symptom experience of young college men, one must consider the possibility that some "posttraumatic" symptoms may occur among football players independent of injury; that is, these symptoms reflect the nature of contact sports. To address this question, we conducted a separate symptom incidence study during the last study season. Three teams from the Atlantic Coast Conference participated: Georgia Tech University, the University of Maryland, and Wake Forest University.

The primary question to be addressed by this study was: What is the incidence of various "posttraumatic symptoms" among football players in general? *More than 300 players participated in this study.* The protocol was simple and involved completion of a symptom checklist at the beginning and end of summer session practice, at the end of the fourth and seventh games of the season, and again at the end of the season. The in-season observation times were chosen at random.

DESCRIPTIVE FINDINGS

Total Series

Table 22-9 presents the distribution of player characteristics based on the entire population of players studied. Offensive team positions were filled by 50% of the players, the remaining 50% of participants playing defensive team or other specialty positions. Nearly one half (48.5%) of the players were 18 years of age on enrollment in the study, and most players were in their sophomore or junior years of college. The oldest player was 26

TABLE 22–9.

Player Characteristics: Total Series

A. Position Usually Played

Position	Frequency	%
Offensive		
Center	81	3.65
Guard	154	6.94
Tackle	145	6.53
Tight end	131	5.90
Receiver	226	10.18
Runningback	252	11.35
Quarterback	127	5.72
Defensive		
Tackle	132	5.95
Noseguard	79	3.56
End	165	7.43
Linebacker	264	11.89
Back/safety	376	16.93
Other		
Punter	29	1.31
Kicker	54	2.43
Other	5	0.24
Total	2,220	100.00

B. Age at Study Entry

Age	Frequency
<18	31
18	315
19	1,078
20	468
21	270
22	54
>22	7
Total	2,223

C. Year in College

Year	Frequency
First	209
Sophomore	1,268
Junior	452
Senior	266
Fifth	30
Total	2,225

D. Previous Head Injuries by Result of Injury

Number of Head Injuries	Confusion No.	Confusion %	Unconscious No.	Unconscious %	Hospitalized No.	Hospitalized %
0	1,280	57.53	1,946	87.34	2,083	93.91
1	434	19.51	210	9.43	126	5.68
2	250	11.24	57	2.56	6	0.27
3	130	5.84	11	0.49	2	0.09
4+	131	5.88	4	0.18	1	0.05
Total	2,225	100.00	2,228	100.00	2,218	100.00

years of age. Only a small proportion of players (1.4%) were fifth-year college students. Of special note is Section D of Table 22–9, which indicates that approximately 42% of the players reported a history of at least one mild head injury resulting in confusion before participation in the study. Slightly more than 11% (11.34%) reported two prior mild head injuries, and 11.6% reported three or more such injuries. A much smaller proportion of these injuries resulted in loss of consciousness or hospitalization. The consequences of this prior history of mild head injury on neurobehavioral test scores is currently being explored in our continuing analyses of the data.

Head Injury Series

When Injuries Occurred—Table 22–10 describes when the players sustained mild head injuries. Slightly more than one half of the injuries (55.8%) were game injuries. The distribution of injuries across quarters of the game indicates no apparent "effect due to fatigue late in the game" situation. There is also no apparent fatigue effect related to the practice injuries. With the exception of the early

TABLE 22–10.

When Player Was Injured

A. When Injured?	No.	%
Game	106	55.79
Practice	84	44.21
Total	190	100.00
No information	6	

B. Quarter Injured?	No.	%
First	28	27.45
Second	23	22.55
Third	26	25.49
Fourth	25	24.51
Total	102	54.84
Not a game	84	45.16
Total	186	100.00
No information	10	

C. Practice Session?	No.	%
First	55	77.46
Second	16	22.54
Total	71	40.11
Not practice	106	59.89
Total	177	100.00
No information	19	

D. Segment of Practice Session?	No.	%
First third	13	22.03
Second third	17	28.81
Last third	29	49.15
Total	59	35.76
Not practice	106	64.24
Total	165	100.00
No information	31	

part of the season practice schedule, there is only one practice session. The 16 players injured in the second practice session probably reflect about half of the players injured at the end of summer practice sessions. Only the University of Pittsburgh had three practice sessions a day during the summer practice sessions. There does appear, however, to be an effect or risk late in the practice sessions. Almost one half (49.2%) of the practice injuries, for which information was available, occurred during the last one third of the practice session the player was injured in. This could be related to fatigue, or it may be that scrimmages or drills occurring later in a practice session involve activities that place players at greater risk.

Mechanisms of Injury

Table 22–11 describes the primary mechanism of injury classified by direct impact to the head and injuries in which there was no apparent impact to the head. Two thirds (67.6%) of the injuries involved direct impacts to the player's head, while 21.6% involved no apparent impact. In 10.8% of the injuries, it was not clear what the mechanism of injury was; that is, there was no identifiable collision that could be pointed to. This was confirmed by the team trainers in a review of the game films where possible.

The majority of injuries involving direct impacts to the head were helmet-to-helmet contacts (21.1%). Collision to the head in which an opponent's torso or body struck the injured player's head caused 11.89% of injuries, and 9.19% of the injuries were the result of players being kicked in the head. A small proportion of injuries (2.16%) occurred when players were kneed in the head. The primary nonimpact head injury involved collision with another player that probably involved some form of rotational injury. We carefully reviewed the narrative descriptions of each of the injuries, and we have provided a selection of these descriptions so that the reader may gain an appreciation for how these injuries have occurred.

HELMET-TO-HELMET IMPACT

Case 1.—I was blocking downfield on a running play and I collided with an opponent and we made contact with our helmets. His face mask hit my helmet on the side, right above the ear. I blacked out for an instant then I was all right.

Case 2.—It was string out drill and I had to fight off three blockers and tackle the

TABLE 22–11.

Injury Characteristics

A. Mechanism of Injury	No.	%
Impact to head	125	67.56
Helmet-to-helmet	39	21.08
Definite collision to head	22	11.89
Probable collision to head	19	10.27
Kicked in head	17	9.19
Head struck ground	7	3.78
Headfirst tackle	6	3.24
Knee hit head	4	2.16
Head hit opponent's torso	4	2.16
Forearm to chin	2	1.08
Speared on ground	3	1.62
Speared in air	2	1.08
No impact to head	40	21.62
Collision to own torso	5	2.70
Nonspecific contact (no head impact)	23	12.43
Hard tackle	9	4.86
Hard block	3	1.62
Unclear	20	10.81
Total	185	100.00
No information	11	

B. Type of Play	No.	%
Running play	96	51.61
Passing play	32	17.20
Kickoff	24	12.90
Punt	8	4.30
Punt return	4	2.15
Broken play	6	3.23
Tackling drill	6	3.23
Blocking drill	3	1.61
Missing	4	2.15
Does not know	3	1.61
Total	186	100.00
No information	10	

C. Player's Activity	No.	%
Being tackled	9	4.95
Tackling	29	15.93
Running with ball	15	8.24
Running after catch	3	1.65
Tackling receiver	4	2.20
Being blocked	31	17.03
Blocking	46	25.27
Catching ball	5	2.75
Pulling to block	1	0.55
Tackling drill	4	2.20
Contact drill	12	6.59
Running drill	1	0.55
Does not know	22	12.09
Total	182	100.00
No information	14	

D. Position When Injured	No.	%
Center	8	4.52
Guard	15	8.47
Tackle	8	4.52
Tight end	10	5.65
Receiver	14	7.91
Runningback	23	12.99
Quarterback	4	2.26
Tackle	11	6.21
Noseguard	2	1.13
End	11	6.21
Linebacker	19	10.73
Back/safety	28	15.82
Kicker	1	.56
Other	5	2.82
Punt coverage, return	5	2.82
Kick coverage, return	13	7.34
Total	177	100.00
No information	19	

fourth. When I came up to make contact I struck down with my head and his helmet caught me on the side the head; then there was a brite [sic] flash. I took off my helmet and my head was pounding. I fell back and waited for help.

Case 3.—I was leading downfield on a screen pass, and saw a defensive back coming upfield. I went to block him and we hit helmets square. I didn't feel hurt at the time, but [after] the next series I was in I didn't remember any of the plays once I [returned to] the sideline.

Case 4.—I was running down on kickoff, first I saw an opponent setting up to block me,

I tried to put a move on so as to miss him. Unfortunately he followed my block and we collided, he was much taller than I and apparently hit his head with my own. I did not lower my head into him though but he put his helmet into my head (forehead) or side I'm not sure it was a very hard hit, probably the hardest hit I've ever encountered.

Case 5.—Pulling to corner Z 50 screen. Rover fire stunt. [Teammate] should have checked over, he didn't. Boy did I find out the hard way. [Opposing player] met me helmet to helmet. [Opposing team color] paint chips from his helmet flew in my face. Nausea followed but I could not puke!

KICKED IN HEAD

Case 6.—I tackled a ball carrier and I think his knees hit me on the forehead. Immediately after the contact I became very dizzy. When I looked up at the opposing team, my vision was very blurred. Gradually, my vision became clearer. It took me approximately 3 to 4 minutes before I could get up and jog off the field. After the game I had a slight headache which lasted about 7 hours.

Case 7.—Sweep play right, fell off block and was kicked in the head by fullback behind me.

Case 8.—Well, it seemed we were in 2-deep coverage. Since I'm F/S [Free Safety] I was away from formation. [Opposing team] ran an option to the strong side. I came across the field to make the play. It was an open field tackle, therefore I was slightly off balance when I made contact. I put my head into the RB's [Running Back's] midsection and caught a knee in the helmet.

Case 9.—We were running a goal line scrimmage at the end of practice. After shedding the block of the tackle I lost my footing. As I was going down to the ground the fullback kneed me in the helmet and then fell on the back of my neck and head.

Case 10.—I was covering a kickoff, a wedge-bust Monday. Someone pushed me on my right shoulder sending me to my left. As I was falling someone else, running put his thigh and knee into my right side of my head.

HEAD HIT GROUND

Case 11.—We threw an interception, I tackled the player and came down on my head.

Case 12.—I ran a pass play across the middle of secondary when one of my teammates came up under me and I landed on my head. It was all I could remember.

COLLISION TO TORSO

Case 13.—As I went to throw the ball, I was hit from behind and then hit from the front.

Case 14.—I was running an off tackle play and got hit from the side. I was stunned for a couple of seconds and got up and ran back to huddle.

COLLISION WITH PROBABLE IMPACT TO HEAD

Case 15.—I ran a pass pattern to the outside about 15 yards downfield. I came back for the ball and was hit with another player's helmet as we dove for the ball.

Case 16.—First play of the game I block down on a double team with the tackle and then slide off to the LB [linebacker]; the [defensive] tackle stunted to his one gap. So the tackle took rain [sic] by himself; I stepped out to get the LB who had a full head of steam and he knocked the [expletive deleted] out of me. It was a head-on hit.

Case 17.—I was hit in the head several times during a drill and then all of a sudden I was standing around and my head began to ache. It was a "serious" hard pounding feeling upon and all around the top of my head.

Case 18.—The play was run to the opposite side of the field. I was being blocked by the guard and as I slid off that block I was hit head-on by someone else.

Case 19.—Hit head-on, saw stars briefly, disoriented for a while.

COLLISION WITH NO IMPACT TO HEAD

Case 20.—I caught a pass at about 25 yards, streaking down the sideline. Just after I caught the ball, I was hit at the top of the chest and everything went blank.

Case 21.—I was crossing the rear of the end zone when the [opposing quarterback] decided to run the ball. I then spotted a defender who would have made the tackle. I cut the defender off with a lunging block and the QB scored!!!!!

COLLISION WITH DEFINITE IMPACT TO HEAD

Case 22.—I was rushing and had just cleared my offensive lineman when the back hit me in the head. I felt dizzy and then I fell down. They took me to sideline and I got dizzy there and fell down again—they took me in.

Case 23.—The last play I remember was a running play up the middle and I made the first hit on the running back (It was a hard hit and I used the front of my helmet to make the hit). Next thing I knew I was taken off the field because I lined up wrong three consecutive plays.

Case 24.—It was a running play and I was blocking a defender. I knocked him backwards and as we were falling others fell around us. Sometime from when I hit him to when we fell on the ground I got hit right above the left eye. I'm not sure what it was that hit me.

Case 25.—I collided with another player as we were going after the same ball. I felt some hot flash through my upper shoulder. After returning to the sideline I experienced some déjà vu feelings. [While covering receiver, he was struck in head by another player.]

HEADFIRST TACKLE

Case 26.—An opposing linebacker intercepted an errantly thrown pass. I was pursuing from the right hash mark to the left hash and made a headfirst tackle in the middle of the field. My face mask was down lower than usual after the play. I experienced blurred vision in my left eye, with accompanying ringing in the ears.

HARD TACKLE

Case 27.—Was collisioned [sic] simultaneous to the reception of a punt; contact was predominantly upper body–chest to chin. The head-on tackle put me on my back. I don't remember the rest.

Case 28.—From left tackle position I came across to middle of formation and made tackle. When I made tackle my body became numb and I became disoriented.

KNEE HIT HEAD

Case 29.—In a running drill, I slipped and was falling when I was hit in the side of the head by a knee. I was stunned for a few seconds.

Case 30.—I was blocking (cut block) the outside men on a 134 counter bootleg. I remember seeing two defenders and identifying the man I was going to destroy. The picture goes blank about 5 yards from the man's right knee.

HEAD HIT OPPONENT'S TORSO

Case 31.—I tackled a running back going as hard as I could; my helmet made contact with his chest and I was dazed by the impact.

Case 32.—I think during a block, I was coming across the field and met the opposing player hitting him with my head, obviously jamming my head and neck. I did not realize the injury until after the game in the locker room when I could not remember things such as our record, who we had played, etc. The next day, Sunday, I had trouble remembering specifics in the past such as names, etc. I was in a daze for at least 3 hours after the injury occurred.

UNABLE TO DETERMINE

Case 33.—Ball was punted. I ran to the ball carrier (40 yards). He ran toward his sideline and pursued. I remember being 2 yards from the ball carrier who was now running up the field. That's all. The next thing I remember is walking from "our" sideline to our bench. I don't remember being hit or how I got from their sideline to ours. After I sat on the bench a minute, I tried to remember things in general. After about 20 minutes I could remember a little, but still don't remember getting hit or how I got to our sideline.

Type of Play When Injured

Just a little more than one half of the injuries (51.6%) involved running plays, 17.2% passing plays, and 22.6% in kicking situations or broken plays (see Table 22–11, section B). There was a small proportion of injuries related to drills during practice sessions. It is interesting that during practice sessions, scrimmage type of plays may have been involved in practice injuries. The general interpretation is that it is a higher speed collision that produces these types of injuries.

Player's Activity When Injured

As we might expect, tackling and blocking are the primary activities of players when they are injured (see Table 22–11, section C). There is slightly more risk for the player who is blocking or tackling an opponent; nearly 44% of the injuries involved these activities, compared with the player who is being blocked or tackled, nearly 32%. The majority of "other" activities, comprising 24% of injured players' activity, is largely special team activities and injuries occurring during practice drills. The injuries appear more likely to occur when the player is proactive (i.e., tackling or blocking) than "reactive" (i.e., when they're being tackled or being blocked).

Player's Position When Injured

Table 22–11, section D presents the injured players' position. The group of players that seem to be at somewhat greater risk appear to be those who perform on special team functions (e.g., kickoff and punt return teams), as well as receivers and defensive backs and linebackers. The injury rates for other player positions seem consistent with the distribution of all players across the various team positions (see Table 22–9, section A). It is likely that there is a differential risk to players in certain positions, depending on the number of plays in a game situation that players in those specific positions may be involved in. We are currently exploring several strategies for estimating this risk factor.

Severity of Injuries

Few of the injuries apparently involved loss of consciousness (4.7%) (Ta-

ble 22–12). This inference should be accepted with considerable caution, since it is virtually impossible to rule out very brief periods of unconsciousness that could go unnoticed. The overall impression provided by this information is that the 50th percentile of the length of time players were disoriented after injury is slightly less than 5 minutes. The duration of loss of consciousness was also brief, generally for less than 1 minute. In game-related injuries, about half of the players were disoriented only for a single series of plays.

There were 13 multiple injuries, which was not a sufficient number to answer our question about the cumulative effect of mild head injuries. We did make some preliminary attempts to look at the consequences of the second/third injuries, but were unable to draw firm conclusions. Suffice it to say here that if the second injury occurred some time after the first there was no apparent relationship between the test scores after each injury.

TABLE 22–12.

How Long Was Player Confused or Disoriented?

A. Unconscious or Stunned?	No.	%
Unconscious	9	4.71
Stunned	182	95.29
Total	191	100.00
No information	5	

B. How Long Unconscious	No.	%
0 to 1 min	7	5.60
1 to 5 min	2	1.60

C. How Long Disoriented	No.	%
Not at all	1	0.55
5 min or less	100	54.65
0 to 1 min	51	27.87
1 to 5 min	49	26.78
More than 5 min	82	44.82
6 to 10 min	17	9.29
11 to 20 min	18	9.84
21 to 60 min	21	11.48
1 to 5 hr	18	9.84
More than 5 hr	8	4.37
Total	183	100.00
No information	13	

INJURY RECOVERY

Mean plots (with standard errors) of three of the neuropsychologic tests used in the study are described in this section. Fig 22–1 presents results for the Paced Auditory Serial Addition Task, series 4 (PASAT4) for head-injured players, student controls, and orthopaedic injuries; Fig 22–2 displays the same results for PASAT3 (series 3), and Fig 22–3, for the Symbol Digit Test. The profiles of scores for the three groups in Fig 22–1 (PASAT4 scores) display the rather typical pattern found when comparing head-injured players and student controls. The average scores from preseason score to 24 hours post-injury score for the head-injured players are not significant, while the comparable change for the student controls is statistically significant. The student controls also show statistically significant improvement between 24 hours and 5 days, but there are no significant increments after that, that is, in the 5- to 10-day interval and the 10-day to post-season intervals. On the other hand,

the head-injured players show statistically significant improvement between 24 hours and 5 days and between 5 and 10 days, with no significant improvements in the 10-day post-season interval. To summarize these changes, we can say that the student controls display normal testing behavior that we would expect in the repeated administration of the tests, while the head-injured players maintain a pre-season baseline score (on average) during the 24-hour post-injury period, and then display an apparent recovery in the 24 hours to 5 days post-injury interval. These players continue to recover in the 5- to 10-day interval, and then level off throughout the remainder of the season to the post-season. By 10 days post-injury, the head-injured players and student controls are equivalent as groups. One sees the same pattern in the mean profiles for the PASAT3 and the Symbol Digit Test displayed in Figs 22–2 and 22–3. Trailmaking Tests A and B were less sensitive to the head injuries and are not reported here. One possible explanation is that the practice or learning effect

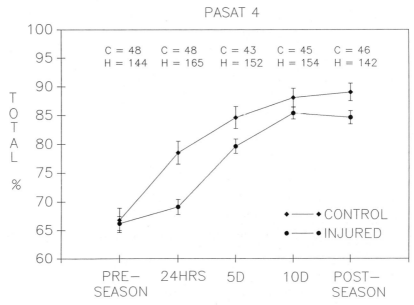

FIG 22–1.
Mean plot (with standard errors) of Paced Auditory Serial Addition Task, series 4 by time of assessment for head-injured players and student controls.

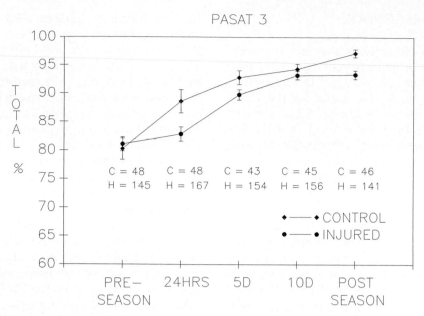

FIG 22–2.
Mean plot (with standard errors) of Paced Auditory Serial Addition Task, series 3 by time of assessment for head-injured players and student controls.

for these two tests is so strong that it dilutes the consequences of the head injury on test performance.

The test score profiles of the orthopaedic injuries have the same general shape as the student control group, a very different profile when we look at the head injury players. While the orthopaedic group may have a different "starting point" (i.e., they are a selected series),

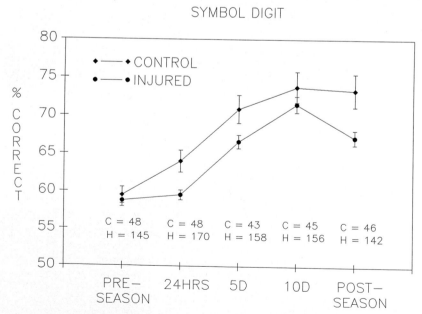

FIG 22–3.
Mean plot (with standard errors) of Symbol Digit Test by time of assessment for head-injured players and student controls.

they do not perform differently than the student controls, whereas both control groups display quite different post-injury performance patterns (measured in terms of test score profiles) than the head injury group.

When we looked at the 95% confidence intervals for these profiles, it was easy to distinguish student controls and players with orthopaedic injuries from the head-injured players. Changes in the test scores appear to be related to the period of confusion, and we are currently examining individual and composite test score changes and injury severity indices and will report these results soon.

Our analyses to date indicate that while an individual player's pre-season score may not be as good as "normative data" based on mean scores for uninjured players (because of motivational and other testing factors), the particular normative criterion we choose (i.e., individual's pre-season, injured player's average, or uninjured player's average), we

are generally going to get the same results.

POSTTRAUMATIC SYMPTOM REPORTING

Fig 22-4 shows the percent of head-injured players, players with orthopaedic injuries, and student controls who reported headaches at each assessment time. Fig 22-5 reports similar distributions for dizziness complaints, and Fig 22-6, for memory difficulties reported after injury. To summarize the findings, we can state that there is a considerable increase in posttraumatic symptom reporting 24 hours after mild head injury, compared with pre-season symptom reporting rates, which then diminish over time to return approximately to the pre-season rate within 10 days post-injury. We do not observe the same pattern of symptom reporting for either the orthopaedic injury group or the student con-

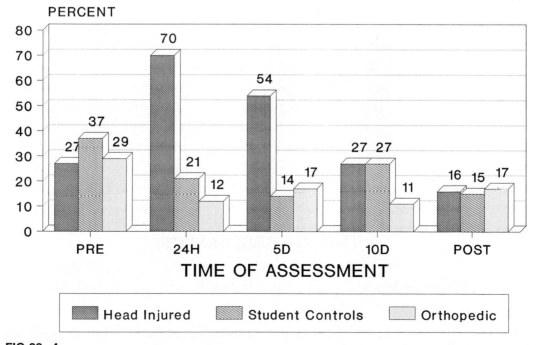

FIG 22-4.
Percent of headache complaints by time of assessment for head-injured players, student controls, and players with orthopaedic injuries.

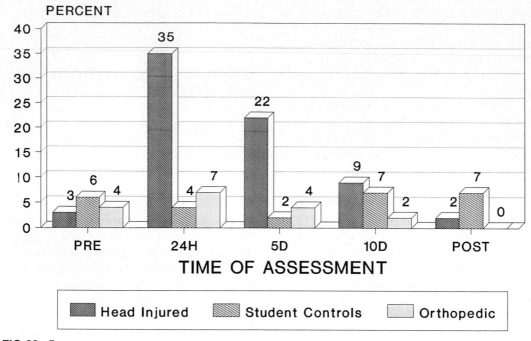

FIG 22–5.
Percent of dizziness complaints by time of assessment for head-injured players, student controls, and players with orthopaedic injuries.

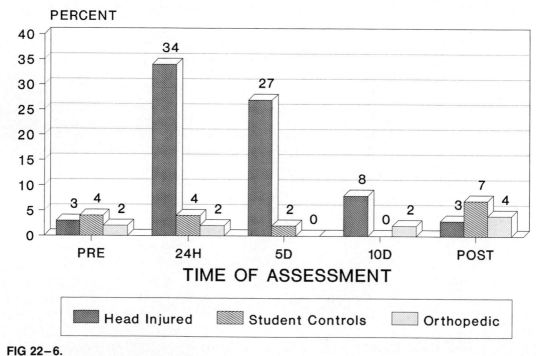

FIG 22–6.
Percent of memory complaints by time of assessment for head-injured players, student controls, and players with orthopaedic injuries.

trols. This gives us rather considerable evidence that the sequelae of minor injury are unique to head injury and not a consequence of trauma per se or a consequence of population-based reporting rates for individuals of similar age and sex. We are currently performing more formal statistical tests in support of these interpretations. The pattern of symptom reporting is consistent with current hypotheses about mild head injury.[1, 4–6, 10]

SUMMARY AND CONCLUSION

We have completed a prospective study of football-induced mild head injuries sustained by players from ten university teams. The study was designed to examine the *frequency of occurrence, how often intellectual functioning is impaired, how long impairment lasts,* and *whether multiple injuries have cumulative effects.* Major objectives were to (1) *estimate* the incidence of football-induced head injuries and determine the extent and nature of neuropsychologic and psychosocial deficits of injured players; (2) *determine* the recovery curve for players with minor head injury and develop guidelines for when players can resume normal activities, including football; (3) *identify* the personal and football-related factors predisposing players to risk of head injury; and (4) *evaluate* the longer-term neuropsychologic and psychosocial consequences of sustaining more than one minor head injury during the player's college career.

On the basis of data analyses conducted to date, and briefly reported in this chapter in a descriptive fashion, we have drawn several initial conclusions. First, recovery from football-induced mild head injuries, as measured by rates of improvement on neurobehavioral test scores, occurs within 5 days after injury. Second, improvements in neurobehav-

ioral test scores and resolution of posttraumatic complaints (such as headaches, dizziness, and memory difficulties) occur together. Third, deficits in sustained attention and concentration may be the most important posttraumatic impairments. This conclusion is drawn cautiously since we were highly selective in the tests chosen for use in this study. Fourth, injured players fully recover from a single mild head injury with no apparent lasting impairments. Fifth, second injuries closely following the first (possibly within the same season) may result in more, possibly lasting, impairments than injuries farther apart. We are currently finishing detailed formal analyses of these data and will report these findings soon in other publications.

Acknowledgments

I acknowledge the following individuals for their support, guidance, and advice throughout the course of this study: Thomas W. Langfitt, M.D., President and CEO, The Glenmede Trust Company, Philadelphia; William F. Collins, M.D., Chairman, Department of Neurosurgery, Yale University; Russell H. Patterson, Jr., M.D., Chairman, Department of Neurosurgery, Cornell University; Joseph S. Torg, M.D., Professor of Orthopaedic Surgery and Director, Sports Medicine Center, University of Pennsylvania; Nicholas T. Zervas, M.D., Chairman, Department of Neurosurgery, Harvard University; Joseph C. Maroon, M.D., Chief, Neurosurgery, Allegheny General Hospital, Pittsburgh, Penn, Bruno Giordani, Ph.D., Department of Psychiatry, University of Michigan, Ann Arbor.

I retain sole responsibility for any errors in the presentation or interpretation of the findings of this study as reported in this chapter.

REFERENCES

1. Alves WM, Colohan ART, O'Leary TJ, et al: Understanding posttraumatic symptoms after minor head injury. *J Head Trauma Rehab* 1986; 1:1–12.

2. Alves WM, Jane JA: Mild brain injury: Damage and outcome, in Becker DP, Povlishock JT (eds): *Central Nervous System Trauma Status Report*. Washington, DC, National Institute of Neurological and Communicative Disorders and Stroke, 1985, pp 255–270.

3. Alves WM, Rimel RW, Nelson WE: University of Virginia prospective study of football-induced minor head injury: Status report. *Clin Sports Med* 1987; 6:211–218.

4. Alves WM: New directions for research on the neurobehavioral consequences of mild brain injury, in Hoff JT (ed): *Mild to Moderate Head Trauma*, Boston, Blackwell Scientific, 1989, pp 187–202.

5. Alves WM, Jane JA: Post-Traumatic syndrome, in Youmans JR (ed): *Neurological Surgery*, ed 3. Philadelphia, WB Saunders Co, 1990, pp 2230–2240.

6. Barth JT, Alves WM, Ryan TV, et al: Mild head trauma in sports: Neuropsychological sequelae and recovery of function, In Levin HS, Eisenberg HM (eds): *Mild Head Trauma*, New York, Oxford University Press, 1989, pp 257–275.

7. Coonley-Hoganson R, Sachs N, Desai BT, et al: Sequelae associated with head injuries in patients who were not hospitalized: A follow-up survey. *Neurosurgery* 1984; 14:315–317.

8. Grant I, Alves WM: Psychiatric and psychosocial disturbances in head injury, in Levin HS, Grafman J, Eisenberg HM (eds): *Neurobehavioral Recovery From Head Injury*. New York, Oxford University Press, 1987, pp 232–261.

9. Gronwall D, Wrightson P: Delayed recovery of intellectual function after minor head injury. *Lancet* 1974; 2:605–609.

10. Levin HS, Gary HE, Jr, High WM Jr, et al: Minor head injury and the postconcussional syndrome: Methodological issues in outcome studies, in Levin HS, Grafman J, Eisenberg HM (eds): *Neurobehavioral Recovery From Head Injury*. New York, Oxford University Press, 1987, pp 262–275.

11. Levin HS, Mattis S, Ruff RM, et al: Neurobehavioral outcome following minor head injury: A three-center study. *J Neurosurg* 1987; 66:234–243.

12. Lidvall HF, Linderoth B, Norlin B: Causes of the post-concussional syndrome. *Acta Neurol Scand* 1974; 50 (suppl 56):7–144.

13. McLean A Jr, Dikmen S, Temkin N, et al: Psychosocial functioning at 1 month after head injury. *Neurosurgery* 1984; 14:393–399.

14. Rimel RW, Giordani B, Barth JT, et al: Disability caused by minor head injury. *Neurosurgery* 1981; 9:221–228.

15. Rimel RW, Giordani B, Barth JT, et al: Moderate head injury: Completing the clinical spectrum of brain trauma. *Neurosurgery* 1982; 11:344–351.

16. Rutherford WH, Merrett JD, McDonald JR: Sequelae of concussion caused by minor head injury. *Lancet* 1977; 2:1315.

17. Wrightson P, Gronwall D: Time off work and symptoms after minor head injury. *Injury* 1981; 12:445–454.

APPENDIX 22–A

Protocol: A Prospective Study of Minor Head Injuries in Football

Pre-Season Testing

Inclusion Criteria.—All football players engaged in play, either practice or games, at any time during the current season are eligible.

Questionnaire.—Every player must fill in the pre-season questionnaire (blue form) before beginning fall practice. This should take about 5 minutes, and should be completed at the first team meeting.

Tests.—All players are to be tested before the beginning fall practice. The initial test battery should take 15 minutes (blue set). Instructions are attached to each of the test sets. The most complex and difficult portion of this study will be the coordination of the pre-season testing. It is very important to test all players. Each school should have at least ten testers in addition to at least one or two persons from Virginia who will direct and assist in the testing. We will pay these testers at a predetermined rate for their services. Individual rooms will be required for each test giver, as well as a cassette recorder and a stopwatch. These are to be provided by the participating institutions. We will provide the testing materials, questionnaires, and testing tapes. The psychology department at your school will be contacted, and an attempt to obtain the necessary examiners will be made.

Data Handling.—At the end of preseason testing, all questionnaires and testing material will be sent to Virginia via Federal Express in prepaid packages. It is important that data forms be filled in completely with date, player's name, and school on each form.

Before shipping completed materials to us, each of you should verify that each form has been completed (e.g., all questions answered).

Post-Injury Testing

Inclusion Criteria.—Any player who sustains a concussion (i.e., injury with a documented loss of consciousness) and any player who is "dinged" is included. If you or another trainer suspect or are unsure if a player has been injured, the following procedures should be initiated on the field immediately. If the player fails to pass these field tests, he should be included for testing.

1. Ask the player his name, the day and year, and the player's present location.
2. Give the player five objects to remember: pencil, elephant, light, truck, book.
3. Ask the player to repeat the following numbers in order: 4-7-3-2-8-1.
4. Ask the player to repeat the five objects he was given in item 2.

An incorrect answer to any one of these questions constitutes a "ding" for purposes of this study. If the player is able to answer all questions correctly but you are still concerned that he has been injured, include him in the post-injury testing. The basis for inclusion should be briefly specified on the 24-hour post-injury questionnaire you will complete.

These instructions are printed on the 3 × 5 cards we have provided, and the player's response can be quickly calculated and filled in later on the post-injury questionnaire you will fill out.

24 Hours Post-Injury

Questionnaire.—Twenty four hours post-injury, the 24-hour post-injury questionnaire should be completed by the trainer (green form). Data collected on the 3 × 5 card should be attached to the questionnaire.

Testing.—The testing of players should be done after completion of the questionnaire (green set). This testing should take about 10 to 15 minutes.

5 Days Post-Injury

Questionnaire.—At 5 days post-injury, the 5-day post-injury questionnaire should be completed by the player (orange form).

Testing.—The testing of players should be done after completion of the questionnaire (orange set). This testing should take about 10 to 15 minutes.

10 Days Post-Injury

Questionnaire.—At 10 days post-injury, the 10-day post-injury questionnaire should be completed by the player (purple form).

Testing.—The testing of players should be done after completion of the questionnaire (dark blue set). This testing should take about 10 to 15 minutes.

Data Handling.—Data forms should be forwarded to Virginia on a weekly basis in the preaddressed envelopes that will be provided. It is important that the data forms be filled in completely with the players' names, dates of testing, and school. Each trainer will verify the completeness of each form before sending the materials to Virginia. Tests should not be scored.

Post-Season Testing

Inclusion Criteria.—All players who were injured during the season must be tested. In addition, a control sample of players not injured during the season will be tested. The control sample will be one half of the number of players injured. For example, if 24 players were injured during the season, 12 uninjured players and the 24 injured players will be evaluated, for a total of 36 players.

Testing.—The testing of injured and control players is done 2 months after the last game (yellow set). This testing takes about 10 to 15 minutes.

Questionnaire.—The post-season questionnaire is completed by all players (yellow form). These will be mailed by the Charlottesville office to each player, and they are to be returned to the trainers.

Data Handling.—All data are forwarded to Virginia in preaddressed envelopes that will be provided. Trainers will verify data completeness before sending materials to Virginia.

CHAPTER 23

Focal Intracranial Hematoma

Leonard A. Bruno, M.D.

In discussing the occurrence of intracranial hematoma as a result of athletic injury, two major points must be emphasized. First, due to recent developments in clinical evaluation of patients and animal research correlation, we have a satisfactory understanding of the mechanism of occurrence of focal intracranial hematoma, which is somewhat different from older concepts of patients with head injuries. Second, management of patients with head injuries has advanced rapidly and changed dramatically during the last decade from management that was accepted medical practice in the past.

DIAGNOSIS

In general, athletic head injuries tend to be dynamic injuries that occur from impact with contact phenomena. These injuries tend to be focal in nature, and are generally less severe than diffuse injuries resulting from acceleration and deceleration. In the unconscious patient, the task is to differentiate between the role played by focal and diffuse strains developed within the head as a result of trauma.

The biologic response to mechanical trauma consists of four basic components: focal concussion; generalized cerebral concussion; primary brain lesions, such as contusions or hematoma; and skull fracture. It is important to realize that each of these four components of biologic response can occur in isolation. The severity of head injury is determined by the relative contributions of these four components plus the added deleterious effects of secondary responses and injury developing after the primary traumatic event. Secondary brain injury, caused by cerebral ischemia or hypoxia resulting from increased intracranial pressure from hemorrhage or brain swelling, or the indirect consequence of hypotension or respiratory compromise, has come to be recognized as the important problem in the care and treatment of patients with head injuries.

In the 1960s it was neurosurgical dogma that patients brought to the hospital unconscious as a result of head injury, who were either deeply comatose or showed signs of neurologic deterioration under observation, required burr hole surgery, often bilateral, as an emergency procedure to assess and treat the possibility of significant intracranial hematoma. Patients were assumed, for all intents and purposes, to have subdural hematoma or epidural hematoma until proved otherwise.

In the early 1970s, computed tomography (CT) of the brain provided a distinct advance in the diagnostic evaluation of patients with severe head injuries. Before the development of CT scanning, the procedures most often used in diagnosing the pathologic process in severe head injuries were carotid angiography and ventriculography. These procedures were time-consuming, somewhat difficult to perform, and involved a certain intrinsic risk from the test procedure alone.

Since 1973 these procedures have been replaced by the CT scan. Since 1983 MRI scanning, or magnetic resonance imaging, has been available in some centers for evaluation of patients with head injuries. At present it is best utilized for follow-up evaluation in stable clinical situations rather than acute trauma management. CT of patients with head injuries can be performed quickly, is noninvasive, and carries essentially no risk.[1] In addition to these logistical advantages, CT scanning provides much information never before available for these patients. Focal lesions such as acute subdural hematoma, epidural hematoma, contusion, and intracerebral hemorrhage are easily diagnosed and visualized. Their distribution and contribution to the overall mass effect of any brain injury can be assessed. Just as important, the large number of patients with diffuse lesions can be classified. Currently, the CT scan is the primary and often only neuroradiologic procedure performed on severely injured patients. Obtaining adequate skull roentgenograms delays the time before the patient can be taken to the intensive care unit for monitoring necessary treatment. The most important information obtained from the plain skull roentgenogram is definition of depressed skull fractures and the presence of linear fractures over meningeal vessels or venous sinuses. The CT scan identifies not only depressed skull fractures but also the extent of depression, the presence or absence of an underlying clot, and the state of the underlying brain. Therefore in this regard it is superior to skull roentgenograms. Linear fractures may not be demonstrated on CT scan. However, more importantly, the presence of epidural hematoma is easily identified. For these reasons, routine skull roentgenograms in comatose patients after head injury are no longer obtained. If the CT scan is not available, many patients may require angiography. These include those with focal neurologic deficit and coma, those who show progressive neurologic deterioration, and those deeply comatose patients in whom it is impossible to differentiate between the primary, diffuse cerebral injury and the late effects of an expanding intracranial mass.

Whenever possible a CT scan should be performed to avoid the use of exploratory burr holes as the primary treatment for patients in whom such surgery frequently results in negative findings. After a normal CT scan, if progressive deterioration of the patient's level of consciousness occurs or if intracranial hypertension develops, a repeat CT scan ensures that there has not been the delayed development of intracranial hematoma.[1]

An accurate picture exists of the frequency of intracranial mass lesions that occur after head injury of all types. As determined by CT scan in a series of 146 children and 171 adults, the incidence of acute epidural, subdural, and intracerebral hematoma and hemorrhagic contusions totals 24% in children and 51% in adults.[1] Thus the majority of patients with head trauma admitted to the hospital do not have an acute intracranial hematoma as the major cause of coma.

The entire spectrum of traumatic intracranial hematomas occurs in sports injuries. These include cerebral contusions, intracerebral hematomas, epidural hematomas, and acute subdural hematomas. The presentation of athletes with head injuries who have had serious trauma is similar in most instances. Management depends on definitive diagnosis and varies depending on the underlying pathologic process.

Head injuries in sports occur in a variety of ways. Many of these injuries involve significant impact to the skull or cranium by a bat, racquet, or club. Other injuries have components of impulse because athletes are often hurling themselves through space or moving at velocities significant enough to cause sizable impulse inertial loading of the brain to occur, with rapid deceleration. Even in athletic contests such as baseball, basketball, or soccer, in which head contact or injury is unlikely, serious brain injury can result from a slip, a fall, accidental collision, or contact with playing equipment.

Head injuries in the athletic setting tend to be of the impact type, with translational or unidirectional application of force and minimal amounts of rotation. In these situations it is not unusual for patients to suffer significant head injury without loss of consciousness. It is known from experimental work that the development of cerebral contusion or small intracerebral hematoma is related to head movement in an interesting manner.[2] If an athlete's head is stable and not moving at the time of impact, he most likely will develop cerebral contusion or a small hematoma under the site of contact. On the contrary, if the athlete is moving in space with a certain velocity and strikes an immovable object with his head, he will develop, in many instances, cerebral contusion or intracerebral hematoma on the side opposite to the area of contact. This is the present explanation of the cause for coup versus contrecoup contusion and hematoma. By their very nature, these types of impact or minimal impulse injuries rarely cause significant unconsciousness.

As outlined by Ommaya and Gennarelli,[2] the degree of alteration of consciousness is directly related to the amount of inertial loading and the rotational component induced at the time of injury, which then cause shear strains in the brain. In precise animal experiments carried out on rhesus monkeys, researchers have clearly demonstrated that the same degree of accleration, deceleration, and inertial loading, when applied to animals in a purely translational mode versus the same inertial loading applied to animals permitted to rotate their heads through 45 degrees, gave the startling but reproducible result that all animals in the rotated group exhibited neurologic evidence of cerebral concussion, defined as the sudden onset of paralytic coma or traumatic unconsciousness. In contrast, none of the translated group showed this effect. Thus it was possible to produce cerebral concussion only when the moving head was allowed to angulate or rotate. When rotation was prevented and the head allowed to move in a straight line only, cerebral concussion did *not* occur.

Conversely, the only animals to develop intracerebral hematoma were those that had received inertial loading in a translational or straight line manner. Petechial hemorrhage of the gray-white interfaces in the brain was present in a bilaterally symmetric fashion in every member of the rotated group of animals, but in only two of the translated group in a sparse asymmetric fashion. These experimental analogs have a clinical analog in athletic head injuries. Most athletic injuries are caused by impact and translational loading. Loss of consciousness in this situation is unusual, whereas development of intracerebral hematoma or contusion without loss of consciousness and without severe neurologic deficit is likely to result from this mechanism of injury.

Intracerebral Hematoma and Contusion

Athletic injuries of this type occur in patients with impressive intracerebral pathology who have never suffered loss of consciousness or focal neurologic deficit, but who do have persistent headache or periods of post-head-injury confusion and posttraumatic amnesia. As with any patients with head injuries, athletes with head injuries who have such symptoms should have a CT scan to permit early differentiation between solid intracerebral hematoma and hemorrhagic contusion with surrounding edema.

Case 1.— A 13-year-old boy was injured while playing ice hockey. At practice, he was struck with a hockey puck in the right temporal region. He fell to the ice, had a momentary episode of confusion, but recovered almost immediately except for complaints of shoulder pain. He was brought to the emergency room for evaluation of possible shoulder separation and was noted by the examining physician to be complaining of pain over the site where he was struck with the puck. Neurologic examination was completely within normal limits, but, because of the location of the impact, skull roentgenograms were obtained,

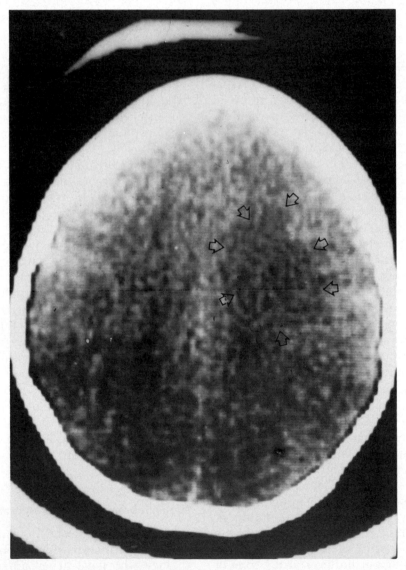

FIG 23–1.
Case 1. Arrows surround a focal area of cerebral edema, which on CT scanning is hypodense or blacker than brain tissue. This localized area of edema in the right temporal lobe represents a small contusion.

which demonstrated a linear fracture in the right temporal region. A CT scan (Fig 23–1) showed an area of radiolucency or decreased density in the right temporal region indicative of edema, which most likely represents a small contusion with surrounding swelling.

Intracerebral hematoma and contusion can be caused by a combination of impact and impulse injury.

Case 2.—While playing basketball on a macadam court at home, a 15-year-old youngster slipped, fell backwards, and struck the back of his head on the hard surface. The CT scan (Fig 23–2) demonstrates diffuse bifrontal edema with multiple areas of small hemorrhagic contusion.

This is an example of a severe contrecoup type of injury; that is, his decelerating head struck the immovable court floor, causing his frontal lobes to strike the frontal bone of his skull. This type of injury occurs in sports in which the participant often has some type of induced body velocity. It happens to riders falling from horses, skiers, skaters, and, occasionally, boxers, basketball players, or

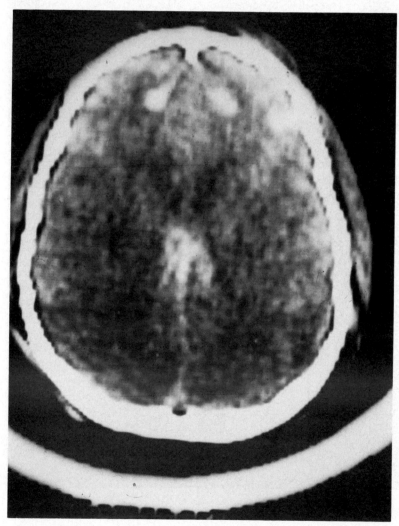

FIG 23–2.
Case 2. CT scan demonstrating diffuse bilateral frontal lobe edema with multiple areas of small hemorrhagic contusion. Blood is hypodense or whiter than brain tissue. This represents a severe contrecoup type injury.

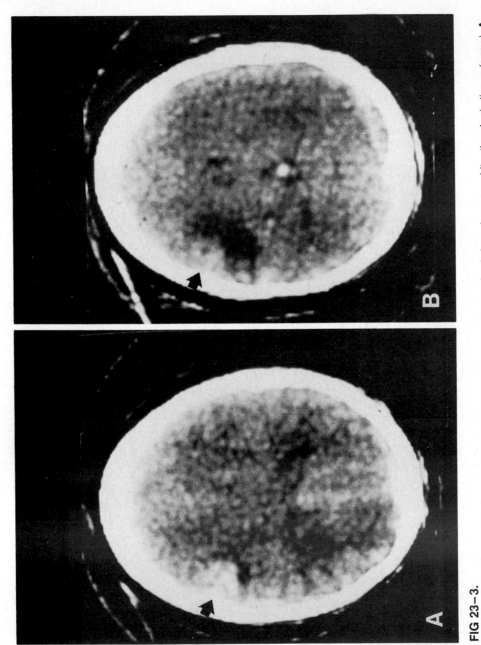

FIG 23–3.
Case 3. CT scan demonstrating a small left frontal intracerebral hematoma that is hypodense or whiter than brain tissue *(arrow)*. **A,** CT scan showing the lesion immediately after initial injury. **B,** CT scan taken 9 days post-injury. Post-beginning resolution of the hematoma.

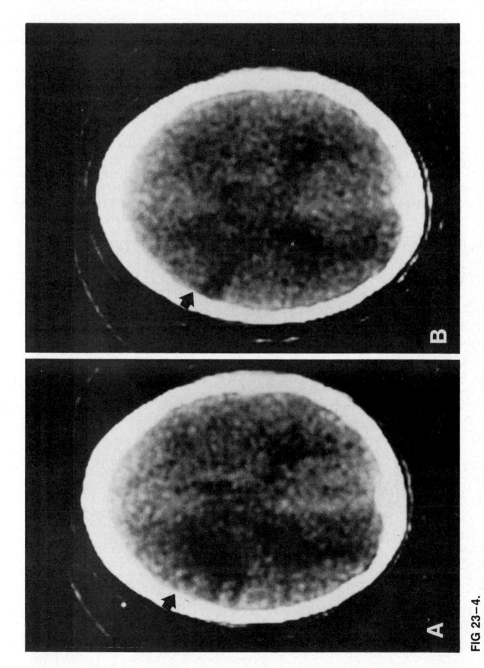

FIG 23–4.
Case 3. **A,** CT scan 16 days post-injury, while **B** was taken 3 months post-injury. Note the marked resolution of the intracerebral hematoma with appropriate conservative (nonoperative) management.

hockey players who fall onto the hard playing surface.

Case 3.—A 16-year-old boy was struck in the left frontal region with a baseball. After his injury he did not lose consciousness, had a fairly severe headache, was a bit lethargic and confused, but never went into coma, and came to the hospital because of persistent headaches and nausea. The CT scan (Fig 23–3) shows his initial picture (Fig 23–3,A), and one obtained 9 days post-injury is shown in Fig 23–3,B. What can be seen is a small frontal intracerebral hematoma, which, with appropriate conservative management, proceeds to its natural history of resolution. A scan of the same patient at 16 days post-injury (Fig 23–4,A) and again 3 months later (Fig 23–4,B) shows that while the brain is some-

what slower than other organs to resolve such injuries, it does recover nicely. What would be anticipated if the scan were repeated a year later is that there would be no abnormalities whatsoever.

Case 4.—A 14-year-old boy was allegedly struck with a soccer ball. He did not fall to the ground and had no loss of consciousness. He had no focal or easily recognizable neurologic deficit, and was brought to the hospital because of confusion, nausea, and headache. On neurologic examination he was found to have diffuse right-sided visual field deficit that could not be well defined. A CT scan (Fig 23–5) demonstrated the intracerebral hematoma in the left occipital lobe. Because of the unusual location of the hematoma, the patient also underwent an arteriogram to determine if he had an underlying arteriovenous

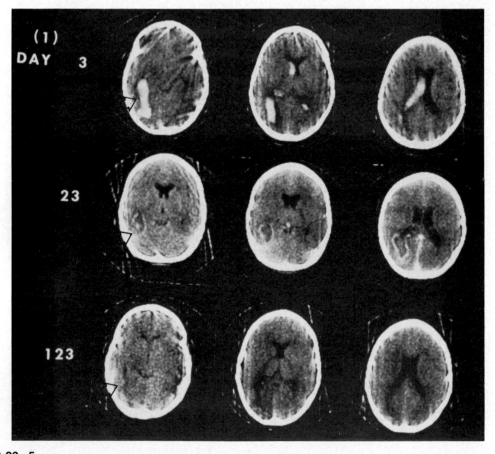

FIG 23–5.
Case 4. Serial CT scans taken at 3, 23, and 123 days post-injury demonstrating presence and subsequent resolution of a left occipital lobe intracerebral hematoma. Patient had been treated conservatively and made a complete recovery without neurologic deficit.

malformation or other predisposing condition. The findings were negative. His CT scan from day 23 post-injury shows beginning resolution of the hematoma, and, with administration of sufficient amounts of corticosteroids, no evidence of spreading cerebral edema or brain shift. By day 123, represented by the bottom series of scans, the hematoma had almost resolved. The patient made a complete recovery with no residual deficit.

Epidural Hematoma

Epidural hematomas are readily correctable lesions if they are identified and removed before secondary injury to the brain stem has occurred from increased intracranial pressure. A review of 300 patients with head injuries who were in a coma at the time of evaluation revealed epidural hematoma present in only 4% to 5%. Because they occur as a result of impact, epidural hematomas develop more often than usual in athletic head injuries, although statistics on their incidence are not readily available.

The pathophysiology of epidural hematoma is that the middle meningeal or other meningeal arteries are often embedded in bony grooves in the skull, and skull fractures, crossing this bony groove, frequently tear the blood vessel at that site. Because bleeding in these instances is arterial, accumulation of clot continues under high pressure and will not tamponade early enough to prevent serious brain injury.

The classic picture of an epidural hematoma is that of loss of consciousness at the time of injury, followed by recovery of consciousness in a variable period, after which the patient is lucid. This is followed by the onset of increasingly severe headache, decreased level of consciousness, dilatation of one pupil (usually on the same side as the clot), and decerebrate posturing and weakness (usually on the side opposite the hematoma). In our experience, however, only one third of

the patients with epidural hematoma have this classic history at initial presentation. Another one third of patients do not become unconscious until late in the course of development of the hematoma, and the other one third are unconscious from the time of injury and remain unconscious throughout its course.

The absence of a classic clinical picture of an epidural hematoma cannot be relied upon to rule out this diagnosis, and the best diagnostic test for evaluating these patients is CT scan (Fig 23–6). If this is unavailable, angiography is necessary. Epidural hematoma can be a clinical diagnosis, however, and in a rapidly deteriorating patient, a plain skull roentgenogram is often adequate for planning surgery. Epidural hematoma is almost always associated with fracture, and since fracture is not uncommon in sports-related head injuries, should be considered as part of the differential diagnosis in all instances. Despite the ready availability of CT scan in our institution, 15% of our patients, both adults and children with epidural hematomas, have been operated on with no special diagnostic tests. These patients had deteriorated so rapidly that immediate surgical decompression was necessary. The treatment of epidural hematoma is surgical removal of the clot.

Postoperatively, about 80% of patients with epidural hematomas do not have elevated intracranial pressure. However, all patients should be monitored and treated expectantly. Therefore, an intracranial pressure monitor is inserted at the time of surgery.

Acute Subdural Hematoma

Athletic head injuries result from lower inertial loading than serious head injuries caused by vehicular accidents or falling from heights. Thus an acute subdural hematoma also occurs much more frequently than epidural hematoma in athletes. In patients with head injuries in

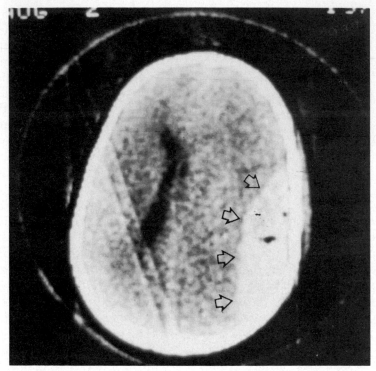

FIG 23–6.
Epidural hematoma is a contained lenticular-shaped collection of blood at the periphery of the brain *(arrows).*
Also demonstrated is associated compression of the ipsilateral lateral ventricle.

general, approximately three times as many acute subdural hematomas occur as do epidural hematomas.

Acute subdural hematomas have been clearly identified as two main types: (1) those with a collection of blood in the subdural space, which are apparently not associated with underlying cerebral contusion or edema (Fig 23–7), and (2) those with collections of blood in the subdural space, but associated with an obvious contusion on the surface of the brain and hemispheric brain injury with swelling (see Fig 23–8). The mortality rate for simple subdural hematomas is approximately 20%, but this increases to more than 50% for subdural hematomas with an underlying brain injury.

Patients with an acute subdural hematoma are typically unconscious, they may or may not have a history of deterio-

ration, and they frequently display focal neurologic findings. Patients with simple subdural hematomas are more likely to have a lucid interval after their injury, and are less likely to be unconscious at admission than those patients with hemispheric injury and brain swelling. It is necessary to obtain a CT scan or angiogram to diagnose an acute subdural hematoma. The size of the subdural clot relative to the size of the midline shift of the brain structures can be evaluated best by CT scan. Of patients with acute subdural hematoma, 84% also have an associated hemorrhagic contusion or intracerebral hematoma with associated brain swelling.

Case 5.—A 21-year-old intercollegiate football player was admitted to the hospital of the University of Pennsylvania on Sept 2,

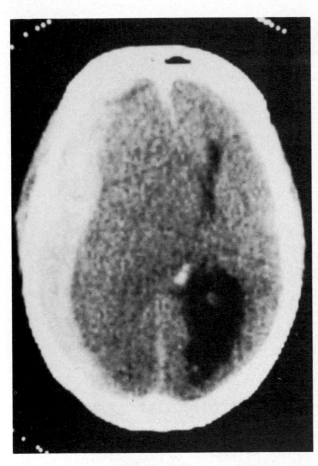

FIG 23–7.
CT scan of a large left subdural hematoma. There is compression of adjacent brain tissue, and cerebral edema is not evident. Such a collection requires surgical decompression. The contrast between this lesion, which requires surgical intervention, and that demonstrated in Figure 23–8, which responded to conservative management, vividly illustrates the difference in the pathomechanics of an acute subdural hematoma, frequently seen as a result of athletic injuries, and the more subacute lesion seen in the older population.

1978, after collapsing during an intrasquad scrimmage. Upon arrival at the emergency room approximately 15 minutes after his collapse, he was unresponsive to painful stimuli, had a fixed dilated nonreactive left pupil, and showed episodic decerebrate rigidity. His vital signs were normal. Motion pictures of the contact activity during a live scrimmage the day before his admission showed that the player, an offensive guard, was kicked on the right side of his helmet by the knee of a linebacker. That evening and the following morning he complained to his teammates of headaches and ringing in his ears, but he participated in the morning noncontact workout. Motion pictures of the afternoon live scrimmage did not demonstrate a significant blow to his head. After the eighth play of that scrimmage, he returned to the huddle confused and disoriented and was helped to the side of the field, where he collapsed and lost consciousness. A CT scan demonstrated a small, acute, subdural hematoma on the left with marked left cortical edema that caused displacement of the ventricles to the right (Fig 23–8). Treatment consisted of large intravenous doses of mannitol, dexamethasone (Decadron), and pentobarbital. After initiation of treatment his left pupil became reactive, and intracranial pressure, which was monitored by an intracranial pressure (ICP) bolt, could then be maintained within the normal range. During an induced coma that was maintained for 10 days, respirations were controlled and supported by a respirator. The patient's hospital course during this time was satisfactory, demonstrated on CT scans by resolution of the left hemispheric edema and subdural hematoma, and by the maintenance of normal vital signs. Three weeks after admission he was transferred to a rehabilitation center. Five weeks after his injury he was discharged from

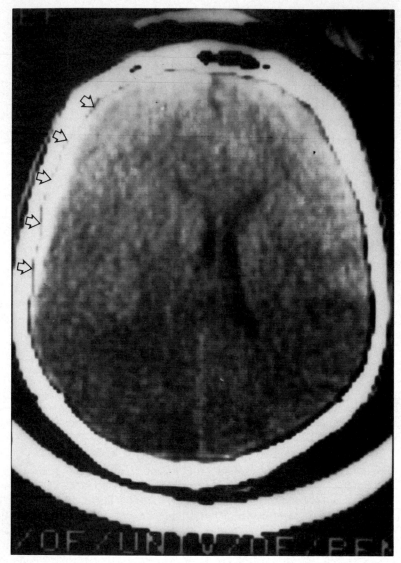

FIG 23–8.
Case 5. CT scan demonstrating a small, acute subdural hematoma in the left temporoparietal area *(arrows).* There is associated marked left cortical edema that has caused displacement of the ventricles to the right.

the center without apparent residual neurologic impairment, and has subsequently graduated from the university (Fig 23–9).

The term *acute subdural hematoma* raises the image in most physicians' minds of a large collection of clotted blood in the intracranial cavity, compressing the brain substance and causing compromise because the hematoma occupies space (see Fig 23–7). While this is

not an infrequent consequence of closed head trauma, this type of subdural hematoma is more common in adults who have a degree of cortical atrophy.

Young athletes, and especially children, frequently develop only minimal subdural hematomas with underlying cerebral hemispheric swelling (see Fig 23–8). This type of brain injury is not the result of a space-occupying mass from clotted blood, causing brain compression,

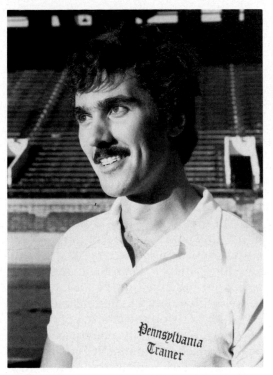

FIG 23–9.
Intercollegiate football player (case 5) after nonoperative treatment for a subdural hemorrhage. He has made a complete recovery. Although not permitted to participate in contact sports after his injury, his interest in football has been sustained by his participation as a member of the university training staff.

but rather swollen brain tissue causing consequent rises in intracranial pressure. The advent of CT scanning permits accurate differential diagnosis between these two conditions, which frequently cause similar clinical pictures. The modalities of treatment for these two distinct types of acute subdural hematomas are quite different.

PRINCIPLES OF MANAGEMENT

As our knowledge of physiology and pathophysiology increased, we have progressed through stages of development and gained the ability to resuscitate seriously ill or severely injured people successfully. We began in the 1950s to treat acute respiratory and postoperative problems successfully, followed by satisfactory cardiac resuscitation and emergency cardiac care in the 1960s. We have extended innovations in critical care medicine in the form of brain resuscitation in the 1970s. Such care is based on the concept that the degree of permanent neurologic, intellectual, and psychologic deficits after brain trauma with coma is only partly the result of the initial injury, and is certainly in part due to secondary postinsult changes, which can be worsened or improved by the quality of the supportive care. Head injuries by their very nature require resuscitation, that is, therapy initiated after the insult. The proper care of patients with head injuries, athletic or otherwise, depends on a full appreciation and use of brain resuscitation measures in an intensive care setting.

Present management of focal intracranial hematoma resulting from athletic injury includes not only treatment for, and removal of, hematoma, but also recognition of, and treatment for, the underlying brain injury that results from severe head trauma. Included in this concept of treatment for the underlying brain injury is that of resuscitation of the brain. This is therapy designed to have specific neuron-saving potential once general resuscitation methods and supportive care have begun. Our concerns in management of the athletic-injured patient are the same as those for any patient who has received severe head injuries. Our current management and treatment protocol is outlined in Table 23–1.

First aid should consist of getting the patient safely into a supine position and determining vital signs and the significance of any associated injuries. Initial treatment should consist of establishing an adequate and useful airway and beginning hyperventilation maneuvers. This can be accomplished by using a manual resuscitation bag with supplemental oxy-

TABLE 23–1.

Head Injury

First Aid—Hyperventilation Diagnosis—CT Scan	
Surgery	**No Surgery**
Epidural hematoma	Small subdural hematoma
Large subdural hematoma	Contusion
	Diffuse injury
Large Intracerebral hematoma	Most intracerebral hematomas

ICP Monitoring and Treatment
Goal modalities
Keep ICP less than 15 mm Hg
Hyperventilation (P_{CO_2} 22 to 30 mm Hg)
Corticosteroids (1 mg/kg of dexamethasone q 6 hr)
Mannitol (1 g/kg; keep serum osmolality <320 mOsm/L)
Barbiturates (30 mg/kg loading and 0.5–3 mg/kg/hr maintenance)

gen, if it is available. The patient should then be transferred as quickly as possible to a medical facility where diagnosis and treatment of brain injury can begin. While these measures are important for all patients who have suffered concussion, they are of extreme importance for the patient who remains comatose after trauma. The use of an initial dose of corticosteroids given parenterally is specifically indicated, and 100 mg dexamethasone or 1 mg methylprednisolone sodium succinate can be administered to the average adult. Once the patient arrives in the emergency room and it is determined that he or she is stable from a cardiorespiratory point of view, endotracheal intubation is immediately performed on comatose patients and a CT scan is obtained as soon as possible. The CT scan provides an immediate diagnosis of the intracranial situation, and, as can be seen from the management schema, patients are then divided into either a surgical or nonsurgical category, depending on the size of intracranial hematoma present.

Initial evaluation of all head trauma patients includes determination of their coma state by numerical ranking on the Glasgow Coma Scale (Table 23–2). This coma scale is based on the patient's response to stimulation by eye opening, best motor response, and best verbal response. Scores of 15 to 3, from normal neurologic status to deeply comatose, are possible.

Patients with a Glasgow Coma Scale of 7 or lower should have immediate intracranial pressure (ICP) monitoring as part of their treatment. Intracranial hypertension, defined as a pressure of more than 15 mm Hg, is seen in 50% or more of patients with severe head injuries. The correlation between alterations in ICP and the patient's neurologic status has been well described in the past. Therapy to treat intracranial hypertension can be given correctly only when the pressure is known. We are firmly convinced of the usefulness of continuous ICP monitoring in the intensive care of the patient with severe head injuries. Because intermittent waves of increased pressure, which commonly occur without other signs or symptoms, can be diagnosed and treated before significant neurologic deterioration occurs, ICP monitoring facilitates titration of therapy.

When muscle paralysis or barbiturates are used to control elevated ICP, it is impossible to follow the patient's neurologic state. Other than brain stem–evoked potentials, ICP is the only parameter that can be followed. It would be inappropriate to use muscle paralysis or barbiturates without continuously recording ICP. Ideally, the ICP should be monitored from the earliest possible time after the patient's arrival in the hospital. In our unit it is usually possible to obtain a CT scan within 1 hour of admission in all severe head injuries. The ICP monitor is usually inserted after the CT scan and within 2 hours of admission.

However, if any delay in diagnosis is foreseen or if the patient is rapidly deteriorating, an ICP bolt is inserted immedi-

TABLE 23–2.

Glasgow Coma Scale*

Eyes	Open	Spontaneously	4
		To verbal command	3
		To pain	2
		No response	1
Best motor response	To verbal command	Obeys	6
	To painful stimulus†	Localizes pain	5
		Flexion-withdrawal	4
		Flexion-abnormal (decorticate rigidity)	3
		Extension (decerebrate rigidity)	2
		No response	1
Best verbal response‡		Oriented and converses	5
		Disoriented and converses	4
		Inappropriate words	3
		Incomprehensible sounds	2
		No response	1
Total			3–15

*The Glasgow Coma Scale, based on eye opening, verbal, and motor responses, is a practical means of monitoring changes in level of consciousness. If response on the scale is given a number, the responsiveness of the patient can be expressed by summation of the figures. Lowest score is 3; highest is 15.
†Apply knuckles to sternum; observe arms.
‡Arouse patient with painful stimulus if necessary.

ately after emergency resuscitation. This early insertion is especially important in patients with signs of shock from other injuries who require rapid fluid replacement. In these cases, we begin to monitor pressure in the emergency room with a portable recording system.

The ICP monitoring system must be simple, easily inserted, and reliable. The subarachnoid bolt, which can be easily inserted and maintained and does not require an operating room procedure, can be accomplished at bedside with local anesthesia.

We monitor ICP in comatose patients with head injuries whether they are operated on initially for decompression or not. We rarely intervene surgically to remove contused brain, believing that if ICP can be controlled, the removal of potentially functional brain tissue is unacceptable because it may limit the patient's recovery. After surgical intervention in patients with hematoma, we routinely insert subarachnoid bolts and monitor ICP for possible further therapy.

The following principles of management of patients with head injuries apply to those who do not have indications for surgical intervention, and to those postoperative. This management is guided by the monitored variables, and its goals are to prevent three major complications that cause most deaths if the patient is alive on arrival at the hospital: (1) intracranial hypertension, (2) inadequate cerebral oxygenation, and (3) systemic medical complications. These must be attacked vigorously for optimum results. Treatment for intracranial hypertension is also designed to maximize cerebral oxygenation, and the modalities are those previously listed.

Of all therapies for high ICP, hyperventilation is the first one that we use, and it is extremely effective. With the patient intubated, we keep the Pco_2 at 22 to 30 mm Hg and note that a fall in ICP is rapid after hyperventilation; in some instances hyperventilation is all that is necessary for control.

Corticosteroids in large doses (1 mg/

kg of dexamethasone every 6 hours) are given routinely. Hyperosmotic agents decrease ICP by removing brain water resulting from an induced osmotic gradient from the brain to the intravascular component. Although slightly less rapid in its action, 20% to 25% mannitol has largely replaced 30% urea in this country because of less rebound after administration. Two forms of hyperosmotic therapy are available: intermittent bolus use and continuous infusion therapy. High-dose bolus therapy, 1 to 2 g/kg of mannitol, is reserved for initial emergency control of ICP, usually in patients who have a rapid decrease in level of consciousness, dilating pupils, or decerebration. Maintenance therapy can then be carried out with smaller boluses of 0.15 to 0.3 g/kg of mannitol every 1 to 2 hours, or whenever the ICP exceeds 15 mm Hg. Close attention must be given to the serum osmolality so that it does not rise above 320 mOsm/L. Significant cardiopulmonary and renal complications are frequent and often irreversible with serum osmolality above these levels. Clinicians utilizing this therapy should have a thorough understanding of the hyperosmolar state.

The most recent contribution to ICP control is the use of barbiturates. When initially used to protect the brain by lowering metabolism, it became apparent that reductions of ICP occurred regularly. Although the mechanism of barbiturate action on elevated ICP is not known, its successful use when other forms of therapy have failed to lower ICP is encouraging. The doses of barbiturates required have varied. Pentobarbital has been the most widely used agent, usually with loading doses of 10 to 30 mg/kg. Thereafter, infusions of 0.5 to 3 mg/kg/hr are maintained. We have been impressed with the wide variation of serum levels obtained by similar doses in different patients and no longer rely solely on serum levels as criteria. We prefer to titrate the dose until a burst-suppression pattern is present on the electroencephalogram monitor. Therapy is then closely regulated to keep the burst-suppressions of equal length. At this physiologic end point, the serum pentobarbital level may vary from 2.5 to 5.0 mg/dl. Care must be taken to prevent barbiturate cardiac toxicity and subsequent hypotension. This has not been a problem except in older patients, and the cerebral perfusion pressure can be adequately maintained without the use of pressor agents.

For the duration of barbiturate therapy, monitoring must be intensive because neurologic signs are abolished. Spontaneous respiratory activity is not present, and all other neurologic signs are generally absent. Although we have continued barbiturate therapy for as long as 21 days, the usual course is less than 5 days. By this time the ICP rarely rises when an attempt is made to discontinue the barbiturate infusion. Once a patient's ICP is less than 15 mm Hg for longer than 48 hours, we discontinue therapy in a sequential manner, stopping barbiturates first, then decreasing hyperosmolar therapy, and, finally, ceasing hyperventilation.

The accepted treatment of a patient with acute subdural hematoma remains controversial. Some neurosurgeons believe that the majority of patients with acute subdural hematomas are not helped by an operation, and that the major problems are the control of brain swelling and elevated intracranial pressure. Others believe that because of obvious deterioration of the patient, evacuation of the hematoma, no matter how large, improves intracranial compliance and the neurologic state.

In those patients whose CT scans show a large localized subdural clot with an equal or larger shift of the midline structures, we surgically evacuate the hematoma. In patients with a "smear subdural hematoma," a few millimeters thick over the entire lateral aspect of one hemisphere, with the midline shift greater than the thickness of the subdural hematoma, we probably would not operate but would aggressively control ICP. Disagreements arise when a state between these two is seen. The argument against surgical intervention is that the major cerebral problem is brain injury, which cannot be helped by an operation. If there is a disruption of the blood-brain barrier with vasogenic edema, craniotomy decreases tissue pressure, increases hydrostatic pressure gradients between capillaries and tissue, and may therefore cause a marked increase in edema in the decompressed hemisphere. Thus, even if the clot is removed, the increased edema may cause swelling of the hemisphere, which rapidly returns the intracranial volume-pressure relationships to where they were before the operation.

If an operation is performed, we recommend a large temporofrontoparietal craniotomy flap with evacuation of the clot and control of the hemorrhage from bridging veins and cortical laceration. The patient with a sizable subdural hematoma, as seen in Figure 23–7, should have an operation for evacuation of the clot followed by management of ICP. A patient with a subdural hematoma along the outside of the left hemisphere, such as that seen in Figure 23–8, is best managed by aggressive treatment of brain swelling and therapy for increased ICP.

The mortality rates for the surgical treatment of acute subdural hematoma reported in the last 10 years vary from 42% to 63%. One important variable seems to be the level of consciousness of the patient at the time of the operation. We do not believe that an operation is necessary in all patients with acute subdural hematoma, but we do believe it is vital that all patients, including those who have had surgical intervention, have postoperative ICP monitoring and control. Of patients who died after surgical intervention, 25% died from uncontrollable elevated ICP. Thus postoperative ICP monitoring plays a major role in the care of patients with acute subdural hematomas. We believe strongly that this will improve not only mortality rates but also quality of life.

In conclusion, we have come to recognize that in all patients with serious head injuries, including athletic head injuries, pathologic damage is usually diffusely distributed throughout the cerebral hemispheres and brain stem. Ideally, therapy should prevent secondary damage rather than modify any secondary injury once it occurs. With this approach it should be possible to limit patient disability to the results of the primary biomechanical injury alone. Theoretically, no patient who is conscious after injury should die or suffer major disability.

Comatose patients require immediate and intensive therapy after their injury. The triage must include transport to a medical facility where rapid diagnosis and intensive care are available and routine.

Early effective diagnosis of surgically correctable lesions by CT scanning has decreased mortality from epidural and surgically treatable subdural hematomas. With no mass lesion, aggressive management can be started without undue concern that a mass lesion has been missed, and negative exploratory surgery can be avoided. The use of ICP monitoring and monitoring of the systemic arterial pressure and blood gases, serum osmolality, and electrolytes allow any trend away from normal to be detected and corrected at the earliest possible time. The use of barbiturates is an effective way to control intracranial hypertension when other more common modes of treatment have failed.

Any athlete who has suffered loss of consciousness from head injury for more than 1 minute, or who has persistent headache with confusion or any disorientation that persists longer than 1 hour after trauma, or an athlete who has more than one episode of unconsciousness, however momentary, during any one playing season should be referred for neurologic examination and CT scan evaluation. With the proper diagnosis and management of patients with head injuries, we are convinced that the present distressingly high mortality and morbidity from severe head injury can be lowered without a decrease in the quality of life.

REFERENCES

1. Bruce DA, Gennarelli TA, Langfitt TW: Resuscitation from coma due to head injury. *Crit Care Med* 1978; 6:254.

2. Ommaya AK, Gennarelli TA: Cerebral concussion and traumatic unconsciousness: Correlation of experimental and clinical observations on blunt head injuries. *Brain* 1974; 97:633.

CHAPTER 24

Criteria for Return to Competition After a Closed Head Injury

Robert C. Cantu, M.D.

Head injury is the most frequent catastrophic sports injury,[24] and it takes on a singular importance because the brain is incapable of regeneration. Also, there is unequivocal evidence that repeated brain injury of concussive or even subconcussive force results in characteristic patterns of brain damage and a steady decline in the ability to process information efficiently.[3, 7, 14, 16, 32] Furthermore, the effects of repeated head injury are cumulative, and this can be shown immediately at the time of the second injury, not years later. While some blows to the head may be more severe than others, none is trivial and each has the potential to be lethal. Blunt head trauma causes shearing injury to nerve fibers and neurons in proportion to the degree the head is accelerated, and these acceleration forces are imparted to the brain.[11, 12, 21] Blows to the side of the head tend to produce greater acceleration forces than those to the face, while those to the chin, which acts as a lever, produce maximal forces. Shearing of blood vessels may lead to epidural and intracerebral hematomas, with rapid death.[27]

The late or chronic effects of repeated head trauma of concussive or even subconcussive force lead to anatomic patterns of chronic brain injury with correlating signs and symptoms. The characteristic symptoms and signs of this traumatic encephalopathy that may occur in anyone subjected to repeated blows to the head from any cause include slow appearance of a fatuous or euphoric dementia, emotional lability, and the victim's displaying little insight into his deterioration. Memory deteriorates considerably, and speech and thought become progressively slower. There may be intense irritability, mood swings, and sometimes truculence leading to uninhibited violent behavior. The most common prevailing mood, though, is a simple fatuous cheerfulness. Occasionally there is depression with a paranoid coloring. The neurologist may encounter almost any combination of cerebellar, pyramidal, and extrapyramidal signs, with tremor and dysarthria being two of the most common findings.

CONCUSSION

What are the definitions and grades or severity of concussion? It must first be stated that universal agreement on the definition of concussion does not exist. This fact renders evaluation of epidemiologic data extremely difficult. A working definition of concussion that has gained general acceptance is the one proposed by the Committee on Head Injury Nomenclature of the Congress of Neurological Surgeons.[6] As stated, a concussion is "a clinical syndrome characterized by immediate and transient post-traumatic impairment of neural function, such as alteration of consciousness, disturbance of vision, or equilibrium, due to brain stem involvement."[6] Maroon et al., in attempting to simplify the clinical problem, divided concussion into three grades based on duration of unconsciousness, that is, mild (no loss of consciousness); moderate (loss of consciousness with retrograde amnesia); and severe (unconsciousness longer than 5 minutes).[20] Others have classified concussion according to duration of posttraumatic amnesia,[16] and, finally, concussion severity has been graded by using both the duration of unconsciousness and posttraumatic amnesia, that is, mild (transient or no loss of consciousness with posttraumatic amnesia less than 1 hour); moderate (unconscious less than 5 minutes with posttraumatic amnesia 1 to 24 hours); severe (unconscious more than 5 minutes with posttraumatic amnesia more than 24 hours).[13] A practical scheme for grading the severity of a concussion based on the duration of unconsciousness or amnesia, or both (retrograde plus posttraumatic) is as follows:

- Grade 1 (mild): No loss of consciousness; posttraumatic amnesia <30 minutes.
- Grade 2 (moderate): Loss of consciousness; <5 minutes or posttraumatic amnesia >30 minutes.
- Grade 3 (severe): Loss of consciousness; > 5 minutes or posttraumatic amnesia >24 hours.

In football a concussion most often occurs while making a tackle (43%), being tackled (23%), blocking (20%), or being blocked (10%).[9] Football head injuries are twice as frequent as neck injuries.

Nearly nine of ten football head injuries are concussions,[2] and one of five high school varsity athletes can anticipate a concussion each season.[9] The incidence of reported concussion may be unquestionably low, because many athletes do not associate a brief loss of awareness or a few minutes of amnesia with concussion. The comment from a player, "The coach took me out of the game to see if I had a concussion but I did not" is not unique. Furthermore, in his desire to play the athlete may deny or minimize symptoms. Since, after a "concussion," catastrophic brain injury is known to occur after a second apparently minor head impact in the same game, especially football, accurate documentation and treatment are of paramount importance.[29, 31, 32]

Recognition and Management of Concussion

There is certainly little difficulty in recognizing a grade 3 or severe concussion, that is, unconscious more than 5 minutes. Initial treatment should be the same as for a suspected fracture of the cervical region of the spine. If the airway is adequate, the helmet should not be removed on the playing field for fear of worsening a cervical fracture dislocation. The face mask can be removed with bolt cutters or left intact if the athlete is stable. The athlete should be transported on a fracture board, with the head and neck immobilized, to a hospital with neurosurgical coverage. There x-ray films of the cervical region, including lateral flexion-extension views if the initial neutral view is normal, should be obtained. Skull x-ray films should be taken to rule out fractures. A computed tomography (CT) scan of the head should be done on all athletes in whom (1) the neurologic examination shows abnormal findings; (2) a skull fracture is identified; (3) the athlete is still unresponsive; or (4) if associated symptoms such as headache, nausea, vomiting, visual impairment, or dysequilibrium persist for 12 hours.[14] Even if an initial CT scan shows normal findings, if these associated symptoms are not markedly improved in 24 to 48 hours, a repeat CT scan should be considered. In this time interval microscopic hemorrhages may coalesce, forming a brain contusion, or a subacute subdural hematoma may be in evolution. It is recommended that all players having severe concussions be admitted for neurologic observation for intracranial bleeding.*

With a grade 2 or moderate concussion, unconscious less that 5 minutes, the athlete should initially be managed as with a grade 3 concussion. Here, though, clinical judgment may dictate that if the period of unconsciousness is brief, and if the now conscious athlete had no neck complaints, removal on a fracture board may not be necessary. It is recommended that the athlete be removed from the contest and evaluated at a neurosurgery staffed medical facility with a thorough neurologic examination and x-ray films of the skull and cervical spine. Results of these examinations and associated symptoms will dictate whether a CT scan of the head is necessary. A period of neurologic observation for most athletes is recommended, and for all who have any central neurologic abnormality by examination, or who have persistent symptoms such as headache or skull fractures.

It is the grade 1 or mild concussion that is the most difficult to recognize and when the greatest clinical judgment must be exercised. Here there is no lapse of consciousness, but an impairment of cortical function, especially for recent memory and assimilating and interpreting new information, is present. This grade of concussion is the most frequent (more than 50%), and not infrequently it escapes medical recognition (see Chapter

*References 2, 9, 13, 19, 29, 31, and 32.

21). It is not uncommon for a player to be "dinged" or have his "bell rung" and continue playing. As described, "your memory is affected although you can still walk around and sometimes continue playing. If you don't feel pain, the only way other players and the coaches know that you have been dinged is when they realize you can't remember the plays."[23]

The initial treatment of the condition involves immediate removal from the game and observation on the bench. In those instances in which the athlete, after a period of time, has no headache, tinnitus, dizziness, nor impaired concentration, including orientation to person, place, and time and full recall for events just before injury, return to the contest can be considered.[37] Before return the athlete not only should be asymptomatic at rest but also should demonstrate that he can move with his usual dexterity and speed. If an athlete has any of the preceding symptoms or signs either at rest or with exertion, he should not be allowed back into the game. Close neurologic observation is essential.

Return to Competition After a Concussion

Just as with the definition of concussion, there are presently no universally accepted criteria for when to allow the athlete to return to competition. Many physicians are more conservative because it has been shown that ability to process information is reduced after a concussion,[10] and the severity and duration of functional impairment are greater with repeated concussions.[10, 11, 35] Although subject to confirmation, these studies suggest that the damaging effects of the shearing injury to nerve fibers and neurons are proportionate to the degree the head is accelerated and that these changes are cumulative.[8, 26, 34] There is also evidence suggesting that once a player has suffered a first concussion, his chances of incurring a second one are more than four times greater than for the player who has not had a concussion.[9] If this is not enough to make the physician wary, the "second impact syndrome" recently reported by Saunders and Harbaugh[30] and also by Schneider[31] most certainly should. In this condition fatal brain swelling may occur after minor head contact in a player still symptomatic from a prior concussion. Although rare, since the consequences are so catastrophic, it suggests that an athlete should not return to competition until he is asymptomatic after a concussion.

The following recommendations for return to competition after concussion are made based on the grade of concussion and prior incidence of concussion. While from a medical standpoint the standards should apply for high school, college, and professional athletes, the implementation may not be as strict in the latter group.

For a first grade 1 concussion, if the athlete is asymptomatic at rest and exertion as discussed, return to the contest as well as subsequent games is permissible. If a second grade 1 concussion occurs in the same game, the player is removed from the game and not allowed to participate for at least 2 weeks provided he is asymptomatic at rest and during exertion. If headache or other associated symptoms either worsen in the first 24 hours or persist longer, a CT scan is recommended. Magnetic resonance imaging (MRI) holds promise to be even more sensitive than CT in detecting inferior frontal lobe and temporal lobe contusions. The electroencephalogram has not been found to be a sensitive indicator of minor neuronal dysfunction. After a second concussion, a thorough review of the circumstances resulting in the concussion should be analyzed. If available, videotapes or game films should be reviewed by the player, coach, and trainer. It should be determined if the player was using the head unwisely, illegally, or both. This review

will also show if the player was wearing his equipment correctly. Finally, neck strength and development, as well as equipment fit and maintenance, should be checked. A player with three grade 1 concussions in one season should not be allowed to play in the remaining games.[28, 36]

After a first grade 2 concussion, return to competition may be as soon as 1 to 2 weeks after the player is asymptomatic at rest and with exertion. After a second grade 2 concussion in the same season, return should be deferred for at least 1 month, and termination of future participation should be considered. An athlete with a history of three grade 2 concussions in 1 year should not be allowed to play a contact sport for 1 year. CT or MRI abnormalities caused by trauma would also preclude future participation.

After a grade 3 concussion the athlete is held out of competition for at least 1 month, and may then return only if asymptomatic at rest and with exercise. A player with two grade 3 concussions should not be allowed to play football. An athlete who has had intracranial surgery for removal of a clot or has developed posttraumatic hydrocephalus should not be allowed to return to competition.[25] A working scheme for number and severity of concussions and disposition is tabulated in Table 24−1.

Postconcussion Syndrome

This syndrome consists of headache, especially with exertion, dizziness, fatigue, irritability, and, especially, impaired memory and concentration have been reported in football players,[13] but their true incidence is not known. The persistence of these symptoms reflects altered neurotransmitter function,[13] and usually correlates with the duration of posttraumatic amnesia.[12] When these symptoms persist, the athlete should be

TABLE 24–1.

Guidelines for Return to Play After Concussion

	1st Concussion	2nd Concussion	3rd Concussion
Grade 1 (mild)	May return to play if asymptomatic*	Return to play in 2 wk if asymptomatic at that time for 1 wk	Terminate season; may return to play next season if asymptomatic
Grade 2 (moderate)	Return to play after asymptomatic for 1 wk	Minimum of 1 mo; may return to play then if asymptomatic for 1 wk; consider terminating season	Terminate season; may return to play next season if asymptomatic
Grade 3 (severe)	Minimum of 1 mo; may then return to play if asymptomatic for 1 wk	Terminate season; may return to play next season if asymptomatic	

*No headache, dizziness, or impaired orientation, concentration, or memory during rest or exertion.

evaluated with CT and neuropsychiatric tests. Return to competition should be deferred until all symptoms have abated and the diagnostic studies are normal.

Intracranial Hemorrhage

Intracranial hemorrage is the leading cause of death in contact sports. This was shown by Schneider[31] and remains true today.[32] The acute subdural hematoma accounts for most head injury deaths.*

Neurologists and neurosurgeons recognize that with an epidural hematoma there is often a lucid period after an initial period of unconsciousness before the athlete starts to experience increasing headache and progressive rapid deterioration in level of consciousness. Conversely, it is conventionally taught that with an acute subdural hematoma the patient will not regain consciousness and the need for immediate neurosurgical evaluation is obvious. This is not correct. A football player or boxer may regain consciousness after a concussion, walk off the field or out of the ring, only to collapse shortly thereafter from a fatal subdural hematoma and associated brain swelling. This is why all players should

*References 8, 10–12, 19, 22, 23, 25, 26, 28, 30–32, 34–37; see Chapter 18.

be observed closely for at least 24 hours after being rendered unconscious, and should be scanned if headache is severe or persistent, if there is any alteration in state of consciousness, or if abnormal neurologic findings are detected.

Rarely, during exercise or with trauma, intracranial hematoma or subarachnoid hemorrhage, or both may result from the rupture of a congenital vascular lesion such as an aneurysm or arteriovenous malformation. There is almost never a lucid period, and neurologic deterioration to death may be extremely rapid. Because of the intense reaction such a tragic event precipitates among fellow athletes, family, students, and even the community-at-large, and, because of the inevitable rumors that follow, it is imperative to obtain a complete autopsy to determine if the cause of death was other than the presumed and ultimately unavoidable. Only by such full, factual elucidation will inappropriate feeling of guilt in fellow athletes, friends, and family be assuaged.

"Malignant Brain Edema"

This condition is found in the pediatric athlete and consists of a rapid neurologic deterioration from an alert conscious state to coma and sometimes death, minutes to several hours after head trauma.[27, 33] While this sequence in adults almost always is due to an intracranial clot, in children the pathologic studies show diffuse brain swelling with little or no brain injury.[1] Rather than true cerebral edema, Schnitker[33] and Langfitt et al[17, 18] have shown that the diffuse cerebral swelling is the result of a true hyperemia or vascular engorgement. Prompt recognition is extremely important since there is little initial brain injury, and the serious or fatal neurologic outcome is secondary to raised intracranial pressure with herniation. Prompt treatment with intubation, hyperventilation, and osmotic agents has helped to reduce the mortality[4, 5]

Second Impact Syndrome

In adults who are still symptomatic from a prior head injury (e.g., persistent headache or dizziness, or both, impaired orientation, concentration, or memory), a second minor blow to the head may produce fatal brain swelling as seen in the "malignant brain edema" syndrome. As mentioned previously, this condition was first described by Schneider[31] and more recently by Saunders and Harbaugh.[29] It carries a 50% mortality rate even with prompt treatment with intubation, hyperventilation, and intravenous osmotic diuretics. Prevention is the only sure cure. It is thus absolutely essential that after a head injury no athlete with residual cerebral symptoms is knowingly allowed to resume participation. Cerebral conditions that absolutely contraindicate contact sports competition are outlined in Table 24–2.

Seizure Disorder

An athlete with a seizure disorder under good control with anticonvulsant medication may be allowed to participate in contact sports. On the other hand, a seizure resulting from head trauma, sin-

TABLE 24–2.

Cerebral Conditions That Absolutely Contraindicate Contact Sports Competition

1. Persistent postconcussion syndrome
2. Permanent cerebral neurologic impairment from a head injury (e.g., dementia, paresis, anopsia)
3. Spontaneous subarachnoid hemorrhage from any cause

gle or multiple, focal or generalized, requires discontinuation of a contact sport for that season. The athlete should be evaluated with an electroencephalogram and CT or MRI head scan in order to exclude any preexisting cerebral abnormality. If none exists, the CT or MRI examination shows normal findings, and the athlete is asymptomatic with regard to cerebral symptoms, return to competition is allowed after 8 weeks.

Reflections

Several cogent points about athletic head injuries bear repeating. There remains a need for:

1. A continuing aggressive educational effort directed not only to team physicians, athletic trainers, and coaches but also to athletes and their parents. The decrease in mortality rates from head injury during the past decade, especially in American football, has resulted not only from improved coaching and training techniques, equipment modifications, and rules changes, but also from the educational programs for coaches, trainers, and team physicians, particularly on the prevention and early recognition of head injuries.

2. Only by constant data gathering and study (research) will the incidence of head injuries be further reduced. Much urgent work remains in the area of the cumulative effects of repeated head injury, especially the once, but not now, lightly regarded concussion.

3. The guidelines for return to competition expressed in this chapter should

be regarded as minimums. In this highly litigious era it is important to remind ourselves, as well as the lawyers who read medical texts, that the final decision regarding returning to competition after a head injury is always a clinical judgment in every case. Deviation from written texts based on the clinical judgment of the treating physician or trainer may be entirely appropriate.

REFERENCES

1. Adams H, Graham DI: Pathology of blunt head injuries, in Critchley M, O'Leary JL, Jennett B (eds): *Scientific Foundations of Neurology.* Philadelphia, FA Davis Co, 1972, pp 478–491.

2. Albright JP, McAuley E, Martin RK, et al: Head and neck injuries in college football: An eight year analysis. *Am J Sports Med* 1985; 13:147–152.

3. Barber HM: Horse-play: Survey of accidents with horses. *Br Med J* 1973; 3:532–534.

4. Bowers SA, Marchall LF: Outcome in 200 consecutive cases of severe head injury treated in San Diego County: A prospective analysis. *Neurosurgery* 1980; 6:237–242.

5. Bruce DA, Schut L, Bruno LA, et al: Outcome following severe head injuries in children. *J Neurosurg* 1978; 48:679–688.

6. Committee on Head Injury Nomenclature of Congress of Neurological Surgeons. Glossary of head injury including some definitions of injury to the cervical spine. *Clin Neurosurg* 1966; 12:386–394.

7. Fekite JF: Severe brain injury and death following rigid hockey accidents. The effectiveness of the "safety helmets" of amateur hockey players. *Can Med Assoc J* 1968; 99:1234–1239.

8. Gennarelli TA, Segawa H, Wald U, et al: Physiological response to angular acceleration of the head, in Grossman RG, Gildenberg PL (eds): *Head Injury: Basic and Clinical Aspects.* New York, Raven Press, 1982, pp 129–140.

9. Gerberich SC, Priest JD, Boen JR, et al: Concussion incidences and severity in secondary school varsity football players. *Am J Pub Health* 1983; 73:1370–1375.

10. Gronwall D, Wrightson P: Delayed recovery of intellectual function after minor head injury. *Lancet* 1974; 2:605–609.

11. Gronwall D, Wrightson P: Memory and information processing capacity after closed head injury. *J Neurol Neurosurg Psychiatry* 1981; 44:889–895.

12. Guthkelch AN: Posttraumatic amnesia, postconcussional symptoms and accident neurosis. *Eur Neurol* 1980; 19:91–102.

13. Hugen HH, Richard MT: Return to athletic competition following concussion. *Can Med Assoc J* 1982; 127:827–829.

14. Hussey HH: Ice hockey injuries. *JAMA* 1976; 236:187.

15. Jennett B: Late effects of head injuries, in Critchley M, O'Leary JL, Jennett B (eds): *Scientific Foundations of Neurology.* Philadelphia, FA Davis Co, 1971, pp 441–451.

16. Krel FW: Parachuting for sport—study of 100 deaths. *JAMA* 1965; 194:264–268.

17. Langfitt TW, Tannenbaum HM, Kassell NF: The etiology of acute brain swelling following experimental head injury. *J Neurosurg* 1966; 24:47–56.

18. Langfitt TW, Kassell NF: Cerebral vasodilatations produced by brainstem stimulation: Neurogenic control vs. autoregulation. *Am J Physiol* 1978; 215:90–97.

19. Lindsay KW, McLatchie G, Jennett B: Serious head injuries in sports. *Br Med J* 1980; 281:789–791.

20. Maroon JC, Steele PB, Berlin R: Football head and neck injuries: An update. *Clin Neurosurg* 1980; 27:414–429.

21. Martland HS: Punch drunk. *JAMA* 1928; 91:1103–1107.

22. McLatchie GR, Davies JE, Caulley JH: Injuries in karate, a case for medical control. *J Trauma* 1980; 2:956–958.

23. Meggyesy D: *Out of Their League.* Berkeley, Calif, Ramparts, 1970, p 125.

24. Mueller FO, Schindler RD: *Annual Survey of Football Injury Research* 1931–1986. American Football Coaches Association, NCAA, and National Federation of State High School Associations, 1987.

25. Murphey F, Simmons JC: Initial management of athletic injuries to the head and neck. *Am J Surg* 1959; 98:379–383.

26. Peerless SJ, Rewcastle NB: Shear injuries of the brain. *Can Med Assoc J* 1967; 96:577–582.

27. Pickles W: Acute general edema of the brain in children with head injuries. *N Engl J Med* 1950; 242:607–611.

28. Quigley TB: Personal communication to RC Schneider, in Schneider RC: *Head and Neck Injuries in Football*. Baltimore, Williams & Wilkins, 1973, p 165.

29. Saunders RL, Harbaugh RE: The second impact in catastrophic contact sports head trauma. *JAMA* 1984; 252:538–539.

30. Schneider RC, Charie G, Pantek H: The syndrome of acute central cervical spinal cord injury. *J Neurosurg* 1954; 11:546–577.

31. Schneider RC: *Head and Neck Injuries in Football*. Baltimore, Williams & Wilkins, 1973.

32. Schneider RC, Kennedy JC, Plant ML: *Sports Injuries*. Baltimore, Williams & Wilkins, 1985.

33. Schnitker MT: A syndrome of cerebral concussion in children. *J Pediatr* 1949; 35:557–560.

34. Strick SJ: Shearing of nerve fibers as a cause of brain damage due to head injury. *Lancet* 1961; 2:443–448.

35. Symonds C: Concussion and its sequelae. *Lancet* 1962; 1:1–5.

36. Thorndike A: Serious recurrent injuries of athletes. Contraindications to further competitive participation. *N Engl J Med* 1952; 247:554–556.

37. Yarnell PR, Lynch S: The "ding" amnestic states in football trauma. *Neurology* 1973; 23:196–197.

PART THREE

Brachial Plexus Injuries

CHAPTER 25

Anatomy of the Innervation of the Upper Extremity

Carson D. Schneck, M.D., Ph.D.

THE PLEXUS CONCEPT

The typical spinal nerve, formed by the union of dorsal and ventral roots, divides outside the intervertebral foramen into a dorsal and a ventral ramus.

In general, the dorsal rami of spinal nerves supply the skin of the medial two thirds of the back from the top of the head to the coccyx, the deep (intrinsic) muscles of the back, and the zygapophyseal vertebral joints. Each dorsal ramus supplies the strip of skin and muscle and the zygapophyseal joint located at the level of its origin.

The ventral rami of spinal nerves supply the rest of the spinally innervated muscles and the skin and joints of the neck, trunk, and extremities. The ventral rami, except those from T2 to T11, form plexuses, that is, they join with higher or lower ventral rami to form networks from which peripheral nerves may arise that contain nerve fibers derived from more than one spinal cord segment. This is in contrast to the dorsal rami, which generally do not form plexuses, and are therefore themselves unisegmental peripheral nerves.

GENERAL MAKEUP OF THE BRACHIAL PLEXUS

The brachial plexus is usually formed from the ventral rami of spinal nerves C5 to T1 (Fig 25–1). The ventral rami of C5 and C6 fuse to form the superior trunk, while the ventral ramus of C7 continues on as the middle trunk, and the ventral rami of C8 and T1 form the inferior trunk. Each trunk separates into an anterior and a posterior division. The anterior divisions of the superior and middle trunks join to become the lateral cord, while the anterior division of the inferior trunk becomes the medial cord. The posterior divisions of all three trunks unite to form the posterior cord. The cords are named according to their relation to the axillary artery. The cords end by dividing into five terminal nerves. The lateral cord gives off the lateral root of the median nerve and then continues as the musculocutaneous nerve. The medial cord gives off the medial root of the median nerve and then continues as the ulnar nerve. The posterior cord terminates by dividing into the axillary and radial nerves. Other nerves arise from the plexus at the levels

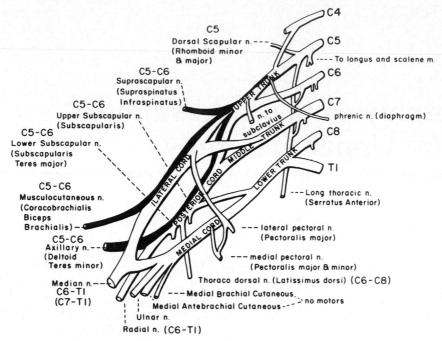

FIG 25–1.
Brachial plexus.

of the ventral rami, trunks, and cords, and the most important of these nerves are indicated in Fig 25–1.

APPLIED ASPECTS OF THE INNERVATION OF THE UPPER EXTREMITY

In considering the innervation of the upper extremity one should think of three general levels of nerve lesions and the resulting motor and sensory deficits.

Injuries may occur distal to the plexus and involve one or more peripheral nerves somewhere along their course. Depending on the level of injury, a complete or partial deficit occurs in the distribution of that peripheral nerve. To identify this type of involvement one must appreciate the general distribution of the peripheral nerves derived from the brachial plexus.

Note that the anterior divisions of the trunks formed the lateral and medial cords, which in turn gave rise to the musculocutaneous, median, and ulnar nerves. These terminal nerves innervate all of the anterior (flexor) muscles of the arm, forearm, and hand.

The musculocutaneous nerve innervates the muscles of the anterior or flexor compartment of the arm (major elbow flexor muscles and major supinator muscles of the forearm) and the skin of the lateral aspect of the forearm.

The median nerve innervates all the muscles of the forearm (major wrist and finger flexor muscles and forearm pronator muscles) with the exception of the musculus flexor carpi ulnaris and the ulnar half of the flexor digitorum profundus. It also innervates the radial two lumbrical muscles, all the intrinsic muscles of the thumb (thumb opposition) except the adductor pollicis, and the skin on the thumb side of the palm of the hand and the palmar aspect of the radial 3½ digits, as well as the dorsal surfaces of their terminal phalanges.

The ulnar nerve innervates the flexor carpi ulnaris, the ulnar half of the flexor digitorum profundus, all the intrinsic muscles of the little finger, the ulnar two lumbrical muscles, the adductor pollicis, and all the interossei muscles (major abductor and adductor muscles of the fingers). It also innervates the skin on the ulnar side of the palm, the dorsum of the hand, and the palmar and dorsal aspects of the ulnar 1½ digits.

The radial nerve, which is the major continuation of the posterior cord, supplies all the posterior or extensor muscles of the arm and forearm and the skin of the posterior aspect of the arm, forearm, and lateral two thirds of the hand distally to about the distal interphalangeal joints.

The axillary nerve supplies the deltoid muscle (major shoulder abduction and hyperextension muscles), the teres minor, and the skin over the insertion of the deltoid muscle.

The pectoral nerves innervate pectoralis major, and the medial pectoral also supplies musculus pectoralis minor.

The medial brachial and antebrachial cutaneous nerves supply their indicated skin areas.

The upper subscapular nerve supplies the upper part of the subscapularis muscle. The lower subscapular nerve supplies the lower part of subscapularis muscle and teres major. The thoracodorsal nerve innervates latissimus dorsi; the suprascapular nerve, musculus supraspinatus and infraspinatus; the dorsal scapular nerve, the rhomboid muscles (and levator scapulae); and the long thoracic nerve, serratus anterior.

Lesions may occur proximal to the plexus either at the spinal cord, root, or spinal nerve and cause sensory and motor deficits on a segmental basis. The cutaneous area innervated by one spinal cord segment is called a dermatome.

Since there is considerable overlap between adjacent dermatomes, a given dermatomal loss may be difficult to identify unless adjacent spinal cord segments are also involved. The general dermatomal distribution in the upper extremity is as follows:

C4	Shoulder pad area
C5	Lateral aspect of arm
C6	Lateral aspect of forearm, hand, and radial two digits
C7	Middle finger
C8	Ulnar two digits and medial aspect of hand and wrist
T1	Medial aspect of forearm
T2	Medial aspect of arm

The segmental motor innervation in the upper extremity is the following:

C5, C6	Deltoid and other intrinsic muscles of shoulder (abduction, hyperextension, and external rotation at shoulder)
C5, C6	Biceps, brachialis, and supinator (elbow flexion and supination of forearm)
C6, C7	Pronators of forearm
C7 (C6, C8)	Triceps and extensors of wrist and of fingers at metacarpophalangeal joints
C8, T1	Intrinsic muscles of hand

The segmental levels of deep reflexes are as follows:

Biceps	C5 (C6)
Triceps	C7 (C6)
Radial jerk (supinator reflex)	C5 (C6, C7)
Ulnar jerk (pronator reflex)	C6 (C7, C8)

Lesions may also involve the plexus itself. For example, the upper plexus may be injured in forcible separation of the head and shoulders during collision; the lower part of the plexus may be injured in forcible abduction of the arm; or mixed types of plexus injuries may follow any type of traction trauma to the extremity. Depending on whether rami, trunks, or cords are injured, these types of injuries cause various segmental deficits.

The ventral rami and trunks of the plexus, as well as the subclavian artery, emerge from the narrow triangular interval between the anterior and middle scalene muscles and the clavicle below. At this point the plexus and the artery may be encroached upon by a number of lesions, such as a cervical rib or an anterior scalene muscle spasm, that narrow this interval. These lesions may cause a neurocirculatory compression (anterior scalene) syndrome with peripheral paresthesia, hypoesthesia, weakness, and vascular insufficiency. To test for this syndrome, the head is turned to the side of the symptoms and extended, and a deep inspiration is taken (Adson's test). This narrows the interval, stretches the neurovascular structures, reproduces the symptoms, and obliterates the radial pulse.

MAJOR EXTRINSIC MUSCLES OF THE SHOULDER

The major extrinsic muscles of the shoulder are the muscles that arise from the axial skeleton and insert on the shoulder girdle or humerus.

The latissimus dorsi is innervated by the thoracodorsal nerve (C6, C7, C8). This muscle extends from the region of the lower portion of the back to the front of the upper end of the humerus. It participates in extension, adduction, and internal rotation at the shoulder, and its downward pull resists upward displacement of the humerus and scapula as in crutch walking. It may also act to pull the trunk upward as in climbing. Its function can be checked by performing its movements against resistance and palpating its contraction over the lower part of the back or in the posterior axillary fold.

The rhomboid muscles (dorsal scapular nerve, C5) are primarily adductor muscles of the scapula.

The course of the serratus anterior (long thoracic nerve, C5, C6, C7) over the apex of the lung exposes it to involvement by apical lung disease. Then its course along the medial axillary wall exposes it to trauma in axillary surgery. This muscle is an abductor and upward rotator of the scapula, and it keeps the vertebral border of the scapula closely applied to the thoracic wall. Paralysis causes winging of the scapula, which can be accentuated by pushing with the arms against a wall.

The pectoralis major (medial and lateral pectoral nerves, C5–T1) is the principal adductor muscle of the arm and also flexes and internally rotates the arm. It draws the chest upward as in climbing, and prevents upward displacement of the humerus and the scapula as in crutch walking.

INTRINSIC MUSCLES OF THE SHOULDER

The intrinsic muscles arise from the shoulder girdle and insert on the humerus. They are all innervated by C5, C6 cord segments.

The axillary nerve (C5, C6) winds around the surgical neck of the humerus and thus may be traumatized in shoulder dislocations or fractures of the surgical neck. The deltoid muscle's primary function is abduction of the arm, but its posterior part is also an important hyperextensor, and its various parts may participate in all movements of the arm. In paralysis, the normal shoulder contour may be flattened and normal abduction and hyperextension are considerably weakened.

The teres minor (axillary nerve) is primarily an external rotator and functions as part of the rotator cuff mechanism.

The supraspinatus (suprascapular nerve, C5, C6) abducts and participates in rotator cuff functions. Its function is more commonly impaired by tendinitis and tendon rupture than by denervation.

The infraspinatus (suprascapular nerve) is the primary external rotator muscle and functions as part of the rotator cuff.

The subscapularis (upper and lower subscapular nerves, C5, C6) is an internal rotator and a cuff muscle.

Like the latissimus dorsi, with which this muscle helps to form the posterior axillary fold, the teres major (lower subscapular nerve) is an internal rotator, extensor, and adductor muscle of the arm.

A C5–C6 lesion of the plexus or spinal cord causes loss of abduction and all external rotation, so that the arm is held in adduction and internal rotation.

CHAPTER 26

Injuries to the Brachial Plexus

Elliott B. Hershman, M.D.

ANATOMY

The anatomy of the brachial plexus has been discussed in Chapter 25. A few pertinent aspects should be well understood in order to diagnose and treat plexus injuries accurately, however. Cervical roots 5, 6, 7 and 8 and thoracic root 1 contribute to the brachial plexus (Fig 26–1). The ventral rami of these roots, formed from a dorsal (sensory) and ventral (motor) root, join together to form the plexus. At each level a dorsal or posterior ramus also exists and supplies innervation to the skin and muscles of the posterior aspect of the neck.

The cords, roots, and rami must be understood to allow one to state the preganglionic or postganglionic site of injury. The sensory and motor axons have ganglia that contain the cell bodies for the nerves. An important fact to bear in mind is that the sensory ganglia are *outside* of the spinal canal, usually within or near an intervertebral foramen. These sensory or dorsal root ganglia remain attached to their distal axons, with lesions occurring proximal to the ganglion (so-called preganglionic lesions). The motor ganglia are the anterior horn cells and are within the spinal cord. If a root is avulsed from the cord, the motor component will undergo wallerian degeneration, but the sensory neurons will remain in continuity with the afferent nerve. Sensation is, of course, lost because the connection between the dorsal root ganglion and the cord is disrupted. This is a preganglionic lesion. If the lesion occurs distal to the dorsal root ganglion, the lesion is considered to be postganglionic, affecting both motor and sensory axons beyond their ganglion. Clinically, preganglionic, root avulsion type injuries are untreatable and have a hopeless outlook, while postganglionic lesions can have spontaneous recovery depending on the grade of the lesion.[67]

The ventral or anterior rami lie between the anterior and middle scalene muscles, where they run adjacent to the subclavian artery. The plexus continues distally, passing over the first rib. It is deep to sternocleidomastoid muscle in the posterior triangle of the neck.[89]

Just above the clavicle, the five ventral rami unite to form three trunks. The upper trunk is composed of roots C5 and C6. The middle trunk is a continuation of C7. The lower trunk consists of the C8 and T1 roots. After passing below the clavicle, each trunk divides into an anterior and a posterior division. Each of these divisions contributes to the formation of three cords.

The three posterior divisions combine to form the posterior cord. The posterior cord thus has contributions from all five original roots (C5, C6, C7, C8, T1). The anterior divisions of the upper and middle trunks form the lateral cord (C5,

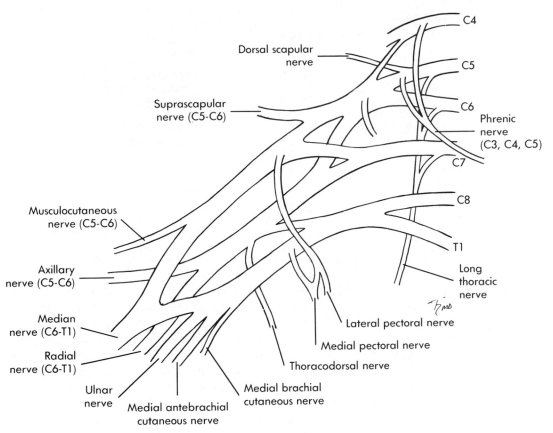

FIG 26—1.
Anatomy of the brachial plexus. *(From Pianka G, Hershman E: Neurovascular injuries, in Nicholas JA, Hershman EB:* Upper Extremity Injuries in Sports Medicine. *St Louis, Mosby—Year Book, 1990.)*

C6, C7 contributions). The medial cord is the continuation of the anterior division of the lower trunk and has contributions from C8 and T1. The cords, medial, lateral, and posterior, are named for the position in relaxation to the axillary artery. The artery and nerves course behind the pectoralis minor muscle in the axillary sheath.

The three cords divide to create five terminal branches that innervate the upper extremity. Other branches emanate from the cords, trunks, and roots and supply neural control to the shoulder and scapular muscles. These branches are outlined in Table 26—1.

The radial nerve is the terminal branch of the posterior cord, middle trunk, and C7 ventral ramus. It receives,

in addition, contributions from the upper and lower trunks. The posterior cord sends out a major branch, the axillary nerve, before it becomes the radial nerve. Other branches from the posterior cord are the thoracodorsal nerve and the upper and lower subscapular nerves.

The ulnar nerve is the terminal branch of the medial cord and lower trunk, arising from the C8 and T1 ventral rami. The medial pectoral nerve, the medial brachial cutaneous, and the medial antebrachial cutaneous nerves are also terminal branches of the medial cord.

The median nerve is created by parts of the continuing segments of the medial and lateral cords. The lateral cord, which arose from the upper and middle trunks, contributes mainly sensory fibers from

TABLE 26–1.

Major Branches of the Brachial Plexus

Peripheral Nerve	Root Composition	Origin
Long thoracic	C5, C6, C7	Cervical root
Dorsal scapular	C5	Cervical root
Suprascapular	C5, C6	Upper trunk
Upper subscapular	C5	Posterior cord
Lower subscapular	C5, C6	Posterior cord
Thoracodorsal	C7, C8	Posterior cord
Lateral pectoral	C5, C6, C7	Lateral cord
Medial pectoral	C8, T1	Medial cord
Medial brachial cutaneous	C8, T1	Medial cord
Medial brachial cutaneous	C8, T1	Medial cord
Axillary	C5, C6	Posterior cord
Radial	C6, C7, C8	Posterior cord
Median	C5, C6, C7, C8, T1	Medial and lateral cords
Musculocutaneous	C5, C6	Lateral cord

the ventral rami of C5, C6, and C7. These fibers join with the primarily motor contribution to form the medial cord, consisting of C8 and T1 fibers.

The suprascapular nerve is the branch arising from the upper trunk, consisting of the C5 and C6 ventral rami. The C5 ventral ramus sends contributions to the phrenic nerve and also has another branch, the dorsal scapular nerve. The long thoracic nerve is formed from contributions of the ventral rami of C5, C6, and C7 nerve roots.

HISTORY

At initial presentation a complete medical history should be obtained from the athlete who has a brachial plexus problem. The exact mechanism of injury and the position of the head, neck, shoulder, and extremity should be elicited if possible. Often, however, athletes cannot recall the exact details of the inciting event. Particular attention should be paid to obtaining the exact distribution and timing of symptoms. Whole arm burning lasting a few seconds after a hard tackle is a different problem than tingling in the thumb and lateral aspect of the forearm that occurs during a golf swing follow-

through and that can at times also be noted to be present at night. The first situation may represent upper trunk stretch neurapraxia or "burner," while the latter may signify a herniated cervical root with C6 radiculopathy. The general health of the athlete should also be noted. Metastatic tumors can involve the lymphatics about the brachial plexus, as can primary lymphoma. Both these situations will lead to signs of plexus compression. A viral illness may precede the onset of acute brachial neuropathy. A review of the athlete's equipment may also be appropriate in these situations. Ill-fitting pads with straps that compress the neural elements can contribute to compression or traction lesions. Complete resolution of symptoms will not occur unless equipment modification is included in the therapeutic program.

PHYSICAL EXAMINATION

The physical examination plays a crucial role in the identification of brachial plexus problems. Localization and classification of lesions can be accomplished by thorough and repeated clinical evaluation.

The athlete should be observed with

the neck, both shoulder girdles, and upper extremities disrobed. In this manner, subtle areas of atrophy or deformity can be observed. Any skeletal deformity should be documented. The scapula position at rest and during a push-up against a wall should be noted: movement of the scapula away from the thorax during the push-up is indicative of scapula winging resulting from weakness in the serratus anterior or occasionally the trapezius muscle. Abnormal appearance in the clavicle should also be documented. The clavicle should be palpated for acute fracture or exuberant callus formation. The supraclavicular fossa and axilla also should be palpated for masses or swelling. A Tinel's sign should be sought in the supraclavicular fossa.[29, 68]

The active and passive range of motion of the neck, shoulders, elbows, wrists, and hands should be measured. Contracture must be identified to assist in rehabilitation prescription. Stability of the shoulder joint should also be ascertained because chronic instability can contribute to plexus pathology.

The motor examination is one of the most important components of the neurologic examination. A complete and accurate motor evaluation can often define the site of the lesion. It is important to differentiate between root lesions, supraclavicular injury, infraclavicular pathology, diffuse plexus involvement, and peripheral nerve problems.[112] This can often be done on the basis of a complete motor evaluation.

In athletes, strength measurement should be performed by standard manual muscle testing. In particularly strong athletes, however, manual muscle testing may be difficult because of the tremendous strength of many athletes. Occasionally the examiner cannot overcome an athlete's strength in an injured extremity because of the great strength of the athlete. In this setting, quantifiable strength measurement may be of value. This can

be accomplished with dynamometers (such as Cybex isokinetic equipment) or by using hand-held measuring devices such as the Nicholas manual muscle tester (MMT). The types of muscle contractions performed during each testing procedure should be borne in mind. Manual muscle testing and the Nicholas MMT device (NISMAT, Nicholas Institute for Sports Medicine and Athletic Trauma, New York) measure eccentric strength, whereas isokinetic devices like the Cybex are determining concentric strength. Strength testing does, of course, have limitations, and these must be recognized at all times. Pain and the test subject effort will greatly affect results, and these factors should be noted and documented at the time of evaluation.

Weakness of the shoulder girdle may also be directly related to rotator cuff pathology rather than to intrinsic neural injury. The integrity of the rotator cuff should be evaluated by appropriate techniques such as arthrography or magnetic resonance imaging (MRI) if external rotation or abduction weakness is present.

The reflexes of the upper extremities should be elicited. They should be judged in terms of their quality, not simply whether present or absent, in order to evaluate for subtle abnormalities.

Sensory evaluation is an important aspect of the physical examination as well. Differentiation between preganglionic and postganglionic lesions can be made with adjunctive testing because of the extraspinal location of the sensory ganglia.

The presence of a Horner's syndrome should be noted by examination of the face. This would indicate a preganglionic lesion of T1.

Vascular evaluation, including both venous and arterial function, must also be performed. The close proximity of the elements of the brachial plexus to the axillary vessels makes combined injuries possible, particularly with penetrating trauma.

ADJUNCTIVE TESTING

Radiography/Imaging

Radiographs of the neck and, if clinically indicated, the shoulder girdle should be obtained on all athletes with trauma to the brachial plexus. Cervical spine injuries are often associated with root injury, and upper extremity neurologic findings may represent the clinical presentation of cervical spine trauma. Avulsion of a cervical transverse process or significant cervical scoliosis is frequently seen in severe plexus injuries. The presence of a cervical rib should be noted, as these can contribute to plexus compression and thoracic outlet syndrome.[93] The appearance of the first rib should be assessed, since the lower portion of the plexus is associated with it. Shoulder radiographs would be important in athletes with a history of previous trauma involving the shoulder girdle. Specific traumatic injuries to be ruled out would include fracture of the clavicle, scapula, or proximal humerus, glenohumeral dislocation, or acromioclavicular separation. Particularly severe trauma might include first rib fracture or lateral dislocation of the scapula (scapulothoracic dislocation).

These films would also be indicated if pain, localized tenderness, or swelling is apparent in the shoulder region at the time of evaluation. On rare occasions, a chest radiograph, apical lordotic film, or computed tomography (CT) scan will be required if a superior sulcus or Pancoast tumor is suspected.[74]

If plain radiographs of the cervical spine show negative findings and a preganglionic cervical root lesion is suspected, MRI, plain myelography, or CT-myelography can be valuable in identifying the site of injury. Disk herniation, foraminal narrowing, and extradural intraspinal masses can all create root compression, with concomitant neurologic findings. Root avulsion can be identified on a cervical myelogram by the presence of traumatic meningocele or pseudomeningocele.[126] CT myelography has proved particularly useful in evaluating avulsion at the C5 and C6 levels. This would be an important finding since the prognosis for root avulsion is poor. MRI can also be useful in examining the plexus to rule out mass lesions (Fig 26-2).

Electrodiagnostic Evaluation

Electrodiagnostic studies are often indicated in the evaluation of brachial plexus injury.[28, 47, 64, 108, 113] A complete electromyographic (EMG) examination, including both nerve conduction studies and a needle electrode examination, should be obtained. It is important to have the examiner sample muscles in the contralateral extremity during needle electrode examination, since subclinical but EMG-positive involvement is frequently found in the "normal" extremity in acute brachial neuropathy.[121] Electromyography should always be delayed for 3 to 4 weeks from the time of the initial injury to allow wallerian degeneration to occur, or nondegenerative lesions to recover spontaneously. Nerve conduction studies should include both routine nerve conduction tests and sensory nerve action potential (SNAP) evaluation. Special studies such as H-responses, F-waves, and repetitive stimulation studies are not of value in evaluating sports injuries.[122] Electrode evaluation of the cervical spine musculature also must be performed to differentiate between preganglionic or root injuries and plexus pathology. The absence of fibrillation potentials in the cervical paraspinal muscles never excludes a root-level lesion, however.[122]

A number of problems are encoun-

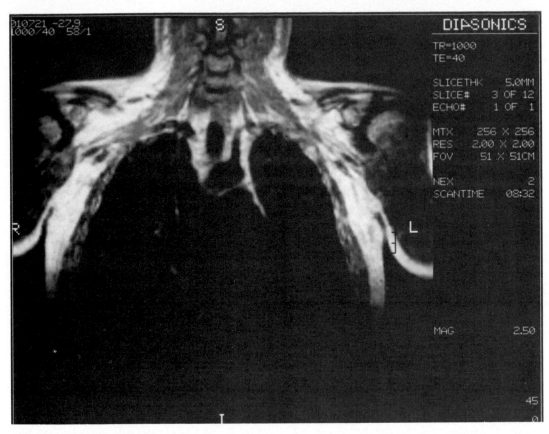

FIG 26–2.
MRI can be used to evaluate the brachial plexus for the presence of a mass lesion.

tered when assessing the shoulder girdle with electrophysiologic testing.[122] Routine nerve conduction studies do not adequately evaluate the upper trunk or the peripheral nerves derived from it. Therefore, "unusual" sensory nerve conduction studies (such as median sensory, recording thumb, and lateral antebrachial cutaneous) must be performed. The needle electrode examination is also more difficult and frequently less helpful for a number of reasons, as Wilbourn et al.[122] have pointed out:

1. Some muscles (e.g., serratus anterior) are often difficult if not impossible to evaluate in heavily muscled men because of the overlying muscle mass and the resultant problem in being certain of needle placement.

2. Many of the muscles innervated by the upper trunk of the brachial plexus are grouped about the shoulder, frequently overlie one another, and are often activated by the same patient movement. Hence it becomes very difficult to be certain of the particular muscle being assessed, a problem that is much less troublesome when evaluating forearm and hand muscles.

3. A proximal upper extremity muscle that has been partially denervated by an axon loss lesion can become reinnervated fairly rapidly because of the short length of nerve over which regeneration must advance; consequently, EMG examinations performed just a few months after injury often are misleading because, depending on the distance of their motor points from the site of nerve in-

jury, some muscles may have reinnervated completely, whereas others may still be partially denervated. As a result, what was actually an upper trunk brachial plexopathy may be mistaken for a proximal mononeuropathy.

AXON RESPONSES

An often described, but seldom clinically used, test involves the skin reaction to histamine injection.[15, 68] Normally, after injections of 1% histamine into the skin, a triple response occurs: vasodilation, wheal formation, and flare (vasodilation). This reaction occurs in normal skin and in anesthetic areas caused by root avulsion. The phenomenon is present because the cell body in the sensory root ganglion (outside the spinal canal) is intact and attached to the distal nerve in both those instances. However, in a postganglionic lesion, that is, a lesion distal to the distal root (sensory) ganglion, the distal nerve undergoes wallerian degeneration and the flare response is absent. Hence a normal triple response would imply a poor prognosis, indicating a preganglionic lesion, while an absent flare response would indicate a postganglionic lesion, with better prognosis.

The histamine response test has been supplanted by electrodiagnostic testing with sensory nerve action potentials (SNAPs). If the lesion in question is preganglionic, the SNAP will be normal to a region that is actually anesthetic, since the dorsal root ganglion and distal affluent axon are intact. This would imply a poor prognosis—high probability of a root avulsion. If the SNAP is abnormal to an anesthetic area, the lesion is postganglionic and recovery may be possible.

CLASSIFICATION

Brachial plexus injuries can be classified by the nerve injury staging system described by Seddon.[105, 106] This classification was designed to correlate histologic findings, clinical findings, and prognostic indications. Many nerve injuries in clinical practice are found to be mixed lesions with varying damage to different nerve fiber populations.[30] This is because of variations in susceptibility to nerve injury based on fiber size and intrafascicular topographic and anatomic position at the time of injury.[71] The classification is, however, still quite useful to permit general analysis of the extent of injury. Recovery from a mixed nerve lesion is characteristically biphasic in that it can be rapid at first, reach a plateau (recovery of neurapraxic fibers), and then be slow thereafter, as axons that have undergone wallerian degeneration slowly regenerate.[114]

Neurapraxia is the mildest lesion and corresponds to demyelination of the axon sheath without intrinsic axonal disruption.[48] This leads to a conduction block at the site of injury. Repair generally proceeds quickly, and function returns as remyelination is completed. This usually occurs within 3 weeks from the time of injury.

The next level of nerve injury is axonotmesis. In this situation there is axon loss, that is, injury severe enough to cause obvious disruption of the axon and myelin sheath. The epineurium, however, is intact. After injury, wallerian degeneration occurs from the point of injury distally. The entire distal axon will degenerate, and complete regeneration must occur for function to return. Because of the integrity of the neurotubes, regeneration can occur. This injury is associated with an abnormal needle electrode examination (fibrillations and positive waves) 2 to 3 weeks after injury in the muscles innervated by the damaged nerves. Recovery is dependent on the quality of axonal regeneration and reestablishment of contact with the denervated muscles or sensory receptors. Since the growing axons are guided by their original tubes, the prognosis is good with respect to regeneration to correct targets. Often motor units are reiterated by "sprouting" of the proximal, intact nerve, and the resultant needle electrode examination shows large (increased duration/amplitude) motor unit potentials.

The most severe injury is neurotmesis. This corresponds to a nerve laceration or an injury to the nerve by crushing or stretching, such that the endoneurium, perineurium, and epineurium are all disrupted. The nerve and its fibrous sheath are completely interrupted, and axonal regeneration is frequently impossible because of the extent of injury and discontinuity of the nerve. If the perineurium remains intact, the healing response at the site of injury is highly disorganized and characterized by extensive scar formation. The differentiation between axonotmesis and neurotmesis is important, because in the former recovery is possible, but in the latter recovery is highly unlikely. Electrophysiologic testing in this injury will show acute and subsequently chronic enervation patterns. Authors such as Leffert find it useful to classify injuries to the brachial plexus into supraclavicular and infraclavicular components.[69] This can be helpful in determining prognosis. The supraclavicular portion of the plexus includes the region from the intradural spinal roots to the divisions; the infraclavicular portion encompasses the cords and terminal branches (peripheral nerves).

INJURY PATTERNS

Brachial plexus injuries are statistically infrequent in sports with the exception of American football. Hirasawa and Sakakida[56] reviewed their 18-year experience with peripheral nerve injuries and found that 66 of a total of 1,167 injuries (5.7%) were related to sports.[56] They also reported that Takazawa et al.[109] found only 28 cases of peripheral nerve injury among 9,550 cases of sports injuries treated over a 95-year period at the clinic of the Japanese Athletic Association. In Hirasawa and Sakakida's[56] patients the most frequently involved site was the brachial plexus (16/66). The overwhelming majority of these patients were injured with heavy backpacks while mountain climbing. North American style football injuries were not described, so the epidemiologic picture, as it pertains to American athletes, may be misleading.

This is confirmed by noting that Clancy et al.[25, 26] reported that 33 of 67 college football athletes sustained at least one significant episode of the "burner" syndrome during their playing career. The frequency of this problem in football makes the "burner" syndrome the most common neural injury sustained by these athletes.

A number of reports in the literature have dealt with mononeuropathies of single peripheral nerve injuries occurring in sports. Authors frequently collect two or three cases and then summarize their findings in a case report. Large series of patients with a single lesion are generally not available. The more common mononeuropathies include injury to the axillary, suprascapular, and long thoracic nerves. Less commonly, musculocutaneous and spinal accessory (although not truly a peripheral nerve) injuries have been discussed with relation to athletic injury.

THE "BURNER" SYNDROME

The "burner" syndrome receives its name from the characteristic symptoms described by the affected athlete. These symptoms are also described as stingers or a pinched nerve by those affected. The injury commences with contact between the shoulder of the affected individual and another object, such as an opposing player, a wall, or a mat. The most common event creating this mechanism is tackling in football. Thus the incidence of the "burner" syndrome is highest in defensive football players such as linebackers and defensive backs. The shoulder is driven downward (caudal) and the neck may be flexed to the contralateral side. The mechanism, driving the shoulder downward from direct contact, is similar to that of an acromioclavicular separation. Concomitant acromioclavicular joint sprain and "burner" syndrome are rare, however. Bergfeld et al.[10] have postulated that this is because of the difference in the point of contact during the injury—over the acromion in acromi-

oclavicular injuries and over the clavicle in "burner" syndrome injuries (Fig 26–3).

The athlete immediately feels a sharp, burning pain radiating from the supraclavicular area down the arm.[98] The pain is associated with paresthesias and anesthesias. The distribution of pain and sensory disfunction is circumferential and does not correspond to any dermatome. Often the athlete will try to shake the arm to "get the feeling back." If severe, the athlete will come off the playing field holding the arm supported by the contralateral arm (Fig 26–4). The burning pain, paresthesias, and anesthesias frequently resolve in minutes. Often a complete motor examination of the upper extremities will reveal normal findings in the period immediately after the injury. Weakness, when it develops, be-

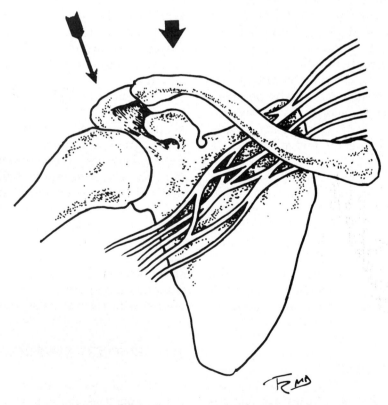

FIG 26–3.
Point of contact in "burner" syndrome is usually over the shoulder girdle *(arrowhead)*, while the area of contact during an acromioclavicular injury is on the point of the acromion *(arrow)*.

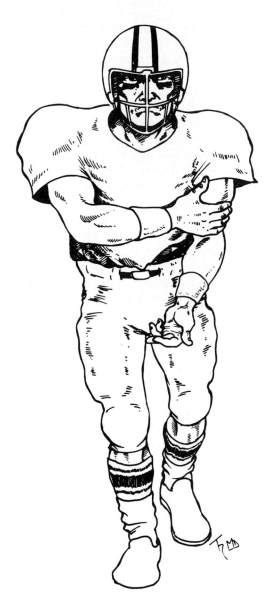

FIG 26–4.
Typical appearance of an athlete who just sustained a "burner."

comes apparent in the hours to days after the initial injury; hence diligent, repeated neurologic examination is mandatory after the traumatic event.

The first discussion of these injuries in the literature was by Chrisman et al in 1965.[24] They analyzed 22 cases (17 football, 2 basketball, 1 wrestling, 1 pit fall in track, and 1 squash wall collision). In half the cases the mechanism of injury

could not be determined, while in the remainder the injury occurred when force was applied to the shoulder and the neck flexed laterally away from the contact point. Because of the mechanism of injury the term *cervical nerve pinch syndrome* was applied to these injuries.

Clancy et al.[25] reported their experience with this clinical syndrome and added electrophysiologic testing to their evaluations. They concluded that the upper trunk of the brachial plexus was the site of the lesion. This was based on an absence of EMG abnormalities in the rhomboid and serratus anterior muscles and involvement of multiple terminal branches of both C5 and C6. A later study confirmed these EMG findings in acute injuries.[97] Other authors have studied athletes with similar clinical problems and concluded that the injury was more likely to be at the root rather than at the plexus level.[73, 90] The conclusions were often based on the presence of muscular fibrillation potentials in the cervical spine.

The brachial plexus is tethered proximally by the attachment of the roots to the spinal cord, the investing cervical fascia, and the surrounding osseous and muscular structures.[89] Traction occurs to the plexus when the shoulder is depressed and the distance between the shoulder and the neck is increased.[6] The force of distraction exerted between the neck and the shoulder is the cause of the traction injury that initiates the "burner" syndrome.

Stevens,[103] in a mechanical analysis, theorized on the ways in which forces applied to the plexus would be distributed among the components. He believed that a weight falling on the shoulder from above would create tension forces in the upper roots. Barnes,[8] in a clinical study, concurred with this concept, stating that with the upper limb by the side, when the shoulder is forcibly depressed, the greatest stress is on the upper roots, and it is impossible to put the lower roots under tension.

The "burner" syndrome is therefore a traction injury to the brachial plexus. The point of plexus injury in the "burner" syndrome is most commonly the upper trunk. There is, however, great variability in the degree of injury and the location of damage. Root involvement, partial or exclusive, can occur with this mechanism of injury. In fact, root avulsion injuries occur with similar traction forces but most likely greater degree of force. Factors that will enter into the degree and location of injury include the force applied to the neck and the position of the upper extremity in relation to the shoulder girdle. Prominent neck symptoms, such as pain and muscle spasm, will be associated with root injury. In addition, the EMG in the presence of root injury will be abnormal in the posterior cervical musculature, although results are variable in this regard.[21, 32] Prominent neck symptoms should also alert the treating individual to assure that neck pathology, such as cervical disk herniation or fracture, is not present.[1, 2, 5] Initial examination of a pure upper trunk lesion would reveal no neck symptoms, and EMG activity in the posterior cervical musculature and clinical and EMG findings in the rhomboid (C5 branch) and serratus anterior muscles (C5, C6, C7 branches) would be normal.

Brachial plexus "burner" injuries were classified by Clancy[26] according to the criteria developed by Seddon. Grade I corresponds to Seddon's definition of neurapraxia—transient loss of motor and sensory deficits without axonal injury. The important point of this group is that complete recovery occurs within 2 weeks by Clancy's criteria. A grade II injury produces significant motor deficits and perhaps some sensory deficits lasting at least 2 weeks. At 3 to 4 weeks after injury, EMG would demonstrate some axonal injury. This level correlates with Seddon's definition of axonotmesis. Clancy's grade III injury produces motor and sensory deficits of at least 1 year's duration, with no appreciable clinical improvement during this period. EMG at that time would show persistent denervation. This corresponds to Seddon's definition of neurotmesis. The "burner" injury is frequently a mild but variable injury to the plexus, with different levels of injury affecting the various areas; thus a clinical classification such as Clancy's can be useful in guiding management.

Although Clancy studied the early EMG changes after these injuries, late findings were not reported until a follow-up EMG and clinical analysis were performed on 20 athletes with "burner" syndrome.[10] This group of athletes was selected for their relatively severe involvement, having both EMG abnormalities and an easily identifiable neurologic deficit at the time of initial evaluation. In these individuals, by EMG criteria, the lesion was localized to the upper trunk in the majority of athletes. In some athletes with "burner" syndrome symptoms and findings, however, the EMG localized the lesion to the root or peripheral nerve level. This may be attributed to difficulty electrophysiologically differentiating between C5/C6 root injury and upper trunk injury.[69] Clinically, none of the athletes had scapula winging, identifiable rhomboid weakness, or distal motor involvement, consistent with an upper trunk lesion. The period to follow-up in these patients was, on average, 53 months. Strength parity was the more likely outcome, but occasional symptoms were present in roughly half of the individuals. Most striking were the EMG changes, which showed increased amplitude motor unit potentials in 80% of the athletes, consistent with the severity of the injury. Even in asymptomatic, normal-strength individuals, the EMGs remained abnormal. Waiting for the EMG to return to normal would not be an appropriate criterion for returning to sports activities. Rather, the clinical examination should be used as a guideline.

The management of the athlete with "burner" syndrome should be thoughtful and well organized. The on-the-field or sideline evaluation will demonstrate weakness and anesthesia while the burning pain is present, but the athlete quickly returns to normal once the "burner" has passed. A true upper trunk "burner" is not generally associated with neck pain or restriction of neck mobility. If examination reveals decreased neck mobility and neck pain, the athlete should be removed from competition pending further evaluation.[5, 85] Evaluation and treatment of neck injuries are discussed elsewhere in this text, but at the minimum, radiographs should be obtained. Often, after resolution of the "burner," full strength can be elicited and the athlete can be permitted to return to participation. It must, however, be emphasized that the athlete must be reexamined again after the game, during the week, and again the following week, since weakness can become apparent for some time after the injury.

Since the "burner" originates from the upper trunk, those muscles innervated by nerve fibers passing through the upper trunk should be closely evaluated. Muscles most commonly affected include the shoulder external rotators, deltoid, and biceps.[89] Persistent sensory deficit is very unusual with brachial plexus "burners," and persistent anesthesia should alert the clinician to the possibility of other injuries. In general, it is common to observe greater motor loss than sensory loss in traction injuries. If persistent weakness is detected, routine cervical radiographs should be obtained to rule out cervical spine pathology. This includes anteroposterior, lateral (neutral, flexion, and extension), oblique, and open mouth views. When weakness or pain persists beyond 3 weeks, an EMG examination is in order to help identify the site of the lesion. If a root level is found, cervical spine MRI may be appropriate to evaluate the possibility of a disk herniation. If the EMG shows an upper trunk plexopathy, the athlete's clinical progress can be used as a guideline to return to sports.[10]

Return to activity criteria are based on clinical findings. Ideally, strength parity should be achieved before allowing return. A mild degree of weakness may be tolerable if strength has been improving up to that point. Weakness that will clearly make participation risky is not tolerable, and the athlete is prohibited from activity until appropriate strength return has been achieved. Athletes can participate with recurrent "burners" as long as strength remains relatively normal. The onset of weakness in the setting of recurrent "burners" should prompt the clinician to remove the athlete from participation until strength returns to normal. Although a prolonged period of refrain from the sport may alleviate further symptoms, this does not occur consistently, and the athlete may have further "burners" even after the time spent out of sports. Ultimately, stopping contact sports will stop "burners." Repeat EMG is not necessary to guide return to activity. Rather, the clinical examination of strength should be used to determine the appropriateness of participation.

A number of anecdotal measures have been advised to prevent recurrence of "burners."[118] Certainly, a neck and shoulder strengthening program is extremely important. Many have advocated the use of neck rolls and pads to prevent lateral and posterior (extension) neck excursion (Fig 26–5). These can be tried on an individual basis. Built-up or high shoulder pads can also be of value in some individuals.[54] Straps that bind the helmet to the shoulder pads should probably be avoided.[118]

Despite these measures, an athlete may have recurrent "burners." In this sit-

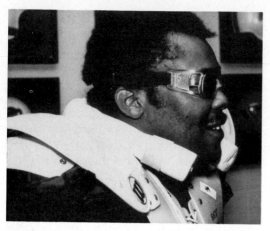

FIG 26–5.
Neck rolls can be added to football gear to help prevent lateral head deviation during contact.

uation, if they are attributable to brachial plexus injury, participation can be guided on the basis of the athlete's strength. Transient, short duration "burners," without associated weakness, can be tolerated without obvious permanent deficits ensuing. However, athletes should never be permitted to participate with significant weakness present.

ACUTE BRACHIAL NEUROPATHY

Acute brachial neuropathy is a clinical entity of unknown cause, characterized by the acute or subacute onset of shoulder pain, weakness, and atrophy of various forequarter muscles. It has been described by a variety of names, including multiple neuritis,[22] localized neuritis of the shoulder girdle,[75, 101] hereditary neuritis,[51, 59, 110] acute brachial radiculitis,[34, 115] neuralgic amyotrophy,[39, 86, 116] shoulder girdle syndrome,[75, 86] Parsonage-Turner syndrome,[86] serum brachial neuritis,[3, 36, 82] brachial plexus neuropathy,[7, 17, 100] and paralytic brachial neuritis.[41, 62, 72, 120] It was initially described in 1942 among the servicemen in the second New Zealand Expeditionary Force.[22]

The importance of understanding the presentation and clinical cause of acute brachial neuropathy is in recognition of the problem so that effective therapy and counseling can be given to the affected individual.

The predominant feature of this problem is pain localized to the shoulder. Characteristically the pain is intense, and may continue for several hours or 2 to 3 weeks despite rest and analgesics. In patients the onset can be associated with athletic activity, although the cause of acute brachial neuropathy is not truly an athletic injury.[53] Weakness either appears with the pain or, more often, develops as the pain recedes. Weakness often becomes apparent during athletic activity.

Involvement is often diffuse and characteristically includes the deltoid, supraspinatus, infraspinatus, serratus anterior, biceps, and triceps muscles. Bilateral involvement can occur clinically but is more often demonstrated to occur bilaterally on electrodiagnostic studies. In contrast to prominent motor findings, sensory loss is usually minimal and typically limited to a small area of diminished sensation over the axillary distribution.

Laboratory studies, including sedimentation rate, blood count, and others, generally show normal findings and are not helpful in establishing the diagnosis.[33] Similarly, radiographs of the neck and shoulder region do not reveal any abnormalities.

Diagnosis is frequently made by EMG evaluation.[43, 53] Involved muscles demonstrate fibrillation potentials. Differentiation of this entity from a traumatic upper trunk or plexus lesion is made from a number of EMG findings, which include[53]: (1) involvement of muscles that are not innervated via the brachial plexus (e.g., serratus anterior, diaphragmatic, trapezius); (2) severe enervation limited to muscles innervated by a single peripheral nerve, or two peripheral nerves (e.g., suprascapular nerve, axillary nerve, anterior interosseous nerve); (3) severe enervation restricted to a single muscle, with sparing of muscles innervated by the same portion of plexus, or even the same nerve trunk (e.g., substantial axon loss in [a] pronator teres with normal biceps, triceps, and abductor pollicis brevis and [b] supraspinatus with normal infraspinatus, or vice versa); and (4) EMG examination that reveals (a) severe motor involvement in a plexus or peripheral nerve distribution, with sparing of the sensory nerve action potentials mediated over the same mixed nerve (e.g., severe enervation of biceps and deltoid muscles with normal lateral antebrachial cutaneous sensory nerve action potentials), and (b) dissociated involvement of sensory fibers that travel over the same portions of the plexus (e.g., a low-amplitude lateral antebrachial cutaneous sensory nerve action potential in the presence of a normal amplitude median sensory, recording thumb sensory nerve action potential). With unequivocal axon loss upper trunk plexopathies, these two studies (lateral antebrachial cutaneous and median sensory nerve action potentials) are almost always affected to the same degree. For these reasons many investigators now consider acute brachial neuropathy as a single or multiple axon loss mononeuropathy multiplex and not a brachial plexopathy.

Once identified, treatment can be divided into two phases.[53] The initial period (phase 1) includes the time from the onset of symptoms until the resolution of the pain. During this phase the extremity is rested because activity may be associated with increased symptoms. Analgesics and a sling are used to help control pain. Rehabilitation (phase 2) commences when pain is relieved. The entire extremity and upper body must be rehabilitated to regain strength in the denervated/reinnervated muscles. All the muscles of the upper part of the body must be rehabilitated, since subclinical involvement is common. The trunk-scapula relationship must be considered as serratus anterior, and rhomboid involvement frequently occurs.

The prognosis for functional recovery is fairly good. Most patients have substantial recovery within 3 years.[110] Residual neurologic deficits with incomplete strength recovery are common, and patients are frequently found to have long-term weakness, scapula winging, and sensory loss. Scapula winging in particular often persists, and athletes who are noted to have winging on their initial presentation should be informed of the probability of its persistence.

For return to sports, athletes should reach a plateau in their strength recovery before return is considered.[53] Athletes who do not regain sufficient strength to control the extremity should be encouraged to limit their athletic endeavors. In addition, athletes should be advised that a permanent strength deficit may be produced by acute brachial neuropathy and that, in particular, scapula winging will probably not resolve. Sports participation guidelines depend on strength recovery. Absolute strength parity may be difficult to achieve, so that permission to participate in athletics must be made on a case-by-case basis, considering individual abilities.

COMPRESSION INJURIES

Compression of the brachial plexus may arise from both intrinsic and extrinsic factors. Both of these mechanisms may occur in association with athletic endeavor.

According to Lundborg and Dahlin,[71] the severity of the nerve lesions induced by acute or chronic compression is a result of the magnitude as well as the direction of the compressive trauma. The onset of symptoms as well as rate of recovery may be variable and reflects the pathophysiologic basis of the lesion.

The basic pathophysiology of acute as well as chronic compression lesions is controversial; ischemia and mechanical factors have been proposed as primary underlying causes for impaired function. Generally slight or moderate compression, resulting in functional disorders immediately reversible after decompression, is based on a microvascular insufficiency, while mechanical factors, resulting in local myelin damage, might constitute primary etiologic factors in lesions requiring a longer time to recover.

The most common external agent creating compressions on the brachial plexus is a knapsack.[68, 119] In Hirasawa and Sakakida's[56] series, 94% of their brachial plexus lesions were described as "backpack paralysis." These lesions occur when large, heavy backpacks are carried for long periods (Fig 26–6). The axillary straps create a compression force around the plexus, with the clavicle as a firm strut against which compression can occur. In addition, the shoulder girdle is pulled posteriorly by the heavy pack, adding perhaps a component of traction. Injury by the same mechanism can also be restricted to the axillary or radial nerve.

Treatment of backpack paralysis is conservative. Physical therapy is appropriate as strength returns in order to allow complete recovery. In one series, 15 patients had complete resolution within 3 months with conservative treatment.[56]

Fractures of the clavicle with exuberant callus formation can also be a source of brachial plexus compression.[40, 77, 81] Progressive neurologic complaints in the extremity as clavicle fracture healing matures represent the initial presentation of this problem. Treatment should consist of resection of the offending callus and appropriate postoperative rehabilitation.

Hypertrophic clavicle nonunions generally in the middle of the clavicle

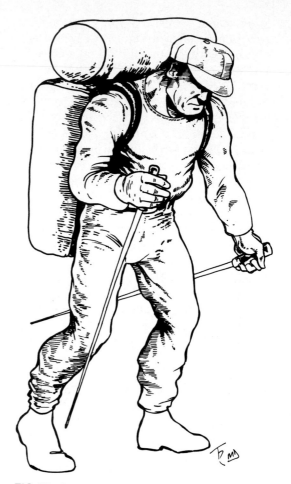

FIG 26–6.
Heavy backpacks create compression over the plexus.

can also create brachial plexus compression. Kay and Eckardt[61] noted that the medial cord can be affected in this situation, producing ulnar nerve symptoms.[61] Treatment options include resection of the callus to decompress the plexus and open reduction and internal fixation to achieve fracture union.

Early treatment of acute clavicular fractures with a figure eight bandage can also create brachial plexus compression. Close attention to the neurovascular evaluation of athletes with clavicular fractures is mandatory to avoid serious neurovascular compromise. Adjustment or removal of the figure eight strap is necessary if neurologic symptoms indicating plexus compression develop. If release of the figure eight strap does not improve the clinical situation, the possibility of fracture fragment encroachment on the plexus and its associated major vasculature should be evaluated and treated.[58, 125] This might require operative treatment of the clavicular fracture to remove the fragment compressing or lacerating the neurovascular structures, reduce the fracture fragments, and stabilize the fracture with internal fixation to allow safe and uncomplicated healing.

ROOT AVULSIONS

Root avulsions are the result of severe traction injuries. The mechanism is similar to that in the "burner" syndrome—forces driving the shoulder downward and the neck away from the shoulder. Fortunately these injuries are relatively rare in most contact sports. The majority of patients are hurt in motorcycle and other high-velocity, high-impact accidents. The position of the arm at impact will determine the portion of the plexus damaged. If the arm is abducted, traction develops in the lower roots, while if the area is adducted or at the side, the upper roots are affected[8, 16, 68] (Fig 26–7).

Diagnosis of root avulsions can be confirmed by a number of studies. Plain radiographs of the cervical spine may demonstrate a fracture of a transverse process.[68] Fractures of these processes are associated with root avulsions as the deep cervical fascia invests both the nerve roots and the cervical transverse processes.[67] Cervical myelography will frequently demonstrate pseudomeningoceles at the level(s) of injury. Sensory nerve conduction studies will show normal response in anesthetic areas (preganglionic lesion), with corresponding muscle paralysis. Histamine skin testing will also demonstrate a preganglionic lesion

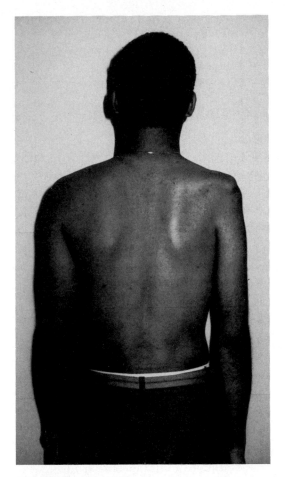

FIG 26–7.
Young man who sustained C5 and C6 root avulsions during sandlot football. Notice deltoid, supraspinatus, rhomboid, and infraspinatus atrophy.

by a normal (3-phase) response. On electromyography the posterior cervical muscles will be denervated, indicating a lesion that includes the posterior primary ramus.

Current treatment for root avulsions is based on supportive and later reconstructive measures. Newer microsurgical techniques may offer hope for acute repair of these lesions, but dependable, reproducible repair of root avulsions has not yet been demonstrated.[65, 83] Spontaneous healing does not occur, and treatment of individuals with these lesions requires extensive early rehabilitation to maintain joint motion and later reconstructive surgery to provide motor units to paralyzed areas.[69, 99] The extent of surgery will depend on the nerves affected and the goals of the patient.

PERIPHERAL NERVE INJURY

Spinal Accessory Nerve

The spinal accessory nerve (eleventh cranial nerve) is the sole motor nerve to the trapezius muscle. The superficial course of this nerve makes it susceptible to injury (Fig 26–8). The nerve lies in the subcutaneous tissue on the floor of the posterior cervical triangle in its course to innervate the trapezius muscle.[89] Blunt trauma and surgery in the posterior cervical triangle are the two predominant causes of injury to this nerve, resulting in paralysis of the trapezius muscle. This lesion, although uncommon, is painful, deforming, and disabling.

A number of events can lead to spinal accessory nerve injury. A direct, forceful blow to the neck in the area of the posterior cervical triangle can cause a crushing injury to the nerve where it passes under the upper border of the trapezius muscle. This can be the result of contact between an athlete and a piece of equipment. Bateman[9] has described these injuries from a hockey stick or a lacrosse stick. Another mechanism is an injury that depresses the shoulder while the head is forced in the opposite direction, resulting in a traction injury to the nerve.[70, 124]

Manifestations of this injury include a dull ache or pain, with drooping of the shoulder and noticeable weakness in arm elevation and abduction. On examination the patient is unable to shrug his shoulders, and shows rotatory winging of the scapula when viewed from behind. Atrophy of the trapezius muscle leads to visible asymmetry about the neck. The scapula is rotated downward and displaced laterally because of the lack of the suspensory action of the trapezius muscle. This results from the paralysis of the upper and central portion of the muscle, which, attached to the acromion, normally pulls the shoulder upward and inward. In addition, the scapula is normally stabilized on the chest wall by the lower portion of the trapezius muscle, and this function, which prevents rotation and translation, is lost. The trapezius muscle not only helps suspend the shoulder but also provides a firm base from which the deltoid muscle acts in elevating the arm. The pain is thought to be due to overuse of the levator scapulae and rhomboid muscles and to be from brachial radiculitis caused by stretching of the brachial plexus.[12] Bigliani et al.[12] have described a triad of findings to alert the examiner to this condition—asymmetric neckline, winging of the scapula, and weakness of forward elevation of the scapula. Evaluation of these aspects will avoid misdiagnosis and inappropriate intervention.

Electrophysiologic studies will reveal injury to the sternocleidomastoid muscle and all three portions of the trapezius muscle. Initial treatment is conservative. The arm is put into a sling, and physical therapy for active and passive exercise is provided to avoid contractures in the arm and shoulder. Paralysis may persist for 3 to 12 months in closed injuries. The function of the trapezius muscle is so vital that even strengthening adjacent muscle groups is often inadequate to compensate for the extensive lost functions.

For lesions caused by open trauma or iatrogenic injury, neurolysis and nerve grafting have given variable results, but generally are more successful when performed within 6 months. After 1 year, reconstructive procedures, with use of muscle transfers, are done to improve shoulder function in isolated injuries,[12] while stabilization procedures are preferred for more widespread weakness and neuromuscular disorders.

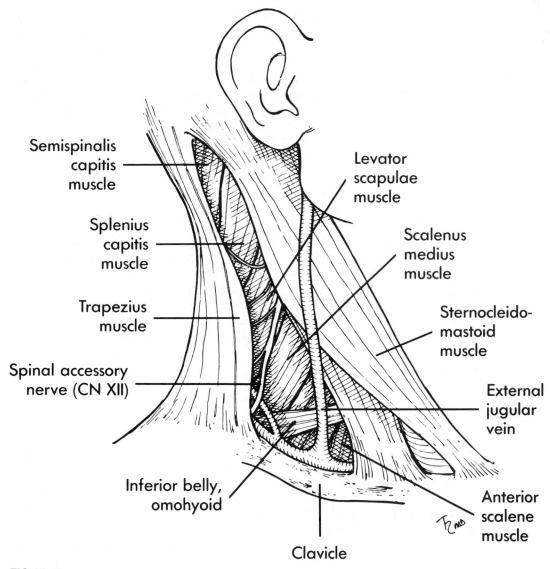

Semispinalis capitis muscle

Splenius capitis muscle

Trapezius muscle

Spinal accessory nerve (CN XII)

Levator scapulae muscle

Scalenus medius muscle

Sternocleido-mastoid muscle

External jugular vein

Inferior belly, omohyoid

Anterior scalene muscle

Clavicle

FIG 26–8.
Superficial course of the spinal accessory nerve makes it vulnerable to injury. *(From Pianka G, Hershman E: Neurovascular injuries, in Nicholas JA, Hershman EB:* Upper Extremity Injuries in Sports Medicine. *St Louis, Mosby–Year Book, 1990.)*

Dynamic procedures described include lateral transfer of the levator scapulae and rhomboid muscles on the scapula, the Eden-Lange procedure.[66] Bigliani et al.[12] achieved satisfactory results with this procedure in their series of patients. Static fixation of the scapula to the spinous processes has been done using fascia lata grafts.[31]

If the lesion is mild and reversible, athletic participation can be attempted when healing has occurred. If trapezius muscle weakness persists, dynamic stabilization of the scapula can be achieved through muscle rehabilitation and reeducation, although frequently this is unsuccessful. For severe lesions with little or no functional return, athletic participation will be restricted insofar as the involved extremity is concerned.

In patients in whom symptoms warrant surgical intervention, the lateral rhomboid/levator scapulae transfer can improve scapular stability and shoulder function so that strenuous activity can be pursued. Long-term physiotherapy is often necessary to maintain maximum function, however.[12]

Suprascapular Nerve

The suprascapular nerve originates from the upper trunk of the brachial plexus and consists of contributions from the fifth and sixth cervical roots. The nerve runs in the posterior triangle of the neck, passing under the body of the omohyoid muscle and anterior border of the trapezius muscle to the scapular notch, where it is firmly fixed in a fibrosseous tunnel.[89] The nerve runs through the scapular notch, a groove in the scapula that is covered by the transverse scapular ligament. It then supplies innervation to the supraspinatus muscle and gives off sensory fibers to the capsular and ligamentous structures of the shoulder and acromioclavicular joint. The nerve continues around the lateral border of the spine of the scapula, through the spinoglenoid notch, to innervate the infraspinatus muscle. Approximately 50% of individuals have a spinoglenoid ligament, an aponeurotic band that separates the supraspinatus and the infraspinatus muscles.[42, 80] The nerve has no cutaneous distribution. Entrapment of the suprascapular nerve has been reported in both the scapular notch and in the region of the spinoglenoid notch[27] (Fig 26–9). A number of mechanisms of injury have been implicated in suprascapular nerve injury.[94–96] Suprascapular nerve injury has been associated with traction injuries to the shoulder, as when the shoulder and neck are separated and the origin of the nerve is damaged.[9] Direct trauma to the shoulder, including shoulder dislocation or fracture, is a more common cause

of suprascapular nerve injury.[128] Repetitive trauma, such as throwing, may also contribute to chronic suprascapular nerve injury.[20] Activities such as weightlifting,[45] volleyball,[42] and backpacking have been found in association with suprascapular nerve injury, with repetitive cross-body shoulder adduction implicated in the mechanism of injury.

Suprascapular nerve entrapment is often described at the scapular notch. The pathology leading to this entrapment syndrome is varied, and includes ganglion cysts compressing the nerve,[91] pressure on the nerve from the "sling effect" of the transverse scapular ligament,[94] a bifid transverse scapular ligament impinging on the nerve,[4] and healed scapular fractures[38] through the scapular notch, with nerve compression from scar tissue or callus formation.

The scapular notch can be visualized on radiographs and imaging studies. Plain radiographs in the anteroposterior projection with the beam directed 15 to 30 degrees caudally can visualize the notch.[94, 95] This view may demonstrate a narrow scapular notch when a fracture has created deformity in the notch. If a ganglion cyst or other mass is suspected, CT scan or MRI may be of value in identifying the lesion. Nerve lesions may also occur distal to the capsular branches, in the region of the spinoglenoid notch.[13, 111] These lesions will affect the infraspinatus muscle only and may not be associated with any discomfort in the shoulder. Asymptomatic isolated infraspinatus muscle paralysis, caused from cocking of the arm and follow-through while serving, has been found in volleyball players.[42]

Clinical findings include atrophy of the supraspinatus or infraspinatus muscle, or both, and poorly localized pain in the posterolateral aspect of the scapula (Fig 26–10). The specific site of the lesion will dictate whether both the supraspinatus and infraspinatus muscles

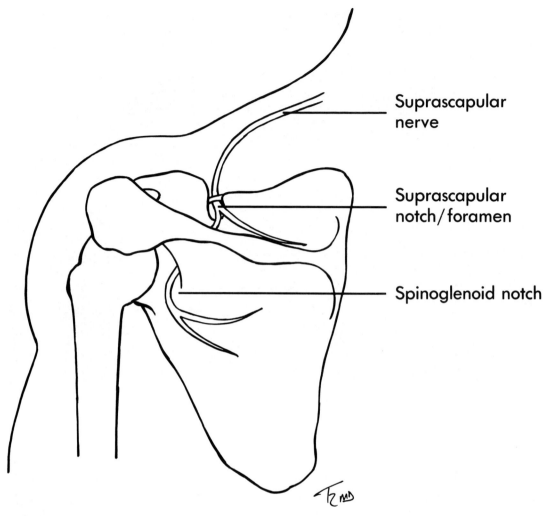

Suprascapular
nerve

Suprascapular
notch/foramen

Spinoglenoid notch

FIG 26–9.
Potential points of compression of the suprascapular nerve. *(From Pianka G, Hershman E: Neurovascular injuries, in Nicholas JA, Hershman EB:* Upper Extremity Injuries in Sports Medicine. *St Louis, Mosby–Year Book, 1990.)*

(suprascapular notch) or the infraspinatus muscle alone (spinoglenoid notch) is involved. Often there is a loss of strength in abduction and external rotation of the arm.[104] Sensation is normal as the suprascapular nerve has no cutaneous distribution. Atrophy in the supraspinatus or infraspinatus fossa is frequently present. Rotator cuff pathology must be considered in the differential diagnosis in addition to cervical radiculopathy, myopathy, and acute brachial neuropathy.[35, 37] At times glenohumeral arthrog-

raphy may be indicated to help eliminate rotator cuff pathology from consideration.

Electromyographic and nerve conduction studies will confirm the suprascapular nerve entrapment and identify the site of the lesion at the suprascapular or spinoglenoid notch. An injection test has been described.[46] A small amount of local anesthetic is injected into the scapular notch. A positive test is present when the shoulder pain is relieved, confirming the site of injury. Traction inju-

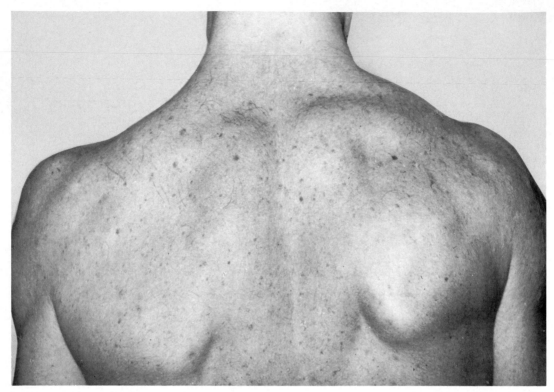

FIG 26–10.
Observe atrophy of muscle in supraspinatus and infraspinatus fossae.

ries from acute trauma to the shoulder or neck usually carry a good prognosis and can be managed conservatively. Rest, analgesia, and progressive return to activity may be all that is necessary. For more severe injuries, physical therapy may be required to restore strength. Conservative therapy with rest, anti-inflammatory medication, and physical therapy may fail to relieve the symptoms, and surgical decompression may be necessary. This is best carried out when an identifiable lesion, either anatomically or electrophysiologically, can be identified.[52, 107] Explorations of the suprascapular nerve have revealed hypertrophy of the transverse scapular ligament and anomalies of the suprascapular notch. Compression of the nerve at the spinoglenoid notch has also been identified.[13, 20] The surgical procedures described have ranged from excision of the transverse scapular ligament

or spinoglenoid ligament to deepening the suprascapular notch.[92] Often ganglion cysts have been found to compress the suprascapular nerve at the notch of the scapula.[57, 84, 111] The clinical response to decompression of the nerve has varied from no improvement to full restoration of muscle bulk and power, and resolution of pain.[52, 117]

If return of supraspinatus and infraspinatus function occurs, athletic participation can be resumed. However, since the infraspinatus muscle supplies 90% of the external rotation power of the shoulder and the supraspinatus muscle stabilizes the humeral head in the glenoid fossa during elevation, residual weakness will often preclude safe return to athletics because the deficits make safe participation difficult to achieve. Isolated infraspinatus weakness resulting from a lesion in the femoral branch of the nerve may not lead to a significant functional deficit. This has been reported in elite volleyball players[42] and a professional baseball player in whom asymptomatic infraspinatus atrophy and weakness have been documented.[20] Correlation of functional ability and physical findings is recommended to judge the ability of the athlete in this situation to continue with sports.

Long Thoracic Nerve

Isolated paralysis of the serratus anterior muscle has been described in a wide variety of sports, including tennis, golf, gymnastics, soccer, bowling, weightlifting, ice hockey, wrestling, archery, basketball, and football.[9, 49, 50, 79, 102, 123] The long thoracic nerve originates from the ventral rami of C5, C6, and C7 cervical nerves and travels beneath the brachial plexus and clavicle over the first rib. The nerve then travels along the lateral aspect of the chest wall to innervate the serratus anterior muscle (Fig 26–11). Its superficial course and length make it especially vulnerable to injury. Damage to the nerve may be caused by blows to the shoulder or lateral thoracic wall. Excessive use of the shoulder or prolonged traction, such

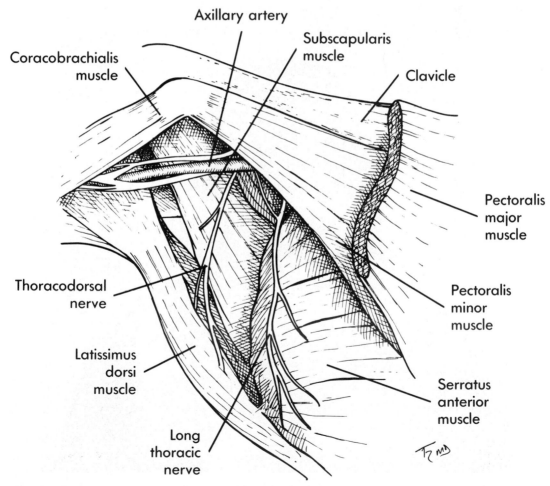

FIG 26–11.
Course of the long thoracic nerve along the chest wall.

as in cycling, has been found to cause this nerve injury.

The serratus anterior muscle stabilizes the scapula on the posterior thoracic wall, therefore providing a firm point for muscles arising from the scapula to move the arm. The serratus anterior muscle, together with the trapezius and levator scapulae muscles, act to rotate the scapula upward, thereby allowing greater glenohumeral motion.

The clinical features include dull ache or pain around the shoulder girdle, a winged scapula, and decreased active shoulder motion.[44, 60] Pain may be increased when the head is tilted to the contralateral side or by raising the ipsilateral arm over the head. Often painless winging of the scapula may be the clinical presentation of someone involved in any of the sports mentioned (Fig 26–12). Winging of the scapula is especially prominent during forward pushing as in push-ups. More severe pain is usually indicative of an acute brachial neuropathy. Patients with acute brachial neuropathy will generally have clinical involvement of ipsilateral proximal muscles such as the deltoid, biceps, infraspinatus, and supraspinatus. At times, however, clinical involvement may be limited to the serratus anterior muscle, and electromyography will be needed to identify subclinical but definite electrical dysfunction in

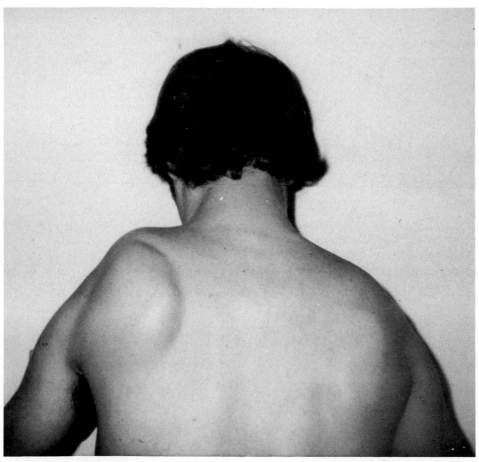

FIG 26–12.
Winging of the scapula associated with long thoracic nerve injury.

other muscles of the shoulder girdle. If a long thoracic nerve injury is suspected, a detailed history, physical examination, and EMG are in order to differentiate between an isolated long thoracic nerve injury and a case of acute brachial neuropathy.[53, 87]

Other conditions, such as polymyositis, muscular dystrophy, and cervical spondylosis, must also be ruled out if the clinical picture is not clear.[60]

There is no consensus on treatment of this condition, but generally conservative measures, such as rest from the associated sport and physical therapy, are advised.[127] The prognosis for serratus anterior muscle paralysis is fair, and recovery can occur up to 2 years after injury.[49, 127] Often some degree of winging persists.

Return to sports can be considered when the shoulder girdles have symmetric strength parity. The likelihood of complete resolution of scapular winging is low and should not be used as a criterion for athletic return.

Axillary Nerve

The axillary nerve branches from the posterior cord of the brachial plexus and contains fibers from the C5 and C6 nerve roots. The nerve then travels laterally and downward, passing just below the shoulder joint and into the quadrilateral space.[19] The axillary nerve next curves around the posterior and lateral portions of the proximal humerus, dividing into anterior and posterior branches, and innervates the deltoid and teres minor muscles. A cutaneous sensory branch of the nerve supplies the lateral aspect of the upper arm.[89]

The usual mechanism of injury to the axillary nerve is trauma, either a direct blow to the shoulder,[11] fracture of the proximal humerus,[14] or a shoulder dislocation,[14] all of which cause stretching of the nerve. Axillary nerve injuries occur

in many sports, such as football, wrestling, gymnastics, mountain climbing, and Rugby.[9] When the arm is displaced away from the trunk, tension is placed on the nerves. This tension or stretch is more severe for the nerves with the shortest distance from the brachial plexus to their muscle insertion. This would help explain the frequent involvement of the axillary nerve in injuries to the shoulder.

Chronic axillary nerve entrapment may also occur. In this situation, entrapment of the nerve arises in the quadrilateral space, and this entity has been termed *quadrilateral space syndrome*.[23, 78] Nerve entrapment arises insidiously in association with compression of the posterior humeral circumflex artery.

The degree of injury to the axillary nerve can vary. The initial presentation may be weakness in elevation and abduction of the arm, with or without numbness along the lateral aspect of the upper arm. Weakness in abduction may not be readily apparent since the supraspinatus muscle alone may effectively abduct the arm. Subsequently, wasting of the deltoid muscle develops (Fig 26–13). Whenever an axillary nerve injury is considered, one must rule out a posterior cord injury by testing the latissimus dorsi muscle, whose nerve branches proximal to the axillary nerve, and by testing the muscles innervated by the radial nerve.[79]

Electrophysiologic testing can be used to determine whether there has been a partial or complete axillary nerve injury. If the injury is partial, the treatment is rest, physical therapy, and a sling. Daily passive range of motion exercises are indicated to prevent stiffness. Because of the short course of the axillary nerve, some degree of recovery should be expected within 3 months. When rehabilitating the athlete, it is important to recall that there are three heads to the deltoid muscle, anterior, middle, and posterior. These must be restored to normal strength to achieve satisfactory return to

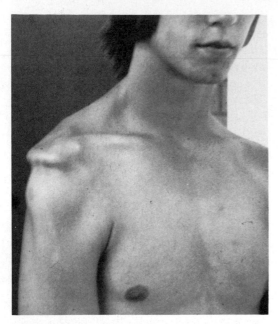

FIG 26–13.
Severe wasting of deltoid muscle resulting from an axillary nerve injury.

participation. Surgical intervention is recommended if there is no sign of improvement by 3 to 4 months.[9, 11] Entrapment in the quadrilateral space may also be treated by surgical decompression.[23, 78] Often exploration and neurolysis or nerve grafting give good results.[88] With any form of treatment, athletic participation can resolve when strength parity has been achieved.

Musculocutaneous Nerve

The musculocutaneous nerve is a mixed motor and sensory peripheral nerve arising from the lateral cord of the brachial plexus, and contains fibers from the C5, C6, and C7 nerve roots. The nerve pierces the coracobrachialis muscle below the coracoid process and travels down the arm between the biceps and brachialis muscles, which it also supplies. The sensory component then continues lateral to the biceps and becomes superficial anterolaterally as it penetrates the deep brachial fascia above the elbow.

Here it becomes the lateral cutaneous nerve of the forearm. In its superficial course the nerve travels through the antecubital fossa between the median cubital vein and the cephalic vein. The anterior division of the nerve supplies sensation to the radial one half of the volar aspect of the forearm, while the posterior branch supplies the radial one third of the dorsal aspect of the forearm.[89]

The presentation of musculocutaneous nerve compression varies according to the site of the lesion.[63] In addition to shoulder dislocation, injury to the nerve proximal to its innervation of the coracobrachialis muscle has been reported by Kim and Goodrich[63] in an athlete after throwing a football. The findings consisted of weakness in elbow flexion, atrophy of the brachialis and biceps brachia muscles, a dull ache in the distal aspect of the forearm with dysesthesia, and an absent biceps reflex. Electrophysiologic studies confirmed the location of the lesion. After 4 months the neurapraxia resolved, with resolution of the symptoms.

Weightlifting has also been associated with musculocutaneous neuropathy, but below the level of the coracobrachialis muscle.[18] The presentation occurred with painless weakness and atrophy of the biceps muscle and dysesthesia in the volar radial aspect of the forearm. Strenuous exercise is thought to cause either repetitive injury to the nerve by the coracobrachialis muscle or chronic compression due to muscle hypertrophy.[18, 76] Cessation of weightlifting resulted in resolution of the symptoms up to 2 months later.

Positioning the arm in abduction, external rotation, and extension during general anesthesia has also resulted in musculocutaneous nerve injury. This syndrome may be confused with a C5 or C6 radiculopathy, brachial plexus injury (especially one involving the lateral cord), and rupture of the biceps tendon. Differentiation is based on careful clinical examination of other muscle groups innervated by the C5 and C6 nerve roots, sensory examination, and electrophysiologic testing.

In general, injuries to the proximal musculocutaneous nerve that occur during athletic endeavor have a favorable prognosis. Identification of the lesion site by examination and EMG is important to differentiate this isolated lesion from other problems. Once confirmed, these lesions can be treated conservatively, with frequent resolution of symptoms occurring after a trial of rest and rehabilitation.

SUMMARY

Brachial plexus injuries are not uncommon in sports. Knowledge of anatomy and neurophysiology is important to permit accurate diagnosis and institution of comprehensive treatment. Traumatic injuries can be caused by traction and compression. Unusual conditions, such as acute brachial neuritis, may also occur. Safe return to sports is permitted when strength parity is achieved and rehabilitation is completed after neural recovery.

REFERENCES

1. Albright JP, McAuley E, Martin RK, et al: Head and neck injuries in college football. An eight year analysis. *Am J Sports Med* 1985; 13:147–152.

2. Albright JP, Moses JM, Feldick HG, et al: Non-fatal cervical spine injuries in interscholastic football. *JAMA* 1976; 236:1243.

3. Allen IM: The neurological complications of serum treatment. With report of a case. *Lancet* 1931; 2:1128–1131.

4. Alon M, Weiss S, Fishel B, et al: Bilateral suprascapular nerve entrapment syndrome due to an anomalous transverse scapular ligament. *Clin Orthop* 1988; 234:31–33.

5. Andrich J, Bergfeld JA, Ramo RA: A method for the management of cervical injuries in football. A preliminary report. *Am J Sports Med* 1977; 5:89–92.

6. Archambault JL: Brachial plexus stretch. *Injury* 1983; 31:256–260.

7. Bale JF Jr, Thompson JA, Petajan JH, et al: Childhood brachial plexus neuropathy. *J Pediatr* 1979; 95:741–742.

8. Barnes R: Traction injuries to the plexus in adults. *J Bone Joint Surg [Br]* 1949; 31B:10–16.

9. Bateman JE: Nerve injuries about the shoulder in sports. *J Bone Joint Surg [Am]* 1967; 49A:785–792.

10. Bergfeld JA, Hershman EB, Wilbourn AJ: Brachial plexus injury in sports—a five year follow-up. *Orthop Trans* 1988; 12:743–744.

11. Berry H, Bril V: Axillary nerve palsy following blunt trauma to the shoulder region—a clinical and electrophysiological review. *J Neurol Neurosurg Psychiatry* 1982; 45:1027–1032.

12. Bigliani LU, Perez-Sanz JR, Wolfe IN: Treatment of trapezius paralysis. *J Bone and Joint Surg [Am]* 1985; 67-A;871–877.

13. Black KP, Lombardo JL: Suprascapular nerve injuries with isolated paralysis of the infraspinatus. *Am J Sports Med* 1990; 18:225–230.

14. Blom S, Dahlback LO: Nerve injuries in dislocations of the shoulder joint and fractures of the neck and humerus. *Acta Chir Scand* 1970; 136:461–466.

15. Bonney G: The value of axon responses in determining the site of the lesion in traction injuries of the brachial plexus. *Brain* 1954; 77:588–609.

16. Bonney G: Prognosis in traction lesions of the brachial plexus. *J Bone Joint Surg [Br]* 1959; 41B:4–35.

17. Bradley WG, Madrid R, Thrush DC, et al: Recurrent brachial plexus neuropathy. *Brain* 1975; 98:381–398.

18. Braddon RL, Wolfe C: Musculocutaneous nerve injury after heavy exercise. *Arch Phys Med Rehabil* 1978; 59:290–293.

19. Bryan WJ, Schauder K, Tullos HS: The axillary nerve and its relationship to common sports medicine shoulder procedures. *Am J Sports Med* 1986; 14:113–116.

20. Bryan WJ, Wild JJ: Isolated infraspinatus atro-

phy: A common cause of posterior shoulder pain and weakness in throwing athletes. *Am J Sports Med* 1989; 17:130–131.

21. Bufalini C, Prescatori G: Posterior cervical electromyography in the diagnosis and the prognosis of brachial plexus injuries. *J Bone Joint Surg [Br]* 1969; 51B:627–631.

22. Burnard ED, Fox TG: Multiple neuritis of shoulder girdle. Report of nine cases occurring in second New Zealand expeditionary force. *NZ Med J* 1942; 41:243–247.

23. Cahill BR, Palmer RE: Quadrilateral space syndrome. *J Hand Surg* 1983; 8:65–69.

24. Chrisman OD, Snook GA, Stanitis JM, et al: Lateral flexion neck injuries in athletic competition. *JAMA* 1965; 192:613–615.

25. Clancy WG, Brand RL, Bergfeld JA: Upper trunk brachial plexus injuries in contact sports. *Am J Sports Med* 1977; 5:209–214.

26. Clancy WG Jr: Brachial plexus and upper extremity peripheral nerve injuries, in Torg JS (ed): *Athletic Injuries to the Head, Neck and Face.* Philadelphia, Lea & Febiger, 1982, pp 215–220.

27. Clein LJ: Suprascapular entrapment neuropathy. *J Neurosurg* 1975; 43:337–342.

28. Collins D, Storey M, Petersank, et al: Nerve injuries in athletes. *Phys Sportsmed* 1988; 16:92–100.

29. Copeland S, Landi A: Value of the Tinel sign in brachial plexus lesions. *Ann R Coll Surg* 1979; 61:470.

30. Denny-Brown D, Doherty MM: Effects of transient stretching of peripheral nerve. *Arch Neurol Psych* 1945; 54:117–129.

31. Dewar FP, Harris RI: Restoration of function of the shoulder following paralysis of the trapezius by fascial sling fixation and transplantation of the levator scapulae. *Ann Surg* 1950; 132:1111–1115.

32. DiBenedetto M, Markey K: Electrodiagnostic localization of traumatic upper trunk brachial plexopathy. *Arch Phys Med Rehabil* 1984; 64:15–17.

33. Dillin L, Hoaglund FT, Scheck M: Brachial neuritis. *J Bone Joint Surg [Am]* 1985; 67A:878–880.

34. Dixon GJ, Dick TBS: Acute brachial radiculitis. Course and prognosis. *Lancet* 1945; 2:707–708.

35. Donovan WH: Rotator cuff tear versus supra-

scapular nerve injury: A problem in differential diagnosis. *Arch Phys Med Rehabil* 1974; 55:424–428.

36. Doyle JB: Neurologic complications of serum sickness. *Am J Med Sci* 1933; 185:484–492.

37. Drez D: Suprascapular neuropathy in the differential diagnosis of rotator cuff tear. *Am J Sports Med* 1976; 4:43–45.

38. Edeland HG, Zachrison BE: Fracture of the scapular notch associated with lesions of the suprascapular nerve. *Acta Orthop Scand* 1975; 46:758–763.

39. England JD, Sumner AJ: Neurologic amyotrophy. An increasingly diverse entity. *Muscle Nerve* 1967; 10:60–68.

40. Enker SH, Murphy KK: Brachial plexus compression by excessive callus formation secondary to a fractured clavicle. A case report. *Mt Sinai J Med* 1972; 37:678–682.

41. Evans HW: Paralytic brachial neuritis. *NY J Med* 1965; 65:2926–2928.

42. Ferretti A, et al: Suprascapular neuropathy in volleyball players. *J Bone Joint Surg [Am]* 1987; 69A:260–263.

43. Flaggman PD, Kelly JJ Jr: Brachial plexus neuropathy: An electrophysiologic evaluation. *Arch Neurol* 1980; 37:160–164.

44. Foo CL, Swann M: Isolated paralysis of the serratus anterior. *J Bone Joint Surg [Br]* 1983; 65B:552–556.

45. Ganzhorn RW, Hocker JT, Horowitz M, et al: Suprascapular nerve entrapment. *J Bone Joint Surg* 1981; 63A:492–494.

46. Garcia G, McQueen D: Bilateral suprascapular nerve entrapment syndrome. *J Bone Joint Surg [Am]* 1981; 63A:491–492.

47. Gerstner DL, Omer GE: Peripheral entrapment neuropathies in the upper extremity. *J Musculoskeletal Med* 1988; 45:14–29.

48. Gilliatt RW, Ochoa J, Rudge P, et al: The cause of nerve damage in acute compression. *Trans Am Neurol Assoc* 1974; 99:71–74.

49. Goodman CE, Kenrick MM, Blum MV: Long thoracic nerve palsy. A follow-up study. *Arch Phys Med Rehabil* 1975; 56:352–355.

50. Gregg JR, Labosky D, Harty M: Serratus anterior paralysis in the young athlete. *J Bone Joint Surg [Am]* 1979; 61A:825–832.

51. Guillozet N, Mercer RD: Hereditary recurrent brachial neuropathy. *Am J Dis Child* 1973; 125:884–887.

52. Hadley MN: Suprascapular nerve entrapment. *J Neurosurg* 1986; 64:843–848.

53. Hershman EB, Wilbourn AJ, Bergfeld J: Acute brachial neuropathy in athletes. *Am J Sports Med* 1989; 17:655–659.

54. Hershman EB: Brachial plexus injuries. *Clin Sports Med* 1990; 9(2).

55. Hershman EB: The team physician's bag. *J Musculoskeletal Med* 1986; 3:4.

56. Hirasawa Y, Sakakida K: Sports and peripheral nerve injury. *Am J Sports Med* 1983; 11:420–426.

57. Hirayama T, Takemitsu Y: Compression of the suprascapular nerve by ganglion at the suprascapular notch. *Clin Orthop* 1981; 155:95–96.

58. Howard FM, Shafer SJ: Injuries to the clavicle with neurovascular complications. A study of fourteen cases. *J Bone Joint Surg [Am]* 1965; 47A:1335–1346.

59. Jacob JC, Andermann F, Robb JP: Heredofamilial neuritis with brachial predilection. *Neurology* 1961; 11:1025–1033.

60. Johnson JTH, Kendall HO: Isolated paralysis of the serratus anterior muscle. *J Bone Joint Surg [Am]* 1955; 37A:567–574.

61. Kay SP, Eckardt JJ: Brachial plexus palsy secondary to clavicle non-union. Case report and literature survey. *Clin Orthop* 1986; 206:219–222.

62. Kennedy WR, Resch JA: Paralytic brachial neuritis. *Lancet* 1966; 86:459–462.

63. Kim SM, Goodrich JA: Isolated proximal musculocutaneous nerve palsy. Case report. *Arch Phys Med Rehabil* 1984; 65:735–736.

64. Kimura J: *Electrodiagnosis in Diseases of Nerve and Muscle*. Philadelphia, FA Davis Co, 1984, pp 452–454.

65. Kline DG, Judice DJ: Operative management of selected brachial plexus lesions. *J Neurosurg* 1983; 58:631–649.

66. Langenskiold A, Ryoppy S: Treatment of paralysis of the trapezius muscles by the Eden-Lange operation. *Acta Orthop Scand* 1973; 44:383.

67. Leffert RD: Lesions of the brachial plexus revisited, in American Academy of Orthopaedic Surgeons: *Instructional Course Lectures*, vol 38. St Louis, Mosby–Year Book, 1989.

68. Leffert RD: Brachial plexus injuries. *New Engl J Med* 1974; 291:1059–1066.

69. Leffert RD: *Brachial Plexus Injuries.* New York, Churchill Livingstone, 1985.

70. Logigian EL, McInnes JM, Berger AF, et al: Stretch-induced spinal accessory nerve palsy. *Muscle Nerve* 1988; 11:146–150.

71. Lundborg G, Dahlin LB: Pathophysiology of nerve compression, in Szabo RM (ed): *Nerve Compression Syndromes.* Thorofare, NJ, Slack, Inc, 1989.

72. Magee KR, DeJong RN: Paralytic brachial neuritis. Discussion of clinical features with review of 23 cases. *JAMA* 1960; 174:1258–1262.

73. Maroon JC: "Burning hands" in football spinal cord injuries. *JAMA* 1977; 238:2049–2051.

74. Marshall RW, DeSilva RD: Computerized tomography in traction injuries of the brachial plexus. *J Bone Joint Surg [Br]* 1986; 68:734.

75. Martin WA, Kraft GH: Shoulder girdle neuritis. A clinical and electrophysiological evaluation. *Milt Med* 1975; 139:21–25.

76. Mastaglia FL: Musculocutaneous neuropathy after strenuous physical activity. *Med J Aust* 1986; 145:153–154.

77. Matz SO, Welliver PS, Welliver DI: Brachial plexus neuprapraxia complicating a comminuted clavicle fracture in a college football player. *Am J Sports Med* 1989; 17:581–583.

78. McKowen HC, Voorhies RM: Axillary nerve entrapment in the quadrilateral space. *J Neurosurg* 1987; 66:932–934.

79. Mendoza FX, Main K: Peripheral nerve injuries of the shoulder in the athlete. *Clin Sports Med* 1990; 9:331–342.

80. Mestdagh H, Drizenko A, Ghestem P: Anatomical basis of suprascapular nerve syndrome. *Anat Clin* 1981; 3:67–71.

81. Miller DS, Boswick JA Jr: Lesions of the brachial plexus associated with fractures of the clavicle. *Clin Orthop* 1969; 64:144–149.

82. Miller HG, Stanton JB: Neurological sequelae of prophylactic innoculation. *QJ Med* 1954; 23:1–27.

83. Millesi H: Surgical management of brachial plexus injuries. *J Hand Surg* 1977; 2:367.

84. Neviaser TJ, Ain BR, Neviaser RJ, et al: Suprascapular nerve denervation secondary to attenuation by a ganglionic cyst. *J Bone Joint Surg [Am]* 1986; 68A:627–628.

85. Nicholas JA: Injuries in football, in Nicholas

JA, Hershman EB (eds): *The Lower Extremity and Spine in Sports Medicine*. St Louis, Mosby–Year Book, 1984.

86. Parsonage MJ, Turner JWA: Neurologic amyotrophy. Shoulder girdle syndrome. *Lancet* 1948; 1:973–978.

87. Petrera JE, Trojaborg W: Conduction studies of the long thoracic nerve in serratus anterior palsy of different etiology. *Neurology* 1984; 34:1033–1037.

88. Petrucci FS, Morelli A, Raimohdi PL: Axillary nerve injuries: 21 cases treated by nerve graft and neurolysis. *J Hand Surg* 1982; 7:271–278.

89. Pianka G, Hershman EB: Neurovascular injuries, in Nicholas JA, Hershman EB (eds): *The Upper Extremity in Sports Medicine*. St Louis, Mosby–Year Book, 1990.

90. Poindexter DP, Johnson EW: Football shoulder and neck injury: A study of the stinger. *Arch Phys Med Rehabil* 1984; 65:601–602.

91. Post M, Mayer J: Suprascapular nerve entrapment. *Clin Orthop* 1987; 223:126–136.

92. Rask MR: Suprascapular nerve entrapment. A report of two cases of treated suprascapular notch resection. *Clin Orthop* 1978; 134:266–267.

93. Rayan GM: Lower trunk brachial plexus compression neuropathy due to cervical rib in young athletes. *Am J Sports Med* 1988; 16:77–79.

94. Rengachary SS, Neil JP, Singer PA, et al: Suprascapular entrapment neuropathy. A clinical, anatomical and comparative study. Part 1. Clinical study. *Neurosurgery* 1979; 5:441–446.

95. Rengachary SS, Burr D, Lucas S, et al: Suprascapular entrapment neuropathy. A clinical, anatomical and comparative study. Part 2. Anatomical study. *Neurosurgery* 1979; 5:447–451.

96. Rengachary SS, Burr D, Lucas S, et al: Suprascapular entrapment neuropathy. A clinical, anatomical and comparative study. Part 3. Comparative study. *Neurosurgery* 1979; 5:452–455.

97. Robertson WC, Eichman PL, Clancy WG: Upper trunk brachial plexopathy in football players. *JAMA* 1979; 241:1480–1482.

98. Rockett F: Observations on the "burner." Traumatic cervical radiculopathy. *Clin Orthop* 1982; 164:18–19.

99. Rorabeck CH, Harris WR: Factors affecting the prognosis of brachial plexus injuries. *J Bone Joint Surg [Br]* 1981; 63B:404–407.

100. Shaywitz BA: Brachial plexus neuropathy in childhood. *J Pediatr* 1975; 86:913–914.

101. Spillane JD: Localized neuritis of shoulder girdle. Report of 46 cases in MEF. *Lancet* 1943; 2:532–535.

102. Stanish WD, Lamb H: Isolated paralysis of the serratus anterior muscle. A weight training injury. *Am J Sports Med* 1978; 6:385–386.

103. Stevens JH: Brachial plexus paralysis, in Codman EA (ed): *The Shoulder*. Melbourne, Fla, Robert E. Krieger Publishing Co, 1934.

104. Strohm B, Colacis SC Jr: Shoulder joint dysfunction following injury to the suprascapular nerve. *Phys Ther* 1965; 45:106–111.

105. Sunderland S: *Nerves and Nerve Injuries*. ed 2. Edinburgh, Churchill Livingstone, 1978.

106. Sunderland S: Traumatic injuries of peripheral nerves, simple compression injuries of the radial nerve. *Brain* 1945; 68:56–72.

107. Swafford AR, Lichtman DH: Suprascapular nerve entrapment. Case report. *J Hand Surg* 1982; 7:57–60.

108. Swash M: Diagnosis of brachial root and plexus lesions. *J Neurol* 1986; 233:131–135.

109. Takazawa H, Sudo N, Akoi K, et al: Statistical observation of nerve injuries in athletes (in Japanese). *Brain Nerve Injury* 1971; 3:11–17.

110. Taylor RA: Heredofamilial mononeuritis multiplex with brachial predilection. *Brain* 1960; 83:113–137.

111. Thompson RC Jr, Schneider W, Kennedy T: Entrapment neuropathy of the inferior branch of the suprascapular nerve by ganglia. *Clin Orthop* 1982; 166:185.

112. Tsairis P, Dyck PJ, Mulder DW: Natural history of brachial plexus neuropathy. Report on 99 patients. *Arch Neurol* 1972; 27:109–117.

113. Tsairis P: Differential diagnosis of peripheral neuropathies, in Omer GE, Spinner M, et al (eds): *Management of Peripheral Nerve Problems*. Philadelphia, WB Saunders Co, 1980.

114. Tsairis P: Peripheral nerve injury in athletes, in Jordan BD, Tsairis P, Warren RF (eds): *Sports Neurology*. Rockville, Md, Aspen Publishers, 1989, pp 180–192.

115. Turner JWA: Acute brachial radiculitis. *Br Med J* 1944; 2:592–594.

116. Turner JWA, Parsonage MJ: Neurologic amyo-trophy (paralytic brachial neuritis). With special reference to prognosis. *Lancet* 1957; 2:209–212.

117. Vastamaki M: Suprascapular nerve entrapment. AAOS 54th Annual Meeting. Scientific Program Paper No. 192, 1987.

118. Warren RF: Neurologic injuries in football, in Jordan BD, Tsairis P, Warren RF (eds): *Sports Neurology*. Rockville, Md, Aspen Publishers, 1989, pp 235–244.

119. White HH: Pack palsy. A neurological complication of scouting. *Pediatrics* 1968; 41:1001–1003.

120. Wiekers NJ, Mattson RH: Acute paralytic brachial neuritis. A clinical and electrodiagnostic study. *Neurology* 1969; 19:1153–1158.

121. Wilbourn AJ, Hershman EB, Bergfeld JA: Brachial plexopathies in athletes: The EMG findings. *Muscle Nerve* 1986; 9:254.

122. Wilbourn AJ: Electrodiagnostic testing of neurologic injuries in athletes. *Clin Sports Med* 1990; 9:229–245.

123. Woodhead AB: Paralysis of the serratus anterior in a world class marksman. *Am J Sports Med* 1985; 13:359–362.

124. Wright YA: Accessory spinal nerve injury. *Clin Orthop* 1975; 108:15–18.

125. Yates DW: Complications of fractures of the clavicle. *Injury* 1979; 7:881–883.

126. Yeoman PM: Cervical myelography in traction injuries of the brachial plexus. *J Bone Joint Surg [Br]* 1968; 50B:253–260.

127. Zeier FG: The treatment of winged scapula. *Clin Orthop* 1973; 91:128–133.

128. Zoltan JD: Injury to the suprascapular nerve associated with anterior dislocation of the shoulder. Case report and review of the literature. *J Trauma* 1979; 19:203–206.

PART FOUR

Cervical Spine and Cord Injuries

CHAPTER 27

Anatomy of the Cervical Spine and Its Related Structures

Robert J. Johnson, M.D.

THE CERVICAL SPINE

The seven cervical vertebrae stand as a slender articulated column between the head and the thorax. Thus the cervical spine connects an approximately 15 lb object (the head) to a relatively immobile mass (the thorax). For its motions of flexion, extension, rotation, and lateral bending, the cervical spine must supply both flexibility and stability. To deliver these two requirements there are 17 diarthroses and 6 synarthroses between the skull and the thoracic spine. In addition, there are many more unions created by ligaments binding various elements of the cervical vertebrae together. In this enumeration the uncovertebral joints (of Luschka) are not considered to be distinct from the intervertebral disks. Thus a large number of individual joints and ligaments contribute to the flexibility and stability of the cervical spine. The musculature of the neck is an additional important system that also aids in flexibility and stability.

There are many different anatomic aspects of the cervical spine that give it special functions beyond those of the remaining spine. The cervical spine has the smallest bodies, and although these increase in size as we move caudally, the vertebral canal is larger at the cervical level of the spine than at all lower levels. The vertebral or neural foramen is triangular, with rounded corners in each of the cervical vertebrae except the atlas, in which it is more circular. The series of vertebral foramina produces the vertebral or spinal canal. The transverse diameter at individual levels varies, decreasing as one progresses caudally. The sagittal diameter of the canal, which is somewhat smaller than the transverse diameter, decreases slightly down to the third cervical vertebra and then remains nearly constant.

Of the cervical vertebrae, four may be considered typical (the third to the sixth inclusive), and three are referred to as atypical or special (the first, second, and seventh).

Typical Cervical Vertebrae

As previously mentioned, the typical cervical vertebrae have small, rather ovoid bodies, with the long axis transversely oriented. The right and left lateral margins of the superior surface of each body are raised upward as uncinate processes, which relate to equivalent beveled surfaces at the right and left lateral margins of the inferior surface of the next vertebral body above (Fig 27–1). Thus

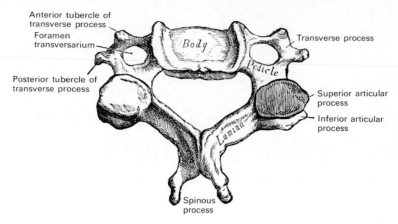

FIG 27–1.
A typical cervical vertebra viewed from above. *(From Goss CM (ed): Gray's Anatomy of the Human Body, 29th American edition. Philadelphia, Lea & Febiger, 1973. Used with permission.)*

the superior aspects of the vertebral bodies of typical vertebrae are curved and resemble somewhat the contour of a bucket seat in a sports car. Stability is gained by this partial interlocking of vertebral bodies. The right and left tilted portions of the intervertebral disk space have long been called the uncovertebral joints, as if they were truly distinct from the intervertebral disk. These ten uncovertebral joints, however, are developmentally lateral parts of the intervertebral joints and disks in which early degenerative change becomes evident after the first decade. These so-called joints acquire particular importance because the posterior part of each forms a part of the margin of the intervertebral foramen, and thus relates to the emergent spinal nerve. Furthermore, they lie immediately medial to the vertebral artery, which ascends through the foramina transversaria. Thus osteophytes may impinge on the artery as well as the nerve.

The right and left transverse processes have a groove on their superior aspect to support the emerging spinal nerve. The transverse foramina, which transmit the vertebral artery, are far enough anterior in the roots of the transverse processes to place the ascending vertebral artery in front of each of the emergent spinal nerves.

The right and left superior and inferior articular processes are situated at the junction of the pedicle (root) with the lamina of the neural (vertebral) arch. Projecting cranially and caudally, these two processes together create a short bony column for each vertebra, and from this column the lamina extends posteromedially to unite with its partner from the opposite side. The several superior and inferior articular processes thus create a posterior column of bones and joints on the right and left. These, together with the anterior column of intervertebral disks and vertebral bodies, create three parallel columns of bones and joints in the cervical spine. The articular facets of the two posterior columns of bones and joints are in a plane that has been tilted from the coronal to an oblique position in such a way that the superior facets face upward and dorsally and the inferior facets face downward and ventrally. Each is nearly flat and is surrounded by an articular capsule.

The spinous processes of the typical vertebrae are usually bifid at their tips and extend dorsally with a slight caudal slant. The long axis of the spinous process is directed so that if a line were extended dorsally from each, these lines would tend to converge at a central point posterior to the cervical spine. Therefore, an abnormality must be suspected at any level where the axes of these processes diverge.

Atypical Cervical Vertebrae

These vertebrae are the atlas (first), the axis (second), and the vertebra prominens (seventh).

The Atlas.—The atlas, which has two superior articular facets that support the condyles of the occipital bone of the skull, is particularly unusual in that it lacks a body. Weight is borne through right and left lateral masses with articular facets above and below on each. The superior articular facets that surmount the lateral masses are ovoid and elongated, with their long axes convergent anteriorly (Fig 27–2). Each of these facets is concave and conforms in size and orientation to the equivalent occipital condyle, so that these condyles may glide and roll on the atlas in nodding (flexion and extension) motions of the head.

The inferior articular facets that face downward on the underside of the lateral masses are rounded in outline to match the equally rounded outline of the superior articular facets of the axis (second cervical vertebra). The plane of the joint formed by these two facets is nearly horizontal and is thus designed for rotatory movements. However, the face of the inferior facet of the atlas is almost flat, while the surface of the superior facet of the axis is slightly convex upward, having a central summit. Accordingly, when the inferior facet of the atlas moves anteroposteriorly on the superior facet of the axis, as in rotation, the lateral mass of the atlas rises slightly as its inferior facet centers over the superior facet of the axis, and the atlas descends slightly as its facet moves anteriorly or posteriorly off the higher central area on the facet of the axis. This telescoping effect can be seen on rotational roentgenograms as a relative narrowing or widening of the joint space. The joint capsules of the atlantoaxial joints are loose, giving these joints the greatest mobility of any between the vertebrae in the spine.

The atlas has anterior and posterior arches, each with a slight median tubercle. The posterior arch is provided with a groove just behind each lateral mass. In this groove, the first cervical (suboccipital) nerve exits from the neural (vertebral)

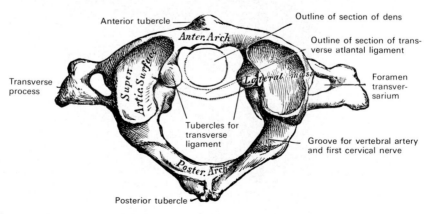

FIG 27–2.
The first cervical vertebra viewed from above. *(From Goss CM (ed):* Gray's Anatomy of the Human Body, *29th American edition. Philadelphia, Lea & Febiger, 1973. Used with permission.)*

canal, and the vertebral artery enters into the neural canal. Here these two structures pierce the atlanto-occipital membrane as they cross the posterior arch. Occasionally the lower border of the membrane is ossified where it bridges over the artery and nerve (the posterior ponticulus), and is therefore discernible on roentgenograms.

The Axis.—The axis, or second cervical vertebra, has a body that supports the upright odontoid process. This process represents the phylogenetically displaced body of the atlas, and serves as a pivot about which the atlas rotates. The superior articular facets of the axis are nearly horizontal to coincide with the inferior articular facets of the atlas (Fig 27–3). However, the inferior articular processes of the atlas have facets that face forward and downward to fit the superior articular facets of the third cervical vertebra. The neural arch of the axis is formed of right and left flattened laminae with a median spinous process projecting dorsally.

The Vertebra Prominens.—The seventh cervical vertebra is a transitional vertebra that has several distinctive features. The spinous process is longer than that of the other cervical vertebrae and is easily palpated clinically. Hence this bone is called the vertebra prominens. Its body is proportionally broader than the bodies of the vertebrae above, and its transverse process is larger and more posteriorly placed. The costal element of the transverse process is less well developed, however, and the anterior tubercle is small or absent. Occasionally the costal element develops excessively and becomes a cervical rib with its potential for producing neurovascular symptoms.

Articulations and Relations Between Cervical Vertebrae

The atlas is held in proper relationship to the axis, not only by the articulation of its right and left lateral masses with the axis, but also by the transverse ligament of the atlas. This ligament forms a sturdy band bridging across the interval

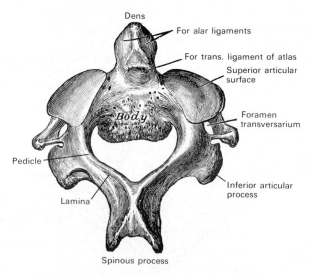

FIG 27–3.
The second cervical vertebra viewed from above. *(From Goss CM (ed):* Gray's Anatomy of the Human Body, *29th American edition. Philadelphia, Lea & Febiger, 1973. Used with permission.)*

between the lateral masses, to each of which it is securely attached. Thus it subdivides the central foramen (or space ringed by the anterior and posterior arches and the lateral masses) of the atlas into a smaller anterior compartment for the odontoid process and a larger posterior compartment for the upper end of the spinal cord. The space relationships here have been schematized by Steel's[4] "rule of thirds," in which the anterior third of the anteroposterior diameter of the central foramen of the atlas is occupied by the odontoid process, leaving one third for the spinal cord and a remaining third that contains only the arachnoid and cerebrospinal fluid. This latter third, however, is distributed both anteriorly and posteriorly to the spinal cord.

Anterior dislocation of the atlas upon the axis, especially when the transverse ligament ruptures but the odontoid process does not fracture, dangerously reduces the available space for the spinal cord and may result in its anteroposterior compression. Since the odontoid process is located anteriorly within the bony ring of the atlas, it is apparent that this process functions as an eccentrically placed pivot, and that rotatory motions of the atlas upon the axis significantly diminish the transverse diameter of the vertebral canal.

When the atlas rotates far to the left on the axis, the right transverse foramen of the atlas moves forward relative to the transverse foramen of the axis, thereby increasing the distance between the two foramina and thus stretching the vertebral artery and increasing its angulation at the transverse foramen of the atlas. In extremes of rotation, as might occur with rotational dislocations and subluxations of the atlas on the axis, the vertebral artery may be so stretched and angulated that circulation to the brain stem and upper spinal cord is impaired.

The major motions that occur in the cervical spine are flexion, extension, lateral bending, and rotation, while minor motions are distraction, anteroposterior translation, and lateral translation in the frontal plane. Although an occasional individual has an essentially straight cervical spine, there is generally a variable degree of lordosis in the cervical spine when it is in the neutral position. About 10 degrees of flexion occur at the atlanto-occipital joint, with further increments being added at the lower joints. In extension, the normal lordosis of the neutral position increases, with about 25 degrees of extension occurring at the atlanto-occipital joint. A slight and variable amount of flexion and extension (up to 15 degrees) also occurs at the atlantoaxial joint. Further increments of extension occur in the lower joints. The full range of extension plus flexion is about 100 degrees in the young adult. Age must be considered, because the range of all cervical spine motions is greater in the child and lesser in the older adult.

The rotational range is approximately 80 degrees to the right and 80 degrees to the left, for a total of 160 degrees. Approximately 50% of this rotational motion occurs at the atlantoaxial articulation, with decreasing increments occurring at joints below this level. The atlanto-occipital joint does not contribute to rotation, but is involved only in flexion and extension.

Because of the oblique plane of the superior and inferior articular facets, lateral bending of the cervical spine is always associated with a certain degree of rotation at all levels. In lateral bending to the right, the upper articular facet of an individual right-sided joint glides downward and posteriorly on the inclined plane of the facet below it, while on the left side the upper facet is gliding upward and forward. This small posterior motion by the right articular process and anterior motion by the left articular process add a rotatory component to lateral bending. A small amount of lateral bending (up to 5 degrees) occurs at the atlantoaxial joint.

Below the axis, intervertebral disks fill each interval between the vertebral bodies. Naturally, the disk follows the same curved contour as does the upper surface of each vertebral body. The disk is thinner at the upcurving right and left margins (the so-called uncovertebral joints of Luschka). It is here that the disk degenerates early, leaving the hyaline cartilage plates intact above and below a fissure, which therefore simulates a diarthrodial joint cavity. As disks are elsewhere, the central, flatter portion of the disk is composed of a peripheral annulus fibrosus and a central nuclear pulposus. In flexion of the cervical spine the anterior part of the disk is compressed and the posterior part is extended. Since in flexion the articular facets of the upper vertebra slide not only upward but also

somewhat forward, the vertebral body also shifts forward to the same degree (anterior translation). In extension there is a comparable posterior translation of the vertebral body.

Ligaments of the Cervical Spine

Ligamentous structures add to the stability of the cervical spine. Space does not permit a complete analysis of all of the ligaments related to this region. Certain ligaments, however, are so unique and important to an understanding of the upper cervical spine that they require discussion.

The right and left alar ligaments extend upward and obliquely laterally from the sides of the apex of the odontoid process (Fig 27–4). Each attaches laterally to the medial aspect of the anterior part of the occipital condyle, thus anchoring the skull to the second cervical vertebra. Each ligament is sturdy and cylindric in

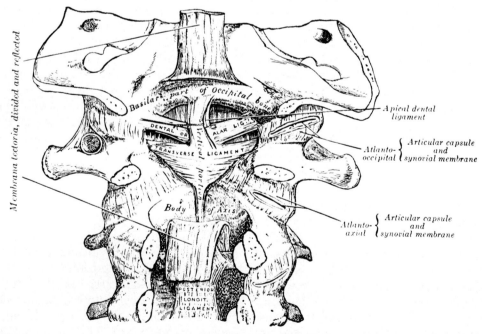

FIG 27–4.
Ligaments of the upper cervical region viewed from behind. The neural arches have been removed. *(From Goss CM (ed):* Gray's Anatomy of the Human Body, *29th American edition. Philadelphia, Lea & Febiger, 1973. Used with permission.)*

form and creates a strong occipitoaxial connection. These two ligaments help check lateral and rotational movement, but play no significant role in restraining flexion and extension movements. After rupture of the transverse ligament of the atlas in dislocations, the alar ligaments become the next structures to resist further forward translation of the atlas upon the axis. When they fail (usually by avulsion from the apex of the odontoid), there is no other significant defense against compression of the cord. There are right and left accessory bands, which extend from the axis to the margin of the foramen magnum, passing behind the transverse ligament of the atlas and functioning somewhat like the alar ligaments.

These accessory ligaments blend with the fibers of both the atlantoaxial and atlanto-occipital joints as they pass beside these capsules.

The transverse ligament of the atlas is a horizontal ligament extending from the medial side of one lateral mass of the atlas to the equivalent site on the opposite lateral mass. As it crosses the central area of the space surrounded by the ring of the atlas, it passes behind the odontoid process, coming into contact with the posterior surface of the process. Here the ligament is flattened and has a fibrocartilaginous surface for apposition against the reciprocal groove on the posterior side of the odontoid process (Fig 27–5). Laterally the ligament is thicker and

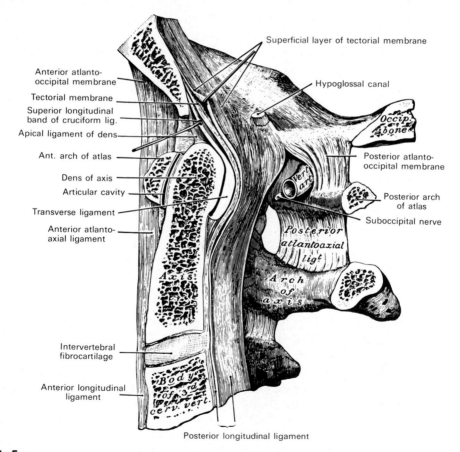

FIG 27–5.
Ligaments of the upper cervical region as seen in midsagittal section. *(From Goss CM (ed):* Gray's Anatomy of the Human Body, *29th American edition. Philadelphia, Lea & Febiger, 1973. Used with permission.)*

more rounded. It is a structure of considerable strength, serving to capture the odontoid process and hold it against the posterior surface of the anterior arch of the atlas, where reciprocal articular facets are found on the apposed surfaces. A joint cavity occurs here as it occurs between the odontoid process and the transverse ligament.

A slender, weak, apical dental ligament ascends from the odontoid tip to the anterior margin of the foramen magnum (see Fig 27–4). Posterior to the apical dental ligament and paralleling it is another vertical bundle of fibers, extending from the odontoid tip to the intracranial aspect of the occipital bone at the anterior margin of the foramen magnum. This bundle has a caudally placed counterpart extending from the odontoid apex downward to attach to the posterior surface of the body of the axis. The cranial and caudal parts of this vertical bundle are in the same plane as, and in part extensions from, the fibers of the transverse ligament. These vertical bands form a cross with the transverse ligament, and all four limbs are collectively called the cruciate ligament of the atlas (see Fig 27–4). The transverse ligament is by far the most important component.

Each of the ligaments on the anterior wall of the vertebral canal is overlaid by the posterior longitudinal ligament, which in the cervical region is broad and obscures the posterior surfaces of all the vertebrae and intervertebral disks (see Fig 27–5). As this ligament ascends behind the axis and atlas, it broadens still more and becomes laminated into a deeper stratum and a superficial stratum. The deeper stratum, called the tectorial membrane, is a strong, flat sheet that lies on the cruciate ligament and extends above through the foramen magnum to attach intracranially to the clivus and adjacent areas of the basilar part of the occipital bone. The superficial stratum is thinner but is not fundamentally distinct, for it

also extends upward to attach to the clivus. The tectorial membrane gives additional support to the atlanto-occipital and atlantoaxial joints, and aids in the prevention of vertical translation or distraction.

Posteriorly the ligamenta flava bridge the gap between the laminae of the neural arches from the axis downward. These are thick membranes of yellow elastic tissue that restrain flexion of the spine. Interspinous ligaments are poorly developed only in the cervical region. The supraspinous ligament does not exist in the cervical region, for its place has been taken by the ligamentum nuchae.

The ligamentum nuchae is a thin septum of collagenous and elastic fibers. When the neck is flexed, its posterior border may be felt to tense under the skin. Its anterior border attaches to the tips of the spinous processes of all the cervical vertebrae and extends in the midline onto the skull to reach the external occipital protuberance. The surfaces of this ligamentous sheet serve as the attachment for a number of muscles.

THE SPINAL CORD

The junction of the medulla and the spinal cord lies approximately at the level of the foramen magnum of the skull. Structures on the neuraxis that mark this junction are the lower limit of the decussation of the pyramids and the upper rootlets of the right and left first cervical nerves. The spinal cord ends below, at, or near the level of the first lumbar intervertebral disk. Below this level the spinal nerve roots, from the second lumbar downward, pass to their respective intervertebral foramina to exit from the vertebral canal. The relatively greater length of the spinal column compared with the spinal cord accounts for the difference in length and the descending obliquity of the ventral and dorsal nerve roots. Only in the cervical region do the spinal nerve roots maintain the nearly horizontal course that they all followed until the third fetal month, when disproportionate growth begins. Even here a slight degree of obliquity develops below the second cervical nerve.

There are eight pairs of cervical nerves. The first is exceptional in that it emerges not through an intervertebral foramen, but through the atlanto-occipital membrane just above the posterior arch of the atlas. The eighth nerve emerges through the foramen between the seventh cervical vertebra and the first thoracic vertebra. Each of the remaining six emerges through an intervertebral foramen formed between cervical vertebrae.

The three white columns of the spinal cord carry the long ascending and descending tracts. In both the ascending sensory pathways and the descending motor tracts there is a laminar pattern of the fibers such that the cervical segment representation is nearest the gray substance, and then moving progressively toward the periphery of the cord, come the thoracic, the lumbar, and the sacral fibers. The latter, therefore, are closest to the surface of the cord (Fig 27–6). This somatotopic laminar pattern of the fibers is seen in the lateral corticospinal tract (motor), the lateral spinothalamic tract (pain and temperature sense), the ventral spinothalamic tract (light touch), and the fibers of the posterior white column (tactile and deep pressure sense, position and motion sense, two-point discrimination, and vibratory sense).

The fibers of the lateral and ventral spinothalamic tracts carry impulses originating in the opposite side of the body (are crossed), while the fibers of the posterior white column are uncrossed. There are two ascending tactile pathways representing any given portion of the trunk or limbs. One of these is uncrossed and in the ipsilateral posterior white column, while the other is crossed and in the con-

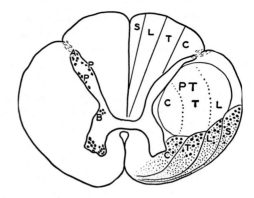

FIG 27–6.
Laminar pattern of the somatotopic arrangement of fiber tracts in the white columns. *(From Goss CM (ed): Gray's Anatomy of the Human Body, 29th American edition. Philadelphia, Lea & Febiger, 1973. Used with permission.)*

tralateral ventral spinothalamic tract. For this reason unilateral spinal cord lesions do not produce a recognizable tactile sensory loss.

The lateral corticospinal tract is also laminated in the same somatotopic fashion as are the sensory pathways. Its fibers terminate ipsilaterally in relation to anterior horn cells. The ventral corticospinal tract, which represents some 10% to 20% of the descending voluntary motor fibers, is uncrossed. Its fibers cross to the opposite side before terminating about anterior horn cells of the cervical and upper thoracic levels only. This ventral motor tract is occasionally absent, and, since it represents only a modest percentage of the descending motor fibers, it is not clinically important in diagnosis of spinal cord injury. The somatotopic laminar patterns of representation of fibers in the long tracts are important clinically because of their localizing value. An encroachment on the spinal cord or other lesion that proceeds from the exterior inward destroys representation of the lower parts of the body first, and, as the damage progresses centrally into the cord, ever higher parts of the body are successively affected. The reverse is also true. A lesion that begins centrally in the cord and expands peripherally produces a sensory or motor loss in higher parts of the body first, with progression caudally, as the lesion expands toward the periphery of the cord.

Throughout the H-shaped gray substance of the cord there is a segmental representation of the muscles supplied by the ventral root of any spinal nerve and an equivalent segmental representation of the sensory fibers that enter over the dorsal root. Thus specific muscle paralysis and dermatomal losses have great localizing value diagnostically. For example, the posture of the upper limbs may be of value in localizing the level of a total transverse injury of the cervical cord. With fracture-dislocations of C6 and C7, the upper limbs are likely to be in a posture with elbows at the sides of the chest, the forearms flexed to 90 degrees, and the hands together in front of the chest. This posture is due to the persisting and unopposed function of the forearm flexors and the arm adductors and medial rotators. With fracture-dislocations of C5 and C6, the upper limbs may assume a posture in which the arms are abducted and the forearms flexed so that the hands lie on the bed alongside the patient's head. This posture is due to the persisting and unopposed function of muscles such as the deltoid and the supraspinatus, the biceps, and the trapezius. With still higher fracture-dislocations, as at C4 and C5, the upper limbs tend to lie flail and at the sides, for now all the roots to the brachial plexus are at or below the cord lesion. If the fracture-dislocation is at the level of C3 and C4, there is also likely to be respiratory paralysis, because the phrenic nerve comes from the third and fourth cervical cord segments, which are probably included in the crushing lesion.

Blood Supply of the Cervical Cord

The entire length of the spinal cord is supplied by longitudinal arteries ar-

ranged as a single median anterior spinal artery and right and left posterolateral arteries. The latter vary greatly, and each is frequently duplicated so that two posterolateral arteries lie on either side of the posterior rootlets of the spinal nerves as these enter the cord. The anterior spinal artery is the largest of the three sets of arteries and forms sulcal branches at fairly regular and close intervals (Fig 27–7). These branches pass alternately to the left and to the right sides. Each sulcal artery supplies the anterior gray horn, the intermediate gray matter, and all but the peripheral or superficial portions of the anterior and lateral white funiculi. At irregular intervals the anterior spinal artery is connected to the posterolateral spinal arteries on either side by slender surface vessels known as the vasa coronaria. It is these anastomosing vessels traversing the surface of the anterior and lateral funiculi that supply the superficial zone of the two white columns. The posterior white column on each side and the associated posterior gray column are supplied by branches of the posterolateral artery.

Occlusion of one sulcal artery is followed by ipsilateral loss of function of the anterior horn cells through approximately one segment of the cord, plus loss of the function of the ventral and lateral spinothalamic tracts and at least the medial (upper limb) portion of the lateral corticospinal tract. Because tactile sensory fibers ascend in both the ipsilateral posterior white column and the contralateral ventral spinothalamic tract, it is evident that tactile sense will not be lost. Thus the major signs of such sulcal artery occlusion in the cervical cord are contralateral loss of pain and temperature sensation below the segment in question, plus ipsilateral upper limb motor loss. Depending on the extent of the damage in the lateral white column, there may be various other deficits such as bladder dysfunction. It must be emphasized that the motor loss is due both to the segmen-

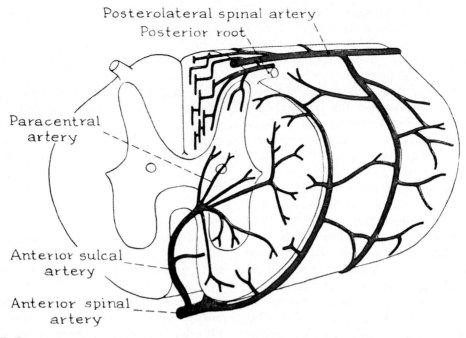

FIG 27–7.
Diagram of the arterial supply of the human spinal cord. *(After Herren and Alexander; from Everett NB:* Functional Neuroanatomy, *ed 6. Philadelphia, Lea & Febiger, 1971. Used with permission.)*

tal damage to anterior horn cells and to destruction of the more medial fibers of the lateral corticospinal tract.

Occlusion of the anterior spinal artery for some of its length is equivalent to obstructing several sulcal arteries, and therefore causes effects such as those described for a single sulcal artery. However, the lesion and signs are bilateral. The three-dimensional pattern of capillaries and smaller arterioles in the gray substance of the cord is a dense plexus with vessels arranged both in the horizontal plane and along the vertical axis. Small vessels in the white substance are arranged more along the longitudinal axis to supply the long ascending and descending tracts. Longitudinal or vertical strain more readily disrupts the plexus of capillaries in the gray substance (with consequent hemorrhage) than it does in the white substance. With compressive forces on the cord, there is not only a horizontal strain at the level of the compression but also a longitudinal strain

above and below this level.[1, 3] This explains why hematomyelia spreads upward and downward beyond the local level of compression.

CERVICAL NERVE ROOTS

Each dorsal root ganglion is found just inside the intervertebral foramen. Immediately beyond and frequently at the level of the ganglion, the ventral and dorsal roots unite to form the spinal nerve, which emerges through the foramen with a sheath of dura mater. This sheath merges imperceptibly into the epineurium, which is the connective tissue sheath that surrounds the entire spinal nerve. The epineurium sends prolongations into the interior of the nerve to invest the various bundles of which the total nerve is composed. These connective tissue investments of the bundles are referred to as the perineurium. Proceeding to a finer level of organization, we find the individual nerve fibers surrounded by a thin reticular connective tissue called the endoneurium. These three levels of connective tissue investments hold the nerve trunk together and give it integrity as a single structure. The ventral and dorsal nerve roots within the dural sheath and spinal canal have no such investments of connective tissue corresponding to the perineurium and epineurium. They possess only the connective tissue prolongations from the pia mater.

At the cervical levels, the ventral and dorsal nerve roots each pierce the dura mater separately, and thus create two small tubes of dura mater that fuse into one as the ventral and dorsal roots fuse together. Each root is surrounded by a sleeve of arachnoid, which is inside the dural sleeve as the roots approach the intervertebral foramen. Thus a short extension of the subarachnoid space briefly follows the ventral and dorsal roots as they penetrate the dural sac (Fig 27–8).

A thin lateral expansion of the pia mater extends like a flange from the midlateral line of the cord and is prolonged by 21 toothlike processes to points of anchorage on the internal aspect of the dural sac. These are the denticulate ligaments, and they serve to tether the spinal cord within the dural tube, resisting lateral and anteroposterior displacements of the cord.

Each spinal nerve promptly divides into anterior and posterior rami. The latter pass backward at once to supply the intrinsic spinal musculature and the overlying skin. The anterior primary rami continue their lateral course, and those from the fifth to the eighth cervical nerves (plus the first thoracic nerve) enter into the formation of the brachial plexus. The epineurium of the anterior primary

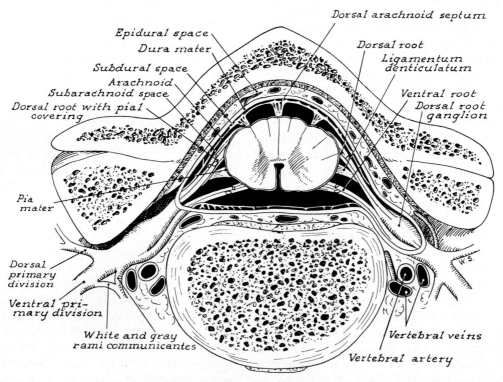

FIG 27–8.
Cross section of spine and cord showing relations of meninges to cord, nerve roots, and intervertebral foramina.
(From Everett NB: Functional Neuroanatomy, *ed 6. Philadelphia, Lea & Febiger, 1971. Used with permission.)*

Color Plates

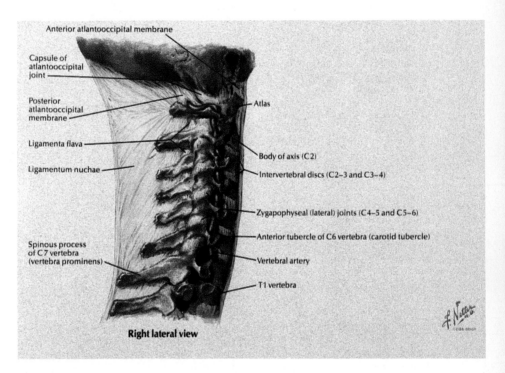

Anterior atlantooccipital membrane

Capsule of
atlantooccipital
joint

Posterior
atlantooccipital
membrane

Ligamenta flava

Ligamentum nuchae

Spinous process
of C7 vertebra
(vertebra prominens)

Atlas

Body of axis (C2)

Intervertebral discs (C2–3 and C3–4)

Zygapophyseal (lateral) joints (C4–5 and C5–6)

Anterior tubercle of C6 vertebra (carotid tubercle)

Vertebral artery

T1 vertebra

Right lateral view

PLATE 7.
External craniocervical ligaments.

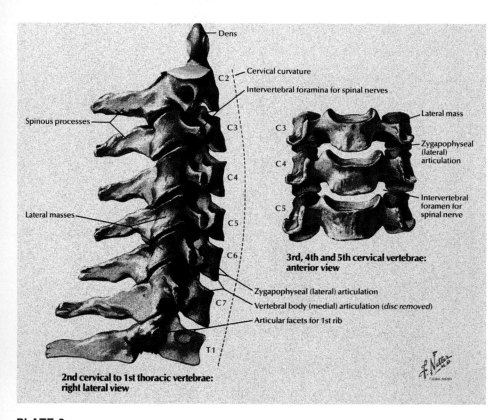

Dens

Cervical curvature

Intervertebral foramina for spinal nerves

C2

Spinous processes

C3

Lateral mass

Zygapophyseal (lateral) articulation

C3

C4

C4

Lateral masses

C5

C5

Intervertebral foramen for spinal nerve

C6

3rd, 4th and 5th cervical vertebrae: anterior view

Zygapophyseal (lateral) articulation

C7

Vertebral body (medial) articulation (*disc removed*)

Articular facets for 1st rib

T1

2nd cervical to 1st thoracic vertebrae: right lateral view

PLATE 8.
Cervical vertebrae.

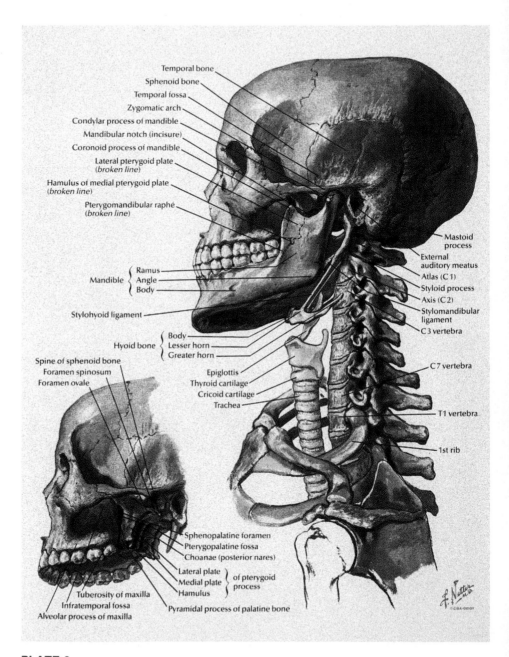

Temporal bone
Sphenoid bone
Temporal fossa
Zygomatic arch
Condylar process of mandible
Mandibular notch (incisure)
Coronoid process of mandible
Lateral pterygoid plate (broken line)
Hamulus of medial pterygoid plate (broken line)
Pterygomandibular raphé (broken line)

Mastoid process
External auditory meatus
Atlas (C 1)
Styloid process
Axis (C 2)
Stylomandibular ligament
C 3 vertebra

Mandible { Ramus
Angle
Body

Stylohyoid ligament

C 7 vertebra

Hyoid bone { Body
Lesser horn
Greater horn

Epiglottis
Thyroid cartilage
Cricoid cartilage
Trachea

T1 vertebra

1st rib

Spine of sphenoid bone
Foramen spinosum
Foramen ovale

Sphenopalatine foramen
Pterygopalatine fossa
Choanae (posterior nares)
Lateral plate } of pterygoid process
Medial plate
Hamulus

Tuberosity of maxilla
Infratemporal fossa
Alveolar process of maxilla

Pyramidal process of palatine bone

PLATE 9.
Bony framework of head and neck.

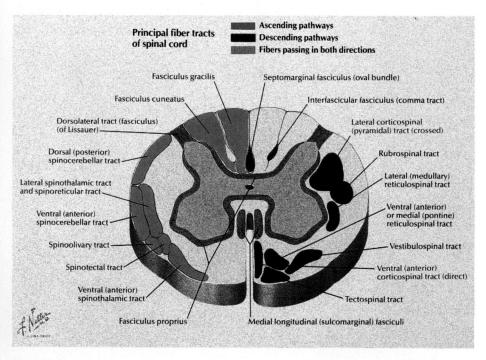

Principal fiber tracts of spinal cord

- Ascending pathways
- Descending pathways
- Fibers passing in both directions

Fasciculus gracilis

Fasciculus cuneatus

Dorsolateral tract (fasciculus) (of Lissauer)

Dorsal (posterior) spinocerebellar tract

Lateral spinothalamic tract and spinoreticular tract

Ventral (anterior) spinocerebellar tract

Spinoolivary tract

Spinotectal tract

Ventral (anterior) spinothalamic tract

Fasciculus proprius

Septomarginal fasciculus (oval bundle)

Interfascicular fasciculus (comma tract)

Lateral corticospinal (pyramidal) tract (crossed)

Rubrospinal tract

Lateral (medullary) reticulospinal tract

Ventral (anterior) or medial (pontine) reticulospinal tract

Vestibulospinal tract

Ventral (anterior) corticospinal tract (direct)

Tectospinal tract

Medial longitudinal (sulcomarginal) fasciculi

PLATE 10.
Spinal cord cross section.

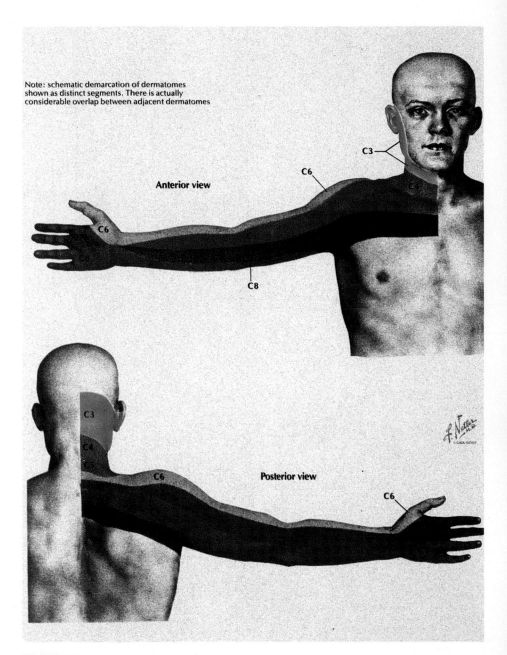

Note: schematic demarcation of dermatomes shown as distinct segments. There is actually considerable overlap between adjacent dermatomes

Anterior view

C3

C6

C6

C6

C8

C3

C4

C6

Posterior view

C6

PLATE 11.
Dermatomes of upper limb.

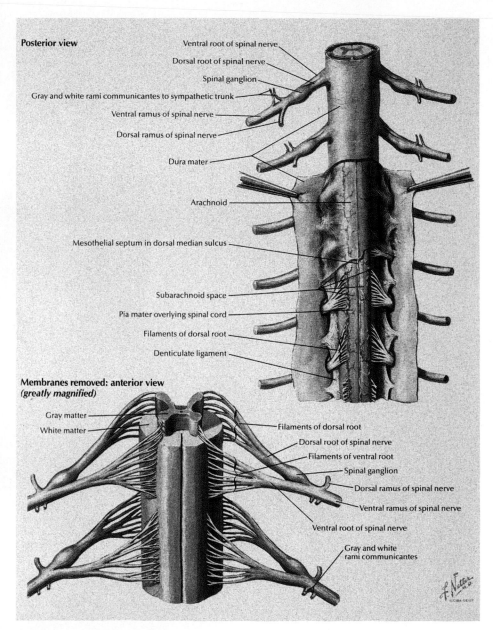

Posterior view

Ventral root of spinal nerve
Dorsal root of spinal nerve
Spinal ganglion
Gray and white rami communicantes to sympathetic trunk
Ventral ramus of spinal nerve
Dorsal ramus of spinal nerve
Dura mater
Arachnoid
Mesothelial septum in dorsal median sulcus
Subarachnoid space
Pia mater overlying spinal cord
Filaments of dorsal root
Denticulate ligament

Membranes removed: anterior view
(greatly magnified)

Gray matter
White matter
Filaments of dorsal root
Dorsal root of spinal nerve
Filaments of ventral root
Spinal ganglion
Dorsal ramus of spinal nerve
Ventral ramus of spinal nerve
Ventral root of spinal nerve
Gray and white rami communicantes

PLATE 12.
Spinal membranes and nerve roots.

rami of the cervical spinal nerves is anchored to the periosteum of the transverse processes. This is especially so at the levels of the fourth, fifth, and sixth cervical nerves.[5] Lateral traction on the nerves is thereby resisted rather than being transmitted along the nerve and its ventral and dorsal roots to the spinal cord.

A further resistance to lateral traction on the nerves is created by the funnel-shaped outpouchings of the dura mater at each level of exit of a nerve root. Under lateral traction, these funnels of dura mater impact into the inner aspect of the intervertebral foramen, and, like a cork in a bottle, offer resistance to further lateral displacement of the nerve.[5] By the two mechanisms cited, the individual nerve fibers of the roots are prevented from having to bear the stress of moderate traction on the brachial plexus. Were it not for these two protective systems, the weakest point in the sequence of spinal cord, nerve roots, and spinal nerve would be torn asunder by traction. This weakest point is at the junction with the spinal cord of the ventral and dorsal roots. Avulsions do occur here when the protective arrangements fail because of excessive traction or injuries to the cervical spine. In this circumstance, the sensory fibers are disrupted on the central side of the dorsal root ganglion cell. Avulsion of the rootlets from the cord, at the level of the first thoracic nerve, interrupts the preganglionic sympathetic fibers destined for the supply of the eye, and the ocular portion of a Horner's syndrome results.

Because of the direction of the nerves in the brachial plexus, downward traction on the arm or shoulder, plus excessive lateral bending of the neck to the opposite side, or severe hyperextension, is likely to stretch the fibers of the fifth and sixth cervical nerves. Disruption of these nerve roots of the brachial plexus would manifest itself primarily by paresis of the muscles supplied by the suprascapular, deltoid, musculocutaneous, and long thoracic nerves. Fiber damage may occur in the roots as an upper radiculopathy or in the superior portion of the trunk as a plexopathy. Minimal damage or strain in fibers of the fifth and sixth nerves may give transitory episodes of burning paresthesia and paresis in the upper limb.[2]

REFERENCES

1. Gosch HH, Gooding E, Schneider RC: Cervical spinal cord hemorrhages in experimental head injuries. *J Neurosurg* 1970; 33:640.

2. Robertson WC, Eichman PL, Clancy WG: Upper trunk brachial plexopathy in football players. *JAMA* 1979; 241:1480.

3. Schneider RC, Cherry G, Pantek H: The syndrome of acute central cervical spinal cord injury. *J Neurosurg* 1954; 11:546.

4. Steel HH: Anatomical and mechanical considerations of the atlanto-axial articulations. *J Bone Joint Surg [Am]* 1968; 50A:1481.

5. Sunderland S: Meningeal-neural relations in the intervertebral foramen. *J Neurosurg* 1974; 40:756.

6. Goss CM (ed): *Gray's Anatomy of the Human Body*, 29th American edition. Philadelphia, Lea & Febiger, 1973.

7. Everett NB: *Functional Neuroanatomy*, ed 6. Philadelphia, Lea & Febiger, 1971.

CHAPTER 28

Radiographic Evaluation of the Cervical Spine and Related Structures

Helene Pavlov, M.D.

The purpose of the radiographic examination of a patient with possible head and neck injuries is to rapidly obtain diagnostic radiographs without further injury. After a brief preliminary clinical examination to determine the vital signs, neurologic status, and possible sites of injury, the radiologic examination is started. Whenever there is a possible cervical spine injury initial radiographs are obtained without moving the patient from the litter. Radiographs taken on the litter are rarely as good as those done on the radiographic table, but they are usually sufficient to diagnose an unstable cervical spine fracture. An anteroposterior and a horizontal cross-table lateral view of the cervical spine, with use of grid cassettes, can demonstrate a fracture or fracture-dislocation. The examination is best performed in the x-ray department with a machine that minimizes the radiographic distortion produced by involuntary patient movement instead of with a portable machine. The technologist must be alerted not to turn the patient's head during the initial examination, because any manipulation of the head and neck in the presence of an unstable cervical spine fracture could damage the spinal cord and result in paralysis or death. Not until an unstable fracture is excluded, or,

if present, properly braced, should the patient be transferred from the litter to the radiographic or computed tomographic (CT) table for additional studies. The vital signs and neurologic status must be monitored continuously, and no patient, especially an unconscious one, should ever be left unattended during the radiologic examination.

RADIOGRAPHIC TECHNIQUES AND ANATOMY

The radiographic examination and interpretation of the cervical spine can be challenging.

As with any body part, the routine radiologic examination requires at least two projections taken at right angles to each other, the anteroposterior (AP) and the lateral views. For the cervical spine, the complete AP study requires two films. The complete lateral study requires one film and is the most important view. Additional plain film examination of the cervical spine includes oblique and pillar views and mobility studies that can be performed after an unstable fracture is excluded. Tomography, fluoroscopy, and CT provide further detail and information about the vertebrae and spinal canal.

The spinal cord and nerve roots are encased by the cervical spine, and are examined by myelography in combination with CT, MRI, or both.

Plain Films

The normal anatomic relationship of the cervical vertebrae must be recognized in order to interpret the abnormal.

The AP view of the cervical spine requires two films. The lower cervical spine, C3 through C7, is demonstrated on the routine view. This view is obtained with the patient sitting, or, with a critically injured patient, with the patient supine on the litter. The atlas and axis are visualized on an open mouth view (Fig 28–1, A and B), usually obtained with the patient supine. On the AP view of the lower cervical spine (Fig 28–1, C), the following structures are examined for integrity and anatomic alignment: the joint of Luschka, the superior and inferior end plates of the vertebrae, the pedicles, and the spinous processes. There is a symmetric undulation of the lateral cortical margins of the articular masses. The tracheal air shadow is midline. On the open mouth view (Fig 28–1, D), the odontoid process is equidistant from the lateral masses of C1, and the lateral masses of C1 and C2 are aligned. Occasionally the posterior arch of C1 projects over the odontoid process, simulating a fracture at the base of the dens. This is known as a Mach effect.[15]

The lateral view of the spine is the most important film in the cervical examination. Optimally, this view is obtained with the patient sitting or standing to maximize the effect of gravity on vertebral body alignment. However, in the critically injured patient with possible cervical spine or spinal cord damage, the lateral view is obtained without moving the patient from the litter by placing the cassette vertically alongside the patient's neck and using a cross-table horizontal

roentgenographic beam, perpendicular to the cassette (Fig 28–2, A). The entire spine, from C1 to C7, should be included on the lateral view. Sometimes the odontoid process is obscured by the mastoid process and the mandible, and C7 (and occasionally C6) may be obscured by the shoulder girdle. The odontoid process can be visualized by tomography or by slightly tilting the head, if an unstable fracture has been excluded. The lower cervical area can be demonstrated by having the shoulders pulled out of the way. If the patient is supine and not fully conscious, someone can gently pull on the patient's arms. If the lower cervical vertebrae are still not demonstrated, a swimmer's view can be obtained. A swimmer's view is a horizontal cross-table view obtained with the patient supine and the arm closest to the cassette raised over the patient's head, simulating a swimming position. The central ray is directed through the shoulder girdle (Fig 28–2, B). If these attempts fail, tomography or CT may be used.

On the lateral view, the prevertebral soft tissues should be examined (Fig 28–2, C). If the lateral cervical spine film is overexposed and only the bones are detailed, the film must be repeated with proper technique factors to delineate the soft tissues. The normal prevertebral soft tissues have specific measurement.[17] The soft tissues at the level of C3 are normally less than one half the AP width of the C3 vertebral body.[38] At the C6 level, the average width of the soft tissues is approximately equal to the AP width of the C6 vertebral body.

On the lateral view, obtained with the patient erect, there is a gentle lordosis to the normal cervical spine. Regardless of the patient's position, the anterior and posterior borders of the vertebral bodies, the posterior cortices of the lateral masses, and the spinolaminar lines of C2 through C7 align to form four uninterrupted parallel lines. The posterior arch

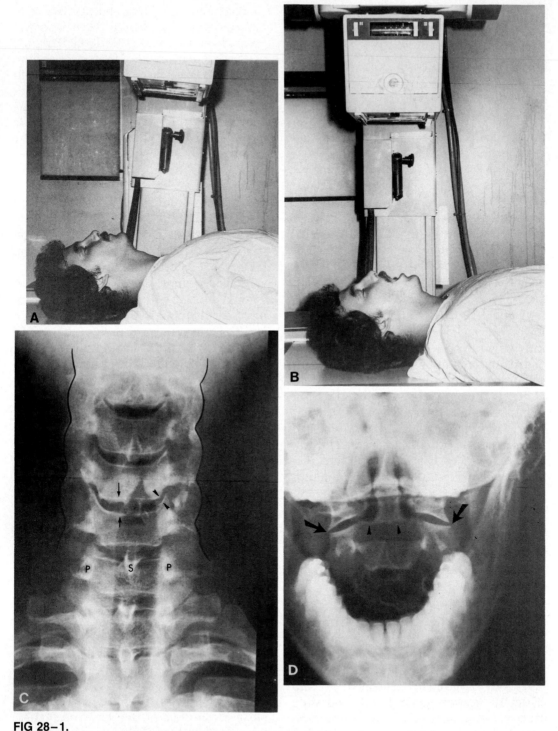

FIG 28–1.
A, an AP view of the cervical spine is obtained with the roentgenographic tube (central ray) angled 5 to 10 degrees cephalad. The cassette is placed behind the patient's neck. The patient may be sitting or supine. **B,** an open mouth view is obtained with the patient supine and the cassette behind the head and neck. The central ray is perpendicular to the cassette and directed through the open mouth. This view may be facilitated in a conscious

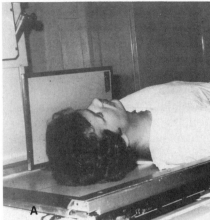

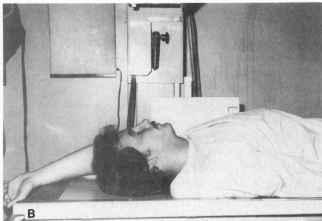

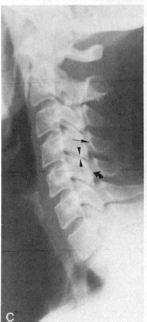

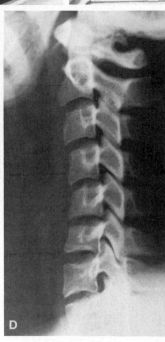

FIG 28–2.
A, a horizontal cross-table lateral view of the cervical spine is the most important film in the examination of an acutely injured patient. The central ray is perpendicular to a vertical cassette, which is placed alongside the patient's neck. **B,** the swimmer's view is obtained with the patient supine. The arm closest to the cassette is raised above the head. This view demonstrates the lower cervical vertebrae through the shoulder girdle. **C,** on the lateral view of the cervical spine, C1 through C7 should be visualized. Gentle lordotic curved lines are formed by the anterior cortical margins of the vertebral bodies, the posterior cortical margins of the articular processes *(short arrow),* and also the spinolaminar lines *(arrow).* The intervertebral disk spaces should be the same height anteriorly to posteriorly and equal in height at each level. The superior and inferior articular facets of the interfacetal joints should be parallel to each other *(arrowheads).* The vertebral body heights are equal. The spinous processes should be almost parallel to each other, and the interspinous distances should be equal. The ADI distance between lines must be less than 3 mm, even in flexion. The prevertebral soft tissues are normal. **D,** the cervical lordosis may be straightened or reversed by spasm or voluntary guarding, and it is a normal variant in 20% of the population. When intact, the reversal should be gradual, and the alignment of the intervertebral spaces, interfacetal joints, and spinous processes is normal. *(D, Courtesy of Jay W. MacMoran, M.D., Director, Department of Radiology, Germantown Hospital, Philadelphia, Penn.)*

---

patient by having the patient chew during the exposure so the mandible is blurred and does not obscure the odontoid process. **C,** an AP view of the cervical spine delineating C3 through C7. The lateral margins of the lateral masses form a gentle undulating line bilaterally. The joints of Luschka *(arrowheads),* the spinous processes *(S),* the vertebral body end plates *(arrows),* the intervertebral disk spaces, and the pedicles *(P)* are identified at each level. The tracheal air shadow is midline. **D,** the atlas and axis are identified on the open mouth view. The lateral margins of the articular masses of C1 and C2 should be in alignment *(arrows).* The odontoid process is equidistant from the lateral masses of C1. Occasionally the posterior arch of C1 overlaps the odontoid process simulating a horizontal fracture. This is known as a Mach effect *(arrowheads).*

of C1 is normally smaller than the rest. The spinous processes converge slightly toward a hypothetic posterior point. The interspinous distances are equidistant at each level, except between C2 and C3, where the distance is greater. The intervertebral disk spaces are uniform in height from anterior to posterior, and the disk spaces are of equal height at each level, except at C2–C3, where they are greater. The interfacetal joints are angled 35 degrees caudally from the vertical plane, and the superior and inferior facets of each joint are parallel to each other. Each vertebral body is equal in vertical height, with the exception of C4, C5, or C6, which on occasion may be slightly smaller. The atlantodens interval (ADI),

the distance between the posterior surface of the anterior arch of C1 and the anterior aspect of the odontoid, normally measures less than 3 mm in adults, regardless of flexion or extension.[11, 18]

The roentgen pattern of the cervical spine in the lateral view can be affected by numerous factors. The cervical lordosis can be reversed or straightened by supine positioning, muscular spasm, voluntary guarding, ligamentous disruption, a fracture, or dislocation. Approximately 20% of the population normally have a straight or kyphotic spine. Twenty degrees of neck flexion will straighten the cervical spine (Fig 28–2, D).[38]

Lateral views of the cervical spine occasionally are inadvertently obtained

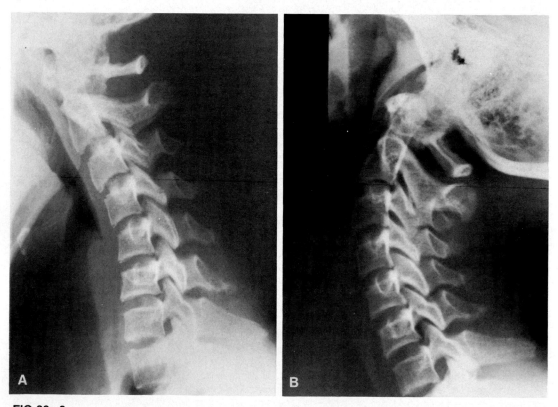

FIG 28–3.
Mobility studies of the cervical spine are lateral views obtained in maximum voluntary flexion and extension. They are useful for determination of ligamentous disruption. **A,** in flexion the cervical lordosis is reversed. Each vertebral body moves slightly anteriorly on the vertebra below. The interspinous distance and the posterior aspect of the interfacetal joints are increased. These changes are present at all levels, but are greatest in the upper segments. **B,** in extension, the cervical lordosis is increased and the changes that occur in flexion are reversed.

with the head or the body slightly rotated. Rotation produces a lack of superimposition of the posterior margins of the vertebral bodies and lateral masses. Rotation of the head or of the body produces a gradual increasing lack of superimposition, which is normal when the lack of superimposition changes gradually at each level.[16]

Mobility studies are lateral views performed with the patient erect and in maximum voluntary flexion and extension. Mobility studies help document and localize ligamentous disruption.[10, 16, 26, 37] In flexion, there is an increase in the intraspinous distances, widening of the posterior aspect of the interfacetal joints and intervertebral disk spaces, and nar-

rowing of the anterior aspect of the intervertebral disk spaces (Fig 28–3, A). The vertebrae may normally slide anteriorly up to 2 mm on the subjacent vertebrae. All these findings gradually increase throughout the cervical spine but are more extreme superiorily. These changes are reduced in extension (Fig 28–3, B).[16] Flexion and extension views must not be performed after trauma until the initial radiographs have been reviewed and an unstable fracture excluded.

Oblique views are important for a complete trauma series. Oblique views demonstrate the interfacetal joints, the lamina, the intravertebral foramina, the pedicles, and the lateral masses (Fig 28–4). The lateral elements of the supe-

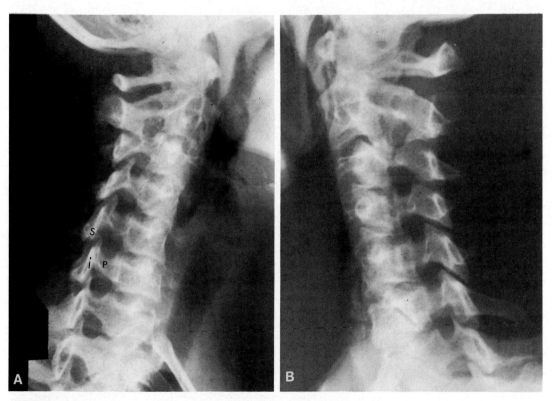

FIG 28–4.
Oblique views of the cervical spine demonstrating the interfacetal joints. **A,** left posterior oblique view demonstrates the right side. The superior facet *(S)* should be lateral to the inferior facet *(i).* The pedicles *(P)* connect the vertebral body to the articular mass and form the border of the intervertebral foramen. The intervertebral foramen should be patent at each level. The laminae are seen en face as corticated oval structures. Each lamina, as each articular process, should be lateral to that of the subjacent vertebra. **B,** the configuration of the articular masses, laminae, pedicles, foramen, and interfacetal joints is slightly different because of a different degree of obliquity.

rior vertebrae are slightly lateral to that of the subjacent vertebrae. The radiographic appearance of these structures depends on the degree of obliquity. The oblique views are usually obtained with the patient sitting, but can be obtained with the patient on the litter by placing the film cassette alongside the neck and angling the central ray 45 degrees toward the cassette from the opposite side of the patient (Fig 28–5).[15]

Pillar views are designed to examine the lateral masses. They are obtained with the patient supine, and with the chin rotated to the direction opposite the side of suspected injury. This position is not recommended for a patient who might have an unstable fracture (Fig 28–6). The tube is angled caudally and centered 2 cm from midline toward the side of interest.[38]

Fluoroscopy and Tomography

The use of fluoroscopy, tomography, or CT is occasionally required in the examination of the cervical spine. Fluoroscopy is an excellent method of obtaining a specific view under direct visual control.

Tomography is useful to demonstrate a part of a vertebra that is otherwise superimposed by an adjacent vertebra. To-mography can be performed in the AP, lateral, oblique, or pillar view.

The CT examination displays the vertebrae in cross section and is especially helpful in determining the integrity of the lamina, pedicles, spinal canal, and spinal cord.[8, 21, 32] CT examination of the cervical spine is discussed in a separate chapter.

Myelography, and CT and MRI

The central nervous system in the region of the cervical spine consists of the spinal cord and nerve roots. These structures are not seen on plain radiographic studies, and require contrast enhancement for radiographic demonstration. A cervical myelogram demonstrates the subarachnoid space, the spinal cord, and the roots of the spinal nerves. A myelogram involves the subarachnoid injection of a radiopaque contrast agent. The contrast can be maneuvered to surround the cord and the nerve roots by adjusting the patient's position (Fig 28–7).[29] A CT examination after a myelogram is extremely helpful in evaluating the spinal cord and spinal canal contents. MRI is a noninvasive technique that does not use X rays to demonstrate the central nervous system structures. CT following myelography

FIG 28–5.
An oblique view can be obtained with the patient supine on the litter, if necessary, by angling the tube 45 degrees from one side of the patient toward a cassette placed on the litter either under or alongside the neck. Both right and left oblique views should be obtained.

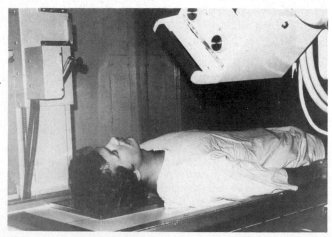

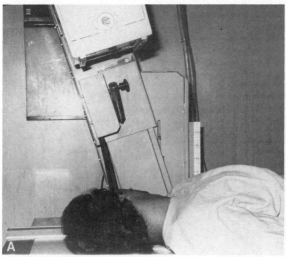

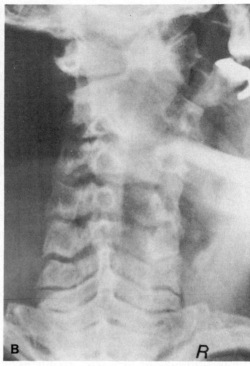

FIG 28–6.

A, pillar views (Weir) are obtained with the patient supine and the head rotated to the opposite side of interest. The head rotation is necessary to eliminate superimposition of the mandible and face on the lateral masses. The central ray is moved 2 cm off midline toward the side of interest and angled 35 degrees caudad. This is an important view but must not be obtained until it has been established that the head can be rotated safely. **B,** pillar view demonstrating the articular masses.

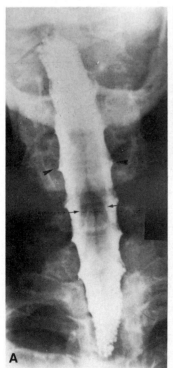

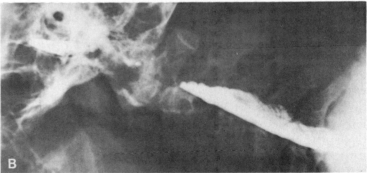

FIG 28–7.

A, AP view of a normal cervical myelogram. The spinal cord *(arrows)* and nerve roots *(arrowheads)* are lucent and surrounded by the white contrast material. **B,** a cross-table lateral view of a normal cervical myelogram, obtained with the patient prone. The radiopaque contrast is adjacent to the posterior aspect of the cervical vertebrae; the cord is dorsal.

and MRI examination of the spinal cord and nerve roots are discussed in another chapter.

CERVICAL SPINE STENOSIS

Cervical spinal stenosis has been determined to be an etiologic factor of transient neurologic symptoms in athletes, specifically, transient cervical spinal neurapraxia. This entity is the sudden sensory loss (numbness, burning, tingling, or parathesias [or all of these]) that may be associated with motor symptoms (weakness or complete paralysis, or both) occurring in both arms or both legs. Symptoms result from hyperflexion, hyperextension, or axial load injuries and last from a few seconds to 36 hours, followed by complete recovery.[36]

Typically, the cervical spinal canal dimension is determined radiographically on the lateral view by measuring the distance from the posterior aspect of the vertebral body at the midpoint to the nearest point of the spinolaminar line.[39] This direct measurement can be misleading because of image magnification. Magnification is produced by two factors: (1) a decrease in the distance between the x-ray tube and the film cassette, the target distance, that is, portable film technique; and (2) an increase in the distance between the cervical spine and the film cassette, that is, a patient with a large shoulder girth. Hence, magnification can be responsible for the spinal canal measurement of a patient with broad shoulders to be in the normal range even though the patient actually has a narrow canal.

The ratio method was devised to determine accurate cervical spinal canal determination without the effects of magnification.[24, 36] The ratio method for determining the spinal canal measurement is the sagittal diameter of the spinal canal, as previously described, divided by the sagittal diameter of the corre-

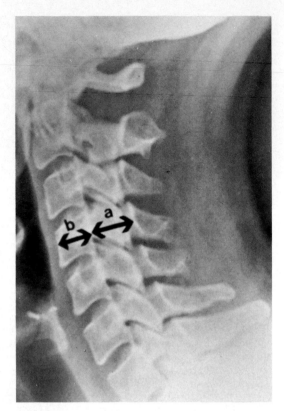

FIG 28–8.
The spinal canal/vertebral body ratio to evaluate the spinal canal dimension is determined on the lateral view. The sagittal canal dimension *(a)* is determined from the midpoint of the posterior vertebral body surface to the nearest point of the corresponding spinolaminar line. The sagittal vertebral body dimension *(b)* is determined at the midbody level. The ratio is a:b. Normally there is a 1:1 relationship.

sponding vertebral body, measured at its midpoint (Fig 28–8). Magnification variables caused by differences in target distance, object to film distance, or body type are eliminated because the sagittal diameter of the spinal canal and that of the vertebral body are in the same anatomic plane.

With use of the ratio method, there is normally a 1:1 relationship between the sagittal diameter of the spinal canal and that of the vertebral body. An average spinal canal/vertebral body ratio of C3–C6 at less than 0.80 indicates a developmentally narrow canal.

FRACTURES AND INJURIES TO THE CERVICAL SPINE

In examining roentgenograms of the cervical spine for trauma, it is important to remember to examine the soft tissues in addition to the bones. On the lateral view, a localized or generalized increase in the prevertebral soft tissues after injury indicates a hematoma or edema. On the AP view, soft tissue swelling is evident by deviation of the tracheal air shadow from the midline (Fig 28–9). In addition to confirming a serious injury and localizing the area of abnormality, soft tissue swelling, in and of itself, can be life threatening. Soft tissue swelling can rapidly obstruct the airway and must not be ignored. If the soft tissues cannot be evaluated on a lateral view of the cervical spine, the radiograph should be repeated.

Cervical spine injuries can be stable or unstable. A stable injury is one in which additional spinal cord or nerve root damage is not anticipated with gentle spine movement. An unstable fracture is one in which there is significant ligamentous damage, and any movement of the spine may further compromise the neurologic status by injuring the nerve roots or the spinal cord or both.[2, 12, 16] Roentgenograms must be evaluated for signs of ligamentous instability in addition to fracture or dislocation (or both).

Radiographically, ligamentous injury and bony fractures and dislocations are evident by a change in the anatomic configuration and alignment. The cervical spine can be divided into anterior and posterior elements. The anterior elements include the vertebral body, intervertebral disks, and the anterior and posterior longitudinal ligaments. The posterior elements include the lamina and pedicles of the vertebral arch, spinous process, the

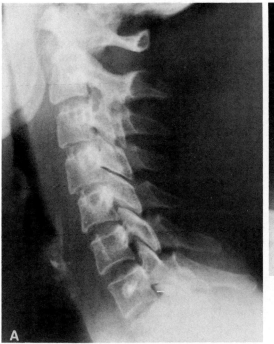

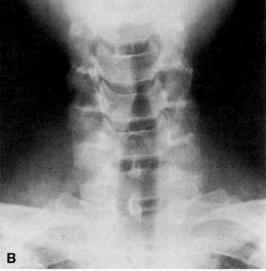

FIG 28–9.
A, the prevertebral soft tissues are swollen anterior to the entire upper cervical spine. **B,** the tracheal air shadow is displaced to the left by a hematoma on the right.

capsule of the interfacetal joints, the ligamentum flavum, and the intraspinous and supraspinous ligaments. Injury to either the anterior or posterior elements is evidenced by impaction or narrowing due to compressive forces, and by separation or widening due to distracting forces. Ligamentous injuries, avulsions, fractures, and dislocations vary according to the position of the cervical spine and the strength and direction of the forces as they are transmitted through its segments. The lower cervical spine (C3 through C7) and the upper cervical spine, the atlas and the axis (C1–C2), are discussed separately.

Lower Cervical Spine

Injuries to the lower cervical spine are divided into three categories: (1) ligamentous injuries, (2) fractures, and (3) dislocations.

Ligamentous Injuries.—Ligamentous injuries are diagnosed indirectly by the malalignment of the osseous structures. An anterior subluxation[7, 16, 19, 37] is the mildest injury that has radiographic manifestations; it is diagnosed on the lateral view. The radiographic findings are localized to one or two levels and include a localized reversal of the normal cervical lordosis, increase in the intraspinous distance or fanning, widening of the intervertebral disk space posteriorly, and loss of parallelism at the interfacetal joints (Fig 28–10, A). All of these findings are more severe when the cervical spine is flexed; flexion views are recommended whenever this injury is clinically suspected and the initial films are normal or inconclusive. The posterior ligaments, interfacetal joint capsule, and occasionally even the posterior aspect of the disk are disrupted; however, the major portion of the disk and the anterior spinous ligament remains intact. When there is disruption of the intervertebral disk and

posterior longitudinal ligament, anterior angulation and anterior translation of the superior vertebrae can occur (Fig 28–10, B).

Fractures.—Fractures of the lower cervical spine are divided into fractures of the vertebral body, isolated or in combination with fractures of the posterior neural elements.

The mildest vertebral body fracture is the wedge fracture.[16, 37] This fracture is diagnosed on the lateral view by a decrease in anterior height of the vertebral body (Fig 28–11). Anterior wedging is due to varying combinations of flexion and axial compression. Pure axial compression produces a comminuted vertebral body fracture with loss of vertebral body stature (Fig 28–12).[25] An isolated wedge or compression fracture of the vertebral body is a stable injury if the anterior longitudinal ligament and the intervertebral disk remain intact. The posterior longitudinal ligament and the posterior ligamentous complex may be lax or disrupted. Disruption or laxity of the posterior ligamentous complex is diagnosed on the lateral view by the following localized changes: "fanning" (an increase in the intraspinous distance), loss of parallelism of the facet joints, and, occasionally, mild anterior subluxation of the involved vertebrae. Lateral views obtained in flexion are helpful to document the extent of posterior ligamentous injury because all of these findings are accentuated in flexion. However, there are several considerations before ordering flexion views: (1) they must not be done if the patient is unconscious; (2) an unstable fracture must be eliminated, requiring excluding a sagittal fracture on the AP view or posterior displacement of the posterior vertebral body fragment, or both. If either of these conditions exists, flexion views are contraindicated.

Occasionally a separate triangular fragment may be identified on the lateral

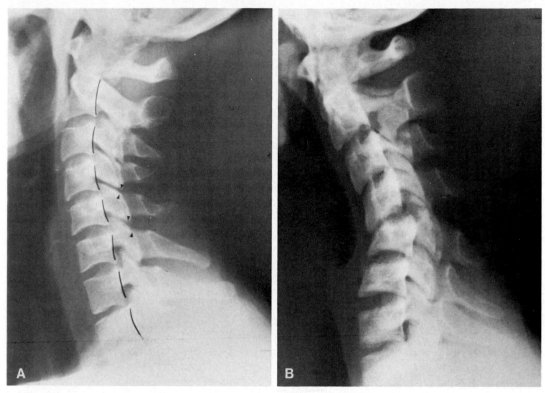

FIG 28–10.
A, an anterior subluxation may be roentgenographically subtle. Interruption of the cervical lordosis at C5–C6, widening of the interspinous distance (fanning), and loss of parallelism of the posterior aspect of the interfacetal joint (lower set of *arrowheads*) are demonstrated. **B,** a more severe anterior subluxation is demonstrated in this patient, in whom, in addition to fanning, there is anterior translation of C4 on C5 and acute angulation of the spine. All of these findings are accentuated in flexion.

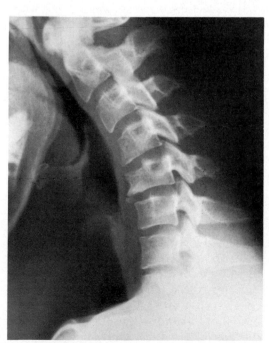

FIG 28–11.
A wedge fracture of C5 with decreased anterior vertebral body height involving both the superior and inferior borders. Localized increased density anteriorly and inferiorly and a small chip fracture are seen. The interspinous distances are normal in flexion, indicating an intact posterior ligamentous complex.

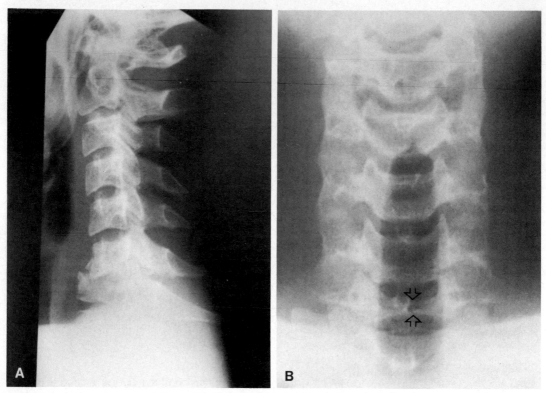

FIG 28–12.
A, a compression fracture of C7 in which only the vertebral body is involved. The superior end plate is fractured and the intervertebral disk space is narrowed. The posterior ligamentous complex is intact, so there is no fanning. **B,** on the AP view, this compression fracture is demonstrated by loss of height of the involved vertebrae *(arrows).* The margins of the lateral masses are normal. This patient was injured during a football game and continued to play. One month later he escorted his brother, who had a broken arm, to the emergency room. While there he mentioned to the doctor that his neck had ached for the past month, and these films were obtained.

view at the anteroinferior corner of the vertebral body. This anteroinferior corner fracture fragment has been termed a "teardrop" because the fragment resembled the tear rolling down the cheek of a patient who had sustained a catastrophic neck injury and was quadriplegic.[22, 27] In the lower cervical spine there are two distinct fracture patterns associated with an anteroinferior triangular "teardrop" fracture fragment, each with a specific neurologic sequela; one is an isolated fracture pattern and the other is a three-part, two-plane fracture pattern. On the lateral view, both fracture patterns have a triangular fracture fragment at the antero-inferior corner of the vertebral body, combined with various degrees of inter-

vertebral disk space narrowing, posterior displacement of the posterior vertebral body fragment, kyphotic angulation at the fracture level, "fanning," and widening of the facet joint. An AP view, in addition to the lateral view, is necessary to distinguish these two injury patterns. The isolated fracture pattern has a normal frontal view and is a stable injury. This injury is similar to a wedge fracture. The patient may experience transient neurologic sequelae of pain or paresthesias, or both, but rarely has permanent neurologic sequelae.

The three-part, two-plane injury[35] consists of a sagittal fracture of the vertebral body combined with fracture(s) of the posterior neural arch and disruption

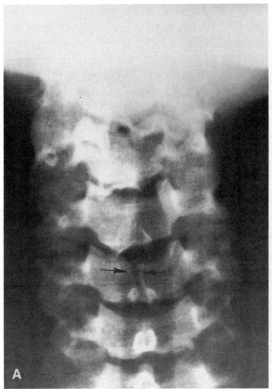

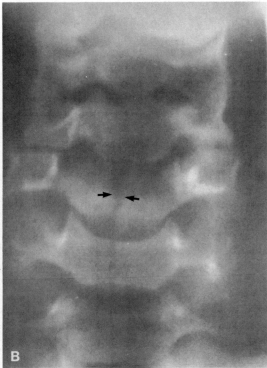

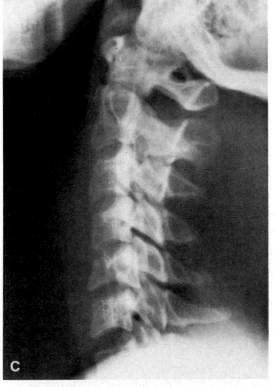

FIG 28–13.

A, a three-part, two-plane fracture of C5 involving the vertebral body and posterior neural arch. On the AP view, a vertical fracture *(arrows)* through the vertebral body is demonstrated. The lateral mass margins are interrupted, indicating a posterior neural arch fracture. **B,** on an AP tomogram, the lateral displacement of the lateral masses, disruption of the undulating curves of the lateral margins, widening of the *interpedicular* distance, and a vertical fracture of the vertebral body are better demonstrated. **C,** on the lateral view, there is a comminuted fracture through the vertebral body involving both the inferior and superior end plates and creating a triangular anterior corner fracture fragment. The posterior fracture fragment is posteriorly displaced without tilting. The interfacetal joint at C5–C6 is widened. There is no fanning. *(Courtesy of Jay W. MacMoran, M.D., Director Department of Radiology, Germantown Hospital, Philadelphia, Penn.)*

of the posterior ligamentous complex, anterior and posterior longitudinal ligaments, and the intervertebral disk. This injury has been referred to in the literature as a flexion "teardrop" or a burst fracture, or both, and the terms are often used interchangeably.[22] The sagittal vertebral body fracture distinguishes this injury from the isolated anteroinferior corner fracture pattern. The sagittal fracture is identified on the AP view as a longitudinal vertical black fracture line extending through the involved vertebral body. Air in the larynx can simulate a sagittal

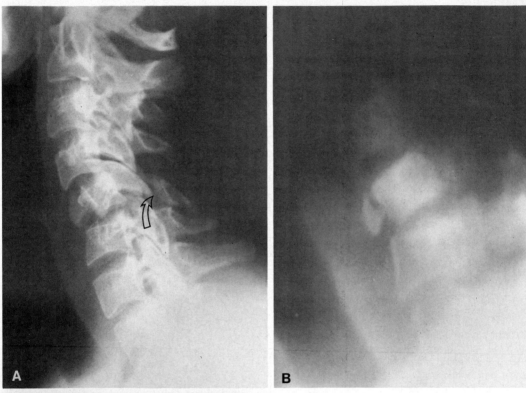

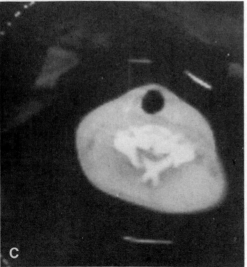

FIG 28–14.
A, a three-part, two-plane fracture of C5. There is a triangular anteroinferior corner fracture. The posterior vertebral fracture fragment is posteriorly displaced and tilted. There is C5–C6 intervertebral disk space narrowing. There is fanning of the C4–C5 spinous processes because of disruption of the posterior ligamentous complex. This patient also has associated fractures of the lamina of C5 *(curved arrow).* **B,** a tomogram of C5 demonstrating the tear-shaped anteroinferior corner fracture fragment. **C,** CT section demonstrates the fracture in cross section. The severe encroachment of the spinal canal from both anterior and posterior fracture fragments is evident.

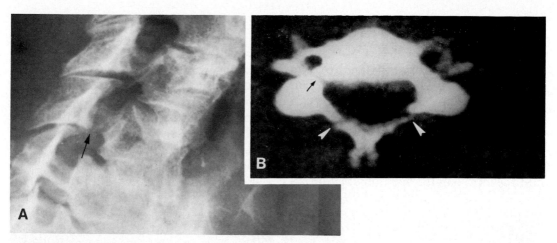

FIG 28–15.
A, a linear nondisplaced pillar fracture *(arrow).* These fractures may be difficult to identify, and usually require multiple oblique views at various degrees of obliquity. **B,** a CT scan demonstrating the nondisplaced pillar fracture *(arrow)* and bilateral lamina fractures *(arrowheads).* The spinal canal integrity is intact.

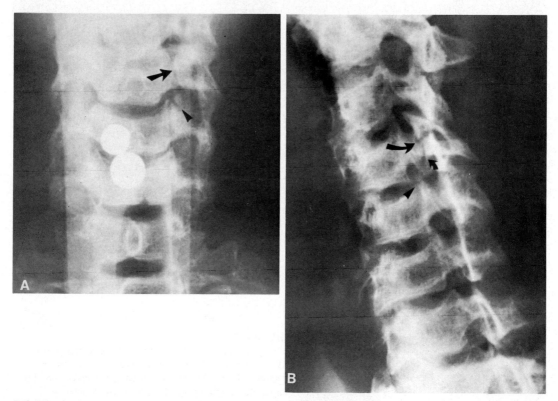

FIG 28–16.
A, AP view of the cervical vertebrae through a cervical collar, demonstrating a fracture of the lateral mass of C4 *(arrow).* The uncinate process of C5 *(arrowhead)* is also fractured. **B,** oblique view demonstrating the position of the fracture fragments of the comminuted lateral mass *(arrows).* The displacement of fracture fragments into the intervertebral foramen *(arrowhead)* may be responsible for nerve root symptoms.

vertebral body fracture, and an AP tomogram or a CT examination may be required to differentiate a sagittal vertebral body fracture from a pseudofracture. The fractures of the posterior neural arch can be suspected on the AP view by the lateral displacement of one or both lateral masses, interruption of the symmetric lateral mass margins, and localized widening of the interpedicular distances. These findings are usually more obvious on an AP tomogram or a CT examination than on the plain AP roentgenogram (Figs 28–13 and 28–14). Spinal cord encroachment by posterior displacement of the posterior vertebral body fracture fragment is best identified on the CT examination.[8, 32] When a sagittal vertebral body fracture or posterior neural arch fractures are present or suspected on the initial radiographic examination, flexion and extension views are contraindicated. The

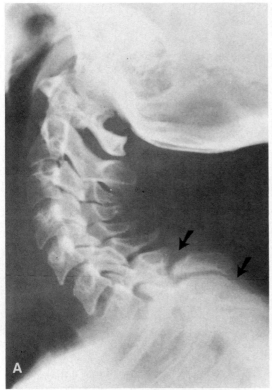

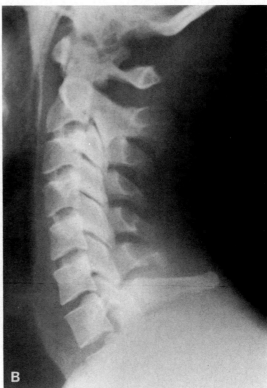

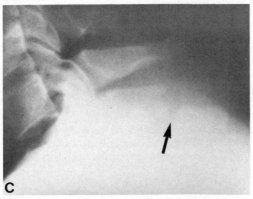

FIG 28–17.
A, clay shovelers' fracture of the spinous process of C7 and T1 *(arrows).* Whenever one spinous process fracture is identified, attention to the spines of the vertebrae above and below is mandatory. **B,** normal lateral view that includes C1 through C7. Broad shoulders obliterate T1, where the patient specifically located his pain. **C,** a coned-down view of the spinous processes of C7 and T1 demonstrating the fracture *(arrow).*

three-part, two-plane fracture pattern is an unstable injury, and the patient is usually permanently quadriplegic.

Posterior neural arch fractures include fractures of the lamina, the pedicles, and the spinous processes. Fractures of the lamina and pedicle are rare and difficult to demonstrate on plain radiographs. These fractures should be suspected from the AP view when the undulating lateral margin is interrupted either unilaterally or bilaterally. Oblique and pillar views better demonstrate these fractures (Fig 28–15, *A*), although a CT scan will optimally visualize them (Fig 28–15, *B*). A fracture of the lateral mass (Fig 28–16) may involve the inferior articular process as well as the superior articular process of the subjacent vertebrae. Isolated posterior neural arch fractures are stable injuries.

A fracture of the spinous process is called a clay shovelers' fracture, and is an avulsion injury. This injury is best seen on the lateral projection. In patients with broad shoulders and short muscular necks, a swimmer's view or lateral tomogram may be required to demonstrate the fracture. The spinous processes of C7, C6, and T1, in decreasing order of frequency, are usually affected, and it is not uncommon to find more than one spinous process fractured (Fig 28–17). These fractures are produced by the abrupt distraction of tensed posterior ligaments, and can occur without impact if the ligaments are voluntarily tensed forcibly. These are stable fractures.

Dislocations.—Dislocations of the cervical spine occur as a result of severe injuries and are usually not associated with significant fractures. Either a unilateral or a bilateral facet dislocation may occur.[4-6, 16]

A unilateral facet dislocation is diagnosed best on the lateral view by the abrupt alteration in the orientation of the posterior cortices of the lateral masses and articular processes at the level of injury and above, compared with those below the level of injury. For example, the posterior cortical margins are superimposed on each other, and the vertebral segments are projected in the lateral position in the lower segments at the level of injury and above, the posterior cortical margins are not superimposed on each other, and the vertebral segments are projected in the oblique position. Minimal anterior displacement of the vertebral body at the level of injury and fanning are present (Fig 28–18). On the AP view, the spinous process of the dislocated facet is displaced toward the side of the locked facet. Oblique views demonstrating the interfacetal joints are necessary to confirm which side is locked. A locked facet is one in which the superior facet of the interfacetal joint (the inferior articular process of the upper vertebra) is displaced upward and over the inferior facet of the interfacetal joint (the superior articular process of the subjacent vertebra) (Fig 28–19,*A*). A subluxed facet is one in which the superior facet is displaced upward and forward, but remains superior to the inferior facet (Fig 28–19,*B*). A unilateral facet dislocation is a stable injury. A unilateral facet subluxation is an unstable injury.

A bilateral facet dislocation is diagnosed on a lateral view by the anterior displacement of the involved vertebra on the vertebrae below, over 50% of its AP width (Fig 28–20, *A* and *B*). In a complete bilateral dislocation, both superior facets of the interfacetal joint (inferior articular processes of the dislocated vertebra) are locked in front of the inferior facets of the interfacetal joint (the superior articulating processes of the lower vertebra). Occasionally one of the facets is also fractured, but this is of little clinical significance in the presence of extensive ligamentous disruption.[4] In a partial bilateral dislocation or a subluxation, the vertebral body is also displaced anteri-

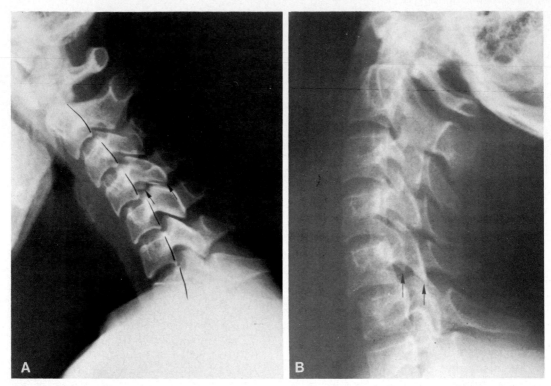

FIG 28–18.
A, lateral view of a unilateral facet dislocation of C4. The C4 vertebra is slightly anteriorly displaced. Both inferior articular processes *(arrows)* of C4 and the higher vertebrae are seen, that is, the vertebrae are oblique; the articular processes of C5 and the lower vertebrae are superimposed on each other, that is, the vertebrae are lateral. **B,** unilateral facet dislocation of C5 demonstrating both articular processes *(arrows)* at this level and above. The articular masses are superimposed normally at C6. There is slight anterior displacement of C5 on C6, and there is fanning of C5–C6 spinous processes.

orly, but less than 50% of its AP width (Fig 28–20, C). Oblique views are necessary to evaluate the facet status. Flexion and extension views are contraindicated. These are unstable injuries in which there is complete disruption of the posterior ligamentous complex, the intervertebral disk, and the anterior longitudinal ligament.[2, 5]

A posterior dislocation should be suspected when a patient is quadriplegic and the radiographs are essentially normal.[3, 13, 16, 23, 33, 34] The radiographic changes, although subtle, are best observed on the lateral view. These findings include prevertebral soft tissue swelling, posterior displacement of the vertebrae above the level of injury, widening of the anterior aspect of the intervertebral disk space, a vacuum in the anterior aspect of the intervertebral disk at the level of injury, and, occasionally, an avulsion fracture of the inferior border of the superior vertebral body or superior corner of the subjacent vertebra. Any one of these signs is a strong indication that this injury has occurred, and the cervical spine should be immediately immobilized. Flexion and extension views are contraindicated.

Upper Cervical Spine

Upper cervical spine injuries include ligamentous injuries, fractures of the at-

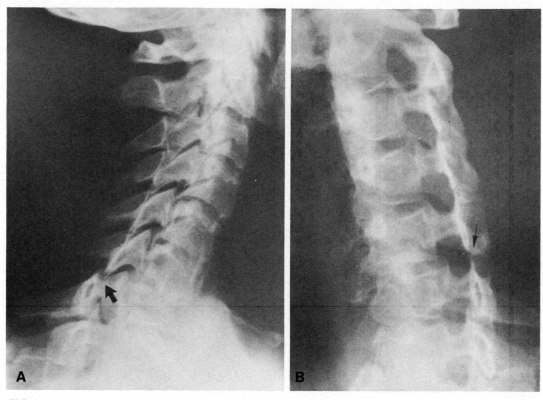

FIG 28–19.
A, demonstration of a locked right facet on the oblique view. The superior facet of C6 is displaced medially to the inferior facet *(arrow).* **B,** oblique view, demonstrating a subluxed left facet joint *(arrow).* The superior facet of C5 is medially displaced but has not fallen over the inferior facet into the intervertebral foramen.

las or axis, or both, and fracture dislocation of C1–C2.

Ligamentous Injuries.—The major ligamentous injury of the upper cervical cord is a tear or disruption of the transverse ligament. This ligament extends between the lateral masses of C1, passes posteriorly to the odontoid process, and maintains the normal atlantodens relationship. A true joint exists between the odontoid process and the anterior arch of C1 and also between the posterior surface of the odontoid process and the transverse ligament. The normal atlantodens interval (ADI) is 2.5 to 3.0 mm. This distance is maximum in flexion. An increase in the ADI indicates disruption or laxity of the transverse ligament.

Fractures of the Atlas.—A Jefferson fracture is a burst fracture of C1 and is diagnosed on the AP open mouth view. On this view there is lateral displacement of the lateral masses of the atlas with respect to the lateral masses of the axis. The odontoid process is usually intact (Fig 28–21). On the lateral view there is an increase in the ADI and prevertebral soft tissue swelling. This is an unstable fracture produced by a compressive force of the occipital condyles into the lateral masses of the atlas, in which both the anterior and posterior elements of the atlas are fractured.[16, 20]

A fracture of the posterior arch of C1 is a stable injury without neurologic symptoms. It is diagnosed on the lateral view. The fracture may be isolated or in

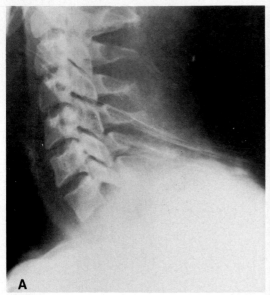

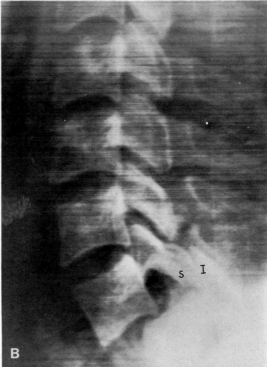

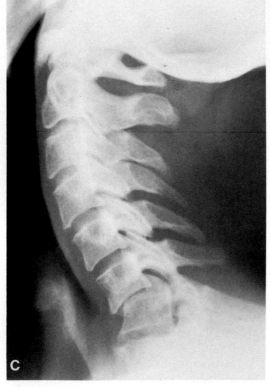

FIG 28–20.
A, cross-table lateral view demonstrating a bilateral facet dislocation with anterior displacement of C7 on T1. **B,** on a grid cassette film, anterior displacement of C7 on T1 more than 75% of its AP width is evident. The superior facets of the interfacetal joints *(S)* (the inferior articular processes of C7) are completely anterior and locked in front of the inferior facets of the interfacetal joint *(I)* (the superior articular processes of T1). **C,** a bilateral facet subluxation of C6–C7. C6 is anteriorly displaced less than 50% of its AP width. The interfacetal joints are subluxed but not locked. The inferior facets of C6 are displaced upward and forward but are not anterior to the superior facets of C7. There is fanning of the spinous processes at this level.

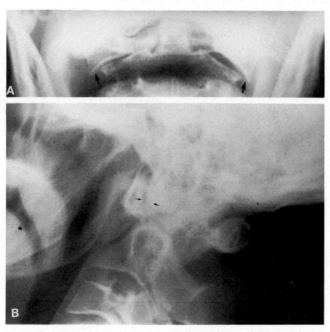

FIG 28–21.
A, a Jefferson fracture is best demonstrated on an open mouth view by the lateral displacement of the masses of C1 *(arrows)* compared with those of C2. **B,** lateral view of a Jefferson fracture demonstrates an increased ADI (distance between arrows).

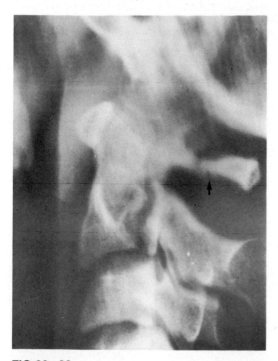

FIG 28–22.
A fracture through the posterior arch of C1 *(arrow)* associated with a hangman's fracture. There is also an avulsion fracture of the anteroinferior corner of C2.

combination with more serious injuries (Fig 28–22).[31]

Fractures of the Axis.—Fractures of the odontoid process have been classified by Anderson and D'Alonzo[1] according to where the dens is fractured. A type I fracture occurs at the tip of the dens and is a rare and stable injury. A type II fracture occurs at the base of the dens where it joins the body of the axis, and is best diagnosed on a lateral-view tomogram (Fig 28–23,A). This is usually initially unstable. A type III fracture extends into the body of the axis and is best seen on an AP open mouth–view tomogram (Fig 12–23,B). This is usually a stable injury. Odontoid fractures can be associated with dislocations of C1.

An avulsion fracture of C2 occurs at the insertion site of the anterior longitudinal ligament on the anteroinferior corner of C2 (Fig 28–24).[4, 16] The posterior ligaments and interfacetal joint capsules are intact, and there is normal vertebral

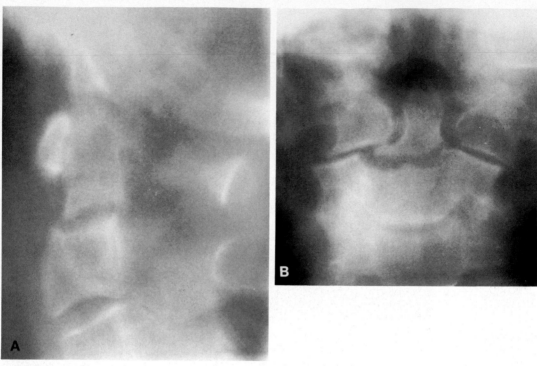

FIG 28–23.
A, type II fracture of the odontoid process. Tomogram demonstrates the fracture at the base of the dens where it joins the body of C2. There is slight posterior displacement of the odontoid process. The ADI is intact. **B,** type III fracture of the odontoid process in which the fracture extends into the body of C2.

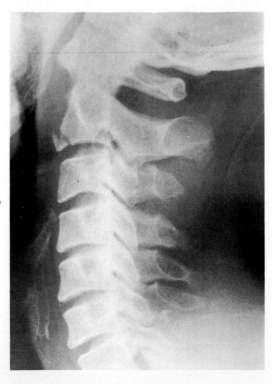

FIG 28–24.
An avulsion fracture of the anteroinferior corner of C2. There is soft tissue swelling. The vertebrae are in normal alignment.

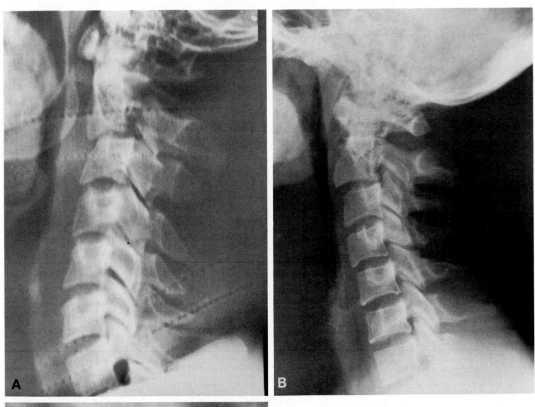

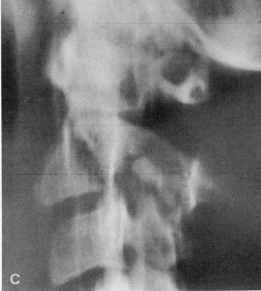

FIG 28–25.
A, a cross-table lateral view of the cervical spine demonstrating a hangman's fracture. There is soft tissue swelling anterior to the upper cervical spine. The pedicles of C2 are fractured. Disruption of the posterior longitudinal ligament and posterior disk is demonstrated by the anterior displacement of C2 on C3 and anterior subluxation of C2–C3. Fanning of the interspinous processes of C1–C2 indicates disruption of the posterior ligamentous complex. This fracture is unstable. **B,** hangman's fracture in this patient is more subtle, but should be suspected by the anterior displacement of C2 on C3 and the narrow posterior aspect of the intervertebral disk space. **C,** a lateral tomogram of C2 **(B)** demonstrates a unilateral pedicle fracture.

alignment. This injury is usually stable in flexion and unstable in extension.

A hangman's fracture is a traumatic spondylolysis or pedicle fracture of C2 with a spondylolisthesis of C2 on C3. It is best diagnosed on the lateral view.[3, 9, 16, 28, 30] There is prevertebral soft tissue swelling, narrowing of the C2–C3 disk, and anterior dislocation of C2 on C3. Occasionally a wedge fracture of C3 is also present (Fig 28–25, A).[3, 12, 28, 30] The ADI remains normal, because the transverse ligament remains intact. A unilateral pedicle fracture should be suspected when there is slight C2–C3 spondylolisthesis. A tomogram should be obtained to confirm or exclude this suspicion (Fig 28–25,B and C). A hangman's fracture is unstable, with the only protection to the cord being the autodecompression resulting from the bilateral pedicle fractures and the increased diameter of the canal in this region.

Fracture Dislocation of C1–C2.—A C1–C2 fracture dislocation is best diag-nosed on the lateral view, while the state of the odontoid process is best identified on the AP open mouth view (Fig 28–26). On the lateral view the ADI should be measured. The ADI is usually increased in anterior dislocations and normal in posterior dislocations.[1, 14] In the open mouth view the odontoid fracture and the degree of odontoid fragmentation can be appreciated. Because the spinal canal is largest in this area the cord is usually not compressed, and the patient may be without neurologic damage.

Central Nervous System

Trauma to the cervical spine can damage the spinal cord, the surrounding ligamentous dural and vascular structures, the intervertebral disk, and the nerve roots. Myelography, especially when combined with CT, and MRI can demonstrate these lesions and are useful before surgery.[29]

Injury to the vessels surrounding the cord most commonly results in an extra-

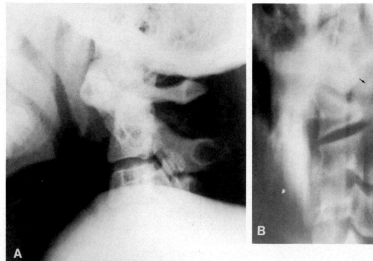
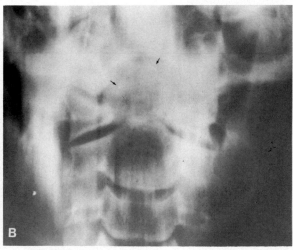

FIG 28–26.
A, lateral view of the upper cervical spine demonstrating an anterior fracture-dislocation of C1 on C2. The top of the odontoid process is not seen, but the ADI measured from a projected line continued cephalad along the anterior cortex of the visualized odontoid process to the anterior arch of C1 is increased. **B,** a tomogram in the AP open mouth view documents the fragmentation of the odontoid process as seen by several cortical surfaces *(arrows).*

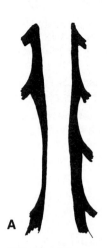 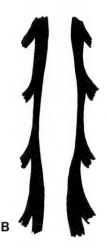

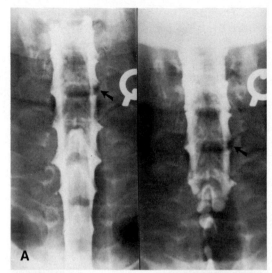

FIG 28–27.
A diagram of a myelogram in AP view. The cord is white and the contrast-filled subarachnoid space is black. **A,** an epidural hematoma narrows the subarachnoid space and displaces the cord to one side. The hematoma is localized but extends over several segments and does not correspond to an intervertebral disk space. **B,** cord swelling, due to hematoma or edema, is seen as a localized widening of the cord. The cord can appear widened when compressed dorsally or ventrally, so true cord swelling must be confirmed by two right-angle films.

dural hematoma. On the myelogram a complete or partial block to the contrast agent may be demonstrated. When this defect is dorsal, it is best seen on the horizontal lateral view performed with the patient prone. A unilateral extradural defect displaces the cord to the opposite side and is best seen on the AP view. The hematoma normally extends over several vertebral segments (Fig 28–27, A).

Injury to the spinal cord caused by fracture or dislocation can result in hemorrhage or localized edema. This can occur immediately or several days after the injury. The injured cord swells and, as indicated on the myelogram, symmetrically narrows the surrounding contrast column or produces a complete block (Fig 28–27,B). AP and lateral views are required to confirm that the cord is actually widened and not compressed from either front or back.

An intervertebral disk herniation can

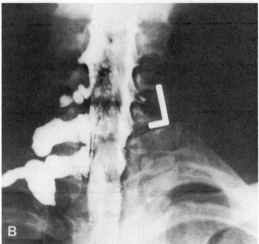

FIG 28–28.
A, an AP cervical myelogram demonstrating a herniated nucleus pulposus (disk). A horizontal lucency at the level of the intervertebral disk space is present, and there is unilateral compression of the nerve root, demonstrated by widening of the nerve root and truncation of the contrast *(arrow).* **B,** an AP myelogram demonstrating an avulsion injury to the right brachial plexus. The contrast material extends along the enlarged and saccular nerve root sheaths.

occur at the time of trauma. A disk herniation is diagnosed on the myelogram as a local defect in the anterior aspect of the contrast column localized at the intervertebral disk space. Occasionally the associated nerve root may be blunted (Fig 28–28, A).

The arachnoid and dura mater accompany the nerve root through the intervertebral foramina. These structures may tear or the nerve root may be avulsed and retract. These injuries result in the formation of a traumatic meningocele, which is an irregular outpouching of the subarachnoid space along the path of the injured nerve root, and can be demonstrated when filled with a contrast agent (Fig 28–28, B).

Further discussion of the radiographic evaluation of the spinal cord and its surrounding soft tissues is presented in the chapter on CT and MRI of the cervical spine.

REFERENCES

1. Anderson LD, D'Alonzo RT: Fractures of the odontoid process of the axis. *J Bone Joint Surg [Am]* 1974; 56A:1663.

2. Apley AL: Fractures of the spine. *Ann R Coll Surg Engl* 1970; 46:210.

3. Babcock JL: Cervical spine injuries. *Arch Surg* 1976; 111:646.

4. Beabrook GM: Stability of spinal fractures and dislocations. *Int J Paraplegia* 1971; 9:23.

5. Beatson TR: Fractures and dislocations of the cervical spine. *J Bone Joint Surg [Br]* 1963; 45B:21.

6. Braakman R, Vinken PJ: Unilateral facet interlocking in the lower cervical spine. *J Bone Joint Surg [Br]* 1967; 49B:249.

7. Cheshire DJE: The stability of the cervical spine following conservative treatment of fractures and dislocations. *Int J Paraplegia* 1970; 7:193.

8. Coin CG, Pennink M, Ahmad WD, et al: Diving type injuries of the cervical spine. Contribution of computed tomography to management. *J Comput Assist Tomog* 1979; 3:362.

9. Cornish BL: Traumatic spondylolisthesis of the axis. *J Bone Joint Surg [Br]* 1968; 50B:31.

10. Evans KD: Anterior cervical subluxation. *J Bone Joint Surg [Br]* 1976; 58B:318.

11. Fielding JW, Van Cochran G, Lowsing JF III, et al: Tears of transverse ligament of the atlas. *J Bone Joint Surg [Am]* 1974; 56A:1683.

12. Fielding JN, Hawkins RJ: Roentgenographic diagnosis of the injured neck, In *AAOS Instructional Course Lectures,* vol 25. St. Louis, Mosby–Year Book, 1976.

13. Forsyth HF: Extension injuries of the cervical spine. *J Bone Joint Surg [Am]* 1964; 46A:1792.

14. Gehweiler JA, Clark WM, Schaaf RE, et al: Cervical spine trauma—the common combined conditions. *Radiology* 1979; 103:77.

15. Harris JH Jr: Acute injuries of the spine. *Semin Roentgenol* 1978; 13:53.

16. Harris JH Jr: *The Radiology of Acute Cervical Spine Trauma.* Baltimore, Williams & Wilkins, 1978.

17. Hay PD: Measurement of the soft tissues of the neck, in *Atlas of Roentgenographic Measurements,* ed 3. Lusted LB, Keats TE (eds): St Louis, Mosby–Year Book, 1972.

18. Hinck VC, Hopkins CE: Measurement of the atlanto dental interval in the adult. *AJR* 1965; 84:945.

19. Holdsworth F: Fractures, dislocations and fracture/dislocations of the spine. *J Bone Joint Surg [Am]* 1970; 52A:1534.

20. Jefferson G: Fracture of the atlas vertebrae. Report of 4 cases, and a review of those previously recorded. *Br J Surg* 1920; 7:407.

21. Kershner MS, Goodman GA, Perlmutter GS, et al: Computed tomography in the diagnosis of an atlas fracture. *AJR* 1977; 128:688.

22. Kim KS, Chen HH, Russell EJ, et al: Flexion teardrop fractures of the cervical spine: Radiographic characteristics. *AJR* 1989; 102:319–326.

23. Marar BC: Hyperextension injuries of the cervical spine. The pathogenesis of damage to the spinal cord. *J Bone Joint Surg [Am]* 1974; 56A:1655.

24. Pavlov H, Torg JS, Robie B, et al: Cervical spinal stenosis: Determination with vertebral body ratio method. *Radiology* 1987; 164:771–775.

25. Roaf R: A study of the mechanics of spinal injuries. *J Bone Joint Surg [Br]* 1960; 42B:810.

26. Scher AT: Anterior cervical subluxation; an unstable position. *AJR* 1979; 133:275.

27. Schneider RC, Kahn EA: Chronic neurologic sequelae of acute trauma to the spine and spinal cord. Part I: The significance of the acute-flexion or "teardrop" fracture dislocations of the cervical spine. *J Bone Joint Surg [Am]* 1956; 38A:985.

28. Schneider RC, Livingstone KE, Cove AJE, et al: "Hangman's fracture" of the cervical spine. *J Neurosurg* 1965; 22:141.

29. Shapiro R: *Myelography.* ed 2. St Louis, Mosby–Year Book, 1968.

30. Sherk HH: Lesions of the atlas and axis. *Clin Orthop* 1975; 109:33.

31. Sinbert SE, Berman MS: Fracture of the posterior arch of the atlas. *JAMA* 1940; 114:1996.

32. Tadmor R, Davis KR, Roberson GH, et al: Computed tomographic evaluation of traumatic spinal injuries. *Radiology* 1978; 127:825.

33. Taylor AR: The mechanism of injury to the spinal cord in the neck without damage to the vertebral column. *J Bone Joint Surg [Br]* 1951; 33B:543.

34. Taylor AR, Blackwood W: Paraplegia in hyperextension cervical injuries with normal radiographic appearances. *J Bone Joint Surg [Br]* 1948; 30B:245.

35. Torg JS: Personal communication.

36. Torg JS, Pavlov H, Genuario SE, et al: Neurapraxia of the cervical spinal cord with transient quadriplegia. *J Bone Joint Surg [Am]* 1986; 68A:1354–1370.

37. Webb JK, Broughton RBK, McSweeney T, et al: Hidden flexion injury of the cervical spine. *J Bone Joint Surg [Br]* 1976; 58B:322.

38. Weir DC: Roentgenographic signs of cervical injury. *Clin Orthop* 1975; 109:9.

39. Wilkenson HA, Le May ML, Ferris EJ: Roentgenographic correlation in cervical spondylosis. *AJR* 1969; 105:370–374.

Computed Tomography and Magnetic Resonance Imaging of Cervical Spine Trauma

Caren Jahre, M.D.

Helene Pavlov, M.D.

Michael D. F. Deck, M.D.

In cases of cervical spine trauma, imaging is required to assess the integrity and alignment of the osseous structures, ligamentous stability, extradural mass effects resulting from osteophytes, herniated disks, fracture fragments and hematomas, and the status of the spinal cord itself. Plain radiographs, sometimes supplemented with tomography, remain the initial diagnostic modality, and further evaluation, if necessary, can be performed with computed tomography (CT) and magnetic resonance imaging (MRI). Recent advances in CT, (including postmyelography CT, sagittal and coronal reformations, and three-dimensional CT) and MRI represent significant improvement in available imaging modalities for evaluating cervical spine injury.

INDICATIONS

Despite the introduction of sophisticated techniques such as CT and MRI, the initial radiographic examination of the patient with cervical spine trauma re-mains the routine radiographic examination. This examination, including lateral, anteroposterior, open mouth (odontoid), and oblique views, is readily available and rapidly obtained, and provides the most important information regarding the presence or absence of unstable fractures, dislocations, and subluxations. Further evaluation with CT or MRI may follow to provide more detailed information, It must be recognized, however, that horizontally oriented fractures and subtle subluxations are often best identified on the routine radiographs.

The choice of imaging technique after plain radiography depends on the findings on the routine examination, the neurologic status of the patient, preference of the individual physician, and availability of imaging modalities.

One approach advocated by Mirvis and Wolf,[5] at the Maryland Institute for Emergency Medical Services, divides the approach according to the presence or absence of neurologic deficits. In the neurologically intact patient with a fracture or suspected fracture on plain radiographs,

CT is performed to better define the extent of fracture. If the initial plain films are unremarkable, flexion and extension lateral views are performed to evaluate for ligamentous instability.

In the patient with neurologic deficit, either MRI or CT myelography must be performed to evaluate the status of the spinal cord and the extradural space. Except for the diagnosis of fracture, MRI is superior to CT myelography for direct visualization of cord pathology and extradural mass effects resulting from herniated disks, osteophytes, and hematomas. The MRI scan can be complemented with CT to further define fractures identified on the initial plain film examination. If MRI is unavailable or contraindicated, CT myelography is indicated.

PRINCIPLES

Computed Tomography

CT involves the use of a series of finely collimated x-ray beams and detectors covering a span of 360 degrees surrounding the patient. The data are relayed to a computer that rapidly constructs axial images of the spine, with use of a gray scale. Radiodense structures such as bone and blood appear white,

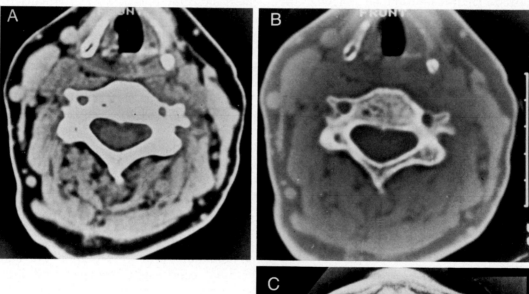

FIG 29–1.
Normal CT anatomy of the cervical spine. **A,** axial CT section through C4 vertebral body demonstrates normal cervical spinal cord with surrounding subarachnoid space. **B,** bone "window" through the same level as **A** provides superior visualization of osseous anatomy, including the lateral masses. **C,** postmyelogram axial CT section through the C5 vertebral body, with contrast opacifying the subarachnoid space and outlining the contour of the spinal cord. The definition of the contents of the spinal canal is much superior to the plain CT.

whereas less radiodense structures such as cerebrospinal fluid (CSF) appear black. Soft tissues are intermediate, and can be represented by various shades of gray. The data can be manipulated on the CT console screen to optimize evaluation of the bone or spinal cord detail, or both ("windowing") (Fig 29–1, *A* and *B*).

With modern CT equipment, each axial image can be obtained in approximately 2 seconds; thus images are obtainable in all but the most uncooperative patients. Because cervical spine fractures and associated injuries (such as herniated disks) occur in relatively small structures, high-resolution CT imaging is required. High-resolution CT imaging involves the use of thin axial sections of 1.5 or 3 mm that can be reformatted by the CT operator to create sagittal or coronal images, or both. These reformatted images are useful for evaluating fractures and spinal alignment. The data from these same axial images can also be used to construct three-dimensional images, with use of special computer software programs. An advantage of three-dimensional imaging is the ability of the computer to rotate the three-dimensional image of the cervical area, thus allowing visualization of fractures and malalignments.

In patients with neurologic deficits, a myelogram is often performed to assess the spinal cord, followed by CT imaging. Myelography after cervical trauma is usually performed with use of C1–C2 puncture. This procedure is performed with the patient in a supine position, avoiding the necessity to place the patient prone. A water-soluble low-osmolality contrast material (such as iohexol, iopamidol) is used. Postmyelography CT, with axial images through the involved area, is then performed.

The myelographic contrast material opacifies the subarachnoid space and outlines the contour of the spinal cord (Fig 29–1, *C*). Focal areas of compression or enlargment of the spinal cord and herniated disks or osseous fragments compromising the spinal cord or the subarachnoid space can be appreciated.

Magnetic Resonance Imaging

Chapter 20 contains a discussion of the basic principles of MRI. It is particularly advantageous in the imaging of cervical spine trauma because of its multiplanar imaging capability, which allows direct sagittal imaging, and also because of its exquisite soft tissue discriminating ability (Fig 29–2). MRI permits the noninvasive diagnosis of impingement on the spinal cord by bone fragments, herniated disks, or hematoma and focal abnormalities within the spinal cord, such as edema or hemorrhage, without the risks of C1–C2 myelography.

Imaging sequences may vary among institutions, depending on individual preference, but generally include all or a combination of short TR, long TR, and gradient echo sagittal images, and long TR and gradient echo axial images. Long TR images are optimal for evaluating spinal cord pathology and produce high signal intensity in the CSF, which reproduces myelogram-like images; gradient echo images (Fig 29–2,*B*) also produce a myelographic effect, require less time, and are highly sensitive to the presence

FIG 29–2.
Normal MRI anatomy of the cervical spine. **A,** sagittal short TR image demonstrates spinal cord anatomy and normal anatomy of the vertebral bodies and disks. **B,** gradient echo sagittal image demonstrates the myelographic effect by turning the CSF white. These images are very sensitive to extradural masses, such as herniated disks and osteophytes, impinging on the subarachnoid space. Long TR images (not shown) are similar and also demonstrate a myelographic effect. Long TR images are more sensitive to signal abnormalities within the spinal cord compared with the short TR images. **C,** gradient echo axial image demonstrates spinal cord surrounded by bright CSF.

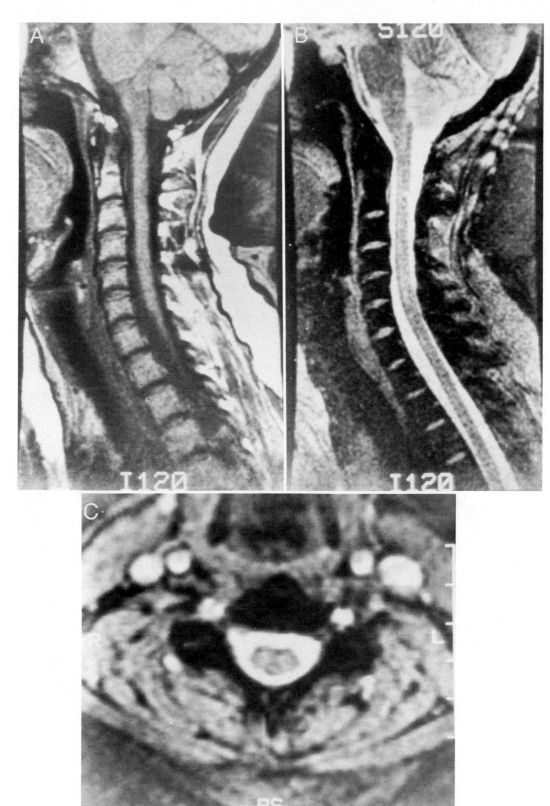

of hemorrhage; however, they are not as sensitive as the long TR images in detecting spinal cord edema.

As mentioned in Chapter 20, there are various contraindications and technical considerations in imaging critically ill patients because of the presence of the strong magnetic field.[5] Spinal immobilization must be accordingly modified, with use of a Philadelphia collar or halo fixation devices made of nonferrous materials. Traction can be performed with special graphite traction tongs, nonferrous pullies, and water bags, or a Sokhoff board and plastic traction weights. Ventilators must be placed beyond the main magnetic field with long connecting hoses to the patient.[3] Cardiac monitors, intravenous infusion pumps, and pulmonary artery pressure monitors cannot be used; this is a problem in critically ill patients with multisystem trauma.

TRAUMATIC LESIONS

Cervical Spine Fracture

The value of CT in the evaluation of fractures of the cervical spine is especially indicated for injuries involving the lateral masses and posterior elements. These areas are difficult to evaluate on plain radiographs where there is extensive overlap of the normal structures. CT is excellent for determining displacement of fracture fragments and subsequent compromise of the spinal canal (Fig 29–3).

A serious limitation of CT involves fractures that are horizontally oriented, such as odontoid fractures. These fractures may be missed when the axial scanning plane coincides with the fracture plane. Coronal and sagittal CT reformations or three-dimensional CT reconstructions may demonstrate these frac-

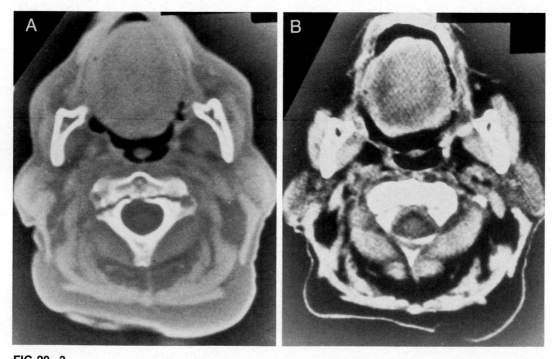

FIG 29–3.
Hangman's fracture. **A,** axial CT section through C2 with use of a bone "window" shows typical configuration of a hangman's fracture. There is minimal displacement. **B,** soft tissue "window" at the same level clearly demonstrates that there is no significant compromise of the spinal canal. The subarachnoid space surrounding the spinal cord is preserved.

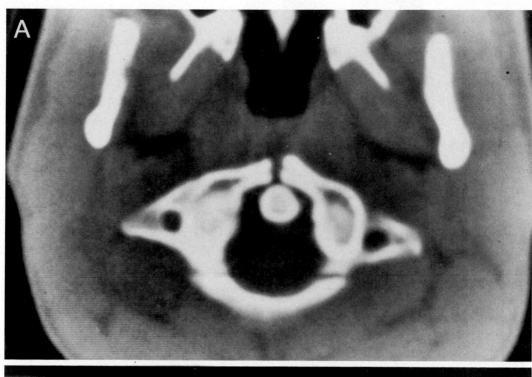

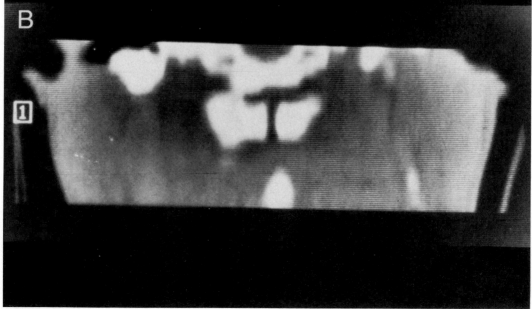

FIG 29–4.
Jefferson fracture. **A,** axial CT section through C1 with use of a bone "window" demonstrates fractures through the anterior arch of C1 and both laminae. **B,** coronal CT reformation with use of bone "windows" demonstrates the vertically oriented fracture through the anterior arch of C1.

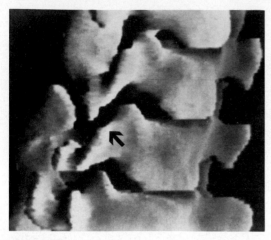

FIG 29–5.
Facet dislocation. Three-dimensional CT reformation rotated into an oblique orientation demonstrates a facet dislocation *(arrow)*.

tures; however, not infrequently these images contain various artifacts produced by patient motion that may obscure or simulate fractures (Fig 29–4).

Three-dimensional CT reformations are performed with use of the data from routine axial scans; therefore they contain no information additional to that obtained from the axial scans. However, the three-dimensional display, which can be rotated, is occasionally easier to interpret than the axial scan. These reconstructed images may be especially useful in complex fractures or dislocations, such as facet dislocation (Fig 29–5).

MRI is extremely limited in fracture evaluation because cortical bone produces a signal void (black). A major dis-

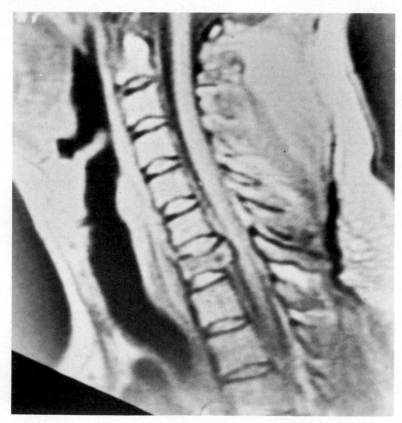

FIG 29–6.
Compression fracture of C7. Sagittal short TR MRI image through the cervical spine demonstrates marked compression of the C7 vertebral body with posterior displacement of fracture fragments, causing spinal cord compression.

ruption or significant alterations in the contours of the vertebral bodies is used to identify an abnormality because the marrow fat produces a relatively bright signal (white) on short TR images. Subtle minimally displaced fractures of the posterior elements will not be readily detected on MRI. Displaced fracture fragments that extend into the spinal canal, with impingement on the spinal cord or subarachnoid space, are well visualized on MRI, however (Fig 29–6).

Ligamentous Injuries

Ligamentous injuries occur with or without associated fractures. Their presence is inferred on plain radiographs or reformatted CT images by malalignment of the vertebral elements. Malalignment may be accentuated on flexion and extension lateral radiographs. A CT examination alone may miss ligamentous injuries because subtle anterior or posterior displacement of the vertebrae will not be demonstrated on a series of axial CT scans, without reformations.

Because of the ability to produce direct sagittal images, MRI can detect evidence of ligamentous injury by visualizing malalignment. In some cases the actual ligament disruption can be directly seen. Fibrous tissues, such as ligaments, normally have a low signal intensity on MRI, because of a relative lack of mobile protons, and appear dark. These dark lines, representing the ligaments, may be seen to be disrupted, as in cases of disk herniation associated with rupture of the annulus fibrosus and the posterior longitudinal ligament. Also, a bright signal within the ligament representing hemorrhage may also be seen in areas of ligamentous injury.

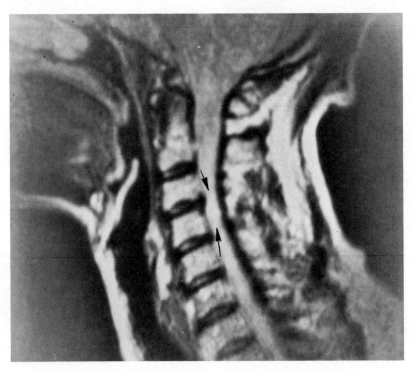

FIG 29–7.
Spinal cord edema after disk herniation. A sagittal proton-density MRI image of the cervical spine demonstrates a focal area of increased signal intensity at C3–C4 at the site of a disk herniation *(arrows)*.

Spinal Cord Injury

MRI is superior to CT in demonstrating spinal cord injury.[1, 2, 4] The CT examination is capable of inferring the presence of spinal cord injury by demonstrating gross compromise of the spinal canal resulting from fractures, dislocations, or herniated disks; CT myelography can show spinal cord compression or expansion resulting from edema or hemorrhage. However, CT cannot detect abnormalities, such as small areas of edema or hemorrhage within the spinal cord, that do not grossly alter the contour of the cord.

MRI is sensitive to subtle abnormalities in the spinal cord because of its excellent soft tissue–discriminating ability and lack of bone artifacts. Areas of edema are seen as hyperintense (bright) on the proton density or long TR images (Fig 29–7) and may be hypointense (dark) on short TR images. Hemorrhage will have varying appearances related to its age; in the acute stages, it will have a decreased signal, which will then increase (becoming brighter) during the next few days. Gradient echo images may be more sensitive in detecting foci of hemorrhage, which will appear dark. Severe injuries, such as cord transection, can be directly visualized with MRI. Early studies have suggested that nonhemorrhagic cord injuries seen on MRI are associated with a better prognosis for neurologic recovery compared with hemorrhagic contusions.[2, 4]

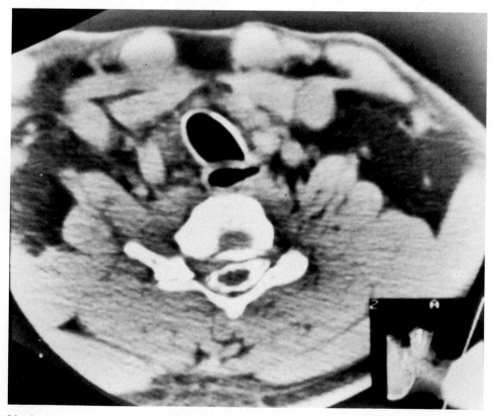

FIG 29–8.
Cervical disk herniation. A postmyelogram axial CT section at C6–C7 demonstrates a right-sided disk herniation compressing the thecal sac and involving the right neural foramen.

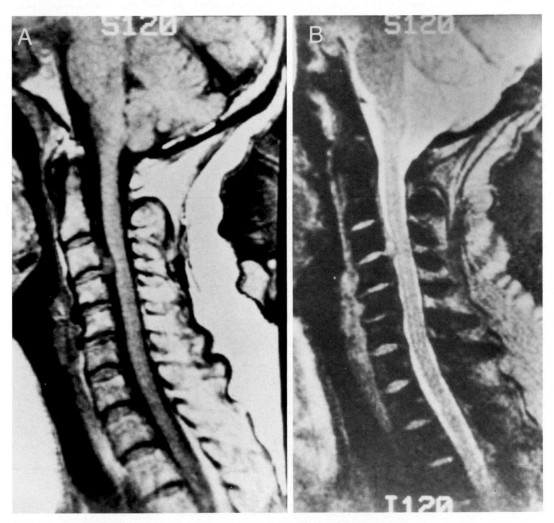

FIG 29–9.
Cervical disk herniation. Short TR **(A)** and gradient echo **(B)** sagittal MRI sections demonstrate a large C3–C4 disk herniation with mild spinal cord compression.

Traumatic Disk Herniation

Thin-section CT is capable of detecting cervical disk herniations; however, images are frequently difficult to interpret because of artifacts, particularly in the lower cervical spine where there is attenuation of the x-ray beam by the shoulders. Diagnostic capability is greatly improved with CT myelography, because the herniated disk is contrasted against the contrast-opacified subarachnoid space (Fig 29–8).

MRI offers comparable ability in diagnosing herniated disks without the invasiveness of myelography. MRI also is advantageous because of its multiplanar imaging capability, producing both sagittal and axial views (Fig 29–9). Gradient echo images and the long TR images are particularly useful. On these images CSF appears white, producing a myelographic effect. The herniated disk is relatively dark, and the CSF is bright (i.e., the herniated disks appear as a protrusion beyond the posterior aspect of the vertebral bodies, which encroach upon the subarachnoid space and may be seen to compress the spinal cord). Normally the posterior aspect of the disk is marked by a thin black line on sagittal images, representing the annulus fibrosus and posterior longitudinal ligament. Disruption of this line on the MRI image confirms a disk herniation.

Axial MRI images are helpful in com-

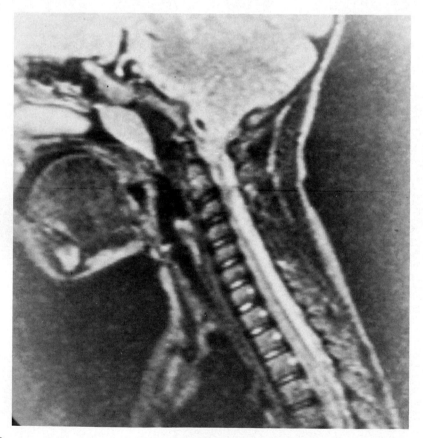

FIG 29–10.
Epidural hematoma in the cervical spine. Long TR sagittal MRI section through the cervical spine demonstrates a large elongated high-signal-intensity mass in the posterior aspect of the spinal canal that compresses the thecal sac. This represents an acute epidural hematoma.

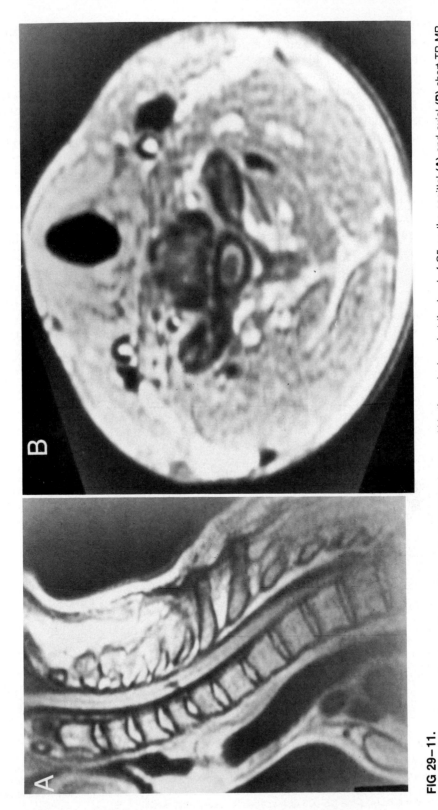

FIG 29–11.
Posttraumatic syringomyelia. A small area of low signal intensity is seen within the spinal cord at the level of C5 on the sagittal **(A)** and axial **(B)** short TR MR images that developed after trauma.

bination with the sagittal images in determining if there is a diffuse bulging of a disk or a focal posterolateral herniation. Osteophytes usually have a lower signal then a disk because they consist of bone. A calcified disk, however, may also have a low signal intensity and may be indistinguishable from an osteophyte on an axial image alone. Therefore, the sagittal images are very useful in determining if there is a protruding osteophyte versus a disk herniation, by demonstrating contiguity of the protruding fragment from the disk, versus contiguity with the bone, which represents an osteophyte.

Other Findings

Epidural hematomas may occasionally occur in the cervical region after trauma. The blood has a dense appearance on computed tomographic examination and may be difficult to detect because of the adjacent bone or streak artifacts, or both. Hematoma may also be indistinguishable from a disk herniation, which may also have a dense appearance on CT. MRI is generally superior to CT in detecting hemorrhagic lesions. On MRI, an epidural hematoma would appear as a mass in the epidural space whose signal intensity would vary depending on the age of the hematoma (Fig 29–10).

Prevertebral edema or hemorrhage is easier to detect with use of MRI than with CT. Edema produces a bright signal on long TR images, and hemorrhage produces a high signal in subacute stages on both short and long TR images.

Associated injuries to the vertebral

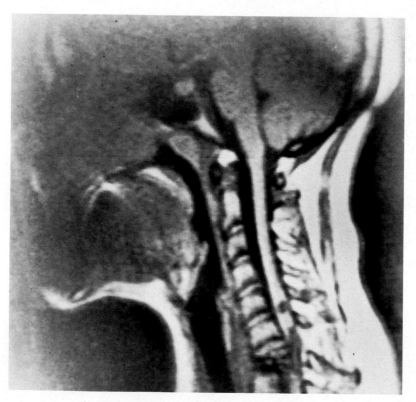

FIG 29–12.
Posttraumatic sequelae. This patient has an extensive fracture of the C7 vertebral body and a flexion deformity. Sagittal short TR image of the cervical spine demonstrates the spinal cord to be markedly thin and distorted at the level of the fracture, representing a near transection. There is also a small cystlike area, possibly representing an early syrinx cavity at the level of the C5–C6 disk space. This patient is quadriplegic.

and carotid arteries, such as dissection, may also be evident on the MRI because these vascular structures normally appear black. The black image is produced secondary to normally flowing blood, which does not produce an MRI signal; however, with thrombosis or dissection, increased signal may be present in the lumen.

Chronic Sequelae

Syringomyelia, a fluid-filled cavity, may form in the spinal cord after trauma. It may extend over many levels and cause progressive neurologic deficits. MRI is an excellent method for detecting syringomyelia. Before MRI myelography was necessary, and diagnosis was made by demonstration of an expanded cord. Delayed post-myelogram CT would occasionally show contrast collecting within the spinal cord. Often, with a small syrinx cavity, myelography and postmyelogram CT would be negative compared with the MRI examination, in which a cavity is detected as an elongated cyst within the spinal cord. The cavity is hypointense on short TR images and hyperintense on long TR images (Fig 29–11, A). If the cavity is small, it may be missed on sagittal images because of the gap between slices; therefore it is impor-

tant to perform and examine axial images for identification of the cavity (Fig 29–11, B). MRI may also document the development of cord atrophy or myelomalacia, after serious trauma with fixed neurologic deficits (Fig 29–12).

Other late findings may include persistent mass effects resulting from fracture fragments and herniated disks (the removal of which may result in further neurologic recovery), arachnoid cysts, and adhesions causing tethering of the spinal cord.[5]

REFERENCES

1. Hackney DB, Asato R, Joseph DM, et al: Hemorrhage and edema in acute spinal cord compression: Demonstration by MR imaging. *Radiology* 1986; 161:387–390.

2. Kulkarni MV, McArdle CB, Kopanicky D, et al: Acute spinal cord injury: MR imaging at 1.5T. *Radiology* 1987; 164:837–843.

3. Mirvis SE, Borg H, Belzberg H: MR imaging of ventilator-dependent patients: Preliminary experience. *AJR* 1987; 149:845–846.

4. Mirvis SE, Geisler FH, Jelinek JJ, et al: Acute cervical spine trauma: Evaluation with 1.5T MR imaging. *Radiology* 1988; 166:807–816.

5. Mirvis SE, Wolf A: Emerging MRI role: Assessing cervical spine trauma. *MRI Decisions*, Jan/Feb 1990, pp 21–31.

CHAPTER 30

Field Evaluation and Management of Cervical Spine Injuries

Joseph J. Vegso, M.S.
Joseph S. Torg, M.D.

The purpose of this chapter is to present clear, concise guidelines for the classification, evaluation, and emergency management of injuries that occur to the cervical spine and its related structures as a result of participation in competitive and recreational activities.

Athletic injuries to the cervical spine may involve the bony vertebrae, intervertebral disks, annulus fibrosus, ligamentous supporting structures, spinal cord, roots and peripheral nerves, or any combination of these structures. The panorama of injuries seen run the spectrum from the "cervical sprain syndrome" to fracture-dislocations with permanent quadriplegia. Fortunately, severe injuries with neural involvement occur infrequently. However, those responsible for the emergency and subsequent care of the athlete with a cervical spine injury should possess a basic understanding of the variety of problems that can occur.

The various athletic injuries to the cervical spine are the following:

1. Brachial plexus neurapraxia
2. Stable cervical sprain
3. Muscular strain
4. Brachial plexus axonotmesis
5. Intervertebral disk injury (narrowing-herniation) without neurologic deficit
6. Stable cervical fracture without neurologic deficit
7. Subluxations without neurologic deficit
8. Unstable fractures without neurologic deficit
9. Dislocations without neurologic deficit
10. Intervertebral disk herniation with neurologic deficit
11. Unstable fracture with neurologic deficit
12. Dislocation with neurologic deficit
13. Quadriplegia
14. Death

In those instances in which the individual complains of neck pain after trauma but is ambulatory, conscious, and without obvious neurologic involvement, significant spinal injury must still be suspected. The presence of the following subtle or perhaps not so subtle findings and symptoms should alert the examiner to the possibility of an injury that precludes further participation pending a definitive radiographic/imaging and neurologic examination. Specifically, they include:

1. Presence of torticollis or wryneck posture (Fig 30–1,*A*)
2. Painful cervical motion
3. Decreased range of cervical motion
4. Persistent paresthesia
5. Persistent weakness

Those responsible for on-the-field management of neck injuries should remember that only a small fraction of the total number of sports-incurred neck injuries result in permanent neurologic injury. It should be emphasized, however, that, if improperly handled, an unstable lesion without neurologic deficit can be converted to one with neurologic deficit.

Stable cervical sprains and strains rarely require extensive treatment, and generally resolve without incident. Yet it is necessary, when injury to the spine is suspected, to perform a thorough neurologic examination and evaluation of the cervical range of motion. This will verify the diagnosis and rule out the possibility of a more serious injury. The presence of torticollis, with or without limited or painful motion, precludes participation and requires that a significant problem be ruled out. Range of motion is evaluated by having the athlete actively nod his head, touch his chin to his chest, touch his chin to his left shoulder, touch his chin to his right shoulder, touch his right ear to his right shoulder, and touch his left ear to his left shoulder (Fig 30–1,*B*–*G*). Inability or unwillingness to perform these motions, while standing erect, is a signal to apply appropriate protection and prohibit further activity. Additional symptoms include persistent paresthesia and weakness. Subsequent evaluation should include appropriate roentgenographic studies, including flexion and extension views to demonstrate fractures or instability, and computed tomography (CT) and magnetic resonance imaging (MRI) scans as appropriate.

The most common and most poorly understood cervical injuries are the pinch-stretch neurapraxias of the nerve root and brachial plexus. Clancy et al.[3] have reported a 50% incidence in college football players during their 4-year exposure. Typically, after contact with head, neck, or shoulder, a sharp, burning pain is experienced in the neck on the involved side that may radiate into the shoulder and down the arm to the hand. There may be associated weakness and paresthesia in the involved extremity lasting from several seconds to several minutes. The brevity of these symptoms, along with the presence of full pain-free range of motion, is the key to the nature of the lesion. Return to activity is permitted when paresthesias have subsided, when full muscle strength in the intrinsic muscles of the shoulder and upper extremity is demonstrated, and when full pain-free range of motion is observed. One cause for concern with regard to this type of injury is the possible development of plexus axonotmesis, which requires a full work-up for neurologic and bony pathology.

Persistence of paresthesia, weakness, or limitation of cervical motion requires that the individual be protected from further exposure and that he undergo neurologic and roentgenographic evaluation.

EMERGENCY MANAGEMENT

Managing the unconscious or spine-injured athlete is a process that should not be done hastily or haphazardly. Being prepared to handle this situation is the best way to prevent actions that could

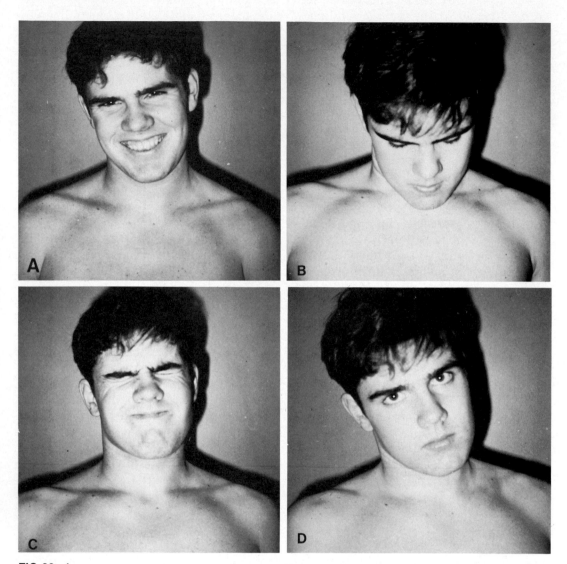

FIG 30–1.
A, examining the athlete with complaints referable to his neck, cervical spine, cervical nerve roots, or brachial plexus first involves observing the postural relationship between the head, neck, and torso. Although apparently comfortable and smiling, torticollis or wryneck posture indicates the possibility of a significant cervical injury. **B,** active flexion of the neck and cervical spine accentuates the torticollis. As a general rule the patient who presents with a wryneck after trauma should have a roentgenographic examination of the cervical spine. **C,** active extension of the neck and cervical spine is markedly limited by pain and muscle spasm. Discomfort is vividly portrayed by his facial expression. **D,** limitation of lateral bend to his right is evident by inability to actively touch right ear to right shoulder. **E,** marked limitation of lateral bend to the left is demonstrated when he attempts to touch his left ear to his left shoulder. The discomfort is vividly portrayed by his facial expression. **F,** rotation of the cervical spine to the right is evaluated by having the patient actively touch his chin to his right shoulder. None of these maneuvers should involve manual assistance on the part of the examiner, nor should the patient be encouraged to attempt to move his neck beyond the point of pain. **G,** rotation of the cervical spine to the left is evaluated by instructing the patient to actively touch his chin to his left shoulder.

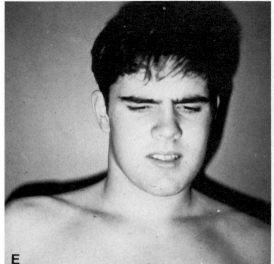

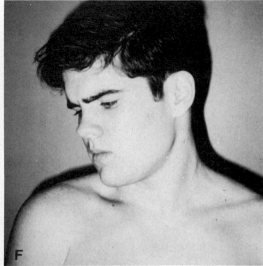

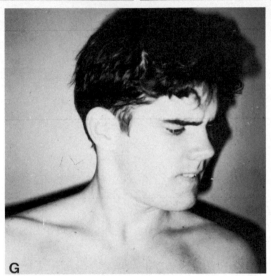

convert a reparable injury into a catastrophe.

Have a "game plan." All the necessary equipment must be readily accessible and in good operating condition. All assisting personnel should have been trained to use it properly. On-the-job training in an emergency situation is inefficient at best. Everyone should know what must be done beforehand, so that on a signal the game plan can be put into effect.

A means of transporting the athlete must be immediately available in a high-risk sport such as football and "on-call" in other sports. The medical facility must be alerted to the athlete's condition and estimated time of arrival so that adequate preparation can be made.

Having the proper equipment is an absolute must. A spine board is essential (Fig 30–2) and is the best means of supporting the body in a rigid position. It is somewhat like a full-body splint. By splinting the body, the risk of aggravating a spinal cord injury, which must always be suspected in the unconscious athlete, is reduced. In football, bolt cutters and a

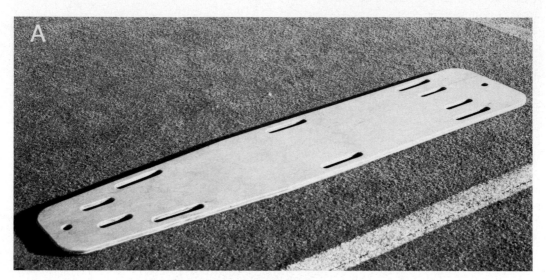

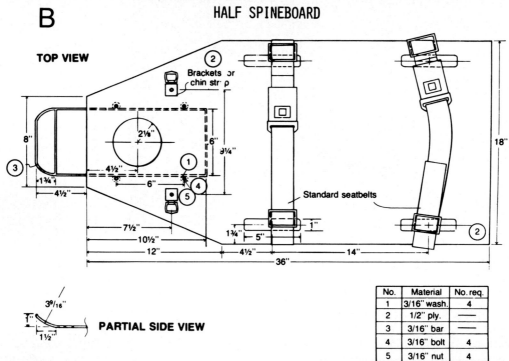

FIG 30–2.
A, standard full-length spine board made of 3/4 in. plywood. Body straps not shown. **B,** the Purdue University (West Lafayette, Ind) spine board can be constructed in any school wood shop. The board is made from 3/4 in. plywood. Body straps are standard seat belts or luggage straps that can be purchased at any Army-Navy surplus store. *(Courtesy of William "Pinky" Newell.)*

sharp knife or scalpel are also essential if it becomes necessary to remove the face mask. A telephone must be available to call for assistance and to notify the medical facility. Oxygen is usually carried by ambulance and rescue squads, although it is rarely required in an athletic setting. Rigid cervical collars and other external immobilization devices can be helpful if properly used. Manual stabilization of the head and neck is recommended even if other means are available, however.

Prevention of further injury is the single most important objective. The first step should be to immobilize the head and neck by holding them in a neutral position (Fig 30–3). Then, in the following order, check for breathing, pulse, and level of consciousness. Do not un-

fasten the chin strap or remove the helmet. With the chin strap fastened, the helmet stabilizes the head and keeps it properly aligned with the body, thereby reducing the risk of spinal cord injury associated with unstable fractures and dislocations.

If the victim is breathing, simply remove the mouth guard, if present, and maintain the airway. It is necessary to remove the face mask only if the respiratory situation is threatened or unstable, or if the athlete remains unconscious for a prolonged period.

Once it is established that the athlete is breathing and has a pulse, evaluate the neurologic status. The level of consciousness, response to pain, pupillary response, and unusual posturing, flaccid-

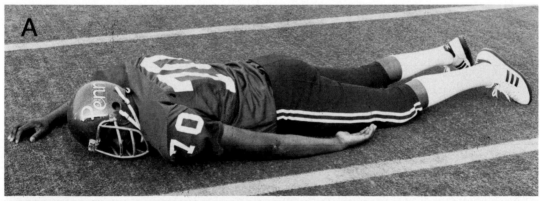

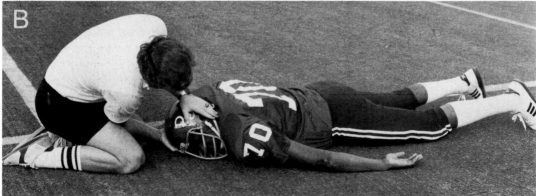

FIG 30–3.
A, athlete with suspected cervical spine injury may or may not be unconscious. However, all who are unconscious should be managed as though they had a significant neck injury. **B,** immediate manual immobilization of the head and neck unit. First check for breathing.

ity, rigidity, or weakness should be noted.

At this point, simply maintain the situation until transportation is available, or until the athlete regains consciousness. If the athlete is face down when the ambulance arrives, change his position to face up by logrolling him onto a spine board. Make no attempt to move him except to transport him or to perform cardiopulmonary resuscitation (CPR) if it becomes necessary.

If the athlete is not breathing or stops breathing, the airway must be established. If he is face down, he must be brought to a face-up position. The safest and easiest way to accomplish this is to logroll the athlete into a face-up position. In an ideal situation the medical support team is made up of five members: the leader, who controls the head and gives the commands only; three members to roll; and another to help lift and carry when it becomes necessary. If time permits and the spine board is on the scene, the athlete should be rolled directly onto it. Breathing and circulation are much more important at this point, however.

With all medical support team members in position, the athlete is rolled "like a log" toward the assistants—one at the shoulders, one at the hips, and one at the knees. They must maintain the body in line with the head and spine during the roll. The leader maintains immobilization of the head by applying slight traction and by using the crossed-arm technique. This technique allows the arms to unwind during the roll (Fig 30–4).[5]

The face mask must be removed from the helmet before rescue breathing can be initiated. The type of mask that is attached to the helmet determines the method of removal. Bolt cutters are used with the older single- and double-bar masks. The newer masks that are attached with plastic loops should be removed by cutting the loops with a sharp knife or scalpel. Remove the entire mask so that it does not interfere with further rescue efforts (Fig 30–5).

Once the mask has been removed, initiate rescue breathing following the current standards of the American Heart Association.[1]

Once the athlete has been moved to a face-up position, quickly evaluate breathing and pulse. If there is still no breathing or if breathing has stopped, the airway must be established.

The jawthrust technique is the safest first approach to opening the airway of a victim who has a suspected neck injury, because in most cases it can be accomplished by the rescuer grasping the angles of the victim's lower jaw and lifting with both hands, one on each side, displacing the mandible forward while tilting the head backward. The rescuer's elbows should rest on the surface on which the victim is lying.[1]

If the jaw thrust is not adequate, the head tilt–jaw lift should be substituted. Care must be exercised not to overextend the neck[1]:

The fingers of one hand are placed under the lower jaw on the bony part near the chin and lifted to bring the chin forward, supporting the jaw and helping to tilt the head back. The fingers must not compress the soft tissue under the chin, which might obstruct the airway. The other hand presses on the victim's forehead to tilt the head back.[1]

The transportation team should be familiar with handling a victim with a cervical spine injury. They should be receptive to taking instructions from the "leader." It is extremely important not to lose control of the care of the athlete; therefore, be familiar with the ambulance crew that is used. In an athletic situation, prior arrangements with an ambulance service should be made.

Lifting and carrying the athlete require five individuals: four to lift, and the leader to maintain immobilization of the head. The leader initiates all actions with clear, loud verbal commands (Fig 30–6).

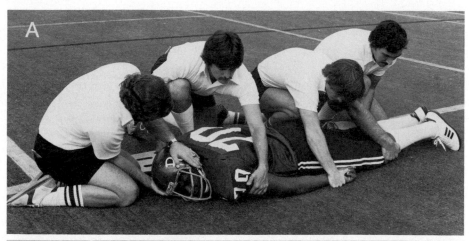

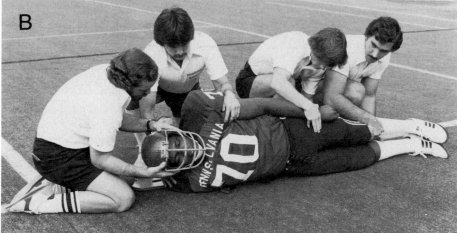

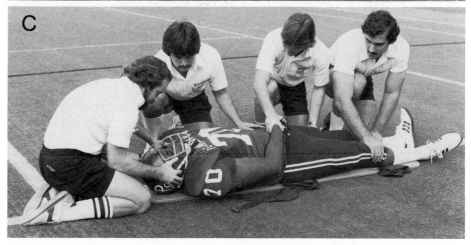

FIG 30–4.
Logroll to a spine board. **A,** this maneuver requires four individuals: the leader to immobilize the head and neck and to command the medical support team, and three individuals who are positioned at the shoulders, hips, and lower legs. **B,** the leader uses the crossed-arm technique to immobilize the head. This technique allows the leader's arms to "unwind" as the three assistants roll the athlete onto the spine board. **C,** the three assistants maintain body alignment during the roll.

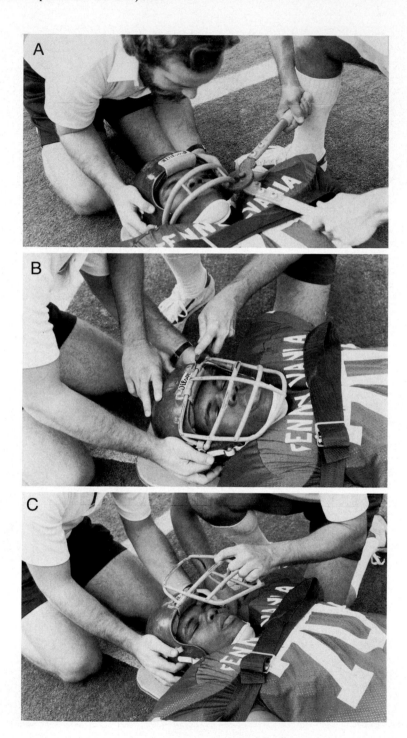

FIG 30–5.
A, remove single- and double-bar masks with bolt cutters. Head and helmet must be securely immobilized. **B,** remove "cage"-type masks by cutting the plastic loops with a utility knife. Make the cut on the side of the loop away from the face. **C,** remove the entire mask from the helmet so it does not interfere with further resuscitation efforts.

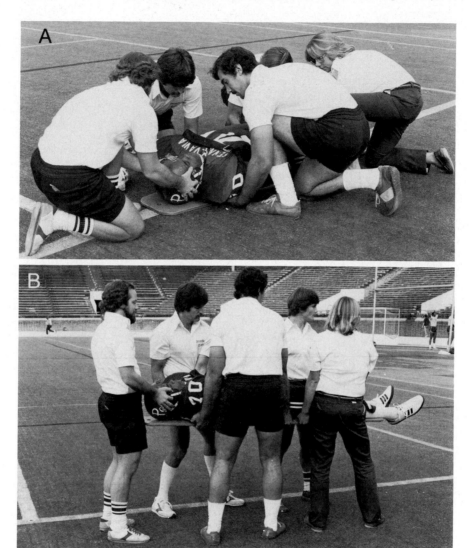

FIG 30–6.
A and **B,** four members of the medical support team lift the athlete on the command of the leader. The leader maintains manual immobilization of the head. The spine board is not recommended as a stretcher. An additional stretcher should be used for transporting over long distances.

The same guidelines apply to the choice of a medical facility as to the choice of an ambulance: Be sure it is equipped and staffed to handle an emergency head or neck injury. There should be a neurosurgeon and an orthopaedic surgeon to meet the athlete upon arrival. Roentgenographic and advanced imaging facilities should be available and standing by.

Once the athlete is in a medical facil-

ity and permanent immobilization measures are instituted, the helmet may be removed. Before removing the helmet, the chin strap must be unsnapped and discarded. In addition, the cheek pads should be removed from the helmet to allow better control of the helmet during removal. Once these preliminary steps have been completed, the athlete's head is supported at the occiput by one person while the leader spreads the earflaps and

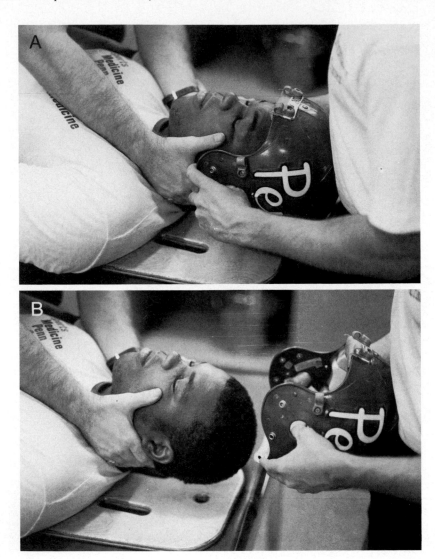

FIG 30–7.
A, the helmet should be removed only when permanent immobilization can be instituted. The helmet may be removed by detaching the chin strap, spreading the earflaps, and gently pulling the helmet off in a straight line with the cervical spine. **B,** the head must be supported under the occiput during and after removing the helmet.

pulls the helmet off in a straight line with the spine (Fig 30–7).

A recent study performed under the auspices of the National Institute of Neurological Disorders and Stroke has demonstrated that patients sustaining spinal cord injury demonstrated significant improvement in muscle function and sensation if administered methylprednisolone intravenously within 8 hours of injury. Specifically, the initial dose of methyl-

prednisolone is administered in a bolus of 30 mg/kg of body weight intravenously with an infusion pump for 15 minutes. Forty-five minutes after this, a maintenance dose of 5.4 mm/kg/hr is administered intravenously with an infusion pump for 23 hours.[2]

Although we do not propose that this regimen be initiated as an immediate emergency procedure, certainly those responsible for the spinal cord–injured athlete have an obligation to ensure that it is administered within the first 8 hours.

It is interesting to note that in the early 1970s Schneider[4] noted:

> Currently there has been a major advance in the treatment of spinal cord injuries. It has been demonstrated definitely in the experimental animal, and is reasonably well supported in man, as of this writing, that *the early use of steroids in the treatment of some spinal cord injuries will cause a diminution of swelling and destruction of the cord with the prevention of neurologic deficit.* Experimental work has shown that the drug probably should be administered within 3 to 6 hours after the spinal cord is injured for the drug to be effective. Therefore the decision whether this form of medical therapy should be instituted should be made by the physician shortly after the player has been taken to the dressing room and the presence of spinal cord damage has been confirmed. It may be withheld if the patient definitely can be transported within 3 hours to the neurosurgeon so he can make the decision. If the time interval is longer than this, then Decadron, 10 mg, should be administered intramuscularly and then 4 mg should be given every 6 hours.

REFERENCES

1. The American Association standards and guidelines for cardiopulmonary resuscitation and emergency cardiac care. *JAMA* 1986; 255:2841–3044.

2. Bracken MB, Shepard MJ, Collins WF, et al: A randomized, controlled trial of methylprednisolone or naloxone in the treatment of acute spinal-cord injury. *N Engl J Med* 1990; 322:1405–1411.

3. Clancy WG, Brand RL, Bergfeld JA: Upper trunk brachial plexus injuries in contact sports. *Am J Sports Med* 1977; 5:209.

4. Schneider RC: *Head and Neck Injuries in Football. Mechanism, Treatment, and Prevention.* Baltimore, Williams & Wilkins, 1972, p 183.

5. Torg JS, Quedenfeld TC, Newell W: When the athlete's life is threatened. *Phys Sportsmed* 1975; 3:54.

CHAPTER 31

Mechanisms and Pathomechanics of Athletic Injuries to the Cervical Spine

James C. Otis, Ph.D.

Albert H. Burstein, Ph.D.

Joseph S. Torg, M.D.

The purpose of this chapter is to describe and illustrate the mechanisms and pathomechanics of the most frequently occurring athletic injuries to the cervical spine on the basis of existing clinical, epidemiologic, and laboratory evidence and our own analysis and experimentation.

HISTORICAL THEORIES

Schneider[4] has observed, "There is probably no better experimental or research laboratory for human trauma in the world than the football fields of our nation." An analysis of available information pertaining to cervical spine injuries resulting in quadriplegia substantiates this thesis.

Accurately describing the mechanism or mechanisms responsible for a particular injury transcends simple academic interests. In order that appropriate measures be implemented to effect prevention, the manner in which injury occurs must be accurately defined. Similarly, erroneous concepts regarding in-

jury causation only act to impede the implementation of proper preventive measures. Consequently, anecdotal examples and unusual case reports must be examined critically, lest inaccuracies become established as "fact."

A variety of mechanisms have been proposed as being responsible for cervical spine injuries occurring in athletics, and, more specifically, tackle football. Two concepts, one that has implicated the face mask as acting as a lever, forcing the head and neck into hyperflexion, and the other that has implicated the posterior rim of the football helmet acting as a "guillotine," have not survived close scrutiny. This discussion of the mechanisms of cervical spine injuries must necessarily dismiss these two concepts as erroneous when evaluated in the light of existing scientific evidence.

Regarding the role of the face mask acting as a lever, causing cervical spine fracture or dislocation with or without quadriplegia, in no instance has this been reported to be a factor in 209 severe injuries that occurred between 1971 and 1975

TABLE 31–1.

Mechanism of Injury Resulting in Permanent Cervical Quadriplegia, 1971–1975

	Injuries Resulting in Quadriplegia (%) (n = 73)	Injuries Not Resulting in Quadriplegia (%) (n = 136)
Hyperflexion	10	11
Hyperextension	3	8
Vertical compression (spearing)	52	39
Knee or thigh to head	15	17
Collision, pileup, or ground contact	11	19
Tackled	7	7
Machine related	3	0
Face mask acting as lever	0	0

[Table 31–1]. The proposal that the upward sweep of a long-lever arm, the face guard, can cause a marked mechanical advantage as the posterior rim of the rigid helmet guillotines the cervical cord has been effectively refuted on the basis of radiographic, biomechanical, and epidemiologic data.

Virgin[7] performed a cineradiographic study to evaluate the possible role of the posterior rim of the football helmet in causing neck injuries. Motion pictures were produced in a series of lateral-view cineradiograms taken to document the path and position of the posterior rim of the football helmet relative to the spinal column of sixteen subjects as they moved their heads from the fully flexed to the fully extended position under several loading conditions. Five different brands of football helmets were used in the study. No contact occurred at any time between the posterior rim of any of the five helmets on the spinous processes of the cervical vertebrae (Fig 31–1). Virgin's conclusion was that the notion of the posterior rim and the helmet striking the cervical spine above the C7 level is without foundation (Fig 31–2).

Carter and Frankel[2] studied the biomechanics of cervical spine hyperextension injuries in football players with use of quasi-static-free body analysis. The study examined the guillotine mecha-

nism of injury. The static-free body analysis was undertaken to determine the forces imposed on the cervical spine when the face guard was struck in such a manner as to create hyperextension of the cervical spine. Three situations that corresponded to the loading conditions created by three different helmet designs were examined. In the first condition it was assumed that the helmet rim was cut high enough posteriorly so that it did not impinge on the posterior cervical spine. In the second condition it was assumed that the helmet rim impacted at the level of the fourth cervical vertebra. In the third case it was assumed that the posterior rim of the helmet struck the shoulder pads. The results of the analysis suggest that the most dangerous hyperextension situation occurs with the first condition, which leads to high forces and possible serious injuries to the upper cervical spine. The impact of the posterior rim of the helmet at the fourth cervical vertebra significantly reduced these forces. This finding directly conflicts with the so-called "guillotine" mechanism of injury. The impact of the posterior rim of the helmet on the shoulder pads is the least hazardous of loading conditions.

Data dealing with the mechanisms of cervical spine injuries resulting from tackle football both with and without neurologic involvement further tend to

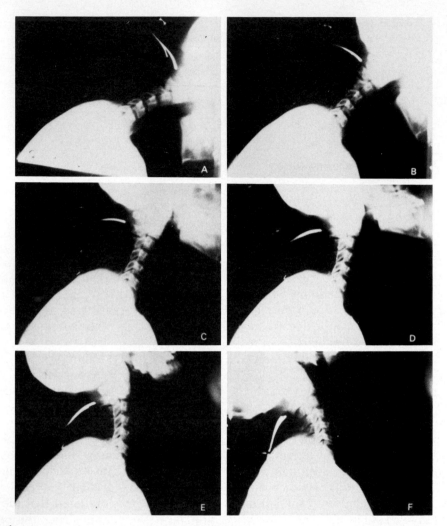

FIG 31–1.
A–F, a series of cineradiograms demonstrating the failure of the posterior rim of one of five different brands of football helmets to impinge on the soft tissue overlying the spinous processes of C1 through C6. *(From Virgin H: Cineradiographic study of football helmets and the cervical spine. Am J Sports Med 1980; 8:310. Used with permission.)*

refute the hyperextension-guillotine concept. Torg et al.[5, 6] noted that only 3% of injuries that resulted in quadriplegia were identified as being due to hyperextension, while 8% of those resulting in fracture or dislocation without quadriplegia were said to be caused by this mechanism.

To reiterate, the concept of the posterior rim of the football helmet acting as a guillotine and incurring injury to the cer-vical spinal cord in extreme forced hy-perextension is without foundation.

RECENT THEORIES

The commonly acknowledged mechanism responsible for fracture-dislocation of the cervical spine is now thought to be axial loading with failure of the spine in a flexion mode, rather than hyperflexion

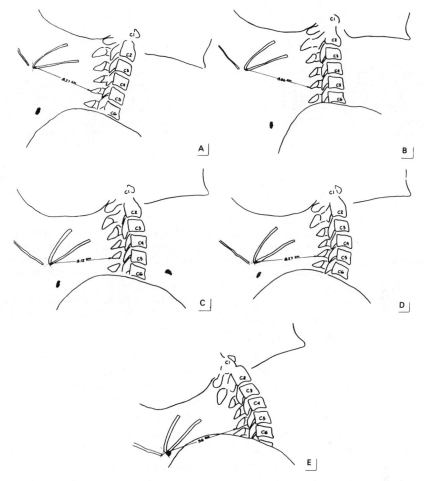

FIG 31–2.
A–E, measurements of the distance from the posterior rim of the helmet to the spinous processes C5 from the neutral position to point of impingement: **A** = 8.27 cm; **B** = 8.06 cm; **C** = 8.12 cm; **D** = 8.27 cm; and **E** = 9.6 cm. Determined from cineradiographic studies, these measurements refute the contention that the posterior rim of the football helmet can act as a guillotine in the extremes of forced cervical extension. *(From Virgin H: Cineradiographic study of football helmets and the cervical spine. Am J Sports Med 1980; 8:310. Used with permission.)*

(Fig 31–3). The subject is an unsuspecting victim of some untoward circumstance, such as an accidental fall, a dive into shallow water, an unexpected large impulse to the head, or, in the case of the athlete, a poorly executed physical act in which the cervical spine is unwittingly forced into compression and flexion, with resulting injury. In the majority of fracture-dislocations of the cervical spine that occur to football players, the major factor differentiating them from the classic in-jury is that the circumstances surrounding the event are often not accidental.

Of those cervical spine injuries resulting in quadriplegia, between 1971 and 1975 at the high school level, 72% resulted from tackling. At the college level, 78% of the quadriplegias resulted from tackling (Table 31–2). At the high school level, 52% of the injured players were defensive backs, 13% were on specialty teams, and 10% were linebackers. At the college level, 73% of those players

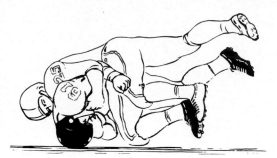

FIG 31–3.
Hyperflexion injury to the cervical spine occurs when it is forced beyond the limits of motion and the applied force exceeds the elastic capabilities of the involved structures. Recent evidence indicates that, contrary to past thinking, this mechanism is an infrequent cause of cervical spine injury in athletes. *(From Melvin WJS: The role of the face guard in the production of flexion injuries to the cervical spine in football. Can Med Assoc J 1965; 93:1110. Used with permission.)*

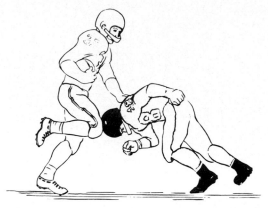

FIG 31–4.
Axial loading of the cervical spine due to impact on the crown of the head or helmet is responsible for the majority of serious injuries that occur in football. The same mechanism is responsible for diving injuries.
(From Melvin WJS: The role of the face guard in the production of flexion injuries to the cervical spine in football. Can Med Assoc J 1965; 93:1110. Used with permission.)

rendered quadriplegic were defensive backs.[6] The data indicated that 52% of all cervical spine quadriplegias that occurred between 1971 and 1975 resulted from "spearing," or direct-compression head-on type collisions, in which initial contact was made with the top or crown of the helmet. These figures clearly identify the individuals at greatest risk of sustaining a cervical spine injury resulting in quadriplegia as the defensive backs, linebackers, or specialty team members who tackle by using their heads as the initial point of contact (Fig 31–4 and Table 31–3).

In the majority of injuries that re-

sulted in quadriplegia, the subject was, of his own volition, executing a maneuver in which the head was used as a battering ram, the initial point of contact being made with the top or crown of the helmet in a high-impact situation. Thus, rather than an accidental, untoward event, a technique was deliberately implemented that placed the cervical spine at the risk of catastrophic injury (Fig 31–5).

When a force applied to the cervical spine exceeds the elastic capabilities of the involved structures, injury results. In the course of a contact activity such as

TABLE 31–2.

Injury by Activity

	Permanent Cervical Quadriplegia, 1971–1975		Cervical Fracture-Dislocations Without Quadriplegia, 1971–1975	
	High School (%) (n = 77)	College (%) (n = 18)	High School (%) (n = 105)	College (%) (n = 46)
Tackling	72	78	59	49
Tackled	14	22	15	24
Blocking	6	0	7	16
Drill	3	0	5	7
Collision pileup	3	0	12	4
Machine related	2	0	2	0

TABLE 31–3.

Injury by Position, 1971–1975

	Permanent Cervical Quadriplegia		Cervical Fracture-Dislocations Without Quadriplegia	
	High School (%) (n = 52)	College (%) (n = 15)	High School (%) (n = 89)	College (%) (n = 47)
Defensive back	52	73	23	33
Linebacker	10	0	18	17
Specialty team	13	7	2	0
Offensive back	12	7	20	21
Defensive line	10	0	28	12
Offensive line	4	13	8	15

tackle football, the cervical spine is repeatedly exposed to potentially injurious energy levels. Fortunately, however, most energy inputs on the cervical spine are effectively dissipated in lateral bending, flexion, or extension by the energy-absorbing capabilities of the cervical paravertebral musculature, the intervertebral disks, and, to a lesser extent, the ligaments. However, the bones, disks, and ligamentous structures can be injured when contact occurs at the top or crown of the helmet, with the head, neck, and trunk positioned in such a way that forces are transmitted along the axis of the cervical spine, obviating the safe modes of energy-absorption of these structures.

Considering the cervical spine from the lateral perspective, with the neck in the neutral position, the normal alignment of the spine is one of extension because of the normal cervical lordosis (Fig 31–6). It is with forward flexion of the neck that the cervical spine is straightened (Fig 31–7). With force exerted along the axis of a straight spine, loading of a segmented column occurs (Fig 31–8). When the energy input exceeds the energy-absorbing capacities of the involved structure, intervertebral disk space injury, vertebral body fracture, ligamentous disruption, or posterior element fracture can ensue. When maximum vertical compressive deformation is reached, acute local cervical spine flexion occurs,

with fracture, subluxation, or unilateral or bilateral facet dislocation. The majority of cervical spine injuries that result in quadriplegia in tackle football are due to purposeful loading along the long axis of the vertebral elements.

INJURY MECHANISM

In order to understand the biomechanics of this injury mechanism, first consider a seemingly unrelated injury, the jammed finger. This is an injury common to basketball players that occurs when the tip of a fully outstretched finger is struck by an oncoming basketball. The resulting injury is a dislocation of the proximal interphalangeal joint. This dislocation occurs because the phalanges behave as a segmented, elastic column. The kinetic energy of the ball is transferred to strain energy in the column, and when sufficient strain energy has been stored to make the column unstable, buckling occurs. Buckling is a mechanism of energy release that can be produced in slender columns subjected to axial compressive loads.

Axial loading fractures, dislocations, and fracture-dislocations of the cervical spine result from the same compressive loading mechanism. Since the typical burst fracture of a cervical vertebral body is produced by direct compressive loads, it is reasonable to expect that axial com-

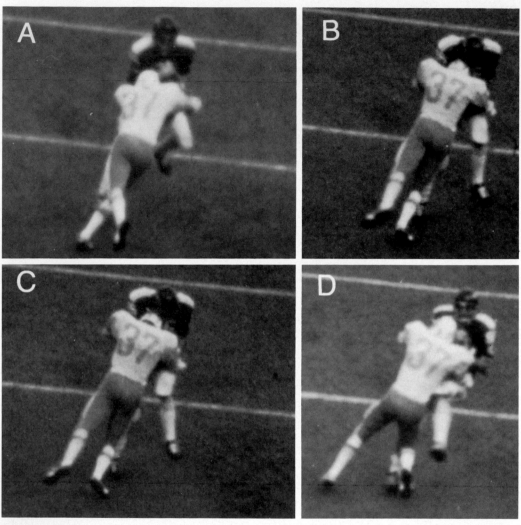

FIG 31–5.
A, subject (37, foreground) lines up in front of ball carrier in preparation for tackling. **B,** preimpact position shows tackler about to ram ball carrier with crown of his helmet. **C,** at impact, contact is made with the top of the helmet. Although the neck is slightly flexed, it is clearly not hyperflexed. The major force vector is transmitted along the axial alignment of the cervical spine. **D,** the tackler recoils after impact.

pression of the cervical spine can result in compressive failures of the vertebral bodies.[8] What then is the mechanism for producing dislocations, which must apparently derive from excessive angulation, that is, hyperflexion of the proximal vertebral body over the contiguous distal vertebral body? As seen in the example of the jammed finger, the buckling phenomenon is really a large local angulation that develops somewhere along the length of the compressed column. This angulation, or buckling, occurs whenever there is more energy due to compression load stored in the column than can be stored in that same column in a bending mode.

Several factors affect the mechanical stability of the system, and, hence, control the point at which buckling occurs. These factors include the size and shape of the vertebral bodies and disks, the

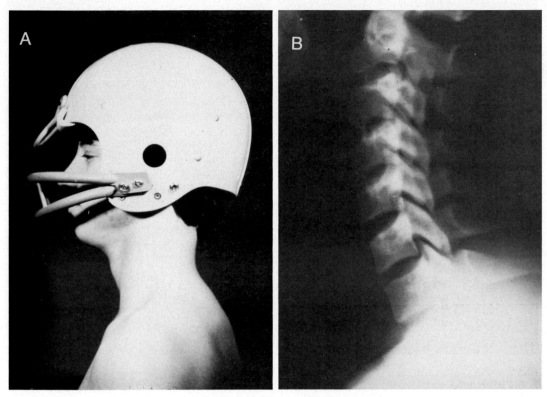

FIG 31–6.
A and **B,** with the head and neck held in the neutral position, because of normal cervical lordosis, the posture of the cervical spine is one of extension. *(From Torg J: National Football Head and Neck Injuries Registry: Report on the cervical quadriplegia from 1971 to 1975. Am J Sports Med 1979; 7:127. Used with permission.)*

elastic characteristics of surrounding ligamentous tissue, and the stabilizing preload imposed by muscles crossing the cervical spine. Under extreme compressive load, damage that occurs in any part of the cervical spine will control the onset of buckling. If, while under compressive load, one vertebral body collapses (compression fracture), the whole system becomes unstable at that point and reverts into a buckling mode failure. The first damage that occurs within the cervical column in many instances is a compression fracture of the vertebral body. After this fracture, local buckling is triggered and hyperflexion occurs in that same region. Buckling may also be triggered by failure of the intervertebral disk. The local hyperflexion that follows often produces a dislocation, and this is the

major damage mode observed. The ability to predict whether a crush fracture or a collapsing disk will be the initiating mechanism has to date eluded exact analytic definition.

The experimental literature contains sufficient information to put critical limits on the magnitude of a compressive load that can be supported by individual vertebral bodies. While most of these data have been accumulated for lumbar and thoracic vertebral bodies, extrapolation of the data gives compressive load limits for cervical vertebral bodies of 3,340 to 4,450 newtons (750 to 1,000 lb).

In order for the cervical spine to carry load under direct compression, it is necessary that the spine be in a straight (anatomically partially flexed) position. In this position the spine is capable of sus-

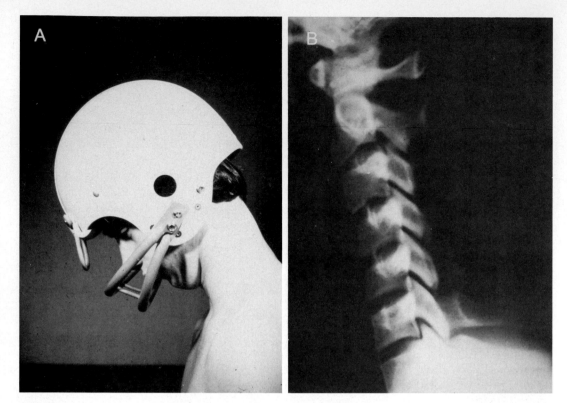

FIG 31–7.
A and **B,** when the neck is flexed approximately 30 degrees, the cervical spine becomes straight; from the standpoint of force, energy absorption, and the effect on tissue deformation and failure, the straightened cervical spine, when axially loaded, acts as a segmented column. *(From Torg J: National Football Head and Neck Injuries Registry: Report on the cervical quadriplegia from 1971 to 1975. Am J Sports Med 1979; 7:127. Used with permission.)*

FIG 31–8.
Axial loading of a segmented column **(A)** initially results in compressive deformation **(B),** and, if the axial load is of sufficient magnitude, more marked deformation occurs **(C).** Absorption of excessive amounts of energy during axial loading can result in buckling, with a resulting fracture or dislocation of the segmented column.

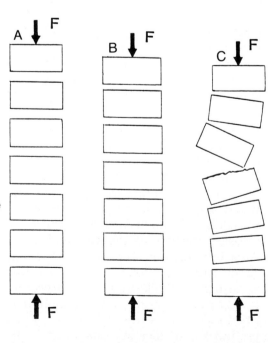

taining compression load directly without assistance from the muscles or supporting ligamentous structures. If the spine is not in a straightened position, axial load simply causes bending moments and bending deformation that result in further asymmetries of loading. Therefore, if a load of 3,340 to 4,450 newtons is reached while the spine is loaded in an axial compressive mode, a compression failure of the vertebral body or disk occurs, and this is the initiating factor in a compression, buckling, local hyperflexion failure mode.

Experimental substantiation of the field observations and subsequent analysis identifying axial loading as the mechanism responsible for the majority of football-related cervical spine injuries have been demonstrated previously by Roaf[3] and Bauze.[1] Roaf published results of studies in which spinal units were subjected to forces differing in magnitude and direction, that is, compression, flexion, extension, lateral flexion, rotation, and horizontal shear. He stated unequivocally that he had never succeeded in producing pure hyperflexion injuries in a normal intact spinal unit, and concluded that hyperflexion of the cervical spine is an anatomic impossibility. Of equal significance is the fact that Roaf[3] was able to produce almost every variety of spinal injury by a combination of compression and rotation.

Bauze[1] reported experimental production of forward dislocation of the cervical spine by subjecting it to pure axial loads. The spine in human cadavers was subjected to loads in a compression apparatus to simulate the clinical situation for dislocation. The movements were recorded by lateral cineradiography. The lower part of the spine was flexed and fixed, and the upper part was extended and free to move forward. Vertical compression then produced bilateral dislocation of the facet joints without fracture. If lateral tilt or axial rotation occurred as

well, a unilateral dislocation was produced. The maximum vertical loading required was 1,420 newtons (319 lb), and coincided with rupture of the posterior ligament and capsule and severing of the anterior longitudinal ligament before dislocation. The low vertical load indicates the peculiar vulnerability of the cervical spine in this position. Bauze[1] concluded that this low load correlated well with the minor trauma often seen in association with forward dislocation.

ANATOMIC MODEL SIMULATION

To determine if an impact loading could cause cervical spine buckling, we constructed an anatomic model of the head, neck, and upper area of the torso with use of a plastic skeleton. Four and one-half kilograms of mass was added to the cranial cavity. Ten kilograms of mass was installed within the thoracic cage. The total mass of the model was approximately 29 kg. The cervical spine segments were assembled in a straight configuration to represent the slightly flexed anatomic position. The intervertebral spaces and the articular facet spaces were filled with silicone (silastic) sealant and allowed to cure. Additional silicone sealant was used to secure the skull to the cervical spine and the cervical spine to the thoracic spine, which was maintained rigid. Further stability and stiffening were achieved by building up Silastic "ligaments" along the anterior surface and around the posterior elements. Stretched latex tubing was used to simulate the extensor muscle forces necessary to maintain a slightly flexed position of the head and neck with the model in a face-down, horizontal attitude. With use of a four-bar linkage system to maintain the horizontal attitude, the model was allowed to swing in a pendular fashion from a height that resulted in an impact velocity of approximately 3 m/sec. The head impacted a vertical barrier, producing a compressive load along the cervical spine. High-speed photography at 9,000 frames per second was conducted to document the motion just before and just after impact.

ANALYTIC MODEL SIMULATION

We then questioned what type of impact situations are capable of generating the compressive loads that will give rise to compression, buckling, local hyperflexion failure. We constructed two analytic models with use of a digital computer to answer this question. The models used measured load vs. deformation parameters for a helmet and approximate load vs. deformation parameters for the neck, in order to examine those situations that could give rise to the aforementioned cervical spine failures.

The two degree-of-freedom model assumed that the cervical spine was in an anatomically straight position and that a football player encountered a fixed object with his helmet while proceeding at some forward velocity. The three degree-of-freedom model allowed for impacting or being impacted by a moving mass. To duplicate actual observed configurations, the model allowed the helmet, head, cervical spine, and a portion of the trunk to move along a straight line coincident with the axis of the neck. It was assumed that contact was made at the top of the helmet in the same area that the central axis of the neck crosses the top of the helmet (Fig 31–9). The mathematic model used either a two or three degree-of-freedom, nonlinear analysis for the dynamic non-steady-state solution. Computation is on the basis of a small time interval approximation with an iterative solution. Two situations were investigated: head-first impact into a rigid barrier, which also simulates impact between two players moving together in a symmetric fash-

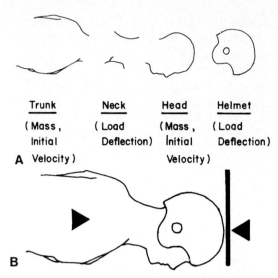

FIG 31–9.
A, the composite model consists of a trunk mass, a nonlinear spring cervical spine, a head mass, and a nonlinear spring-damped helmet load-deflection function. The basic law of dynamics ($F = MA$) characterizes system. **B,** the model, representing the axial loading injury condition, illustrates how the cervical spine is compressed between an abruptly decelerated head mass and the continued momentum of the body.

ion, and impact between two players with one or both moving.

The mechanical load vs. deflection characteristics of several helmets had been determined experimentally by placing the helmets on a rigid head form. An MTS hydraulic servocontrolled test machine was used to apply a ramp displacement to the crown of the helmet (Fig 31–10). The load vs. displacement tests were conducted so that the test cycle was completed in 60 ms. While the final solutions indicate that the actual sequence of events occurs in less than 60 ms, it was nevertheless believed that a 60 ms duration test would portray the characteristics of the helmet with reasonable accuracy. The resulting load vs. deformation curves were recorded on an oscilloscope and then digitized for use in the computer simulation. For each test the helmet was preconditioned by several loading cycles and adjusted on the head form in accordance with the fitting instructions. There-

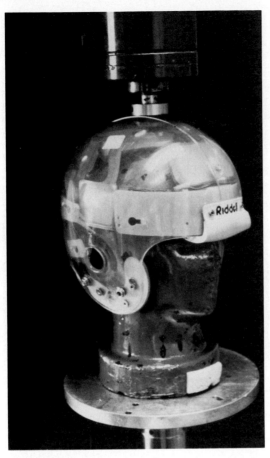

FIG 31–10.
The MTS hydraulic servocontrolled test machine used to apply step displacement to the crown of the helmet in load vs. displacement test.

fore, all data represent reproducible load-deformation cycle curves. For modeling purposes the curve was assumed to be infinitely stiff at that amplitude at which the helmet system starts to display an almost vertical asymptote on the load vs. deformation curves.

In addition to investigating headfirst impact into a fixed barrier and impact of the body of a moving player into the head of a stationary player, three parametric studies were carried out to determine whether conditions existed that would allow development of between 3,340 and 4,450 newtons of compressive force on the neck. The first study examined variations in impact velocity, the second ex-

amined the effect of varying trunk mass, and the third examined the influence of varying helmet performance characteristics.

The parameters that the designer can vary within the helmet are the stiffness and thickness of the lining. These two parameters are responsible for the shape and extent of the load-deformation curve. If a helmet is to be used in football, it must possess reversible deformation characteristics. This limits the material choice to those that either display straight-line load deflection characteristics (the so-called "linear materials") or, in a more realistic representation, those that display curves that may be described as exponential.

The impact velocities examined were 2.3, 4.6, and 6.1 m/sec (7.5, 15, and 20 ft/ sec), which ranged from fast walking speed to about two thirds of the top speed of a well-conditioned athlete.

In football impact situations, since the trunk, legs, and arms are not always traveling along the same axis as the head and neck, the third study was conducted to see what the effect of trunk mass would be on the loading dynamics and load magnitudes that cause catastrophic cervical spine failure. Therefore, three effective trunk masses were considered: 36, 18, and 9 kg. A conservative estimate of the trunk mass (less limbs) was 36 kg, while the 9 kg mass was used to represent that portion of the trunk associated only with the shoulders and upper thoracic region. This last estimate is probably a minimum, since that portion of the trunk is virtually always traveling in almost the same direction as that of the neck at the time of impact.

TEST RESULTS

Anatomic Model

The photographic results of the impact study with use of the anatomic

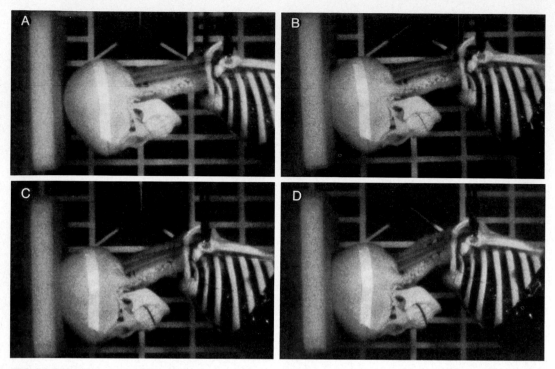

FIG 31–11.
A–D, selected stills from the high-speed photographic study demonstrate the configuration. **A,** at time of initial impact (*t* = 0 m/sec); **B,** when the head has stopped (*t* = 11.1 m/sec); **C,** when the continued motion of the torso compressed the cervical spine (*t* = 16.7 m/sec); and **D,** when buckling resulted in the mechanical destruction of the midcervical spine (*t* = 22.2 m/sec).

model are illustrated in Figure 31–11. The configuration at the time of initial impact (*t* = 0/m/sec) is illustrated in Figure 31–11,*A*. Comparison of Figures 31–11,*B* and *C* obtained at 11.1 m/sec and 16.7 m/sec, respectively, illustrates that the head has stopped at 11.1 m/sec while the torso continues to move toward the head. At 22.2 m/sec it can be seen that the continued motion of the torso compressed the cervical spine and produced mechanical destruction of the midcervical spine because of buckling (Figure 31–11,*D*). This is evidenced from the increased flexion angle locally at the midcervical spine and the increased spacing posteriorly between the spinous processes at this level. Thus the high-speed photographic study with use of the anatomic model permitted the documentation of the events associated with this

impact, which in real time appears to occur instantaneously. The study demonstrated the phenomenon of the head stopping, the cervical spine being compressed as it attempts to decelerate the torso, and the subsequent buckling of the cervical column. Figure 31–12 illustrates the mechanical disruption of the model of the cervical spine that occurred as a result of buckling.

Analytic Model

The simulation results obtained from the model with use of a torso mass of 36 kg, an impact velocity of 4.6 m/sec, and the load vs. deflection characteristics of a Riddell PAC-3 football helmet showed a displacement capability of approximately 3 cm when it develops a resisting load of approximately 7,000 newtons. The simu-

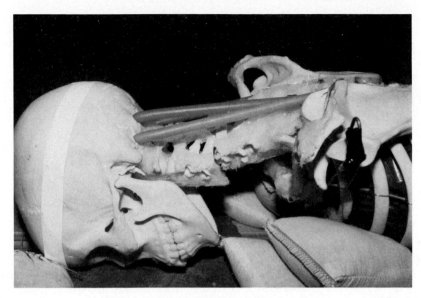

FIG 31-12.
The mechanical disruption of the cervical spine model that occurred as a result of buckling.

lation runs were conducted until the neck force reached 4,450 newtons, the upper load limit identified for failure in compression. The force and displacement curves (Fig 31–13) illustrated that the helmet force increased as the head continued to move further into the helmet, until a time at which the head rebounded (t = 8 m/sec) and the helmet force decreased. Unlike the motion of the head, the displacement of the torso continued at a nearly constant rate such that the distance between the torso and the head was being compromised and the force in the neck increased to 4,450 newtons at 11 m/sec.

Just before impact, all of the energy was the kinetic energy of the moving torso and head masses. Figure 31–14 illustrates that the kinetic energy of the

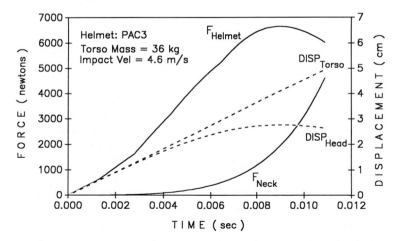

FIG 31-13.
Force and displacement curves after impact with a fixed barrier demonstrate that the helmet force increased until a time at which the head rebounded (t = 8 m/sec). Torso displacement can be seen to continue at a nearly constant rate until the force limit was reached for the cervical spine.

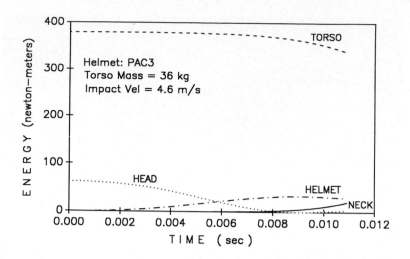

FIG 31–14.
The curves illustrate that the initial energy is that of the moving head and torso. Immediately after impact the kinetic energy of the head is first transferred to the helmet, which bottoms out, and, subsequently, the kinetic energy of the torso is transferred to the neck. Failure of the neck occurs, with nearly all of the kinetic energy of the torso remaining.

head decreased as it was transferred into the helmet liner as stored elastic energy. The head came to a stop at about 8 m/sec as the helmet reached its capacity for absorbing energy and bottomed out. At this time the torso energy began to decrease more rapidly as its energy was being absorbed by the neck. This continued until the neck reached its force limit at 11 m/sec. Only a small percentage of the initial kinetic energy of the torso was dissipated at the time of cervical spine failure, indicating that failure occurred with a large percentage of the initial kinetic energy of the torso remaining. It should be noted that the simulation accounts for only the major energy losses, so that results are approximate.

The forces and displacements resulting from an impact between two players are illustrated in Figure 31–15. The injured player was stationary when impacted by a 36 kg mass moving at a velocity of 4.6 m/sec along a direction coincident with the long axis of the cervical spine. As the helmet was pushed toward the body of the injured player, the helmet force increased directly after impact, and, as a result of the force applied

to it, the head displaced backward toward the torso. The relatively large inertia of the torso resisted motion, thus creating a situation in which, because of the backward motion of the head, the neck force increased until failure occurred. A comparison of Figures 31–15 and 31–13 illustrates the similarity of the helmet force and neck force histories for the case in which the injured player impacted a fixed barrier and this case in which the head of the injured player was impacted while at rest. In both cases neck failure occurred at 11 m/sec, and there is virtually no difference from the viewpoint of the loading history of the cervical spine.

The effects on neck force dynamics were computed for variations in impact velocity and torso mass. Figure 31–16 illustrates the neck force histories for impact velocities of 2.3 m/sec to 6.1 m/sec. The variation in velocity significantly affected the time at which failure occurred, with the fast velocity resulting in a predicted failure at 8 m/sec, whereas the slower velocity resulted in a predicted failure at 17 m/sec. It does remain, however, that with a torso mass of 36 kg, neck failure occurred at all velocities investi-

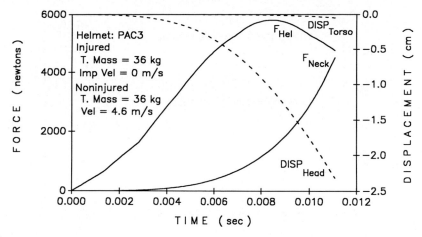

FIG 31–15.
The forces and displacements for a stationary injured player resulting from an impact by a moving opponent illustrate the rapid increase in force at the helmet as it is pushed toward the body of the injured player, and the resulting head displacement against a nearly fixed torso, which results in an increase in neck force until failure occurs.

gated. On the other hand, when varying the torso mass from 36 to 9 kg while maintaining impact velocity of 4.6 m/sec, it is evident from Figure 31–17 that the effect on the neck force history was negligible, with all three predicted failures occurring within 1 ms of each other. Clearly, neck failure occurred for all conditions of velocity and mass that were examined, but with fracture time being more strongly influenced by velocity than torso mass. The results clearly reflect that energy that is responsible for this injury mechanism is proportional to mass raised to the first power and velocity raised to the second power.

The results of incorporating the load-displacement characteristics of five different helmets into the simulation are illustrated in Figures 31–18 and 31–19 for

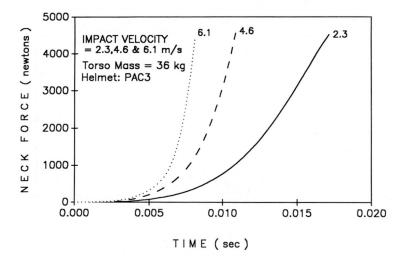

FIG 31–16.
The neck force histories are illustrated for variations in impact velocity from 2.3 m/sec to 6.1 m/sec with use of a constant torso mass of 36 kg.

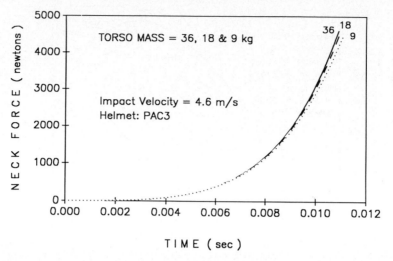

FIG 31–17.
The neck force histories for variations in torso mass from 36 to 9 kg with impact velocity remaining constant at 4.6 m/sec.

conditions of an impact into a fixed barrier at 4.6 m/sec and a torso mass of 36 kg. Although under these conditions neck injury resulted regardless of helmet type, there were some temporal differences in performance with respect to the onset of the failure load (Fig 31–18). The most rapid rate of load transmission to the neck was with the Shoei motorcycle helmet, where neck failure was predicted

to occur by 7 ms. The two Riddell football helmets yielded similar responses. The SK600 hockey helmet was more comparable to the two Riddell football helmets, but with a slightly more rapid loading of the neck, and the Bike football helmet demonstrated the least rapid neck loading response. The simulated head decelerations associated with these five helmets are illustrated in Figure 31–19. The

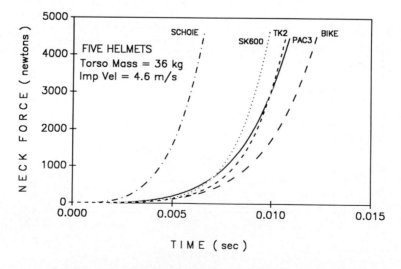

FIG 31–18.
The neck force histories utilizing five different helmet characteristics in the simulation with an impact velocity of 4.6 m/sec and a torso mass of 36 kg, demonstrating temporal differences in performance with respect to the onset of the failure load.

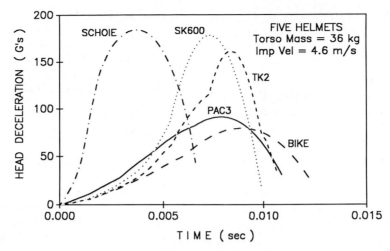

FIG 31–19.
Simulated head decelerations associated with the five different helmets tested are illustrated with use of a constant torso mass and impacting velocity.

Shoei, SK600, and TK2 all demonstrated peak decelerations of greater than 150 g, whereas the head decelerations of the PAC-3 and the Bike were less than 100 g. It is interesting to note that the dynamic loads on the neck for the two Riddell helmets, the TK2 and the newer type PAC-3, were quite similar, yet the PAC-3 displayed lower "g" head loads. The PAC-3 was capable of taking up more energy earlier during the impact, allowing for a more gradual deceleration of the head compared with the TK2 helmet. Thus significant improvements in "g" loads experienced by the head are not associated with major changes in the neck loading dynamics.

Our results demonstrate that the typical helmet was able to bring the head to rest at between 6 and 12 m/sec, depending on the initial velocity of the head. It did this while keeping the head accelerations well within intended limits. Since the kinetic energy of the head is approximately 60 Nm, while the kinetic energy of the torso can easily exceed 380 Nm, it is obvious that the helmet cannot be relied upon to absorb the kinetic energy of the torso. Moreover, since the function of the helmet is to provide protection for

the skull, a redesigned helmet, which would also be capable of absorbing all the kinetic energy of the body, would be a disproportionate and totally useless head protection structure.

The mechanism displayed for the rigid wall impact in the computation model was one of the helmet stopping the head while the trunk continued its motion and transferred its kinetic energy to the neck. Under the alignment conditions previously described, the neck, a relatively fragile structure in compression, cannot absorb the kinetic energy without exceeding its dynamic load limits. Therefore fractures or dislocations occur. Furthermore, these damages also occur under the alignment conditions described even when a player is in a stationary position and is impacted to the top of the head by another player or body segment of that player.

The model that has been examined described the conditions under which cervical spinal fractures or dislocations occur. Based on observed geometry during actual cervical spine injury in football, there was a coincident anatomic axis for the head, neck, and trunk. In addition, the velocity of these segments was parallel to this anatomic axis, and the impact occurred between the helmet and a relatively immovable object. This study showed that the helmet successfully stopped the head. However, in all dynamic conditions examined, the trunk continued to input kinetic energy into the neck in the form of strain energy until a sufficient amount of energy was stored to damage the cervical spine. The damage mode may be (1) compression, which produces crush fractures of the cervical vertebrae; (2) buckling, which produces acute flexion dislocation at one cervical level; or (3) a combination of these two modes. Because of disparity between the kinetic energy of the head, the helmet is not a suitable structure for absorbing all kinetic energies, and therefore is not useful in preventing neck injury.

The one meaningful conclusion to be drawn from the available data is that axial loading of the cervical spine must be avoided if injuries are to be prevented. Cervical spine injuries are a function of technique, that is, head tackling or diving into shallow water, and cannot be prevented by equipment, that is, helmets. The implications of this fact for coaches, game officials, and athletic administrators are obvious.

Acknowledgment

We gratefully acknowledge the effort and expertise of Peter A. Torzilli. Without him the high-speed photographic study would not have been possible.

REFERENCES

1. Bauze RJ: Experimental production of forward dislocations in the human cervical spine. *J Bone Joint Surg* [Br] 1978; 60B:239.

2. Carter DR, Frankel VH: Biomechanics of hyperextension injuries to the cervical spine in football. *Am J Sports Med* 1980; 8:302.

3. Roaf R: A study of the mechanics of spinal injuries. *J Bone Joint Surg* [Br] 1960; 42B:810.

4. Schneider RC: *Head and Neck Injuries in Football.* Baltimore, Williams & Wilkins, 1973.

5. Torg JS, et al: Spinal injury at the level of the third and fourth cervical vertebrae from football. *J Bone Joint Surg* [Am] 1977; 59A:1015.

6. Torg JS, et al: The National Football Head and Neck Injury Registry: 14-year report on cervical quadriplegia, 1971–1984. *JAMA* 1985; 254:3439–3443.

7. Virgin H: Cineradiographic study of football helmets and the cervical spine. *Am J Sports Med* 1980; 8:310.

8. White AA, Panjabi MM: *Clinical Biomechanics of the Spine.* Philadelphia, JB Lippincott Co, 1978.

CHAPTER 32

Upper Cervical Spine Injuries (C1 and C2)

Steven G. Glasgow, M.D.

Traumatic lesions to the upper cervical spine rarely occur in athletic activities. This region, which includes the first and second cervical vertebrae, serves as a transition zone between the cranium and the more typical middle and lower cervical vertebrae. The anatomy of C1 and the upper portion of C2 is unique, while the lower portion of C2 conforms to the more typical cervical vertebrae. Approximately 50% of axial rotation of the cervical spine takes place at the atlantoaxial joint, and 40% to 50% of flexion-extension takes place between the occiput and C2.[15, 21, 23] Just as the anatomy and physiology of C1 and C2 are unique, so are those lesions resulting from trauma.

ATLAS FRACTURES

Jefferson,[10] in 1920, described three different types of atlas fractures: (1) a comminuted burst fracture; (2) a posterior arch fracture, and (3) a fracture of both the anterior and posterior arches.

The burst fracture is a four-part fracture of the ring occurring in approximately 30% of C1 fractures. Jefferson described the mechanism of injury as a blow to the vertex of the head, with its force transmitted through the occipital condyles to the lateral masses of C1 (Figs 32–1 and 32–2). The transmission of the axial load results in a comminuted fracture of the ring of C1, with lateral displacement of the lateral masses. An anteroposterior (AP) open mouth projection of C1–C2 best demonstrates the bilateral overhang of the lateral masses of the atlas in relationship to the axis. These fractures are generally stable when the combined lateral overhang of the atlas measures less than 7 mm. Stable fractures can be treated by rigid cervical orthosis.[11–13, 22, 24] When the transverse diameter of the atlas is 7 mm or greater than the transverse diameter of the axis, a transverse ligament rupture should be suspected[23] (Fig 32–3). These fractures are considered unstable, and treatment includes traction, to improve fracture fragment position, and halo immobilization. Posterior cervical fusion is occasionally indicated[19] (Figs 32–4 and 32–5).

Fractures of the posterior arch are the most common atlantal fractures, and occur at the groove for the vertebral artery where the posterior arch is thinnest. The

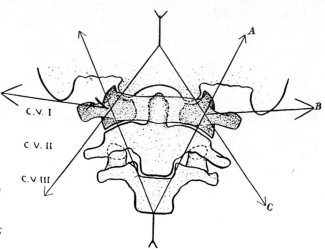

FIG 32–1.
Schematic representation of the force vectors resulting in a comminuted burst fracture of the atlas. Axial load from the vertex of the head through the occipital condyles to the lateral masses of C1 *(C)*. Axial load from below through the axis to the lateral masses of C1 *(A)*. The resultant lateral spread of the lateral masses of C1 *(B)*. *(From Jefferson G: Br J Surg 1919; 7:407–422. Used with permission.)*

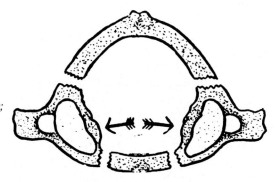

FIG 32–2.
Schematic representation of the four-part comminuted burst fracture of the atlas as seen from above. *(From Jefferson G: Br J Surg 1919; 7:407–422. Used with permission.)*

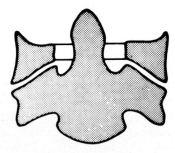

STABLE

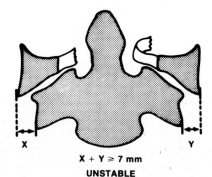

$X + Y \geq 7$ mm
UNSTABLE

FIG 32–3.
Illustration of a comminuted Jefferson fracture with both the transverse ligament intact (stable configuration) and a transverse ligament rupture (unstable configuration). *(From White AA, Penjabi MM: Clinical Biomechanics of the Spine. Philadelphia, JB Lippincott Co, 1978, p 204. Used with permission.)*

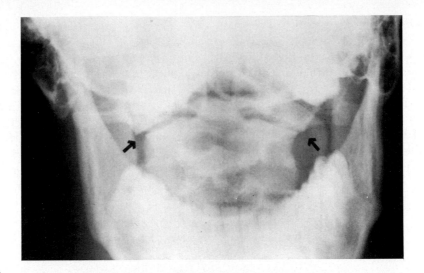

FIG 32–4.
Clinical example of a comminuted four-part C1 fracture with a stable configuration. This is an open mouth view of a 19-year-old football player who injured his neck in delivering a blow with the crown of his head. The patient was examined on the sidelines and was noted to have neck pain with decreased motion and a click with flexion-extension. There were no neurologic findings. The player was not allowed to return to the game, and a subsequent cervical study revealed splaying of the C1 lateral masses less than 7 mm *(black arrows).* He was not permitted to return to tackle football.

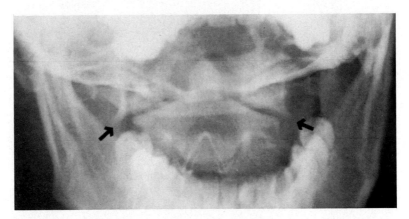

FIG 32–5.
Open mouth view illustrating an unstable C1 burst fracture with rupture of transverse ligament as indicated by lateral overhang greater than or equal to 7 mm *(black arrows).*

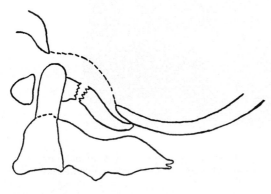

FIG 32–6.
Illustration of vertical compression with extension of the occiput, fracturing the posterior arch of C1 just posterior to the lateral masses in the groove for the vertebral artery. *(From Sherk HH, Nicholson JT: J Bone Joint Surg [Am] 1970; 52A:1017–1024. Used with permission.)*

mechanism of injury is considered to be an extension force, with a vertical compression of the posterior ring of C1 by the occiput[18] (Fig 32–6). They are generally considered to be stable and can be treated with a rigid cervical orthosis.[13, 22]

Simultaneous fractures of the anterior and posterior rings have also been noted. This atlas fracture pattern is the least common, and is occasionally seen with an odontoid fracture. When an odontoid fracture is not present, these fractures are considered to be stable and can be treated in a rigid cervical orthosis. If a fracture of C1 is suspected and not confirmed on the open mouth and lateral-view radiographs, a computed tomography (CT) scan of C1–C2 is indicated (Fig 32–7).

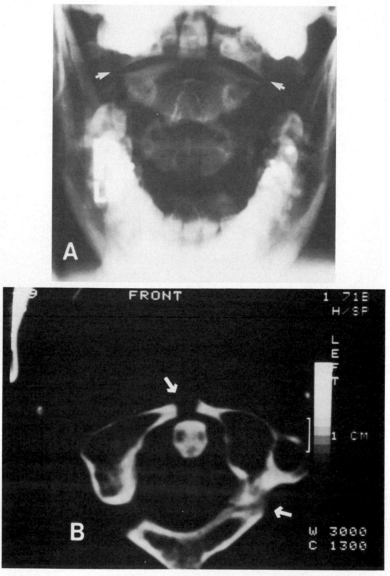

FIG 32–7.
Clinical example of undisplaced anterior and posterior arch fractures. **A,** open mouth view is without abnormality *(arrowheads).* **B,** CT scan illustrates an anterior arch fracture with a concomitant left posterior arch fracture *(white arrows).*

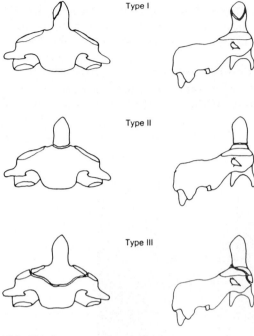

Type I

Type II

Type III

FIG 32–8.
Illustration of the three types of odontoid fractures in both the AP and lateral planes. Type I is an oblique avulsion fracture from the upper portion of the odontoid process. Type II is a fracture of the odontoid process at its base. Type III is an odontoid fracture through the body of C2. *(From Anderson LD, D'Alonzo RT: J Bone Joint Surg [Am] 1974; 56A:1663–1674. Used with permission.)*

ODONTOID FRACTURES

Fractures of the odontoid process have been classified into three types by Anderson and D'Alonzo[1] (Fig 32–8). The mechanism of injury for odontoid fractures has not been clearly delineated. These fractures appear to be due to a head impact with a flexion or an extension force. A blow to the head with forward flexion is thought to be the more common mechanism, because anterior displacement of the odontoid fracture is seen far more frequently than posterior displacement. A high index of suspicion is needed to diagnose this fracture, and all routine cervical spine roentgenographic studies should include an open mouth view to identify these lesions. If these radiographs are negative and a lesion is suspected, tomograms of C1–C2 will further delineate the pathologic process.

The type I fracture is an avulsion of the tip of the odontoid process at the site of attachment of the alar ligaments. This is a rare fracture pattern and is considered a stable lesion. Treatment may range from symptomatic treatment alone to a rigid cervical orthosis.[13, 22]

The type II fracture is a fracture through the base at or just below the level of the superior articular process (Fig 32–9). This is the most common odontoid fracture and the most difficult to

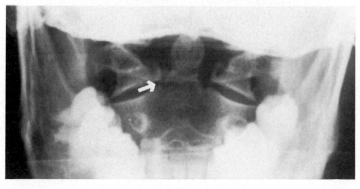

FIG 32–9.
Illustration of a type II odontoid fracture. Open mouth view reveals a fracture at the base of the odontoid process *(white arrow).*

treat. Nonunion rates range from as low as 17% in undisplaced fractures to as high as 64%.[1, 2, 16, 17] In undisplaced or minimally displaced fractures (displacement equal to or less than 4 mm), treatment should consist of halo immobilization. For fractures that are significantly displaced (displacement greater than 4 mm), treatment consists of attempted reduction with traction, followed by halo immobilization, with a possibility of a high nonunion rate, or primary posterior fusion performed after the patient has been placed in halo immobilization.[13, 22]

The type III fracture involves the body of the axis. This is a less common fracture pattern than type II, and it is considered more stable. Treatment

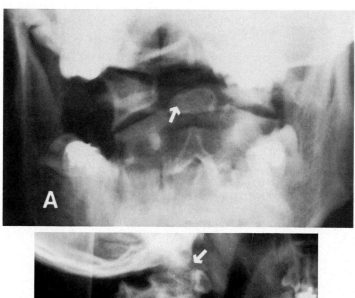

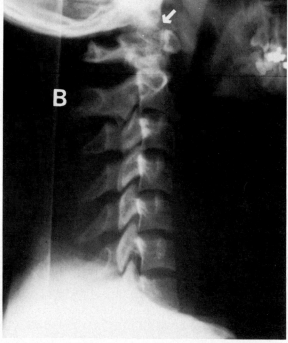

FIG 32–10.
Illustration of os odontoideum. Open mouth view **(A)** and lateral-view **(B)** radiographs illustrating os odontoideum (white arrows).

should consist of traction followed by halo immobilization.[13, 22]

In assessing the possibility of a type II dens fracture, os odontoideum requires consideration[7, 9] (Fig 32–10). The significance of an os odontoideum can range from a spurious finding to the pathologic lesion in question. The stability of the segment can be assessed with voluntary lateral flexion-extension views.

ATLANTOAXIAL DISLOCATIONS

The transverse and alar ligaments are responsible for atlantoaxial stability. With rupture, resulting from a flexion injury, C1 translates anteriorly, and the spinal cord can become impinged between the posterior aspect of the odontoid process and the posterior rim of C1.[8] Such a lesion is very unstable and potentially fatal. At this level of the cervical spine, Steel's rule of thirds applies. One third of the AP diameter of the atlas, respectively, consists of the dens, the spinal cord, and free space. This degree of unoccupied space about the spinal cord is unique to this region of the spine and is protective when serious fracture or dislocation or both occur[8, 20] (Fig 32–11).

Clinically the patient gives a history of head trauma and complains of neck pain, particularly with nodding. Cord signs may or may not be present. Roentgenographically, lateral views of the C1–C2 articulation demonstrate an increase of the atlanto-dens interval (ADI) and a decrease in a space available for the cord (SAC)[8] (Fig 32–12). An atlantodens interval of more than 3 mm in adults and more than 4 mm in children represents instability of the atlantoaxial complex. Fielding et al.[4, 5] determined that the transverse ligament ruptures within a range of 3 to 5 mm. An increase of the atlantodens interval beyond this represents not only rupture of the transverse ligament but also of the alar liga-

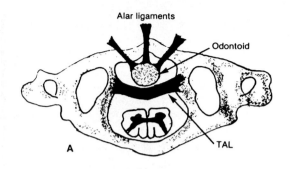

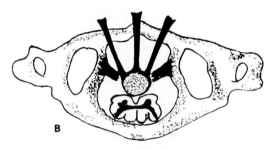

FIG 32–11.
A, illustration of the atlantoaxial complex as seen from above representing Steel's rule of thirds. **B,** disruption of the transverse ligament *(TAL)* with intact alar ligaments, resulting in C1–C2 instability without cord compression. *(From Hensinger RN: Congenital anomalies of the atlantoaxial joint, in The Cervical Spine, ed 2. Philadelphia, JB Lippincott Co, 1989, p 242. Used with permission.)*

ments and, possibly, capsular structures as well. In a clinical study, Fielding et al. noticed that the patients with an atlantodens interval of 5 to 6.5 mm complained of cervical pain and that those patients with an increased displacement of 7.5 to 11 mm complained of neurologic symptoms. Treatment of choice for this lesion is a posterior C1–C2 fusion.

TRAUMATIC SPONDYLOLISTHESIS OF THE AXIS

Fractures through the arch of the atlas are also known as traumatic spondylolisthesis or a hangman's fracture. These are relatively rare lesions that most commonly result from motor vehicle accidents or a fall. The mechanisms

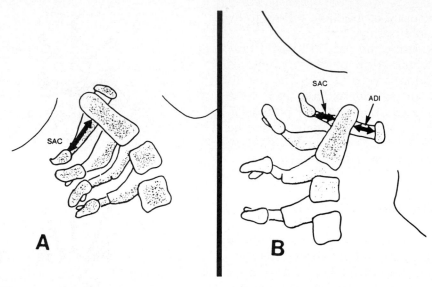

FIG 32–12.
Illustrations representing atlantoaxial instability resulting from transverse and alar ligament rupture. In extension, the atlantoaxial complex is reduced, and the atlantodens interval (ADI) and space available for the cord *(SAC)* appear normal **(A).** With forward flexion the instability becomes apparent. As the odontoid process displaces posteriorly, the atlantodens interval *(ADI)* increases and the space available for the cord *(SAC)* decreases **(B).** *(From Hensinger RN: Congenital anomalies of the atlantalaxial joint, in The Cervical Spine, ed 2. Philadelphia, JB Lippincott Co, 1989, p 238. Used with permission.)*

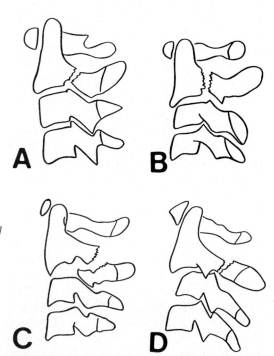

FIG 32–13.
Levine and Edwards' classification of traumatic spondylolisthesis **A,** type I: Mechanism is axial load hyperextension. **B,** type II: Mechanism is axial load hyperextension followed by flexion. **C,** type IIa: Mechanism is a flexion-distraction. **D,** type III: Mechanism is flexion-compression. *(From Levine AM, Edwards CC: The management of traumatic spondylolisthesis of the axis. J Bone Joint Surg [Am] 1985; 67A:217–226. Used with permission.)*

of injury are complex and are still disputed. Multiple classifications of traumatic spondylolisthesis have been proposed. The Levine and Edwards' classification,[14] which is a modification of that of Effendi et al.,[3] is based on the proposed mechanism of injury along with the fracture dislocation pattern[6] (Fig 32–13).

The mechanism of injury of type I fractures is an axial load hyperextension force. These fractures are less than 2 mm displaced, and are considered stable. Stability should be assessed by flexion and extension views when the patient is able. Treatment of choice for this injury is a rigid cervical orthosis.

The proposed mechanism of injury for type II fractures is axial load hyperex-

tension followed by flexion. This mechanism of injury produces a displaced posterior neural arch fracture with anterior subluxation of the body of C2 on C3. Treatment of this unstable fracture pattern consists of traction followed by halo immobilization in the lesser displaced and angulated fractures. For the severely displaced and angulated fractures, traction is maintained until fracture callus is evident.

The proposed mechanism of injury for the type IIa fracture is a flexion-distraction force. Treatment of this unstable fracture pattern consists of reduction by a slight compression, and extension of the neck with application of halo immobilization.

The proposed mechanism of the type

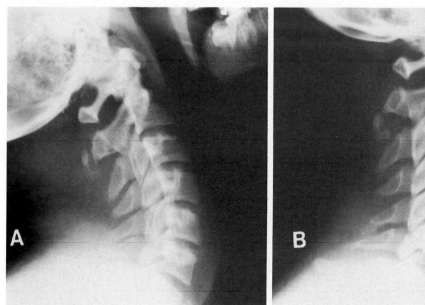
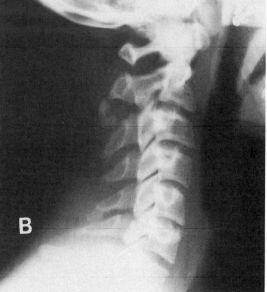

FIG 32–14.
An avulsion fracture of the tip of the spinous process with disruption of the C2–C3 interspinous ligaments. **A,** the lateral-view radiograph of the cervical spine in extension shows reduction of the C2 spinous process into the ossified portion of the interspinous and supraspinous ligaments. **B,** a lateral flexion view displays splaying of the C2–C3 interspinous space. These radiographs were taken 5 days after a minor neck injury that was incurred by a football player while tackling an opposing player. The patient was noted to have paraspinous and trapezius muscle spasm along with soreness and tenderness. On further questioning it was determined that 4 years before this injury while tackling, the patient sustained a more severe cervical "strain" as a result of diving into a swimming pool and striking his head on the bottom. At that point in time radiographs were not taken. The patient's symptoms resolved, and he competed in five seasons of football without further complaints before this injury. The present radiographs illustrate hypermobility of C2 on C3 as a result of an old rupture of the posterior ligaments.

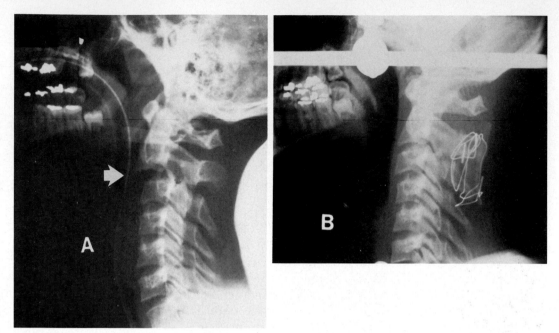

FIG 32–15.
Lateral-view radiographs of a 16-year-old wrestler who sustained a neck injury during a practice, resulting in immediate respiratory difficulty and quadriplegia. **A,** lateral-view radiograph taken in the emergency room reveals a unilateral facet dislocation. **B,** lateral-view radiograph taken in a "halo" status post open reduction and C2–C3 posterior fusion.

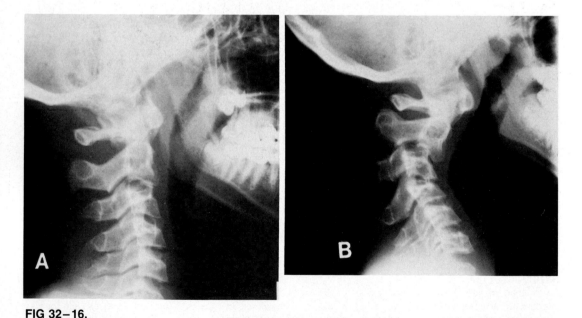

FIG 32–16.
Clinical example of a C2–C3 kyphotic deformity. The lateral-view radiographs were taken of a young high school athlete whose injury resulted from striking a tube while diving into a pool. **A,** lateral-view roentgenogram immediately after injury displays no instability nor loss of normal cervical lordosis, and minimal kyphotic deformity at C2–C3. The patient's acute pain resolved quickly, and he was gradually advanced and returned to football and basketball. The patient had no neurologic complaints, but noted intermittent neck stiffness and pain. Six months after the initial injury he began to notice a prominence in the posterior aspect of his neck. **B,** lateral-view radiograph 6 months after injury illustrates C2–C3 instability with a progressively developed kyphotic deformity.

III fracture is a flexion-compression. These forces can produce bilateral dislocation of facets, with bilateral pars fractures and anterior subluxation of the body of C2 on C3, with severe displacement (average 10.4 mm) and angulation (average, 15.6 degrees). Of the 52 patients with traumatic spondylolisthesis that Levine and Edwards presented, only 5 had the type III fracture pattern at initial presentation. Of note, two of these five fractures occurred during athletic participation. Treatment consists of attempted reduction of facet dislocation utilizing halo traction. If reduction is successful and maintained, the patient may be converted to halo immobilization. If attempted reduction of facets is unsuccessful, open reduction of the facet dislocation followed by posterior C2–C3 fusion should be performed, along with halo immobilization.[14]

TRAUMATIC INJURIES TO THE C2–C3 ARTICULATION

The C2–C3 articulation is the end of the upper cervical spine transition zone, and more closely resembles the middle and lower cervical articulations. As one would expect, its traumatic lesions, other than the hangman's fracture, also more closely resemble lesions found in the middle and lower cervical spine.

Disruption of the posterior elements has not been observed frequently. The least severe injury involves disruption of the supraspinous and interspinous ligaments (Fig 32–14). With increasing severity, involvement of the joint capsule of the facet joints occurs.

With increased disruption of the facet joints, unilateral or bilateral facet dislocations or fractured facets have been observed (Figs 32–15 and 32–16).

As stated, fractures of the upper cervical spine are unusual in athletic participation. A thorough understanding of the unique anatomy and function of this region, as well as the mechanism of injury will allow one to better understand and manage these problems.

REFERENCES

1. Anderson LD, D'Alonzo RT: Fractures of the odontoid process of the axis. *J Bone Joint Surg [Am]* 1974; 56A:1663–1674.

2. Anderson LD, Clark CR: Fractures of the odontoid process of the axis, in Cervical Spine Research Society Editorial Committee: *The Cervical Spine*, ed 2. Philadelphia, JB Lippincott Co, 1989.

3. Effendi B, Roy, D, Cornish B, et al: Fractures of the ring of the axis. *J Bone Joint Surg [Br]* 1981; 63B:319.

4. Fielding JW, Cochran GV, Lawsing JF III, et al: Tears of the transverse ligament of the atlas. *J Bone Joint Surg [Am]* 1974; 56A:1683–1691.

5. Fielding JW, Hawkins RJ, Ratzan SA: Spine fusion for atlanto-axial instability. *J Bone Joint Surg [Am]* 1976; 58A:400–407.

6. Garfin SR, Rothman RM: Traumatic spondylolisthesis of the axis; in Cervical Spine Research Society Editorial Committee: *The Cervical Spine*, ed 2. Philadelphia, JB Lippincott Co, 1979.

7. Fielding JW, Hensinger RN, Hawkins RJ: Os odontoideum. *J Bone Joint Surg [Am]* 62A:376–383.

8. Hensinger RN: Congenital anomalies of the atlantoaxial joint; in Cervical Spine Research Society Editorial Committee: *The Cervical Spine*, ed 2. Philadelphia, JB Lippincott Co, 1989.

9. Hawkins RJ, Fielding JW, Thompson WJ: Os odontoideum: Congenital or acquired. *J Bone Joint Surg [Am]* 1976; 58A:413–414.

10. Jefferson G: Fracture of the atlas vertebra. *Br J Surg* 1919; 7:407–422.

11. Johnson RM, Hart DL, Owen JR, et al: The Yale cervical orthosis: An evaluation of its effectiveness in restricting cervical motion in normal subjects and a comparison with other cervical orthoses. *Phys Ther* 1978; 58:865.

12. Johnson RM, Hart DL, Simmons EF, et al: Cervical orthoses: A study comparing their effectiveness in restricting cervical motion in normal subjects. *J Bone Joint Surg [Am]* 1977; 59A:332.

13. Johnson RM, Owen JR, Hart DL, et al: Cervical orthoses: A guide to their selection and use. *Clin Orthop*, 1981; 154:34.

14. Levine AM, Edwards CC: The management of traumatic spondylolisthesis of the axis. *J Bone Joint Surg [Am]* 1985; 67A:217.

15. Park WW: Applied anatomy of the spine, in Rothman RH, Simeone FA (eds): *The Spine*, vol 1. Philadelphia, WB Saunders Co, 1975.

16. Schatzker J, Rorabeck CH, Waddel JP: Fractures of the dens (odontoid process): An analysis of thirty-seven cases. *J Bone Joint Surg [Br]* 1971; 53B:392–404.

17. Schatzker J, Rorabeck CH, Waddell JP: Non-union of the odontoid process—an experimental investigation. *Clin Orthop Rel Res* 1975; 108:127–137.

18. Sherk HH, Nicholson JT: Fractures of the atlas. *J Bone Joint Surg [Am]* 1970; 52A:1017–1024.

19. Spence KR Jr, Decker S, Sell K: Bursting atlantal fracture associated with rupture of the transverse ligament. *J Bone Joint Surg [Am]* 1970; 52A:543.

20. Steel HH: Anatomical and mechanical considerations of the atlanto-axial articulations. *J Bone Joint Surg [Am]* 1968; 50A:1481–1482.

21. Werne S: Studies in spontaneous atlas dislocation. *Acta Orthop Scan [Suppl]* 1957; 23.

22. Wolf JW, Johnson RM: Cervical orthosis; in Cervical Research Society Editorial Committee: *The Cervical Spine*, ed 2. Philadelphia, JB Lippincott Co, pp 97–105, 1989.

23. White AA, Panjabi MM: *Clinical Biomechanics of the Spine*. Philadelphia, JB Lippincott Co, 1978.

24. Wolf JW, Jones HC: Comparison of cervical immobilization in halo-casts and halo-plastic jackets. *Orthopaedic Transactions* 1981; 5:118.

CHAPTER 33

Middle Cervical Spine Injuries (C3 and C4)

Joseph S. Torg, M.D.
Helene Pavlov, M.D.

Injuries to the cervical spine at the C3–C4 level involving the bony intervertebral disk and ligamentous structures are rare and have been reported infrequently in the literature. The purpose of this chapter is to present a series of traumatic C3–C4 level injuries sustained by young athletes and documented by the National Football Head and Neck Injury Registry (NFHNIR).[14, 18] Review of this material reveals that the response to energy inputs at the C3–C4 level differs from the response to those involving the upper (C1–C2) and lower (C4–C5–C6) cervical segments. Specifically, these lesions appear unique with regard to infrequency of bony fracture, difficulty in effecting and maintaining reduction, and a more favorable response to early aggressive treatment. Also, these lesions resulting from athletic activity are due to axial loading. On the basis of these observations, traumatic lesions of the cervical spine resulting in instability due to subluxation/dislocation or fracture (or both) can be classified according to upper, middle, and lower cervical segment lesions.

REVIEW OF LITERATURE

To date a review of the English literature documented 22 traumatic lesions involving the C3–C4 level. Norton [8] reported on four C3–C4 subluxations in a series of 88 cervical spinal injuries. Burke and Berryman[4] presented two unilateral facet dislocations in a series of 76 cervical spine injuries. Torg et al.[12] reported eight cases of spinal injury at the level of the third and fourth cervical vertebrae resulting from football. Bohlman[3] reported on six C3–C4 lesions in a series of 300 cervical spine injuries, and, most recently, O'Brien[9] documented two C3–C4 lesions in a series of 34 cervical spine injuries.

During the 18-year period 1971 through 1988, the NFHNIR has documented 1,062 injuries that have involved a fracture, dislocation, or subluxation of the cervical spine. Of these injuries, 25, or 2.4%, involved the C3–C4 level.

It has been observed previously that not only are traumatic lesions at the C3–C4 level infrequent, but also that they usually occur without associated fractures.[12] Also, they can be further characterized as involving (1) acute intervertebral disk herniation; (2) anterior subluxation of the third cervical vertebra on the fourth; (3) unilateral dislocation of the joint between the articular processes; and (4) bilateral dislocation of the joints between the articular processes.[12] In addition, a fifth group can be added to include the lesions with involved vertebral body fractures.

Analysis of these injuries included the following parameters: (1) injury mechanisms; (2) lesion type; (3) initial neurologic status; (4) treatment factor, that is, immediate vs. delayed, open, or closed, and (5) final neurologic status.

In the series of 25 cervical spine injuries involving the C3–C4 level, 24 resulted from football and 1 from baseball. The lesion categories were as follows:

Group	Lesion	Number
1.	Acute intervertebral disk herniation	4
2.	Anterior subluxation C3 on C4	4
3.	Unilateral facet dislocation	6
4.	Bilateral facet dislocation	7
5.	Fracture vertebral body C4	4

C3–C4 ACUTE INTERVERTEBRAL DISK HERNIATION

Four football players, one high school, two college, and one professional, sustained acute C3–C4 intervertebral disk lesions, all due to axial loading of the cervical spine. Three experienced an episode of transient quadriplegia. All four were treated surgically, three having an anterior C3–C4 diskectomy and interbody fusion and one a posterior C4 laminectomy and C3–C4 posterior fusion. All four experienced successful fusions and complete neurologic recovery without sequelae.

One of the patients (Case 3) was a 19-year-old college player who was injured during spring practice in a blocking drill. He is described as having "spear blocked" a dummy and experienced an acute onset of quadriplegia. Routine roentgenograms showed negative findings. He was placed in cervical traction, and complete motor and sensory function returned during the next 36 hours. Because of persistent neck pain, a cervical myelogram was done 6 weeks after the initial injury and demonstrated a defect at the C3–C4 level (Fig 33–1). He subsequently underwent a C3–C4 anterior diskectomy and interbody fusion (Fig 33–2). He has remained neurologically intact and has effected a successful fusion with no residual disability.

Review of these four cases reveals remarkable similarity with regard to mechanism of injury, initial neurologic manifestations, and favorable response to surgical treatment. Of note is the fact that of 1,062 cervical spine injuries documented by the registry, there were 31 acute intervertebral disk herniations, 4 of which involved the C3–C4 interspace (Table 33–1).

ANTERIOR SUBLUXATION OF C3 ON C4

Four football players, two high school and two college, sustained lesions due to axial loading of the cervical spine, resulting in anterior subluxation of C3 on C4. All six were neurologically intact.

One of the players was an 18-year-old college wide receiver who became injured while attempting to make a downfield block. Initial examination revealed the patient to have limitation of neck motion; however, he was neurologically intact. Roentgenographic examination demonstrated instability and narrowing of the C3–C4 disk space, with angulation and slight anterior translation of C3 on C4 (see Fig 33–2). Treatment consisted of

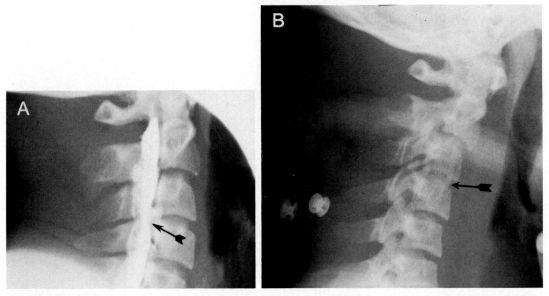

FIG 33–1.
Case 3. **A,** 6 weeks' post-injury, myelogram demonstrating defect at C3–C4 level due to posterior herniation of the intervertebral disk *(arrow).* **B,** lateral roentgenogram after anterior discectomy and interbody fusion *(arrow).* *(From Torg JS, Sennett B, Vegso JJ:* Am J Sports Med, *in press. Used with permission.)*

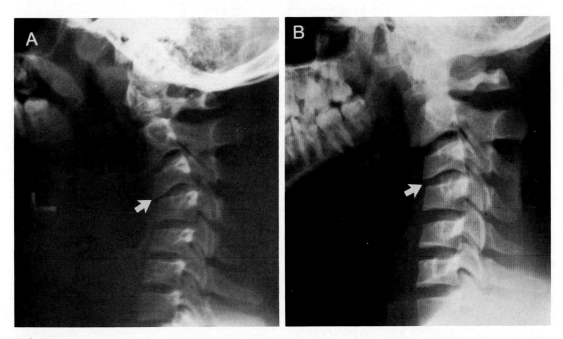

FIG 33–2.
Case 7. **A** and **B,** flexion-extension roentgenograms obtained on the day of injury demonstrate instability at the C3–C4 level *(arrows).* Of note is the intervertebral disk space narrowing, anterior angulation, and displacement of the third cervical vertebra in relationship to the fourth, as well as fanning of the spinous processes. *(From Torg JS, Sennett B, Vegso JJ:* Am J Sports Med, *in press. Used with permission.)*

TABLE 33–1.

Acute Intervertebral Disk Herniations Involving the C3–C4 Interspace

Patient	Age	Date of Injury	Level of Participation	Roentgenographic Findings	Mechanism of Injury	Initial Neurologic Status	Treatment	Current Neurologic Status
1	16	11/24/74	Football (HS)	Herniated nucleus pulposus C3–C4; posterior myelogram	Axial loading	Normal	Anterior C3–C4 discectomy; anterior interbody fusion	Normal
2	25	9/23/84	Football (Professional)	Herniated nucleus pulposus C3–C4; posterior myelogram	Axial loading	Transient quadriplegia	Anterior C3–C4 discectomy; anterior interbody fusion	Normal
3	19	5/30/73	Football (college)	Herniated nucleus pulposus C3–C4; posterior myelogram	Axial loading hyperext.	Transient quadriplegia	Anterior C3–C4 discectomy; anterior interbody fusion	Normal
4	23	11/03/84	Football (college)	Herniated nucleus pulposus C3–C4; posterior myelogram	Axial loading	Transient quadriplegia	C3–C4 discectomy with posterior cervical laminectomy	Normal

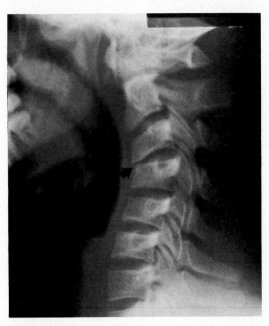

FIG 33–3.
Case 7. Four and one-half months after the injury, conservative management in a four-poster cervical brace has resulted in persistent instability with subluxation and anterior angulation *(arrow). (From Torg JS, Sennett B, Vegso JJ: Am J Sports Med, in press. Used with permission.)*

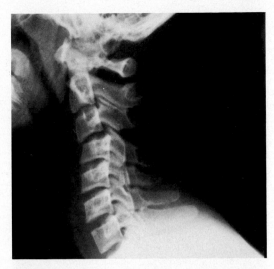

FIG 33–4.
Case 6. Roentgenogram taken 3 days after a "spearing" injury demonstrates anterior subluxation and angulation associated with disk space narrowing at this C3–C4 level *(arrow).* Also, there is increased distance between the spinous processes, indicating disruption of the interspinous ligament. *(From Torg JS, Sennett B, Vegso JJ: Am J Sports Med, in press. Used with permission.)*

traction for 2 weeks, followed by a cervical brace for 12 weeks. There was no neurologic impairment. Roentgenographic examination 4½ months after the injury demonstrated persistence of disk space narrowing with significant angulation and anterior displacement of C3 on C4 (Fig 33–3).

A second injured patient (Case 6) was a 16-year-old high school football player who injured his neck participating in an interscholastic game. He was playing defensive halfback and has been described as "spearing another player" while in the course of making a tackle. Initial roentgenograms of the cervical spine taken 3 days after injury demonstrated angulation and anterior translation of C3 on C4 (Fig 33–4). Also, there was increased distance between the spinous processes of C3 and C4, suggesting disruption of the interspinous ligament. Physical examination revealed full range of cervical spine motion. Neurologic examination showed

negative findings for impairment of sensory or motor function. The patient did complain of experiencing paresthesias in the distribution of C2, C3, and C4, however. He was admitted to the hospital and placed in head halter traction. Roentgenograms in traction demonstrated partial reduction of the subluxation (Fig 33–5). Eight days after admission to the hospital he was placed in a "halo" cast. Fusion of the posterior elements of C2, C3, and C4 was performed 18 days after injury. At surgery, disruption of the interspinous ligament between C3 and C4 was demonstrated. The patient had an uncomplicated postoperative course and went on to a solid fusion. Neurologic findings remained negative, and he was pain free when last examined 5 months postoperatively. Also to be noted is that he regained excellent strength in the paracervical musculature and regained an almost complete range of motion. Flexion-extension films demonstrate solid bony fusion (Fig 33–6).

On the basis of these two well-docu-

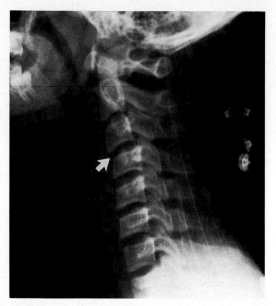

FIG 33–5.
Case 6. Head halter cervical traction affects improvement in the alignment and incomplete reduction of the C3–C4 subluxation *(arrow)*. *(From Torg JS, Sennett B, Vegso JJ, et al: Am J Sports Med, in press. Used with permission.)*

mented cases, it appears that anterior subluxation due to ligamentous injury at the C3–C4 level is disposed to clinical instability as defined by White and Panjabi.[19] Specifically, Case 7 exceeds 3.5 mm anterior translation and 11-degree

angulation in an individual with potential exposure to heavy loading of the cervical spine. In Case 6 the subluxation was initially reduced by skeletal traction. A posterior fusion was performed, and the patient was maintained in a "halo" cast. Although a successful fusion was obtained, there was partial recurrence of the anterior subluxation. This sequence emphasizes the difficulty in maintaining a reduction of anterior subluxation at this level and supports the role of surgical stabilization (Table 33–2).

UNILATERAL FACET DISLOCATION

Six football players, three high school, two college, and one recreational, sustained C3–C4 unilateral facet dislocations. In four the mechanism of injury was identified as being due to axial loading, one to flexion-rotation, and one undetermined. All six were immediately rendered quadriplegic.

These six patients with C3–C4 unilateral facet dislocation were treated by three different methods: (1) immediate reduction by closed manipulation under nasotracheal general anesthesia, followed by anterior diskectomy and interbody fu-

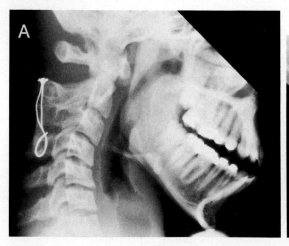
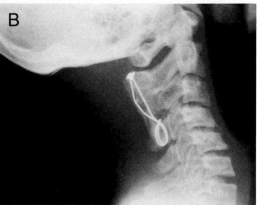

FIG 33–6.
Case 6. **A** and **B,** flexion-extension roentgenograms of the cervical spine, taken 6 months after fusion of the posterior elements of C2 through C4, demonstrate a solid bony fusion. However, slight anterior subluxation persists. *(From Torg JS, Sennett B, Vegso JJ, et al: Am J Sports Med, in press. Used with permission.)*

TABLE 33–2.
Anterior Subluxation of C3 on C4

Patient	Age (yr)	Date of Injury	Level of Participation	Roentgenographic Findings	Mechanism of Injury	Initial Neurologic Status	Treatment	Current Neurologic Status
5	16	10/22/81	Football (HS)	Subluxation C3–C4	Compression; flexion; rotation	Normal	Traction; collar	Normal
6	16	10/4/75	Football (HS)	Subluxation C3–C4	Axial loading	Paresthesia C2–C4	Traction; fusion C2–C4	Normal
7	18	10/12/74	Football (college)	Subluxation C3–C4	Unknown	Normal	Traction; fusion C2–C4	Normal
8	20	10/23/76	Football (college)	Subluxation C3–C4	Axial loading	Unknown	Traction; fusion C2–C5	Normal

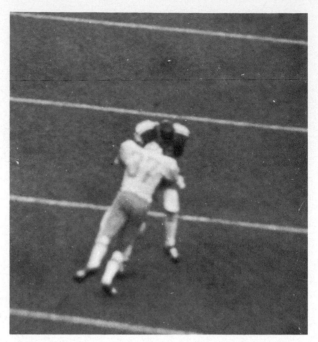

FIG 33–7.
Photograph of the injury in Patient 9 demonstrates the injured player, a defensive halfback, driving the top or crown of his helmet into the chest of the opposing ball carrier. Although there is a slight degree of flexion, this is not a hyperflexion injury, and major impact is directed down the axis of the cervical spine.

sion at 7 days (Case 9) and 2 months (Case 10); (2) open reduction and C3–C4 laminectomy (Cases 11 and 12); and (3) closed reduction with skeletal traction (Cases 13 and 14).

Of these six patients, the two reduced by closed manipulation under general an-

esthesia within 3 hours of their injury had eventual dramatic neurologic recovery. The other four remain quadriplegic.

One of the players (Case 9) was a 19-year-old defensive halfback who was injured while participating in an intercollegiate game. He tackled an opposing ball

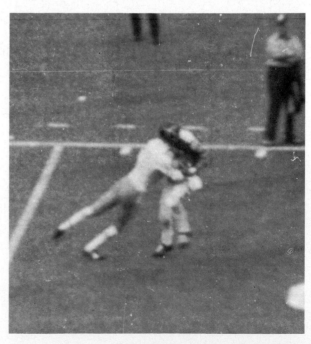

FIG 33–8.
Picture from the lateral aspect demonstrates the helmet to be in axial alignment with the trunk. The head and neck appear to be impacted again in the longitudinal axis, however.

carrier by striking him with the top or crown of his helmet (Figs 33–7 and 33–8) and was immediately rendered quadriplegic for both motor and sensory function distal to C4. There were no reflexes, either physiologic or pathologic, and there was no evidence of sacral sparing. Initial roentgenograms of the cervical spine on admission to the hospital demonstrated a unilateral facet dislocation of C3 on C4 without evidence of fracture (Fig 33–9).

Gardner skull tongs were applied and a reduction of the dislocation attempted by applying a total of 18 kg in progressive increments during a period of one-half hour. A reduction by this method was unsuccessful (Fig 33–10). The patient was then taken to the operating room,

and under nasotracheal anesthesia it was possible to effect a satisfactory reduction by closed manipulation (Fig 33–11).

The following morning neurologic examination revealed persistence of complete motor paralysis. However, there was definite evidence of return of some elements of posterior column function, specifically, position and vibrating sensation.

Four days after injury a cervical myelogram was performed by way of lateral C1–C2 puncture. The myelogram demonstrated a complete block at the C3–C4 level (Fig 33–12). The following day he was taken to the operating room and, under general nasotracheal anesthesia, a C3–C4 diskectomy and anterior interbody fusion were performed (Fig 33–13).

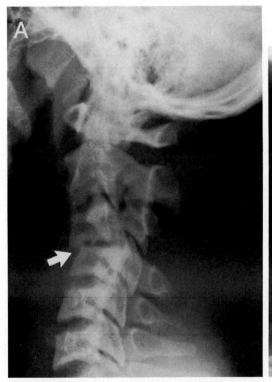
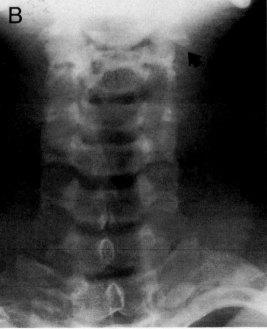

FIG 33–9.
Case 9. **A** and **B,** lateral and anteroposterior (AP) roentgenograms of the cervical spine demonstrated a unilateral facet dislocation of the third cervical vertebra, in addition to anterior displacement and angulation of C3 on C4 *(white arrow).* Of note, the spinous process of C3 has rotated from its normal relationship with the spinous processes of the second and fourth cervical vertebrae and is not seen on the lateral roentgenogram. Also, the dislocated left articular process of C3 *(arrowhead)* is clearly visible on the AP view. *(From Torg JS, Sennett B, Vegso JJ, et al: Am J Sports Med, in press. Used with permission.)*

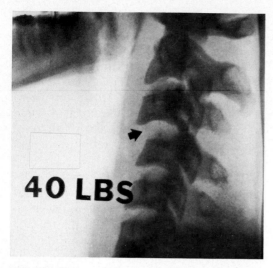

FIG 33–10.
Case 9. Eighteen kilograms of skull-caliper traction distracted the interspace but was unable to disengage the locked facet. *(From Torg JS, Sennett B, Vegso JJ, et al: Am J Sports Med, in press. Used with permission.)*

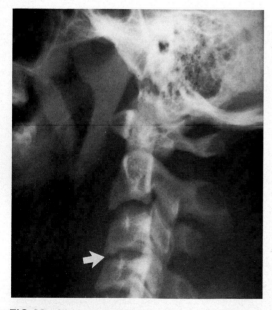

FIG 33–11.
Case 9. Lateral roentgenogram of the cervical spine, obtained after closed manipulative reduction performed under nasotracheal general anesthesia, demonstrates successful reduction of the facet dislocation. There is persistence of intervertebral disk space narrowing at the involved level *(arrow)*. *(From Torg JS, Sennett B, Vegso JJ, et al: Am J Sports Med, in press. Used with permission.)*

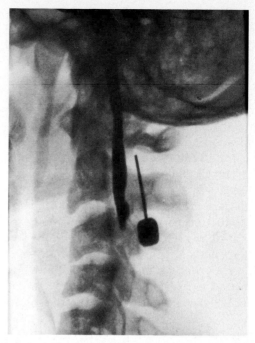

FIG 33–12.
Case 9. A cervical myelogram performed the day after the injury demonstrates a complete block to the flow of panopaque at the C3–C4 level. *(From Torg JS, Sennett B, Vegso JJ, et al: Am J Sports Med, in press. Used with permission.)*

The patient's subsequent course has been quite gratifying, with progressive improvement in both motor and sensory function. Approximately 1 month after injury motor return first became evident in the long toe extensor muscles in the right foot. Roentgenograms 2 months after injury demonstrated a stable fusion (Fig 33–14).

One year after injury he had significant return of motor function to all major muscle groups of the lower extremities. There was return of motor function to muscle groups of both upper extremities; however, this was decidedly less than that of the lower extremities. Also, he had bilateral intrinsic minus hands. In general, motor return on the left side of the body was greater than on the right. He was able to ambulate with bilateral Loftstrand crutches and to manage stairs with one rail and one crutch. Return of sensory function was complete with the

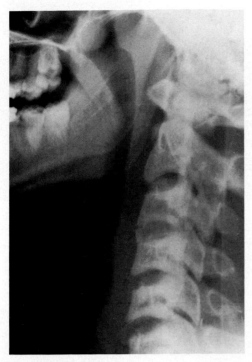

FIG 33–13.
Case 9. Lateral roentgenogram immediately after anterior C3–C4 diskectomy and interbody fusion. *(From Torg JS, Sennett B, Vegso JJ, et al:* Am J Sports Med, *in press. Used with permission.)*

exception of decreased pain and sensation to temperature throughout. His bladder remained neurogenic.

Case 10 involved a 15-year-old high school student who sustained a C3–C4 dislocation while participating in a sandlot tackle football game. Although circumstances surrounding the injury are somewhat obscure, it appeared that he was running with the ball and head-butted a tackler. The patient was immediately rendered quadriplegic and taken to a local hospital, where he was subsequently transferred to the university hospital. Initial examination demonstrated complete motor and sensory quadriplegia below C4. He was conscious, alert, and oriented to time, place, and person. Roentgenographic examination demonstrated a unilateral facet dislocation with anterior translation of C3 on C4 without evidence of fracture (Fig 33–15).

Gardner skull tongs were inserted, and attempts to reduce the dislocation with 18 kg of skeletal traction under x-ray guidance for 30 minutes were unsuccessful (Fig 33–16). General nasotracheal

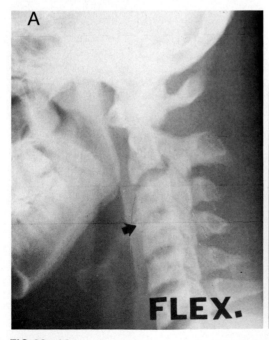

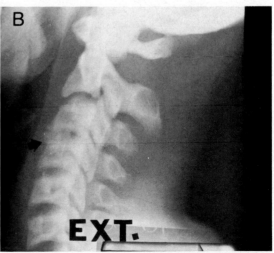

FIG 33–14.
Case 9. **A** and **B,** flexion-extension roentgenograms obtained 2 months after anterior diskectomy and interbody fusion at the C3–C4 level demonstrate solid bony union. *(From Torg JS, Sennett B, Vegso JJ, et al:* Am J Sports Med, *in press. Used with permission.)*

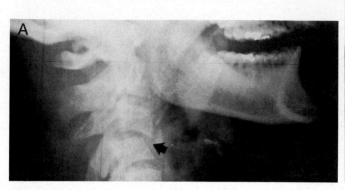
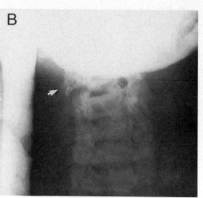

FIG 33–15.
Case 10. **A** and **B,** lateral and AP roentgenograms of the cervical spine taken after injury demonstrate a unilateral facet dislocation at C3–C4 *(arrow).* There is anterior translation of C3, as well as increase in the distance of the C3–C4 spinous processes, indicating disruption of the interspinous ligament. Dislocation of the right articular process of C3 *(arrow)* is demonstrated on the AP view. *(From Torg JS, Sennett B, Vegso JJ, et al: Am J Sports Med, in press. Used with permission.)*

anesthesia was then administered, and reduction of the C3–C4 dislocation was accomplished by closed manipulation (Fig 33–17). Subsequent roentgenograms demonstrated instability of the reduction. The patient was placed on a CircOlectric

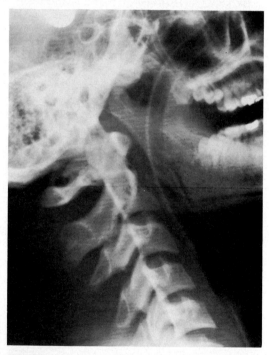

FIG 33–17.
Case 10. After closed manipulative reduction under general nasotracheal anesthesia, the unilateral facet dislocation is reduced; however, there persists a minimal degree of anterior angulation at C3–C4. *(From Torg JS, Sennett B, Vegso JJ, et al: Am J Sports Med, in press. Used with permission.)*

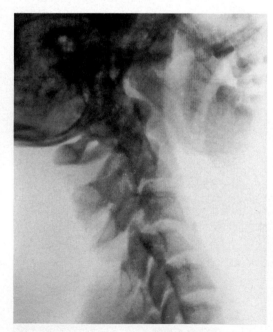

FIG 33–16.
Case 10. Lateral roentgenogram taken with 18 kg of skull traction demonstrates failure to reduce the unilateral facet dislocation. *(From Torg JS, Sennett B, Vegso JJ, et al: Am J Sports Med, in press. Used with permission.)*

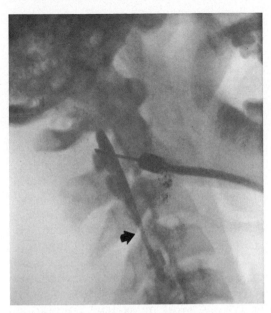

FIG 33–18.
Case 10. Cervical myelogram performed the day after the injury reveals negative findings for intervertebral disk herniation. *(From Torg JS, Sennett B, Vegso JJ, et al: Am J Sports Med, in press. Used with permission.)*

bed, and intravenous steroids were administered. During the subsequent 48 hours there was return of touch, position sense, and vibrating sensations in an inconsistent fashion. Motor function, light touch, and sensation of temperature remained absent. A cervical myelogram showed negative findings (Fig 33–18). Subsequently the patient's course was complicated by development of gastric stress ulcers and protracted delayed gastric emptying, with ensuing debilitating malnutrition requiring hyperalimentation. Subsequent roentgenograms at 4 and 6 weeks after injury demonstrated persistent instability at the C3–C4 levels (Figs 33–19 and 33–20).

Two months after the injury, under general nasotracheal anesthesia, a C3–C4 anterior cervical discectomy and interbody fusion were performed (Fig 33–21). After stabilization of the spine there was progressive increase in motor and sensory function. He was able to ambulate

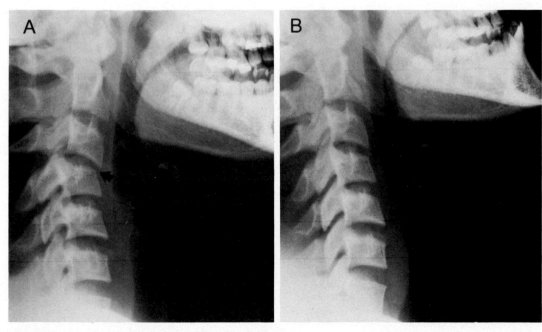

FIG 33–19.
Case 10. **A** and **B**, lateral roentgenograms in traction 4 weeks after injury demonstrate anterior subluxation and angulation of C3 at 2:00 P.M. After adjustment of traction the subluxation is partially reduced, with significant fanning of the spinous process observed at 4:00 P.M. *(From Torg JS, Sennett B, Vegso JJ, et al: Am J Sports Med, in press. Used with permission.)*

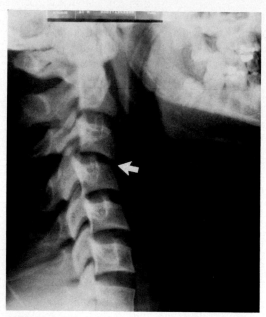

FIG 33–20.
Case 10. Lateral roentgenogram 6 weeks after the injury demonstrates persistent instability at C3–C4. *(From Torg JS, Sennett B, Vegso JJ, et al: Am J Sports Med, in press. Used with permission.)*

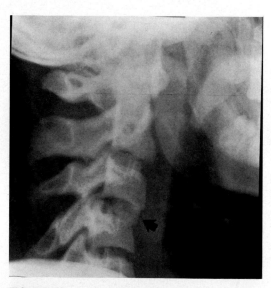

FIG 33–21.
Case 10. Lateral roentgenogram after anterior diskectomy and interbody fusion demonstrates persistence of subluxation and angulation of C3–C4 *(arrow).* The patient went on to a fusion and subsequently experienced almost complete neurologic and functional return. *(From Torg JS, Sennett B, Vegso JJ, et al: Am J Sports Med, in press. Used with permission.)*

on parallel bars 6 months after the injury and independently 8 months post-injury.

Examination 1 year after injury revealed excellent strength of all muscle groups of the lower extremities. Muscle strength of groups in the left shoulder girdle and the left upper extremity were good, whereas those on the right were graded as fair plus. The patient has intrinsic deficiency of hands bilaterally. However, he stated that he "can perform all tasks but is somewhat clumsy." All sensation has returned with the exception of spotty decrease to temperature. He has regained bowel and bladder function.

Our experience in managing these two cases has emphasized the difficulty in reducing unilateral facet dislocation at the C3–C4 level by skeletal traction, as well as the urgency in effecting immediate reduction in order to obtain maximum neurologic return. Also, the protracted period for maximum neurologic recovery is noteworthy (Table 33–3).

BILATERAL C3–C4 FACET DISLOCATION

Of the seven documented C3–C4 bilateral facet dislocations, six resulted from football and one from baseball. Six of these injuries were attributed to axial loading. All seven youngsters were rendered and remained quadriplegic.

Review of these cases reveals that they can be divided into three groups: (1) those who had an open reduction and posterior fusion, (2) those with successful skeletal traction and subsequent anterior interbody fusion, and (3) those who had an unsuccessful attempt at closed reduction.

Two youngsters, Cases 15 and 17, both had open reduction 5 days after their injuries. Two others, Cases 16 and 18, had successful closed reduction by skeletal traction. Of significance is the fact that the three youngsters in whom re-

TABLE 33–3.
Unilateral Facet Dislocation

Patient	Age (yr)	Date of Injury	Level of Participation	Roentgenographic Findings	Mechanism of Injury	Initial Neurologic Status	Treatment	Reduction (Postinjury)	Current Neurologic Status
9	19	11/8/75	Football (college)	Unilateral facet dislocation C3–C4	Axial loading	Quadriplegia C3–C4	Closed reduction: 11/8/75; C3–C4 anterior fusion: 11/13/75	Yes (0 day)	Central cord syndrome
10	15	11/16/75	Football (recreational)	Unilateral facet dislocation C3–C4	Axial loading	Quadriplegia C3–C4	Closed reduction: 11/16/75; C3–C4 anterior fusion: 1/18/76	Yes (0 day)	Central cord syndrome
11	16	10/4/74	Football (HS)	Unilateral facet dislocation C3–C4	Flexion; rotation	Quadriplegia C3–C4	Open reduction: 10/4/74; cervical laminectomy: 10/4/74; anterior fusion: 10/16/74	Yes (0 day)	Quadriplegia C6
12	19	10/7/72	Football (college)	Unilateral facet dislocation C3–C4	Axial loading	Quadriplegia C3–C4	Open reduction: 10/8/72; cervical laminectomy: 10/8/72	Yes (1 day)	Quadriplegia C5
13	17	8/20/76	Football (HS)	Unilateral facet dislocation C3–C4	Flexion; axial loading	Quadriplegia C3–C4	Closed reduction: 9/10/76; Posterior fusion: 9/15/76	Yes (3 wk)	Quadriplegia C3–C4
14	17	10/2/74	Football (HS)	Unilateral facet dislocation C3–C4	Unknown	Quadriplegia C3–C4	Closed reduction: 10/31/74	Yes (4 wk)	Quadriplegia C3–C4

duction was not obtained (Cases 19, 20, and 21) died at 3 days, 9 days, and 20 months.

One of the deceased players (Case 19) was a 15-year-old junior high school varsity football player who was injured participating in a junior varsity, interscholastic game while playing as defensive halfback. Attempting to make a tackle, he sustained a bilateral facet dislocation of C3 on C4, with immediate quadriplegia (Fig 33–22). Initial management consisted of insertion of Crutchfield tongs with attempted reduction of dislocation with 11.2 kg of traction. Although there was improvement in the alignment of the cervical spine, reduction was not successful (Fig 33–23). The patient required a respirator, and, because of precarious status, neither manipulative nor operative reduction was considered. The patient was maintained on a Stryker frame

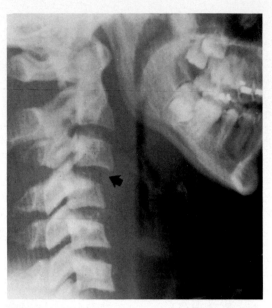

FIG 33–23.
Case 19. Traction, 11.2 kg, mediated through Crutchfield tongs improves the alignment but fails to disengage the locked facet. *(From Torg JS, Sennett B, Vegso JJ, et al: Am J Sports Med, in press. Used with permission.)*

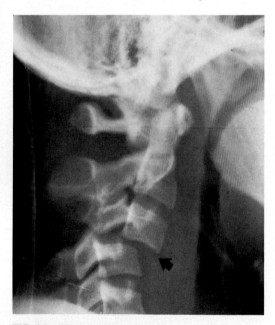

FIG 33–22.
Case 19. Lateral roentgenogram of the cervical spine obtained shortly after the patient's injury demonstrates a bilateral facet dislocation at C3–C4. In addition to marked anterior translation of C3, there is associated anterior angulation as well as increased distance between the spinous processes of C3 and C4. *(From Torg JS, Sennett B, Vegso JJ, et al: Am J Sports Med, in press. Used with permission.)*

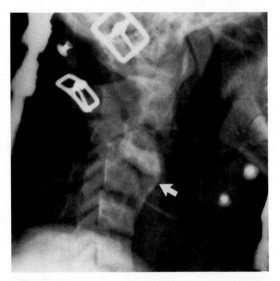

FIG 33–24.
Case 19. Lateral roentgenogram of the cervical spine obtained 3 months after injury demonstrates persistence of the bilateral facet dislocation. The lesion has gone on to an autofusion at C3–C4. Of interest is ossification that has occurred anteriorly within the confines of the anterior longitudinal ligament. *(From Torg JS, Sennett B, Vegso JJ, et al: Am J Sports Med, in press. Used with permission.)*

and went on to an autofusion with persistence of a bilateral facet dislocation (Fig 33–24). Twenty months after injury the patient had remained quadriplegic, without evidence of sensory or motor return below the level of C3–C4 and died of respiratory complications.

Case 21 involved a 19-year-old defensive halfback who, while playing in a practice intercollegiate game during spring practice, sustained a bilateral facet dislocation of C3–C4 while making a tackle. He was immediately rendered quadriplegic. Initial x-ray films demonstrated 60% anterior dislocation of C3 on C4, with some degree of anterior angulation (Fig 33–25). Crutchfield tongs were inserted, and 20 kg of skeletal traction was applied. Roentgenograms demonstrated correction of angulation and widening of the C3–C4 disk space; however, there was persistence of the bilateral facet dislocation (Fig 33–26). The patient died 3 days after the injury.

The third fatal injury (Case 20) involved a 16-year-old high school defen-

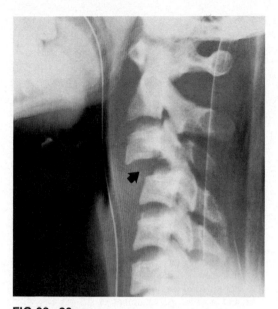

FIG 33–26.
Case 21. Skeletal traction, 20 kg, affects marked distraction of the C3–C4 disk space. The bilateral facet dislocation persists, however. *(From Torg JS, Sennett B, Vegso JJ, et al: Am J Sports Med, in press. Used with permission.)*

sive halfback who sustained a C3–C4 bilateral facet dislocation while making a tackle. The youngster was immediately rendered quadriplegic, with loss of all motor and sensory function distal to C4. Respirations were supported from the site of injury to the hospital, where a tracheostomy was performed before his being placed on a respirator.

Initial reontegenograms of the cervical spine demonstrated bilateral facet dislocation of C3 on C4, with 60% anterior displacement and marked angulation of C3 (Fig 33–27). Cruthfield tongs were inserted. Roentgenograms with the 11.4 kg of traction demonstrated widening of the C3–C4 disk space, with correction of the anterior angulation. The bilateral facet dislocation was not reduced, however (Fig 33–28).

The patient developed a gastric stress ulcer, gastrointestinal stasis, and pneumonia resulting from pulmonary insufficiency. He died 9 days after the injury from respiratory insufficiency (Table 33–4).

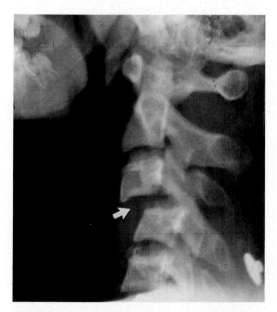

FIG 33–25.
Case 21. Lateral roentgenogram of the cervical spine obtained shortly after injury demonstrates a bilateral facet dislocation of C3–C4. *(From Torg JS, Sennett B, Vegso JJ, et al: Am J Sports Med, in press. Used with permission.)*

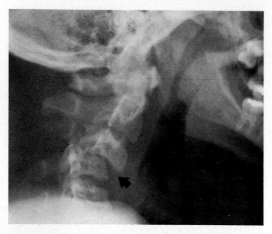

FIG 33–27.
Case 20. Lateral roentgenogram of the cervical spine demonstrates a bilateral facet dislocation, with C3–C4 intervertebral disk narrowing and marked angulation and anterior displacement of C3 on C4. Also, there is increased distance between the spinous processes. *(From Torg JS, Sennett B, Vegso JJ, et al: Am J Sports Med, in press. Used with permission.)*

C4 VERTEBRAL BODY FRACTURES

Four of the injuries in this series involved comminuted fractures of the vertebral bodies of C4. To be emphasized,

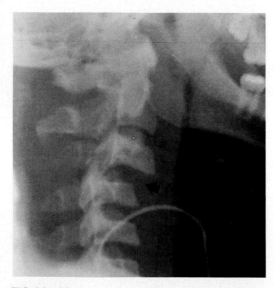

FIG 33–28.
Case 20. Skeletal traction, 11.2 kg, distracted the disk space and corrected angulation. It did not affect a reduction of the bilateral facet dislocation, however. *(From Torg JS, Sennett B, Vegso JJ, et al: Am J Sports Med, in press. Used with permission.)*

these were the only four injuries in which there was fracture of the bony elements. Of the 1,062 football injuries documented, none involved a fracture of C3, and only four involved fracture of the body of C4. And of significance, of the 251 cervical spine injuries with associated quadriplegia that occurred during the 18-year period 1971 to 1988, 62% were associated with comminuted vertebral body fractures.

The four group 5 lesions in this series all resulted from axial loading. Of note, two of the injuries (Cases 22 and 23) involved only the vertebral body and were not associated with neurologic involvement. However, Patients 23 and 25 had associated fracture through the pedicle, with disruption of the supporting posterior ligamentous structures, and were permanent quadriplegia (Table 33–5).

DISCUSSION

The rare occurrence of lesions at the C3–C4 level is apparent in view of the sparse documentation in the literature. Although this is the largest reported series to date, other than to reiterate the established implications of axial loading, the relatively small size of the series precludes other firm conclusion; however, it appears that analysis of these 25 cases affords some new insights into the nature of traumatic injuries at this level.

It is suggested that traumatic lesions of the cervical spine can be classified as involving either the (1) upper (C1–C2), (2) middle (C3–C4), or (3) lower (C4–C7) segments.

This is based on the observations in this series that C3–C4 lesions (1) generally do not involve fracture of the bony elements; (2) acute intervertebral disk herniations are frequently associated with transient quadriplegia; (3) reduction of anterior subluxation of C3 on C4 is difficult to maintain; (4) reduction of unilat-

TABLE 33–4.
Bilateral C3–C4 Facet Dislocation

Patient	Age (yr)	Date of Injury	Level of Participation	Roentgenographic Findings	Mechanism of Injury	Initial Neurologic Status	Treatment	Reduction (Postinjury)	Current Neurologic Status
15	19	9/11/82	Football (college)	Bilateral facet dislocation C3–C4	Axial loading	Quadriplegia C3–C4	Open cervical reduction; bilateral superior facetectomy; fusion C2–C5: 9/16/82	Yes (5 days)	Quadriplegia C3–C4
16	15	4/25/80	Baseball (HS)	Bilateral facet dislocation C3–C4	Axial loading	Quadriplegia C3–C4	Closed reduction: 5/2/80; anterior fusion: 6/3/80	Yes (1 wk)	Quadriplegia C3–C4
17	17	11/12/76	Football (HS)	Bilateral facet dislocation C3–C4	Axial loading	Quadriplegia C3–C4	Open reduction, partial hemilaminectomy, wiring C3–C4: 11/17/76	Yes (5 days)	Quadriplegia C3–C4
18	19	10/26/85	Football (college)	Bilateral facet dislocation C3–C4	Axial loading	Quadriplegia C3–C4	Closed reduction: 10/26/85; anterior fusion: 11/2/85; laminectomy: 11/20/85	Yes (0 day)	Quadriplegia C3–C4
19	15	9/29/75	Football (HS)	Bilateral facet dislocation C3–C4	Axial loading	Quadriplegia C3–C4	Closed reduction unsuccessful	No	Deceased (5/5/77)
20	16	11/14/75	Football (HS)	Bilateral facet dislocation C3–C4	Axial loading	Quadriplegia C3–C4	Closed reduction unsuccessful	No	Deceased (11/23/75)
21	19	3/04/75	Football (college)	Bilateral facet dislocation C3–C4	Tackling another player	Quadriplegia C3–C4	Closed reduction unsuccessful	No	Deceased (3/7/75)

TABLE 33–5.
C4 Vertebral Body Fractures

Patient	Age (yr)	Date of Injury	Level of Participation	Roentgenographic Findings	Mechanism of Injury	Initial Neurologic Status	Treatment	Current Neurologic Status
22	17	10/30/76	Football (HS)	Comminuted fracture C4 body	Axial loading	Normal	Posterior cervical fusion	Normal
23	17	9/22/78	Football (HS)	Comminuted fracture C4 body	Axial loading	Quadriplegia C5	Traction, posterior laminectomy, and fusion	Quadriplegia C5
24	15	9/20/73	Football (HS)	Comminuted fracture C4 body	Axial loading	Normal	Posterior cervical fusion	Normal
25	15	10/17/80	Football (HS)	Comminuted fracture C4 body	Axial loading	Quadriplegia C5	Posterior cervical fusion	Quadriplegia C5

eral facet dislocation is difficult to obtain by skeletal traction and is best managed by closed manipulative reduction under general anesthesia; and (5) reduction of bilateral facet dislocation is difficult to obtain by skeletal traction and is best managed by open methods.

The more favorable results of immediate reduction of both unilateral and bilateral facet dislocations deserve emphasis. In two cases of unilateral facet dislocation reduced within 3 hours of the injury and subsequently fused anteriorly, significant neurologic recovery occurred. The other four patients, two who underwent an open reduction and laminectomy and two treated closed with skeletal traction, remained quadriplegic.

In the four instances of bilateral facet dislocation in which reduction was achieved by either closed or open methods, although there was no neurologic recovery, all four survived their injuries. The three youngsters in whom reduction was not successful died, however.

CONCLUSIONS

1. The response to axial loading energy inputs at the middle cervical segment (C3–C4) differs from response to those involving the upper (C1–C2) and lower (C4–C5–C6–C7) cervical segments. It is suggested that traumatic lesions to the cervical spine be categorized accordingly.

2. The majority of traumatic lesions at the C3–C4 level resulting from athletic activities are due to axial loading of the cervical spine.

3. Reduction of anterior subluxation of C3 on C4, although not generally associated with neurologic involvement, is difficult to maintain, and clinical instability is predictable. Posterior fusion without laminectomy appears to be the treatment of choice in young, physically active patients.

4. Unilateral C3–C4 facet dislocations are difficult to reduce by skeletal traction. Immediate closed manipulative reduction under nasotracheal general anesthesia, followed by anterior diskectomy and interbody fusion, appears to offer the best opportunity for maximum neurologic recovery when the injury is associated with quadriplegia.

5. Bilateral facet dislocation at the C3–C4 level is difficult to reduce by skeletal traction. Early reduction, either by closed or open means, is indicated in order to afford the patient the best chances for survival. Neurologic recovery is not to be expected.

BIBLIOGRAPHY

1. Bauze RJ: Experimental production of forward dislocations in the human cervical spine. *J Bone Joint Surg [Br]* 1978; 60:239–245.

2. Bohlman HH: Pathology and current treatment concepts of cervical spine injuries, in American Academy of Orthopaedic Surgeons: *Instructional Course Lectures*, vol 21, St Louis, Mosby–Year Book, 1972, pp 108–115.

3. Bohlman HH: Acute fractures and dislocations of the cervical spine. *J Bone Joint Surg [Am]* 1979; 61A:1119–1142.

4. Burke DC, Berryman D: The place of closed manipulation in the management of flexion-rotation dislocations of the cervical spine. *J Bone Joint Surg [Br]* 1971; 53B:165–182.

5. Burstein AH, Otis JC, Torg JS: Mechanisms and Pathomechanics of Athletic Injuries to the Cervical Spine. in Torg JS (ed): *Athletic Injuries to the Head, Neck, and Face*. Philadelphia, Lea & Febiger, 1982, pp 139–142.

6. Forsyth HF, Alexander E, Davis C, et al: The advantages of early spine fusion in the treatment of fracture-dislocations of the cervical spine. *J Bone Joint Surg [Am]* 1959; 41A:17–36.

7. Holdsworth F: Fractures, dislocations and fracture-dislocations of the spine. *J Bone Joint Surg [Am]* 1970; 52A:1534–1551.

8. Norton WL: Fractures and dislocations of the cervical spine. *J Bone Joint Surg [Am]* 1962; 44A:115–139.

9. O'Brien PJ, Schweigel JF, Thompson WJ: Dislocations of the lower cervical spine. *J Trauma* 1982; 22:710–714.

10. Roaf R: A study of the mechanism of spinal injuries. *J Bone Joint Surg [Br]* 1968; 42B:810–823.

11. Torg JS, Quedenfeld TC, Thieler ER, et al: Collision with spring-loaded football tackling and blocking dummies. *JAMA* 1976; 236:1270–1271.

12. Torg JS, Truex RC, Marshall J, et al: Spinal injury at the third and fourth cervical vertebrae from football. *J Bone Joint Surg [Am]* 1977; 59A:1015–1019.

13. Torg JS, Quedenfeld TC, Burstein A, et al: National Football Head and Neck Injury Registry report on cervical quadriplegia: 1971–1975. *Am J Sports Med* 1977; 7:127–132.

14. Torg JS, Truex R Jr, Quedenfeld TC, et al: The National Football Head and Neck Injury Registry: Report and conclusions 1978. *JAMA* 1979; 241:1477–1479.

15. Torg JS, Vegso JJ, Yu A, et al: Cervical quadriplegia resulting from axial loading injuries; cinematographic, radiographic, kinematic and pathologic analysis. American Orthopaedic Society for Sports Medicine Interim Meeting abstracts, Atlanta, Feb. 8–19, 1984. Chicago, American Orthopaedic Society for Sports Medicine, 1984, p 18.

16. Torg JS, Vegso SS, O'Neill M, et al: The epidemiology, pathology, biomechanical, and cinematographic analysis of football-induced cervical spine trauma. *Am J Sports Med* 1990; 18:50–57.

17. Torg JS: Epidemiology, pathomechanics, and prevention of athletic injuries of the cervical spine. *Med Sci Sports Exerc* 1985; 17:295–303.

18. Torg JS, Vegso JJ, Sennett B, et al: The National Football Head and Neck Injury Registry 14 Year Report on Cervical Quadriplegia: 1971 through 1984. *JAMA* 1986; 254:3439–3443.

19. White AA, Panjabi MM: *Clinical Biomechanics of the Spine.* Philadelphia, JB Lippincott, 1978.

CHAPTER 34

Management of Lower Cervical Spine Injuries (C4–C7)

Marvin R. Leventhal, M.D.

Injuries to the lower cervical spine (C4–C7) account for most of the fractures and dislocations sustained in athletic events. The most frequently injured levels are C5 and C6.[24] Torg et al.[26] have shown that the mechanism of injury in tackle football is axial loading from improper use of the top of the head during tackling or blocking (Fig 34–1).

CLASSIFICATION

Numerous classifications of lower cervical spine injuries have been formulated, but the mechanistic classification system proposed by Allen et al.[1] appears to be the most complete. In an extensive review of 165 lower cervical spine injuries, they identified six common patterns of injury, each of which is further subdivided into stages based on the degree of injury to osseous and ligamentous structures.

Compressive Flexion (Five Stages)

CF Stage 1.—Blunting of the antero-superior vertebral margin to a rounded contour. There is no evidence of failure of the posterior ligamentous complex.

CF Stage 2.—Obliquity of the anterior vertebral body with loss of some anterior height of the centrum, in addition to the changes seen in stage 1. The anteroinferior vertebral body has a "beak" appearance. The inferior end plate may have increased concavity, and there may be a vertical fracture of the vertebral body.

CF Stage 3.—A fracture line passing obliquely from the anterior surface of the vertebra through the centrum and extending through the inferior subchondral plate and a fracture of the beak, in addition to the characteristics of the stage 2 injury.

CF Stage 4.—Deformation of the centrum and fracture of the beak with mild (less than 3 mm) displacement of the inferoposterior vertebral margin into the spinal canal.

CF Stage 5.—Bony injuries seen in the stage 3 lesion, but with more than 3 mm of displacement of the posterior portion of the vertebral body posteriorly into the spinal canal. The vertebral arch characteristically remains intact. The articular facets are separated and the interspinous process space is increased at the level of injury, suggesting a posterior ligamentous disruption in a tension mode.

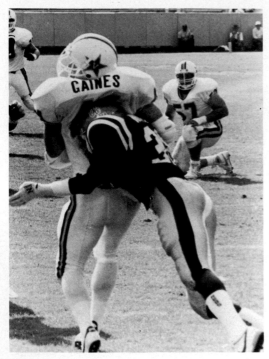

FIG 34–1.
On this tackle, collegiate defensive back sustained an axial loading injury to the neck that resulted in high cervical quadriplegia. (Photo by Randy Green, Vanderbilt Student Communications.)

Vertical Compression (Three Stages)

VC Stage 1.—Fracture of the superior or inferior end plate with a "cupping deformity." Failure of the end plate is central rather than anterior, and there is no evidence of posterior ligamentous failure.

VC Stage 2.—Fracture of both vertebral end plates with cupping deformities. Fracture lines through the centrum may be present, but displacement is minimal.

VC Stage 3.—Progression of the vertebral body damage seen in stage 2. The centrum is fragmented, and the displacement is peripherally in multiple directions. Most commonly the centrum fails with significant impaction and fragmentation. The posterior aspect of the vertebral body is fractured and may be dis-

placed into the spinal canal. The vertebral arch may be intact with no evidence of ligamentous failure, or the arch may be comminuted with significant failure of the posterior ligamentous complex; the level of ligamentous disruption is between the fractured vertebra and the subjacent one.

Distractive Flexion (Four Stages)

DF Stage 1.—Failure of the posterior ligamentous complex as evidenced by facet subluxation in flexion, with abnormal divergence of the spinous process.

DF Stage 2.—Unilateral facet dislocation (the degree of posterior ligamentous failure ranges from partial failure sufficient only to permit the abnormal displacement to complete failure of both the anterior and posterior ligamentous complexes, which is uncommon). Subluxation of the facet on the side opposite the dislocation suggests severe ligamentous injury. In addition, a small fleck of bone may be displaced from the posterior surface of the articular process, which is displaced anteriorly. Widening of the uncovertebral joint on the side of the dislocation and displacement of the tip of the spinous process toward the side of the dislocation may be seen. Beatson[4] serially divided the posterior interspinous ligaments, facet capsule, posterior longitudinal ligament, annulus fibrosus, and anterior longitudinal ligament and found that unilateral facet dislocation can occur with rupture of only the posterior interspinous ligaments and the facet capsule.

DF Stage 3.—Bilateral facet dislocation, with approximately 50% anterior subluxation of the vertebral body. Blunting of the anterosuperior margin of the inferior vertebra to a rounded contour may or may not be present. Beatson demonstrated that rupture of the interspinous ligament, the capsules of both facet joints, the posterior longitudinal ligament, and the annulus fibrosus of the intervertebral disk were necessary to create this lesion.

DF Stage 4.—Full vertebral body width displacement anteriorly or a grossly unstable motion segment, giving the appearance of a "floating vertebra."

Compressive Extension (Five Stages)

CE Stage 1.—Unilateral vertebral arch fracture, with or without anterorotatory vertebral displacement. Posterior element failure may consist of a linear fracture through the articular process, impaction of the articular process, and ipsilateral pedicle and lamina fractures, resulting in the "transverse facet" appearance on anteroposterior radiographs, or a combination of ipsilateral pedicle and articular process fractures.

CE Stage 2.—Bilaminar fractures without evidence of other tissue failure. Typically the laminar fractures occur at contiguous multiple levels.

CE Stage 3.—Bilateral vertebral arch fractures with fracture of the articular processes, pedicles, lamina, or some bilateral combination, without vertebral body displacement.

CE Stage 4.—Bilateral vertebral arch fractures with partial vertebral body width displacement anteriorly.

CE Stage 5.—Bilateral vertebral arch fracture with full vertebral body width displacement anteriorly. The posterior portion of the vertebral arch of the fractured vertebra does not displace, and the anterior portion of the arch remains with the centrum. Ligament failure occurs at two different levels: posteriorly between the fractured vertebra and the one above it and anteriorly between the fractured vertebra and the one below it. Characteristically, the anterosuperior portion of the subjacent vertebra is sheared off by the anteriorly displaced centrum.

Distractive Extension (Two Stages)

DE Stage 1.—Either failure of the anterior ligamentous complex or a transverse fracture of the centrum. The injury is usually ligamentous, and there may be an associated fracture of the adjacent anterior vertebral margin. The radiographic clue to this injury is abnormal widening of the disk space.

DE Stage 2.—Evidence of failure of the posterior ligamentous complex, with displacement of the upper vertebral body posteriorly into the spinal canal, addition to the changes seen in the stage 1 injury. Because displacement of this type tends to reduce spontaneously when the head is placed in a neutral position, radiographic evidence of the displacement may be minimal, rarely greater than 3 mm on initial films with the patient supine.

Lateral Flexion (Two Stages)

LF Stage.—Asymmetric compression fracture of the centrum and vertebral arch fracture on the ipsilateral side, without displacement of the arch on the anteroposterior view. Compression of the articular process or comminution of the corner of the vertebral arch may be present.

LF Stage 2.—Lateral asymmetric compression of the centrum and either ipsilateral vertebral arch fracture with displacement or ligamentous failure on the contralateral side with separation of the articular processes. Both the ipsilateral compressive and contralateral disruptive vertebral arch injury may be present.

INSTABILITY

The spectrum of injury to the cervical spine outlined in the preceding classification system clearly demonstrates that multiple mechanisms of injury exist in the clinical setting; similarly, there are various degrees and different patterns of instability. White and Panjabi[28] defined clinical instability as loss of the ability of the spine under physiologic loads to maintain relationships between vertebrae in such a way that there is neither damage nor subsequent irritation to the spinal cord or nerve roots and, in addition, no development nor deformity with excessive pain.[28–30] Clinical instability may be caused by trauma, neoplastic or infectious disorders, or it may be iatrogenic after surgery. In addition, instability may be acute or chronic. Acute instability is defined as bone or ligament disruption that places the neural elements in danger of injury with any subsequent loading or existing deformity. Chronic instability is

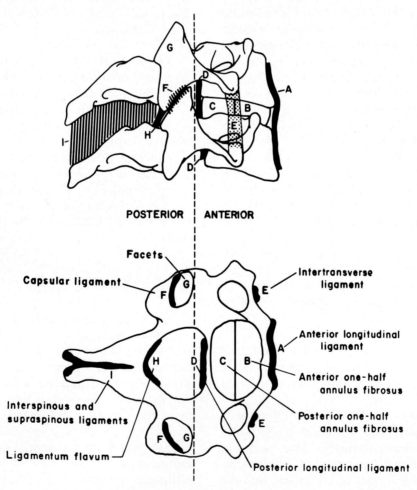

FIG 34–2.
Important anterior and posterior supporting structures of the spine. *(Redrawn from White AA, Southwick WO, Panjabi MM: Spine 1976; 1:15.)*

defined as progressive deformity that may lead to neurologic deterioration, prevent recovery of injured neural tissue, or cause increasing pain or decreased function.

In a series of cadaver studies, White and Panjabi[28] systematically cut the various supporting structures and noted the resulting instabilities in the spine. The supporting structures of the lower cervical spine can be divided into two groups, anterior and posterior (Fig 34–2). The anterior elements are the posterior longitudinal ligament and everything before it (anterior and posterior longitudinal ligaments, intervertebral disk, and annulus fibrosus). The posterior elements include everything behind the posterior longitudinal ligament (facet capsules, ligamentum flavum, and interspinous and supraspinous ligaments). A motion segment is two adjacent vertebrae and the intervening soft tissue. On the basis of the studies of White and Panjabi,[28] if a motion segment has all its anterior elements intact plus one additional structure or all its posterior elements intact plus one additional structure, it will remain stable under physiologic loads. White and Panjabi[28] suggest that any motion segment should be considered unstable if all of the anterior elements or all of the posterior elements are destroyed or are unable to function.[29, 30] They developed a checklist for the diagnosis of clinical instability in the lower cervical spine (Table 34–1). With use of their point value system in the evaluation of a cervical spine injury, a total of five or more indicates clinical instability of the spine.

Radiographically, cervical spine instability is indicated by a horizontal translation of one vertebra relative to an adjacent vertebra in excess of 3.5 mm on the lateral flexion-extension view (Fig 34–3). Instability also is indicated if lateral views demonstrate more than 11 degrees of angulation of one vertebra relative to another (Fig 34–4).

The stretch test may be useful for evaluation of clinical instability in the lower cervical spine, but is unnecessary

TABLE 34–1.

Checklist for the Diagnosis of Clinical Instability in the Lower Cervical Spine*

Element	Point Value
Anterior elements destroyed or nonfunctioning	2
Posterior elements destroyed or nonfunctioning	2
Relative sagittal plane translation >3.5 mm	2
Relative sagittal plane rotation >11 degrees	2
Positive stretch test	2
Spinal cord damage	2
Nerve root damage	1
Abnormal disk narrowing	1
Dangerous loading anticipated	1

*Adapted from White AA, Panjabi MM: Spine 1984; 9:512.

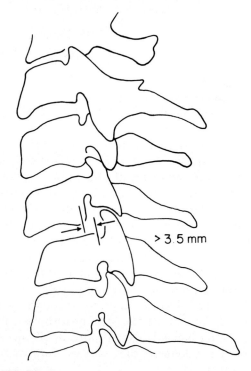

FIG 34–3.
Sagittal plane translation of more than 3.5 mm suggests clinical instability. *(Redrawn from White AA, Johnson RM, Panjabi MM, et al: Clin Orthop 1975; 120:85.)*

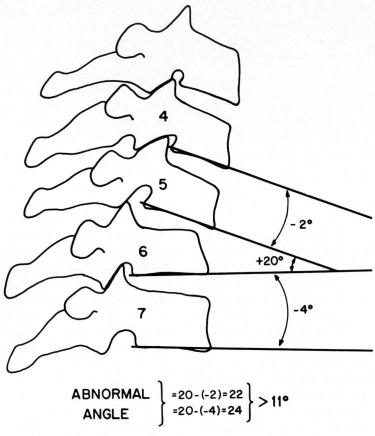

FIG 34–4.
Significant sagittal plane rotation (more than 11 degrees) suggests instability. *(Redrawn from White AA, Johnson RM, Panjabi MM, et al:* Clin Orthop *1975; 120:85.)*

and contraindicated in an obviously unstable injury. This test measures the displacement patterns of the spine under carefully controlled conditions, and identifies disrupted ligaments either anteriorly or posteriorly (Fig 34–5). The procedure for the stretch test is as follows:

1. The test should be done under the supervision of an attending physician.
2. Traction is applied through secured skeletal traction or a head halter. If the latter is used, a small portion of gauze sponge between the molars improves comfort.
3. A roller is placed under the patient's head.
4. The film is placed as closely as possible to the patient's neck. The tube-to-film distance is 72 in.
5. A lateral-view film is made first.
6. Weight is added up to 10 lb.
7. Traction is increased in 5 lb increments, and measurements are made on a lateral-view film after each addition, until either one third of body weight or 65 lb is reached.
8. After each additional weight application, the patient is checked for any change in neurologic status. The test is stopped and considered positive if this occurs or if there is any abnormal separation of the anterior or posterior elements of the vertebrae. At least 5 minutes should be allowed between incremental weight applications for developing the

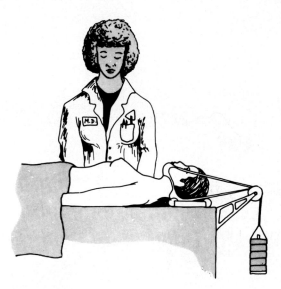

FIG 34–5.
Stretch test to determine cervical spine instability. This test must be closely monitored by the physician and is contraindicated when the spine is obviously unstable. *(Redrawn from White AA III, Panjabi MM: Clinical Biomechanics of the Spine, Philadelphia JB Lippincott Co, 1978.)*

film, necessary neurologic checks, and creep of the viscoelastic structures involved. White et al.[30] suggest that an abnormal stretch test is indicated by either differences of more than 1.7 mm interspace separation or more than 7.5 degrees of change in angle between the pre-stretched condition and that after the application of one third of the patient's body weight.

TREATMENT

Management of fractures and dislocations of the lower cervical spine in the athlete should proceed in an orderly fashion to minimize morbidity and enhance functional recovery. The cervical spine must be immobilized at the time medical stabilization is implemented. Appropriate means for immobilizing the injured cervical spine include a hard cervical collar or sandbags, and the patient should be placed on a spine board. The

patient is then transported to a medical facility where spinal alignment is assessed initially by plain radiographs. In general, a complete cervical spine series includes open mouth odontoid, antero-posterior, lateral (must include C7–T1), and right and left oblique views to assess the lateral masses. If the cervicothoracic junction cannot be adequately seen on initial lateral views, a swimmer's view or computed tomography (CT) scans must be obtained to document absence of pathology at this level.

The goals of treatment of lower cervical spine injuries are to (1) realign the spine, (2) prevent loss of function of uninjured neurologic tissue, (3) enhance neurologic recovery, (4) achieve and maintain spinal stability, and (5) obtain early functional recovery. After initial medical stabilization and documentation of a lower cervical fracture or dislocation, spinal alignment can be obtained in skeletal traction by application of either spring-loaded Gardner-Wells tongs or application of a halo ring through which traction may be applied. Patients who are undergoing reduction of fractures or dislocations in cervical traction must be monitored continuously, and a meticulous neurologic examination must be performed repeatedly to prevent iatrogenic injury from overdistraction of an unstable motion segment. After application of either Gardner-Wells tongs or a halo ring, 10 lb of weight is applied, and a lateral-view cervical spine radiograph is obtained. Then weight is added in 5 lb increments, with lateral-view radiographs obtained after each weight change until spinal realignment is achieved (Fig 34–6). Although disagreement exists concerning the safe upper limit of weight that may be applied to the injured cervical spine, most surgeons do not apply weight in excess of 40 to 50 lb. A general guideline for addition of weight to the cervical spine is 10 lb for the head and 5 lb for each additional level of injury (Ta-

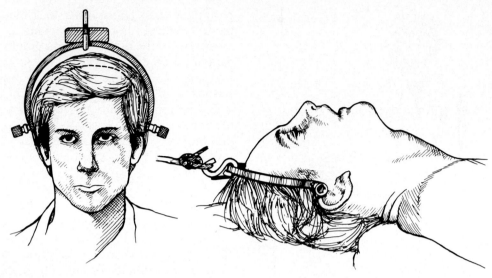

FIG 34–6.
Correct placement of Gardner-Wells tongs just above the ears and below the greatest diameter of the skull.
(From Stauffer ES: Management of cervical spine injuries, in Evarts CM (ed): Surgery of the Musculoskeletal System, *ed 1. New York, Churchill Livingstone, 1983. Used with permission.)*

ble 34–2). If spinal realignment cannot be obtained by traction, the patient is taken to the operating room for open reduction and stabilization, usually through a posterior approach. If spinal realignment is achieved through skeletal traction and is documented on radiographs, weight is reduced by 50% to

TABLE 34–2.
Traction Recommended for Levels of Injury*

Level	Minimum Weight, lb (kg)	Maximum Weight, lb (kg)
1st cervical vertebra	5 (2.3)	10 (4.5)
2nd cervical vertebra	6 (2.7)	10–12 (4.5–5.4)
3rd cervical vertebra	8 (3.6)	10–15 (4.5–6.8)
4th cervical vertebra	10 (4.5)	15–20 (6.8–9.0)
5th cervical vertebra	12 (5.4)	20–25 (9.0–11.3)
6th cervical vertebra	15 (6.8)	20–30 (9.0–13.5)
7th cervical vertebra	18 (8.1)	25–35 (11.3–15.8)

From Freeman BL: Fractures, dislocations, and fracture-dislocations of the spine, in Campbell's Operative Orthopedics, ed 7. St Louis, Mosby-Year Book, 1986, p 3115. Used with permission.

maintain alignment. A decision must then be made concerning nonoperative or operative treatment. In most instances, sophisticated imaging techniques, including tomograms, CT scans, and magnetic resonance imaging (MRI), provide additional information about ligamentous, intervertebral disk, and osseous injuries. To prevent complications, the pathologic anatomy must be defined precisely before therapeutic intervention. Recently, Arena et al.[3] documented the association of intervertebral disk extrusion with cervical facet dislocations. They noted that in 8.8% of their patients posterior herniation of disk material existed in conjunction with cervical facet subluxations and dislocations. They recommend preoperative evaluation of these injuries with either myelography, CT, or MRI. In the presence of associated disk herniation, anterior diskectomy and interbody fusion should be done before posterior cervical wiring and fusion, to avoid neurologic deterioration after open reduction and posterior stabilization.

Indications for Nonoperative Therapy.—Many injuries of the lower cervical spine may be treated successfully without surgical intervention. Immobilization in a rigid cervical orthosis for 8 to 12 weeks may be appropriate. For a stable cervical spine injury with no compression of the neural elements, application of a rigid cervical brace or halo may be expected to lead to a stable, painless spine without residual deformity in most patients. Stable compression fractures of the vertebral body and undisplaced fractures of the lamina, lateral masses, or spinous processes can be adequately treated with immobilization in a cervical orthosis until healing occurs. In addition, a unilateral facet dislocation that is reduced successfully in traction may be treated with immobilization in a halo vest for 8 to 12 weeks. Patients treated nonoperatively for a cervical spine injury must be followed closely. Serial radiographs should be obtained weekly for the first 3 weeks and then at 6 weeks, 3 months, 6 months, and 1 year. Herkowitz and Rothman[19] have demonstrated subacute instability of the cervical spine after initial radiographic evaluation, showing no bony or soft-tissue abnormality. The elastic and plastic deformation of the ligamentous structures and disks of the cervical spine is believed to be responsible for this subacute instability. It is important to realize that instability of the cervical spine may occur despite an adequate initial physical and radiographic examination. A complete follow-up evaluation should be obtained within 3 weeks of injury.

Indications for Operative Therapy.— Unstable injuries of the lower cervical spine, with or without neurologic deficit, require surgical intervention. Many factors influence the timing of operative intervention, but in most patients early open reduction and internal fixation are indicated to achieve stabilization. Surgical stabilization of cervical spine injuries may be done through an anterior or a posterior approach, or may be a combination of procedures carried out simultaneously or in stages. Usually stability is achieved through a posterior approach with use of triple-wire stabilization and fusion with iliac bone graft. This allows rapid mobilization of the patient in a cervical orthosis, and healing usually occurs within 8 to 12 weeks. If the spinal cord or nerve roots are compressed by retropulsed bone fragments or disk material, anterior decompression may enhance neurologic recovery; however, Stauffer and Kelly[25] have shown the disadvantages of anterior decompression and strut grafting in the face of posterior instability. Posterior stability should be obtained first, followed by anterior decompression and fusion if indicated, except in patients who are either neurologically incomplete or normal with subluxations or dislocations that cannot be reduced by traction. In this uncommon situation, MRI, CT scan, or myelography should be used to determine if a herniated disk is present. If it is, anterior diskectomy and interbody fusion are done first, followed by a posterior cervical stabilization procedure. Anderson et al.[2] have recently shown improved neurologic recovery in both cervical incomplete and complete cord injuries after anterior decompression and fusion.

When surgical intervention is indicated either for decompression or for stabilization, several basic principles must be followed:

1. The pathologic anatomy must be clearly defined before intervening surgically. Therefore, evaluation of plain radiographs and high-resolution CT scans, with sagittal and coronal reconstructions and MRI, provides valuable information for determining the proper approach to the injured cervical spine.

2. Laminectomy in the treatment of fractures or dislocations of the cervical spine has a very limited role, and may contribute to clinical instability and increased neurologic deficit. In Bohlman's[7] series of 300 cervical spine injuries, 22%

FIG 34–7.
A, lateral-view radiograph of compressive flexion injury in 20-year-old female patient with complete C5 quadriplegia. **B,** CT scan shows encroachment on subarachnoid space and flattening of cervical cord, with fractures of the left lateral mass. **C,** CT scan with sagittal reconstruction shows fracture of C5 vertebral body with mild displacement of posterior vertebral margin into spinal canal; no widening of inner spinous process space, suggestive of posterior ligamentous instability, is apparent. **D,** postoperative CT scan shows adequate anterior decompression and placement of iliac crest strut graft. *(Continued.)*

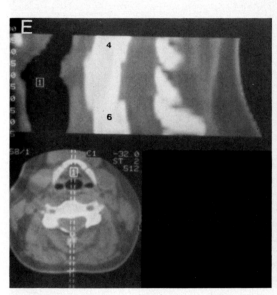

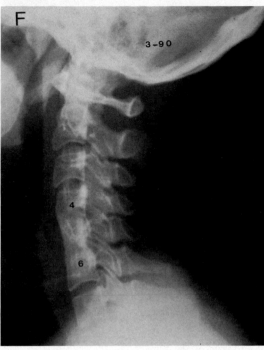

FIG 34–7 (cont.).
E, postoperative CT scan with sagittal reconstruction shows adequately decompressed spinal canal with proper positioning of iliac crest strut graft from C4 to C6. **F,** 3 years after surgery, lateral-view radiograph shows incorporation of iliac crest strut graft and solid arthrodesis from C4 to C6. This patient had single-level root recovery and is a functional C6 quadriplegic.

of the 55 patients who were treated by laminectomy had increased permanent loss of neural function immediately after surgery. In addition, laminectomy caused increased instability and allowed further subluxation or dislocation. In rare instances when compression of the neural elements posteriorly by bone fragments from the vertebral arch is documented, a laminectomy may be indicated.

3. Compression of the cervical cord or roots usually is anterior, and may be caused by retropulsed bone fragments or disk material. In this case an anterior approach for decompression and fusion is indicated.

4. If posterior ligamentous or bony instability is present, stability can best be achieved by posterior triple-wire stabilization and fusion with iliac bone graft.

Operative Procedures.—The choice of surgical approaches for injuries of the lower cervical spine depends on the injury pattern and the goals of treatment. Anterior decompression and fusion are indicated most often for burst fractures of the cervical spine with documented neurocompression from retropulsed bone or disk fragments and an incomplete neurologic deficit (Fig 34–7). Posterior approaches are most often indicated for ligamentous instability (Fig 34–8). Anterior decompression and posterior stabilization are indicated for posterior instability and anterior compression of the neural elements (Fig 34–9). The surgeon must carefully scrutinize all preoperative studies to plan the correct procedures. Again, it must be noted that there is a high incidence of anterior strut graft extrusion

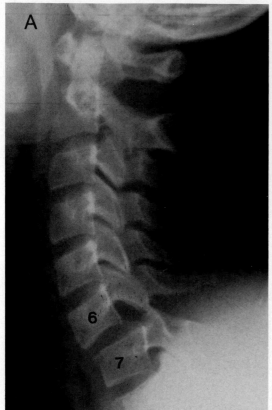

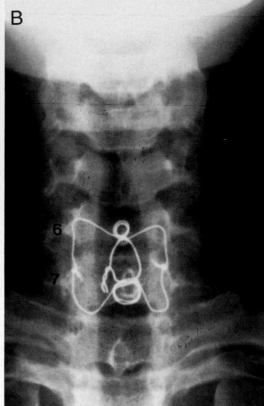

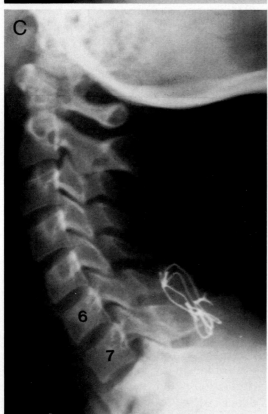

FIG 34–8.
A, lateral-view radiograph of distraction flexion
lesion at C6/C7 in 18-year-old patient. Note
widening of interspinous process space, moderate
anterior subluxation at C6/C7, and perched facets
bilaterally. **B** and **C,** radiographs (anteroposterior
and lateral views) after posterior stabilization, with
use of triple-wire technique and autogenous iliac
bone graft, show restoration of spinal alignment.
The patient was mobilized early in a rigid cervical
orthosis and had a full functional recovery.

when the posterior ligamentous complex is disrupted.

Posterior Fusion.—Numerous techniques have been described for posterior stabilization of the cervical spine. In our experience the triple-wire technique with autogenous iliac bone graft, as described by Bohlman,[11] has been an effective method of restoring stability to the unstable lower cervical spine. Biomechanical studies comparing the rigidity of different stabilization techniques for cervical fractures[21] suggest that the triple-wire technique is significantly stronger in compression and in flexion than are standard wiring techniques.

The procedure may be carried out safely with the patient under general or local anesthesia. In patients with a high cervical quadriplegia, local anesthesia is preferred to avoid the respiratory complications that can be encountered with general anesthesia. Usually the patient is intubated with use of an atraumatic, fiberoptic intubation technique, and is then positioned prone on a Stryker turning frame. Longitudinal traction is applied to the shoulders and maintained with tape. A permanent lateral-view radiograph is obtained in the operating room to document alignment of the cervical spine. The posterior aspects of the neck and the iliac crest are then scrubbed and draped in a sterile fashion. We prefer to sew the towels in place to prevent interference in radiographs from towel clips. A midline posterior skin incision is made, usually extending one spinous process above and one below the segment to be fused. Infiltration of the skin, subcutaneous tissue, and erector muscle of the spine down to the level of the lamina with a 1:500,000 epinephrine solution is helpful in obtaining hemostasis. Subperiosteal exposure is carried down to the level of the lamina with use of electrocautery. Dissection is carried laterally on either side to the lateral margin of the facet joints. A permanent lateral-view radiograph should be obtained, with a marker on a spinous process to confirm accurate localization.

With use of either a small high-speed bur or a towel clip, a hole is then drilled in the base of the spinous process to be wired. To avoid passage of the wire into the spinal canal, care must be taken in the proper placement of the hole posterior to the spinal laminar fusion line. The triple-wire technique uses a midline, 20-gauge wire passed through the hole in the superior spinous process and looped over the top of its superior edge. This same wire is then passed through and around the inferior spinous process of the levels below. The wires are then carefully tightened. Placement of each wire through and around the posterior elements improves stability by increasing the surface area of contact at the bone-metal interface. A 22-gauge wire is then passed through and around the holes in the spinous processes of the superior and inferior vertebrae to be fused, in preparation for securing a thick unicortical cancellous bone graft. The length of the area to be fused is then measured, and a bone graft is harvested from the posterior iliac crest. The graft should be of appropriate length and width so that it can be divided into two pieces for each side of the fusion. Strips of cancellous bone are harvested from the pelvis and placed beneath the thick unicortical cancellous bone graft to provide additional bone for fusion. Holes are placed in the superior and inferior ends of the bone grafts, through which the 22-gauge wires are passed. The bone grafts are held in place against the lamina and spinous processes as these wires are tightened. The wires are cut off and bent upon themselves to prevent protrusion into the soft tissues (Fig 34–10).

As shown by Bohlman,[7] decortication of the posterior elements is not required to obtain a solid arthrodesis. Sta-

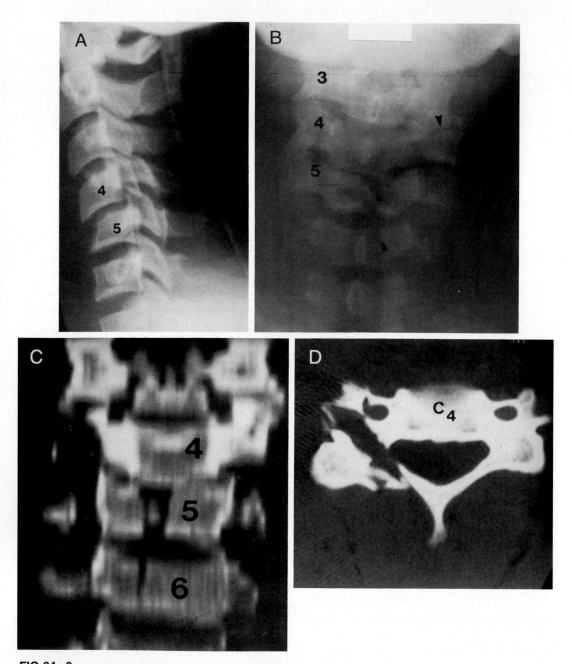

FIG 34–9.
Collegiate defensive back sustained axial loading injury to cervical spine while making a tackle (see Fig 34–1); he was rendered complete C5 quadriplegic. A–G show preoperative images. **A,** on lateral-view radiograph, note mild anterior subluxation of C4 and C5 caused by left unilateral facet dislocation. **B,** anteroposterior view shows significant fractures of lateral mass of C4 on the right and of the bodies of C5 and C6 vertebral bodies (arrows). **C,** CT scan, with coronal reconstruction, shows significant vertical fractures of the bodies of C5 and C6 that were not noted on initial lateral-view films **(A)**. **D,** CT scan through C4 vertebral body shows fractures through ipsilateral right pedicle and lamina with free-floating lateral mass at this level. (Continued.)

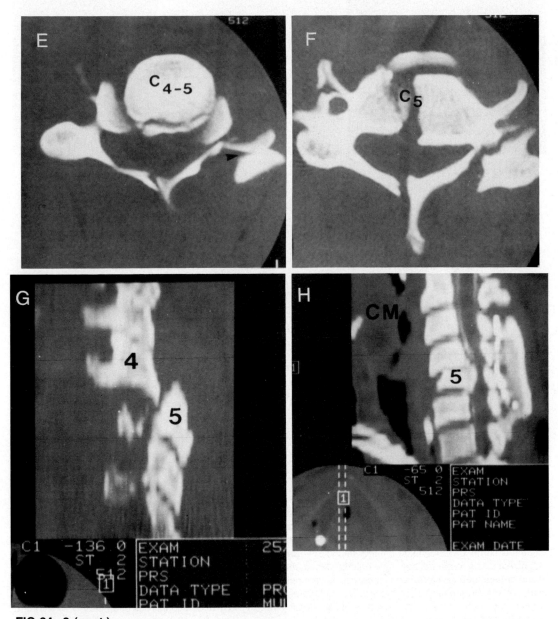

FIG 34–9 (cont.).
E, CT scan through C4/C5 shows unilateral left-sided C4/C5 facet dislocation *(arrow).* **F,** CT scan through C5 vertebral body shows significant fractures of anterior and posterior elements and marked narrowing of spinal canal. **G,** CT scan with sagittal reconstruction shows left-sided unilateral C4/C5-facet dislocation. **H** and **I,** after initial posterior cervical fusion from C3 to C6 with triple-wire technique. **H,** CT scan with sagittal reconstruction shows significant narrowing of spinal canal resulting from retropulsed bone and disk material. *(Continued.)*

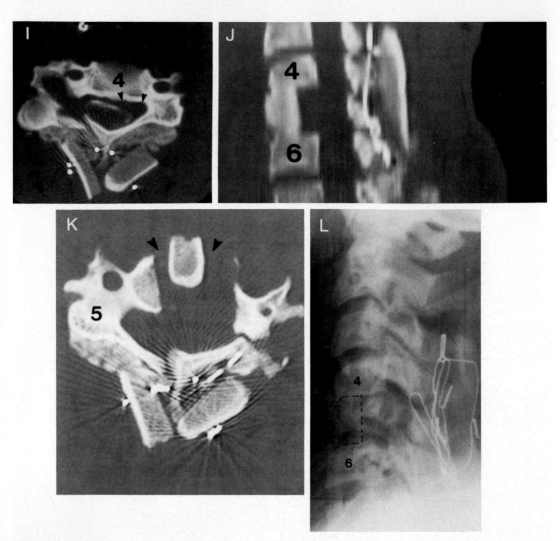

FIG 34–9 (cont.).
I, CT scan with contrast in subarachnoid space shows disk material retropulsed into spinal canal to left of midline behind body of C4. This was believed to impair function of left C4 nerve root and cause paralysis of left hemidiaphragm. Note also large, cortical cancellous bone grafts wired into place posteriorly. **J,** CT scan with sagittal reconstruction shows adequate anterior decompression at C5 level and placement of iliac strut graft from C4 to C6. **K,** Axial scan confirms adequate anterior decompression and proper placement of strut grafts *(arrow)*. Spinal alignment has been restored and stability achieved; patient was successfully weaned from ventilator and showed improved diaphragmatic function of left side. **L,** Lateral-view radiograph shows final alignment of spine after combined anterior and posterior fusions; note oblique facet wire used to give additional rotational stability to standard triple-wire technique.

bility may be determined by grasping the spinous process of one vertebra with a clamp and picking it up. The wired levels should move as a single unit. A permanent lateral-view radiograph is obtained to confirm the position of the wires and fusion of the proper segment.

The wound is then thoroughly irrigated with an antibiotic solution and closed in layers over a suction drain. In most patients skeletal traction can be discontinued and immobilization in a rigid cervical orthosis begun immediately postoperatively; however, the surgeon

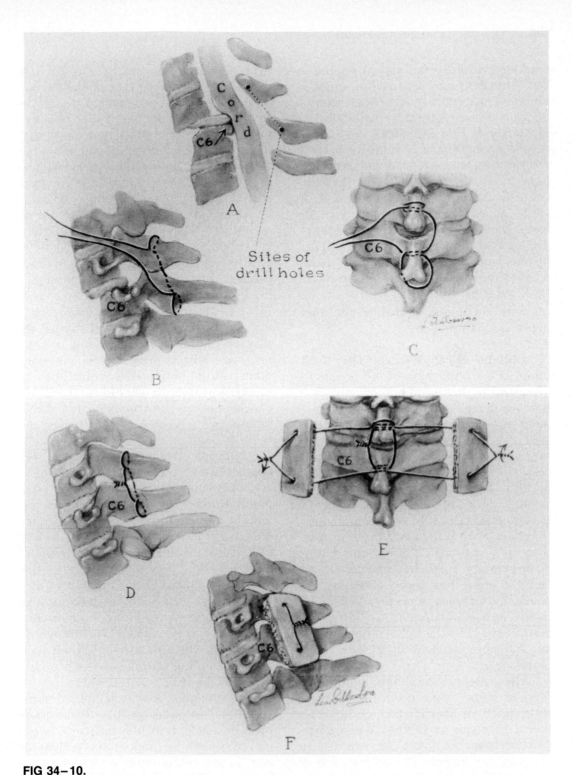

FIG 34–10.
Cervical arthrodesis with use of Bohlman triple-wire technique. **A,** placement of drill holes above spinolaminar fusion line. **B–D,** midline 20-gauge tethering wire wrapped through and around spinous processes above and below. **E,** 2 additional 22-gauge wires are then added to secure thick unicortical cancellous bone grafts against posterior elements. **F,** final position of graft. *(Courtesy of Dr. H.H. Bohlman, Case Western Reserve, Cleveland.)*

may elect to keep the patient supine in bed with light cervical traction for 24 to 48 hours before fitting a cervical orthosis. Perioperative prophylactic antibiotics are recommended for 48 hours.

A cervical brace is worn for 8 to 12 weeks; then lateral flexion and extension radiographs are made. The brace is discontinued when there is evidence of fusion, and stability is documented on lateral flexion and extension views. Analysis of failures of posterior cervical fusions indicates that problems occur when the wire cuts out of the bone. McAffee et al.[21] have shown that the triple-wire technique decreases the incidence of this problem.

Oblique Facet Wiring.—This technique is a modification of the procedure described by Robinson and Southwick.[23] It is indicated when the posterior elements are insufficient for spinous process wiring. The procedure may be performed for fractures of the lamina or spinous processes, or when laminectomy has been performed. It provides excellent rotational stability by serving as a checkrein in unilateral facet subluxation or dislocations, as well as bilateral facet dislocations (Fig 34–11). The oblique wiring technique for rotational injuries of the cervical spine has been shown by Edwards[17] to provide more effective fixation in the face of rotational instability than that provided by the use of a halo vest or an interspinous wiring fixation technique.

The patient is positioned prone on a Stryker frame, with cervical alignment maintained in skeletal traction with either a halo ring or Gardner-Wells tongs. The posterior elements are exposed in the midline subperiosteally with use of the electrocautery as described previously. It is important to expose the lateral margin of the facet joints to permit access to the facets. After accurate radiographic localization of the proper level to be fused, a small 7/64 in. drill is used to drill a hole carefully in the lateral mass at 45 degrees off the horizontal through the inferior facet. The facet joint may be pried open with a small ear, nose, and throat freer or a Penfield-type elevator. A 20- or 22-gauge stainless steel wire is then passed through the hole in the facet joint and grasped with a small hemostat. This procedure should be carried out on each facet bilaterally to create a stable construct. The wires can then be tightened down and around an intact spinous process inferiorly, or passed through a thick unicortical cancellous bone graft (Fig 34–12). The wound is closed in layers over a suction drain, and the patient may be placed into a halo vest or rigid cervical orthosis. Healing of the bone grafts can be anticipated within 8 to 12 weeks, and stability should be confirmed on lateral-view flexion-extension radiographs.

Anterior Decompression and Fusion.—Exposure of the mid and lower cervical regions of the spine is most commonly through an anterior approach medial to the carotid sheath. A thorough knowledge of anatomic fascial planes, as described by Robinson and Southwick,[22] allows a safe, direct approach to this area. The patient is positioned supine, with skeletal traction maintained through either Gardner-Wells tongs or a halo ring. Exposure may be carried out through either a transverse or a longitudinal incision, depending on the surgeon's preference (Fig 34–13).

We generally prefer a left-sided transverse skin incision because of the more constant anatomy of the recurrent laryngeal nerve and less risk of inadvertent injury. In general, an incision 3 to 4 fingerbreadths above the clavicle will be needed to expose from C3 to C5, and an incision 2 to 3 fingerbreadths above the clavicle will allow exposure from C5 to C7. A transverse incision is centered over

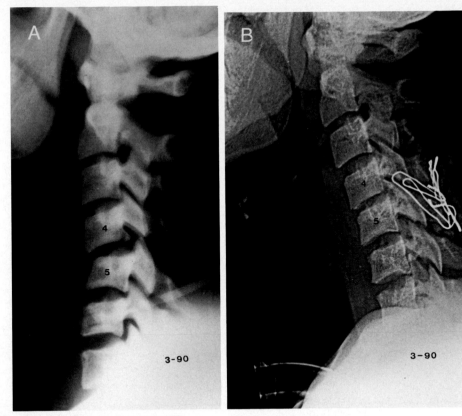

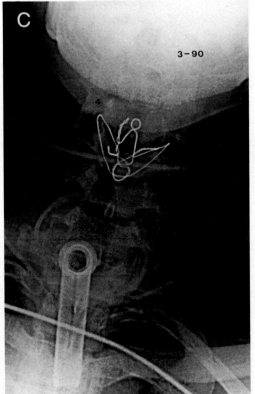

FIG 34–11.
Distractive flexion injury at C4/C5 level causing complete C5 level quadriplegia in 22-year-old patient. **A,** on lateral view, note widening of interspinous process space, mild anterior subluxation, and disruption of facet joints. **B** and **C,** after restoration of anatomic alignment with use of oblique facet wires and traditional midline wiring; patient was mobilized in cervical orthosis, and early rehabilitation was begun.

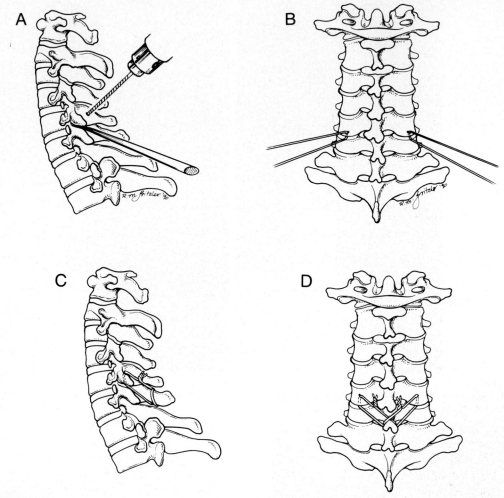

FIG 34–12.
Oblique facet wiring. **A,** placement of drill hole in lateral mass at 45-degree angle to horizontal; note placement of Penfield elevator in facet joint. **B,** oblique facet wires placed through holes in articular masses. **C** and **D,** wires tightened around intact caudal spinous process. *(Modified from Robinson RA, Southwick WO: South Med J 1960; 53:565.)*

the medial border of the sternocleidomastoid muscle. Infiltration of the skin and subcutaneous tissue with a 1:500,000 epinephrine solution will assist in hemostasis. The platysma muscle is incised in line with the skin incision. The anterior border of the sternocleidomastoid muscle is identified, the superficial layer of the deep cervical fascia is incised longitudinally, while the carotid pulse is localized by finger palpation.

The middle layer of the deep cervical fascia that encloses the omohyoid medial to the carotid sheath is divided carefully. As the sternocleidomastoid muscle and the carotid sheath are retracted laterally, the anterior aspect of the cervical spine can be palpated. The esophagus is identified lying posterior to the trachea, and the trachea, esophagus, and thyroid are retracted medially. The deep layers of the deep cervical fascia, consisting of the pretracheal and the prevertebral fascia overlying the musculi longus colli, are divided bluntly. The musculi longus colli are reflected subperiosteally from the an-

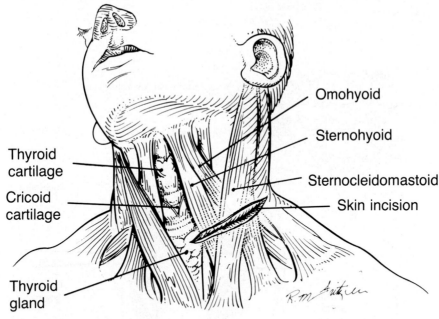

FIG 34–13.
Anterior approach to middle and lower cervical spine through left-sided transverse incision. Dissection is carried medially to carotid sheath and laterally to trachea and esophagus. *(Redrawn from Southwick WO, Robinson RA: J Bone Joint Surg [Am] 1957; 39A:631.)*

terior aspect of the spine laterally to the level of the uncovertebral joints. The resulting exposure is sufficient for wide decompression and bone grafting (Fig 34–14). Usually the fractured vertebra is readily identified; however, accurate localization is suggested by placing a needle into a disk space and obtaining a permanent lateral-view radiograph. After identification of the level to be decompressed, the anterior longitudinal ligament and annulus overlying the adjacent disk are incised with a No. 15 blade, and this material is removed with curets. Using hand-held rongeurs or a high-speed drill, the anterior portion of the fractured vertebral body is removed (Fig 34–15,A and B). Disk material is removed back to the posterior longitudinal ligament. Complete removal of the intervertebral disk is important to provide identification of the posterior longitudinal ligament and to assist in delineating the extent of the carpectomy. The posterior aspect of the vertebral body is then removed carefully

with use of power burs and hand-held curets and pituitary forceps as the posterior cortical wall of the vertebra is approached (Fig 34–15,C and D). Retropulsed bone and disk fragments are removed carefully from the spinal canal. In severely unstable injuries, the posterior longitudinal ligament is usually disrupted.

The lateral margin of the dissection is defined by the uncovertebral joints. Care must be taken not to extend the dissection out too far laterally because of the risk of injury to the vertebral arteries. After completion of the anterior carpectomy, the end plates of the superior and inferior vertebrae must be exposed and seating holes must be fashioned with use of angled curets or a small bur in preparation for placement of the tricortical iliac crest graft or fibular graft (Fig 34–15,E). In general, the seating holes should be centered in the end plate and should allow placement of approximately half the length of the distal phalanx of

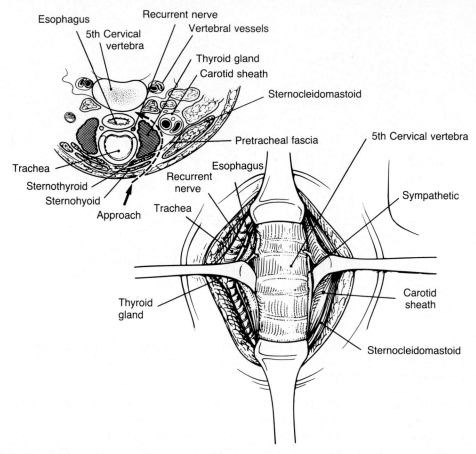

FIG 34–14.
Deep dissection to middle and lower cervical spine. Thorough knowledge of anatomic fascial planes is mandatory to gain adequate exposure of anterior aspect of cervical spine. *(Redrawn from Southwick WO, Robinson RA: J Bone Joint Surg [Am] 1957; 39A:631.)*

the surgeon's little finger. Once the seating holes are fashioned, Gelfoam may be placed over the exposed dura mater, which should be noted to expand anteriorly after a complete decompression. Once the iliac strut graft is harvested, it is fashioned into a T shape, with the cancellous portion of the graft facing anteriorly. Longitudinal traction is then increased, and the graft is locked into the seating holes. The anterior aspect of the graft is then trimmed flush with the front of the vertebral bodies to prevent erosion into the esophagus.

A permanent lateral-view radiograph is obtained to confirm proper positioning of the graft. Recently stability has been enhanced by the use of anterior spinal plates and screws. Although stability is increased by the use of these internal fixation devices, there is also an increased risk of iatrogenic neurologic injury. In our experience, anterior decompression and placement of an iliac or fibular strut graft has been a safe and effective procedure without the need for internal fixation in most instances.

After placement of the graft, a drain is placed along the anterior aspect of the spine to prevent postoperative respiratory compromise from a hematoma in the prevertebral space. The platysma muscle, subcutaneous tissue, and skin are closed in layers. After anterior decompression

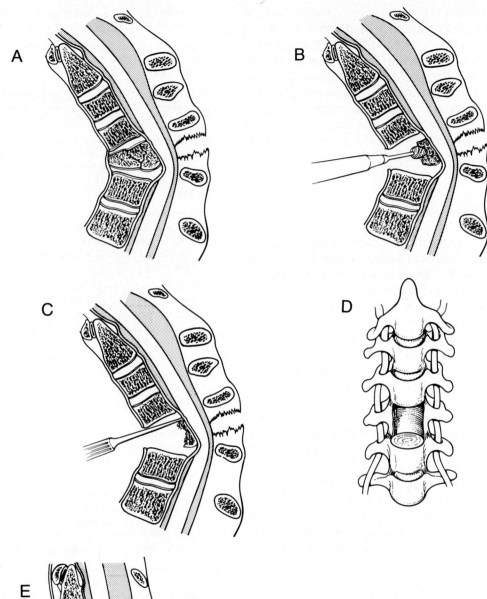

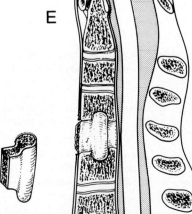

FIG 34–15.
A, typical burst fracture at C5 with retropulsed bone and disk fragments in spinal canal causing compression of neural elements. **B,** material above and below fractured vertebra has been removed and high-speed power bur is used to remove bone back to level of posterior longitudinal ligament. **C,** residual posterior vertebral margin is removed carefully with small curet to decompress the neural elements. **D,** extent of anterior cervical carpectomy. **E,** placement of tricortical iliac crest graft after adequate cervical decompression.(**A** *redrawn from Bohlman HH:* J Bone Joint Surg [Am] *1979; 61A:1119;* **B–E** *redrawn from Bohlman HH, Eismont FJ:* Clin Orthop *1981; 154:57.)*

and strut grafting, the patient may be placed into either a rigid cervical orthosis or a halo vest depending on the degree of stability achieved. Immobilization is continued for 8 to 12 weeks while the bone graft incorporates. In general, the predominantly cancellous iliac strut graft heals rapidly, whereas the predominantly cortical fibular graft may require longer for consolidation.

CONCLUSION

Proper management of injuries to the lower cervical spine is based on a thorough understanding of the pathology involved, including injuries to the soft tissues, osseous structures, and neural elements. The patient must be evaluated carefully before implementation of treatment to prevent complications that may have an adverse effect for the remainder of his/her life. A thorough history and physical and neurologic evaluations must be obtained and documented, and then supplemented with high-quality imaging techniques such as myelography, CT scan, and, most recently, MRI in order to diagnose the injury accurately and implement proper treatment. Goals of treatment should be to achieve realignment and stability, preserve neurologic function, and maximize functional rehabilitation.

BIBLIOGRAPHY

1. Allen BL, Jr, Ferguson RL, Lehmann TR, et al: A mechanistic classification of closed, indirect fractures and dislocations of the lower cervical spine. *Spine* 1982; 7:1.

2. Anderson PA, Bohlman HH, Freehafer A: Anterior decompression and fusion in traumatic quadriplegia: Long term neurologic recovery in 111 patients. *Orthop Trans* 1986; 10:456.

3. Arena MJ, Eismont FJ, Green BA: Intervertebral disc extrusion associated with cervical facet subluxation and dislocation. Presented at the Cervical Spine Research Society Fifteenth Annual Meeting, Washington, DC, Dec 2–5, 1987.

4. Beatson TR: Fractures and dislocations of the cervical spine. *J Bone Joint Surg [Br]* 1967; 49B:249.

5. Bohlman HH, Eismont FJ: Surgical techniques of anterior decompression and fusion for spinal cord injuries. *Clin Orthop* 1981; 154:57.

6. Bohlman HH, Bahniuk E, Raskulinecz G, et al: Mechanical factors affecting recovery from incomplete cervical spinal cord injury: A preliminary report. *John Hopkins Med J* 1979; 145:115.

7. Bohlman HH: Acute fractures and dislocations of the cervical spine: An analysis of three hundred hospitalized patients and review of the literature. *J Bone Joint Surg [Am]* 1979; 61A:1119.

8. Bohlman HH: Complications of treatment of fractures and dislocations of the cervical spine, in Epps CH Jr (ed): *Complications in Orthopaedic Surgery*, ed 2. Philadelphia, JB Lippincott Co, 1986.

9. Bohlman HH: Late anterior decompression and fusion for spinal cord injuries: Review of 100 cases with long term results. *Orthop Trans* 1980; 4:41.

10. Bohlman HH: Pathology and current treatment concepts of cervical spine injuries, in American Academy of Orthopaedic Surgeons: *Instructional Course Lectures*, vol 21. St Louis, Mosby–Year Book, 1972, p 108.

11. Bohlman HH: Surgical management of cervical spine fractures and dislocations, in Stauffer ES (ed): *American Academy of Orthopaedic Surgeons: Instructional Course Lectures*, vol 34. St Louis, Mosby–Year Book, 1985, p 163.

12. Bohlman HH: The neck, in D'Ambrosia RD (ed): *Musculoskeletal Disorders: Regional Examination and Differential Diagnosis*. Philadelphia, JB Lippincott Co, 1977.

13. Bohlman HH: Indications for late anterior decompression and fusion for cervical spinal cord injuries, in Tator CH (ed): *Early Management of Acute Spinal Cord Injury. Seminars in Neurological Surgery*. New York, Raven Press, 1982.

14. Burstein AH, Otis JC, Torg JS: Mechanisms and pathomechanics of athletic injuries to the cervical spine, in Torg JS (ed): *Athletic Injuries to the Head, Neck and Face*. Philadelphia, Lea & Febiger, 1982.

15. Davis D, Bohlman H, Walker AE, et al: The

pathological findings in fatal craniospinal injuries. *J Neurosurg* 1971; 34:603.

16. Ducker TB, Bellegarrigue R, Salcman M, et al: Timing of operative care in cervical spinal cord injury. *Spine* 1984; 9:525.

17. Edwards CC, Matz SO, Levine AM: Oblique wiring technique for rotational injury of cervical spine. *Orthop Trans* 1985; 9:142.

18. Eismont FJ, Clifford S, Goldberg M, et al: Cervical sagittal spinal canal size and spine injury. *Spine* 1984; 9:663.

19. Herkowitz HN, Rothman RH: Subacute instability of the cervical spine. *Spine* 1984; 9:348.

20. Mazur JM, Stauffer ES: Unrecognized spinal instability associated with seemingly "simple" cervical compression fractures. *Spine* 1983; 8:687.

21. McAfee PC, Bohlman HH, Wilson WL: The triple wire fixation technique for stabilization of acute cervical fracture-dislocations: A biomechanical analysis. *Orthop Trans* 1985; 9:142.

22. Robinson RA, Southwick WO: Surgical approaches to the cervical spine, in Reynolds FC (ed): *American Academy of Orthopaedic Surgeons: Instructional Course Lectures,* vol 17. St Louis, Mosby–Year Book, 1960, p 299.

23. Robinson RA, Southwick WO: Indications and technics for early stabilization of the neck in some fracture dislocations of the cervical spine, *South Med J* 1960; 53:565.

24. Shields CL, Fox JN, Stauffer ES: Cervical cord injuries in sports. *Phys Sportsmed* 1978; 6:71–76.

25. Stauffer ES, Kelly EG: Fracture-dislocations of the cervical spine: Instability and recurrent deformity following treatment by anterior interbody fusion. *J Bone Joint Surg [Am]* 1977; 59A:45.

26. Torg JS, Vegso JJ, Sennet B: The National Football Head and Neck Injury Registry: 14 year report on cervical quadriplegia 1971–1984. *JAMA* 1985; 254:34–39.

27. Weiland DJ, McAfee PC: Enhanced immediate postoperative stability: Posterior cervical fusion with triple wire strut technique. Presented at the Cervical Spine Research Society Seventeenth Annual Meeting, New Orleans, La, Dec 5–8, 1989.

28. White AA, Panjabi MM: The role of stabilization in the treatment of cervical spine injuries. *Spine* 1984; 9:512.

29. White AA, Panjabi MS, Posner I, et al: Spinal stability: Evaluation and treatment, in American Academy of Orthopaedic Surgeons: *Instructional Course Lectures,* vol 30. St Louis, Mosby–Year Book, 1981, p 457.

30. White AA, Southwick WO, Panjabi MM: Clinical instability in the lower cervical spine: A review of past and current concepts. *Spine* 1976; 1:15.

CHAPTER 35

Axial Load "Teardrop" Fracture

Joseph S. Torg, M.D.

Helene Pavlov, M.D.

A triangular fracture fragment at the anteroinferior corner of a cervical vertebral body is frequently referred to as a "teardrop" fracture. This anteroinferior corner fracture fragment actually is an integral part of two specific cervical vertebral body compression fractures that occur in the lower cervical spine. One fracture pattern is an isolated anteroinferior fracture, and the other, the more common fracture pattern, is a three-part, two-plane fracture. The three-part, two-plane fracture consists of the anteroinferior corner fracture fragment combined with a sagittal vertebral body fracture and fractures of the posterior neural arch. These two fracture patterns have distinct neurologic sequelae; however, in the medical literature cervical spine fractures with an anteroinferior triangular fracture are often grouped together and referred to as a "flexion teardrop" or a "burst" fracture (or both). Analysis of 55 such injuries reveals that these commonly used terms are an incomplete description of the bony pathology and an inaccurate explanation of the mechanism of injury.

The purposes of this chapter are to delineate the radiographic, neurologic, and biomechanical aspects of two types of vertebral body compression fractures of the lower cervical spine that present, with an anteroinferior corner fracture fragment, (1) an isolated anteroinferior fracture and (2) a three-part, two-plane fracture, in which there is an associated sagittal vertebral body fracture and posterior neural arch fractures.

Schneider and Kahn[81] were the first investigators to describe the anteroinferior or "teardrop" vertebral body fracture and to evaluate the neurologic consequence. In their original description Schneider and Kahn enumerated the fracture findings, emphasizing the anteroinferior corner fracture fragment, posterior displacement of the fractured vertebral body into the spinal canal, and disk space narrowing. All of these observations were made from lateral roentgenograms. Descriptions of the roentgen findings from the anteroposterior view were not reported, and the possibility of a sagittal vertebral body fracture or posterior arch fractures was not mentioned. Essentially, their explanation of the "teardrop" fracture was determined solely on the lateral roentgenogram. Because findings from the anteroposterior view were not presented, Schneider and Kahn did not distinguish between an isolated anteroinferior corner cervical vertebral body fracture and those associated with the sagittal fracture. They concluded that the "teardrop" fracture was caused by "acute flexion" of the cervical spine and resulted in severe neurologic deficits. Subsequently the terms "acute flexion" and "teardrop" have been recognized and accepted as the descriptive label for vertebral body fractures with an anteroinferior corner fracture fragment.* Similar injuries have also been described as "burst" or "compression" fractures,† while other authors use the terms *"flexion teardrop"* and *"burst"* interchangeably.‡

Inherent in the descriptive terminology of these injuries is confusion regarding the mechanism of injury. These fractures have been attributed to flexion,§ hyperflexion, or hyperflexion with compression,‖ axial loading,¶ hyperextension (presumably an avulsion of the anterior longitudinal ligament),** and a combination of hyperextension and hyperflexion.[15, 30, 44, 102] Woodford[105] reported that the sagittal fracture occurs in "burst" fractures caused by an axial force but not with "flexion teardrop" fractures, and stated that the two fractures can be differentiated based on the mechanism of injury. Allen et al.[5] claim that "vertical compression" fractures with an anterior fracture fragment can be differentiated from anteroinferior corner fractures caused by "compression flexion." Lee reported that forceful flexion produces the anteroinferior corner triangular fracture, and strong axial load compression produces the sagittal fracture.[54]

Because of the inconsistency in re-

*References 1, 2, 5, 7, 13, 14, 20, 30, 31, 37, 41, 42, 45, 47–51, 53, 54, 78, 79, 81, 82, 102, 103, 105.

†References 2–6, 10–12, 15, 17, 18, 20–22, 25, 39, 44, 47, 49–50, 52, 59, 62, 67, 69–72, 75, 76, 80, 83, 86, 89–91, 102, 105.

‡References 2, 5, 24, 30, 41, 42, 47, 49.

§References 1–5, 7, 13–17, 20, 22, 26, 30, 31, 35, 37, 41, 42, 45, 47–54, 59, 62, 67, 71, 72, 78, 79, 81, 83, 101–103, 105.

‖References 1, 7, 13, 14, 17, 22, 26, 31, 37, 45, 47, 48, 51, 53, 54, 59, 62, 69, 78, 79, 83, 102, 103.

¶References 2–6, 10–12, 18, 20, 21, 24, 25, 30, 35, 36, 42, 44, 49–54, 56, 63, 66, 69–72, 75, 76, 86, 68–91, 101, 105.

**References 8, 15, 27, 30–32, 41, 42, 44, 58, 74, 102.

gard to both terminology and mechanism of injury, the neurologic sequelae associated with the different fracture patterns have not been clarified.[25, 64, 85, 86] Richmond and Freedman[68] reviewed 17 cases of cervical vertebral body fractures with an associated sagittal fracture in quadriplegic patients and concluded that the sagittal fracture indicated "severe trauma." Lee et al. observed the sagittal fracture in association with a "teardrop" fracture in 51 cases; they reported that 94% had permanent neurologic deficits, and 38 of the 51 were quadriplegic.[54] In another study, Lee reported that 41 (61%) of 61 patients with an anterior triangular fracture fragment without facet locking had an associated sagittal fracture of the vertebral body. Of this group of 61, 53 (87%) sustained a permanent neurologic injury, of which the majority were quadriplegic.[53] Unfortunately no mention of the neurologic status of the patients having only the isolated anteroinferior corner fracture was indicated in either of these studies.

Our analysis of fifty-five fractures indicates that in most instances the prevalent descriptive terms for these fractures inaccurately or incompletely (or both) describe both the bony pathology and the mechanism of injury. The fifty-five cases that are the subject of this communication represent the largest series of anteroinferior corner cervical vertebral body compression fractures to be reported in the orthopaedic literature. The purposes of this chapter are to (1) identify two distinct fracture patterns associated with an anteroinferior corner fracture fragment (i.e., an isolated fragment [Fig 35–1] and a three-part, two-plane fracture in which there is associated sagittal vertebral body fracture and posterior neural arch fracture [Fig 35–2]; (2) demonstrate that both fracture patterns result from axial loading, not hyperflexion, of the cervical spine; and (3) emphasize that when the sagittal fracture is present the lesion is

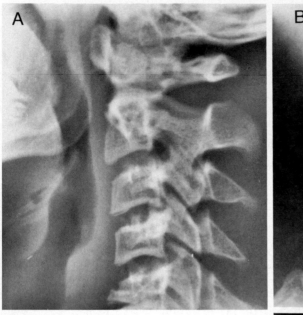

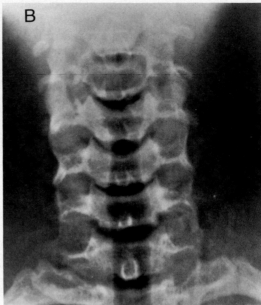

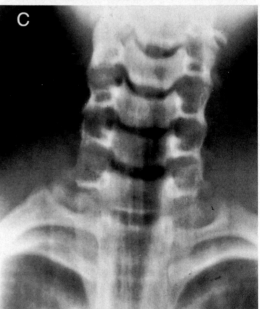

FIG 35–1.
An isolated anteroinferior corner fracture fragment is identified on lateral and frontal views. The patient had no permanent sequelae. **A,** lateral view demonstrates minimal prevertebral soft tissue swelling and a compression deformity of C5 with an anteroinferior vertebral body fracture fragment. There is narrowing of the C5–C6 intervertebral disc space, with capsular disruption and mild "fanning." **B** and **C,** there is no evidence of a sagittal vertebral body fracture on either the routine frontal view **(B)** or on an anteroposterior tomogram **(C).** The gentle undulating margins of the lateral masses are symmetric and normal. *(From Torg JS, Pavlov H, O'Neill MJ, et al: Am J Sports Med, in press. Used with permission.)*

unstable and usually associated with severe spinal cord injury.

Medical records and roentgenograms on 156 athletes with cervical spine injuries were obtained for this study from those reported to the National Football Head and Neck Injury Registry (NFHNIR) between 1971 and 1987.[96] An anteroinferior corner fracture of the vertebral body

occurred in 55 of these patients. All were injured playing football.

Medical records of the 55 patients were reviewed for information pertaining to patient age, mechanism of injury, position and activity of the athlete, treatment received, and extent and duration of motor or sensory neurologic deficit resulting from the injury. The mechanism of injury

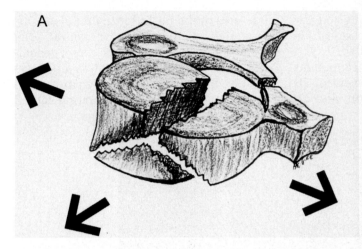

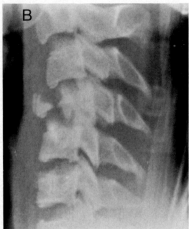

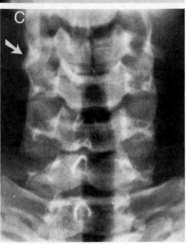

FIG 35–2.
A three-part, two-plane fracture of C4 is identified on lateral **(B)** and frontal **(C)** roentgenograms. **A,** a three-part, two-plane fracture is illustrated, showing an anteroinferior corner fracture fragment and a sagittal fracture through the entire vertebral body. The posterior arch is fractured. **B,** lateral view demonstrates an anteroinferior vertebral body fracture fragment of C4. The fragment is approximately one-fourth the VBW and involves the entire VBH. Marked posterior displacement and angulation of the posterior vertebral body fragment are present, together with narrowing of the C4–C5 intervertebral disk space, marked posterior ligamentous complex disruption with capsular disruption at C4–C5, and "fanning." **C,** frontal view demonstrates a sagittal vertebral body fracture at C4. There is minimal lateral mass displacement on the right *(arrow),* indicating disruption and fracture of the posterior neural arch. *(From Torg JS, Pavlov H, O'Neill MJ, et al: Am J Sports Med, in press. Used with permission.)*

was obtained from injury reports, coaches, hospital records, or game films. Cinematographic records were available for 8 of 55 athletes included in this study. Stop-frame analysis[98] of these game films was utilized to evaluate the mechanism of injury and the type of collision that occurred.

Roentgenograms or roentgenographic reports (or both) of the 55 patients have been analyzed. Both anteroposterior and lateral roentgenograms or reports were available in 37 of these 55 cases. The remaining 18 had only lateral roentgenograms or reports. The lateral roentgenograms or reports (or both) were reviewed for (1) the presence of an anteroinferior corner fracture, sagittal vertebral body fracture; (2) posterior displacement of the fractured vertebral body; (3) disk space widening or narrowing; (4) facet joint capsular disruption; and (5) disruption of the interspinous ligament.

The size of the anteroinferior corner fragment was measured as a fraction of vertebral body height (VBH) and vertebral body (sagittal) width (VBW). Posterior displacement of the fractured vertebral body was determined at both the superior and inferior posterior corners and measured with respect to the adjacent vertebrae. Facet joint capsular disruption was determined by the loss of parallelism of the articular processes. Disruption of the interspinous ligament was determined by an increase in the interspinous distance, as manifested by "fanning" of the spinous processes of the involved vertebrae (Fig 35–3, *A*).

The anteroposterior roentgenograms or reports (or both) were reviewed for (1) a sagittal vertebral body fracture and (2)

fractures of the posterior neural elements. Fractures of the posterior neural arch were determined by either direct visualization or by the lateral mass displacement, which produces an interruption in the symmetric, gentle undulating lateral

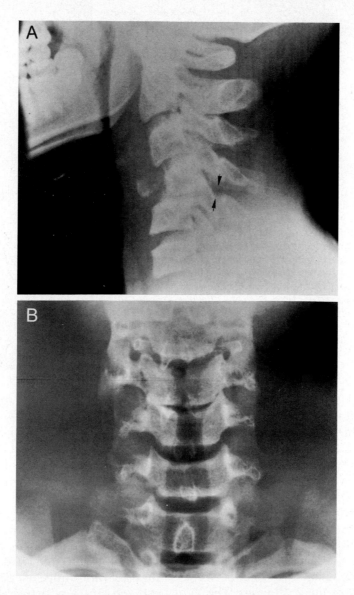

FIG 35–3.
A, the patient was rendered permanently quadriplegic after tackling practice with a spring-loaded dummy. There is a three-part, two-plane fracture of C4. Lateral view demonstrates prevertebral soft tissue swelling. There is an anteroinferior fracture fragment of C4. .The fragment measures one-third VBW and the entire VBH. There are posterior displacement and angulation of the posterior vertebral body segment and there are intervertebral disk space narrowing of C4–C5 and disruption of the posterior ligamentous complex, with loss of parallelism of the facet joint *(arrows)* and mild "fanning." **B,** frontal view demonstrates a sagittal vertebral body fracture of C4. There is lateral mass displacement bilaterally, right greater than left, indicating a fracture of the posterior neural arch. *(From Torg JS, Pavlov H, O'Neill MJ, et al: Am J Sports Med, in press. Used with permission.)*

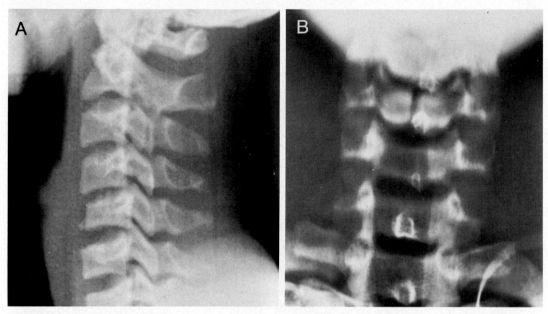

FIG 35–4.
A, three-part, two-plane fracture of C5. The patient was permanently quadriplegic. Lateral view demonstrates minimal anterior prevertebral soft tissue swelling. There are mild compression of C5 and a small anteroinferior fracture fragment. There is minimal posterior displacement of the posterior aspect of the C5 vertebral body. The C4–C5 intervertebral disk space is minimally narrowed. There is no evidence of capsular disruption or "fanning." **B,** an anteroposterior tomogram demonstrates a complete sagittal vertebral body fracture of C5 with lateral displacement of both lateral masses. *(From Torg JS, Pavlov H, O'Neill MJ, et al:* Am J Sports Med, *in press. Used with permission.)*

margins of the cervical spine (Fig 35–3, B). Signs of a vertebral body or posterior neural arch fracture were also examined on tomograms or a CT examination (or both) when available (Figs 35–4 and 35–5).

The average age of the patients was 16.2 years (range, 14 to 24). All patients were injured while playing football, either in a game or at practice. Patients were assigned case numbers in a random sequence. In 7 of the 55 cases the specific activity at the time of injury was unknown. In the remaining 48 patients, 73% (35/48) were attempting to tackle another player at the time of injury, while 25% (12/48) were being tackled, and 2% (1/48) were blocking. Three of the 35 athletes injured while tackling (9%) were participating in tackling drills involving a spring-loaded tackling dummy. Cinematographic records with stop-frame analysis were available in 8 patients and

injury reports in 43. In review of all 8 cinematographic records and 47 injury reports, axial loading was determined to be the predominant mechanism of injury. The mechanism of injury was axial loading in 52 of the patients and was unclear in the remaining 3 patients.

In 52 of the 55 patients, the reported or determined mechanism of injury was axial compression of the cervical spine. Generally the athlete lowered his head before making a head-on tackle or block, or he received a blow to the vertex of the head as a result of being tackled. Stop-frame analysis of films of the 8 patients (all of whom had anteroinferior corner fractures and 3 of whom had documented 3-part, 2-plane fractures) revealed that three basic types of collisions occurred: (1) a direct collision in which two individuals are moving along the same straight line immediately before impact, (2) a direct collision in which one indi-

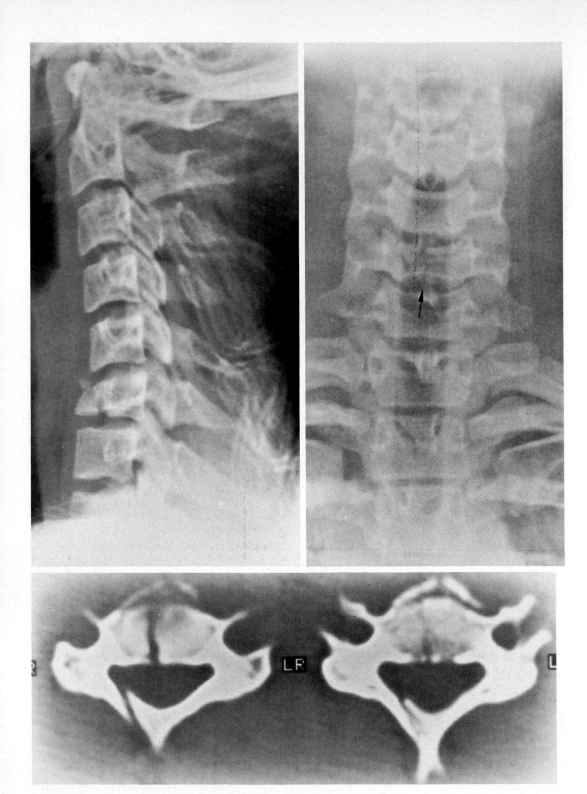

FIG 35–5.
A, a three-part, two-plane fracture of C6. The patient had no permanent neurologic sequelae. Lateral view demonstrates prevertebral soft tissue swelling and an anteroinferior fracture fragment of C6 involving the entire VBH and one third of the VBW. There is approximately 1 mm of posterior displacement of the inferior aspect of the posterior vertebral body. The C6–C7 intervertebral disk space is minimally narrowed posteriorly, with associated

vidual is at rest and the other moves on a line directly toward him, and (3) an oblique collision resulting in the oblique impact of two moving bodies.[94] Two of the eight injuries were type 1, two were type 2, and four were type 3. The posture of the head, cervical spine, and trunk and application of the axial impact to the crown of the helmet, as observed by cinematographic analysis, supports axial loading with failure in the flexion mode as the mechanism of injury. Specifically, impact occurred to the top or crown of the injured player's helmet while his neck was flexed approximately 20 to 30 degrees, normal cervical lordosis was neutralized, and the straightened spine approximated the structure of a segmented column. Axial loading results from either abrupt deceleration of the head with continued momentum of the body, or acceleration of the head with inertia of the body, with the cervical spinal segment being crushed between head and body.[95, 98] Excessive flexion was not seen in any of the 8 cases reviewed by stop-frame analysis.

Radiographically, patients were divided into three groups according to the identified fracture pattern. All 55 patients included in this study had an anteroinferior fracture fragment identified on the lateral roentgenogram or report (or both). Of these 55 patients, 37 had an anteroposterior roentgenogram or report to review. Of these 37 patients, 6 had the isolated anteroinferior fracture pattern and were identified as group I; 31 patients had an anteroinferior fracture fragment plus a sagittal vertebral body fracture, the three-part, two-plane fracture pattern, and were identified as group II. The remaining 18 patients had only lateral roentgenograms or reports to re-

view and were identified as group III.

Of the 55 patients, 45 were permanently quadriplegic, and the remaining 10 had transient neurologic symptoms consisting of either pain or paresthesia (or both) (8 patients) or a central cord syndrome (2 patients) that resolved.

Of the entire group of 55 patients, 8 (14.5%) had a vertebral fracture at two contiguous levels. Three of these patients had an anteroinferior fracture fragment at both levels. The level of the 58 anteroinferior corner fracture fragments was at C4 in 9 (16%), at C5 in 43 (74%), and at C6 in 6 (10%).

Of the 6 patients in group I with the isolated anteroinferior corner fracture pattern, 5 had a vertebral fracture at one level and 1 patient had vertebral fractures at two levels. All 5 patients with the fracture at a single level had transient neurologic symptoms. The 1 patient with vertebral fractures at two levels was quadriplegic.

Of the 31 patients in group II with the three-part, two-plane fracture pattern, 26 had vertebral fracture at one level and 5 had fractures at two levels. Twenty-seven of the 31 patients were permanently quadriplegic (23/26 with a single-level injury and 4/5 with a two-level injury), and four patients had transient symptoms (3/26; 1/5).

Of the eighteen patients in group III, those with an anteroinferior fracture fragment but without an anteroposterior radiograph or report to confirm or exclude a sagittal fracture, 15 had a vertebral fracture at one level and 3 had fractures at two levels. Of the 18 patients, 17 were permanently quadriplegic, and one initially had a mild central cord syndrome that resolved.

In 50 of the 55 patients, lateral x-ray

capsular disruption and "fanning." **B,** frontal view demonstrates a faint, linear radiolucency through the C6 vertebral body, indicating a sagittal vertebral body fracture *(arrow)*. There is mild lateral mass displacement. **C,** CT examination demonstrates the sagittal fracture extending completely through the vertebral body, with disruption of the lamina on the right. *(From Torg JS, Pavlov H, O'Neill MJ, et al: Am J Sports Med, in press. Used with permission.)*

films were available for review. The remaining 5 had lateral x-ray reports to be examined. The size of the anteroinferior corner fragment was measured as a fraction of the VBH and width the VBW. In 3 patients the fragment size was not indicated in the report. The anteroinferior fragment involved the entire height of the vertebral body (VBH) in all but 9 of the patients. In these 9 patients the fragment ranged from one-eighth to one-half the VBH. In the 52 patients, the fragment ranged from one-eighth to three-fourths the sagittal VBW.

Posterior vertebral body displacement was determined at both the superior and inferior aspects and measured with respect to the adjacent vertebra. There was no posterior displacement in 1 patient; straight posterior displacement in 9 patients; angulation, with the inferior displacement greater than the superior displacement, in 35 patients; and angulation, with the superior displacement greater than the inferior displacement, in 6 patients. In 4 of the 5 patients with lateral reports, the amount of posterior displacement was not mentioned. Posterior displacement of the vertebra into the vertebral canal was greater than 2 mm in 40 of the 45 patients who were permanently quadriplegic. Of the patients who were quadriplegic, maximum posterior displacement of the posterior aspect of the vertebral body averaged 5.4 mm (0–18 mm); in patients without permanent neurologic sequelae, the maximum posterior displacement averaged 2 mm (0–4 mm).

Intervertebral disk space narrowing was present in 48 of the 50 patients with lateral x-ray films to be reviewed. The predominant level of narrowing varied according to the level of vertebral fracture, occurring primarily below at C4–C5 with lesions at C4; primarily above at C5–C6 with lesions at C6; and above at C4–C5 and below at C5–C6 with lesions at C5.

Facet joint capsular disruption and fanning of the spinous processes indicates disruption of the posterior ligamentous complex. Facet joint capsular disruption as indicated by loss of parallelism of the adjoining articular facets was present in 49 patients. Disruption of the intraspinous ligament as demonstrated by "fanning,"[30] an increase in the intraspinous distance at the involved level compared with adjacent levels, was present in 44 patients. Damage to the posterior ligamentous complex was in general more severe in those patients who were quadriplegic.

Lateral mass displacement and loss of the gentle undulating symmetric margins of the cervical spine as identified on the anteroposterior roentgenogram indicate fractures of the posterior neural arch.[54, 92] This finding was present in all 31 patients in group II with a documented three-part, two-plane fracture and also in 1 of 6 patients in group I with an isolated anteroinferior fracture. The solo group I patient was the only patient in the group who had fractures at two levels and who was quadriplegic.

While this report is based on the injury pattern occurring in football, a similar fracture pattern associated with quadriplegia has also been reported in Rugby,[16, 73, 76, 83, 104] ice hockey,[90, 91] wrestling,[106] trampolining,[33, 40, 88, 93] parachuting,[17] gymnastics,[40, 93] and water sports.*

Review of the 55 cases presented in this report establishes a distinction between the isolated anteroinferior corner and the three-part, two-plane fracture pattern. The three-part, two-plane fracture defines a cervical vertebral body compression fracture consisting of (1) an anteroinferior corner fracture fragment, (2) a sagittal vertebral body fracture, and (3) various injuries to the intervertebral disk, the facet joints, the posterior neural

---

*References 1, 3–5, 19, 21, 25, 36, 37, 39, 50, 53, 59, 62, 67, 68, 71, 75, 78, 79, 81, 82, 86, 89, 102.

arch, and the posterior ligamentous structures. This particular fracture pattern has not been included in common classifications.[5]

Many reports regarding fractures of the lower cervical spine have relied solely on the lateral roentgenograms.* However, in order to delineate the full extent of the injury associated with the anteroinferior fracture fragment, a minimum of two roentgenograms (an AP and a lateral projection) are required. On the lateral view, in addition to the anteroinferior corner vertebral body fracture fragment, it is essential to determine (1) retropulsion or angulation (or both) of the posterior body fragment, (2) intervertebral disk space narrowing, and (3) loss of parallelism of the interfacetal joints and fanning of the intraspinous processes, indicating a tear or rupture of the posterior ligamentous complex.

On the AP view, it is essential to determine (1) the sagittal fracture of the vertebral body, (2) widening of the interpediculate distance, and (3) asymmetry of the lateral borders, indicating a posterior neural arch fracture. Care must be taken not to confuse the air in the larynx (formed as the tracheal air column narrows to a slit as it projects over the vertebral bodies of C3, C4, or C5) with a sagittal fracture (Figs 35–6 and 35–7).

Anteroposterior tomograms or a CT examination may be necessary to exclude or confirm the presence of a sagittal fracture or posterior neural arch injuries (see Figs 35–4, *B*, and 35–5, *C*; also see references 25, 34, 42, 57, 64, 90. Lee reported that CT and polytomography were necessary to document the presence of a sagittal fracture and the fractures of the posterior arch.[54] In his series posterior arch fractures were present in association with six of seven isolated sagittal vertebral body fractures and in 36 of 51 "teardrop" fractures associated with a sagittal verte-

*References 2, 8, 10–12, 15, 18, 24, 26, 28, 30, 31, 35, 36, 47–49, 58, 67, 72.

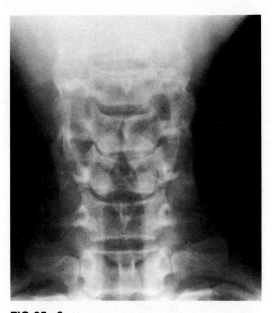

FIG 35–6.
Frontal view demonstrates the normal tracheal air shadow, which narrows gently and symmetrically in the region of the larynx, overlying the C5 vertebra in this patient. This normal slitlike radiolucency produced by air within the larynx can simulate a sagittal vertebral body fracture. Note that the gentle indulating lateral masses are symmetric. *(From Torg JS, Pavlov H, O'Neill MJ, et al: Am J Sports Med, in press. Used with permission.)*

bral body fracture. Of these 42 posterior arch fractures, only 13 were evident on the routine plain films. Posterior arch fractures are an expected occurrence with a sagittal fracture because it is unlikely for a rigid ring structure to fracture in only one site (see references 27, 54, 61, 65, 87, 89).

The isolated anteroinferior corner fracture pattern and the three-part, two-plane fracture pattern have vastly different neurologic sequelae. Of the 31 patients in our series with a documented three-part, two-plane injury, 27 (87%) were quadriplegic. In the remaining 4 patients, all had initial neurologic symptoms of paresthesias or paresis, including one case of central cord syndrome, all of which eventually resolved.

Of the 6 patients with an isolated anteroinferior corner fracture fragment

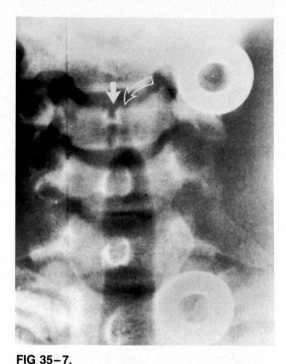

FIG 35–7.
Frontal view demonstrates the tracheal air shadow, which narrows to a slitlike shadow in the region of the larynx as it projects over C5 *(open arrow)*. Just to the right of the laryngeal air shadow, there is a vertical radiolucent line representing a sagittal vertebral body fracture of C5 *(closed arrow)*. There is associated lateral mass displacement bilaterally. *(From Torg JS, Pavlov H, O'Neill MJ, et al:* Am J Sports Med, *in press. Used with permission.)*

without an associated sagittal fracture, 5 (83%) had no serious neurologic sequelae. The one remaining patient had fractures to the posterior elements of the subjacent vertebra and was quadriplegic.

An anteroinferior corner fracture without a sagittal fracture has a less detrimental pattern. This finding has been substantiated by other studies in which the sagittal fracture accompanying an anteroinferior corner fracture fragment has been reported associated with severe cord injury or quadriplegia, or both.* King noted a correlation between the sagittal fracture associated with an anteroinferior corner fracture and cord damage, while patients with an isolated anteroin-

*References 20, 22, 54, 86, 90, 101.

ferior corner fracture did not have cord damage.[52] In a review of 45 patients with an anterior corner "teardrop" fragment, Kim reported that five of six patients with intact neurologic status did not have an associated sagittal fracture, compared with 38 of 39 patients with neurologic deficits who had an associated sagittal fracture.[51]

A sagittal fracture without an anteroinferior corner fracture fragment at the same level occurred in one patient who had a three-part, two-plane fracture at the level above and posterior neural arch fractures at both levels (Fig 35–8). This patient had no permanent neurologic sequelae. Several case reports of a sagittal fracture occurring without an anterior triangular fracture are found in the literature with various patterns of associated neurologic sequelae.[68, 82] Mansfield,[57] Neilson,[65] and Schneider[82] reported isolated sagittal vertebral body fractures of the lower cervical spine without neurologic sequelae. McCoy and Johnson[61] reported a sagittal vertebral body fracture associated with fractures of the lamina and a C3–C4 unilateral facet dislocation in a 15-year-old boy, resulting in a transient episode of paresis and paresthesias in all four extremities. Lee et al.,[54] in a retrospective study of 270 cervical spine injuries, reported 7 cases of "isolated" sagittal vertebral body fractures, all resulting in quadriplegia.

MECHANISM OF INJURY

The most popular description of the mechanism responsible for fracture/dislocation of the cervical spine has been accidental forced hyperflexion. The reports describe the subject as an unsuspecting victim of some untoward circumstance, that is, an accidental fall, a dive into shallow water, an unexpected blow to the head, or, in the case of an athlete, a poorly executed physical act in which the cervical spine is unwittingly forced

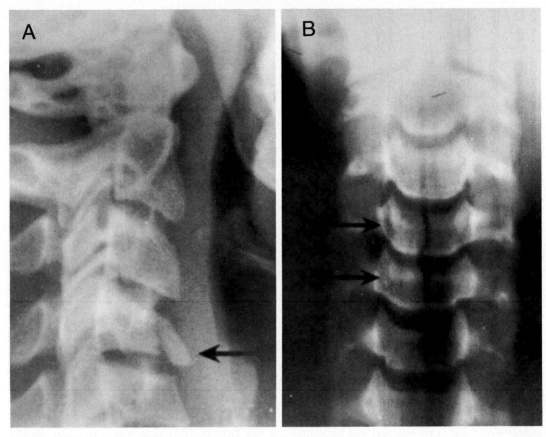

FIG 35–8.
A and **B,** this patient has a two-level injury: a three-part two-plane axial load "teardrop" fracture at C4 and a sagittal vertebral body fracture with associated fractures of the posterior neural arch at C5. The patient had no permanent neurologic sequelae. Lateral view demonstrates an anteroinferior fracture fragment involving one-fourth VBW of C4 *(arrow).* There is minimal straight posterior displacement of the posterior vertebral body fracture fragment. **B,** anteroposterior tomography through the vertebral bodies demonstrates sagittal vertebral body fractures at C4 and C5 *(arrows).* There is minimal displacement of the lateral mass of C5 on the right. *(From Torg JS, Pavlov H, O'Neill MJ, et al:* Am J Sports Med, *in press. Used with permission.)*

into the extreme of motion, with resulting injury. This hyperflexion mechanism was established by Schneider and Kahn as the force responsible for the "acute flexion teardrop" fracture.[81] There are two major factors to differentiate the isolated anteroinferior corner fracture and the three-part, two-plane fracture described in this report from the classical hyperflexion (or hyperextension) injuries. First, the circumstances surrounding the event are usually not accidental. Injury reports and cinematographic analysis have clearly demonstrated that in most instances the subject was executing a ma-

neuver in which the head was used as a battering ram, the initial point of contact being made with the top or crown of the helmet in an impact situation. Second, the principal mechanism of injury is not cervical spine hyperflexion or hyperextension, but, instead, axial loading. The vast majority of injuries occurred as the athlete struck another player or object, attempted a tackle, or performed a block with the crown of his helmet and his neck slightly flexed, reducing the cervical lordosis to a straight line. When the cervical spine is straight it becomes a segmented column. Loading of this segmented column occurs when impact is exerted to the vertex of the head along the vertical axis of the straightened spine. In this situation the forces are transmitted along the vertical axis of the cervical spine, obviating the impact-absorbing capacities of the disks, joints, and paravertebral muscles to the extent that injury occurs to the bones, disks, and ligamentous structures. When the maximum axial compressive deformation is reached, cervical spine flexion or rotation (or both) occurs with fracture, subluxation, or unilateral or bilateral facet dislocation. An excessive axial load is one force that could theoretically produce the components of both the isolated anteroinferior corner and the three-part, two-plane cervical vertebral body fractures.

Multiple authors have supported axial compression as the mechanism responsible for the anteroinferior corner fracture pattern.* Furthermore, other reports have suggested that a pure hyperflexion force cannot produce significant cervical spine fractures or dislocations.[6, 29, 46, 49] The axial loading mechanism of cervical spine injuries has been presented in previous published studies based on data from the NFHNIR.[93-98] These studies have demonstrated a causal relationship between axial loading and serious cervical spine injury based on injury reports, cinematographic analysis, and biomechanical models.

The mechanism of axial loading is supported by several biomechanical studies.† Mertz et al.,[63] Hodgson and Thomas,[43] and Sances,[72] have measured stresses and strains within the cervical spine when axial impulses are applied to helmeted cadaver head-spine-trunk specimens and demonstrated that fractures of the lower cervical spine occur when the impulse is applied to the crown of the helmet. Hodgson and Thomas[43] have de-

termined that a direct vertex impact imparts a larger force to the cervical vertebra than forces applied farther forward on the skull. Gosch et al.[38] have investigated three different injury modes, hyperflexion, hyperextension, and axial compression, in their experiment involving anesthetized monkeys, and conclude that axial compression produces cervical spine fractures and dislocations. Maiman et al.,[38] Roaf,[69] and White and Punjabi[101] have demonstrated vertebral body fractures in the lower cervical spine due to the axial loading of isolated spinal units. Roaf[69] believes it is the failure of the vertebral body−intervertebral disk complex that accounts for the vertical fractures of the vertebral body occurring in burst fractures. He has shown that in the presence of an intact intervertebral disk, a compressive load initially causes end plate failure, with herniation of the nucleus pulposus into the vertebral body, followed by bony failure. White and Punjabi[101] emphasize that axial loading is the major injury vector involved in the production of the "teardrop" fracture in the cervical vertebrae.

Several clinical studies support these findings and emphasize that tackling with the head down is the major cause of serious cervical spine injuries occurring in Rugby and tackle football (see references 23, 60, 76, 84, 97, 99, 100). Based on these studies, it can be concluded that axial loading is the dominant mechanism of injury for the various cervical spine fractures and dislocations occurring in tackle football, including the two types discussed in this report.

The fracture pattern originally described by Schneider and Kahn[48] as the "acute flexion teardrop" fracture was made on the basis of an incomplete roentgenographic analysis of the problem. As the cases that we have reported demonstrate, two types of fractures exist that involve the anteroinferior corner of the vertebral body, an isolated fracture,

---

*References 6, 11, 12, 18, 21, 24, 25, 36, 46, 55, 66, 69, 70, 75−77, 86, 89−91.

†References 9, 63, 38, 43, 69, 72, 101.

and a three-part, two-plane injury in which there is a sagittal vertebral body fracture. Both lesions are primarily produced by an excessive axial load to the cervical spine. An axial load can theoretically and experimentally produce the fractures to both the anterior and posterior elements of the vertebral body, as well as the posterior ligamentous disruption and posterior displacement of the vertebral body that are seen clinically.[9] Hyperflexion or hyperextension mechanisms fail to account for all the pathologic aspects of either the isolated anteroinferior corner fracture or the three-part, two-plane fracture.

In summary, the following points must be emphasized:

1. The terms *"flexion teardrop," "acute flexion teardrop,"* and *"burst fracture"* to describe a comminuted fracture of the cervical vertebral body are incomplete descriptive terms and inaccurately explain the mechanism of injury.

2. There are two fracture patterns associated with the anteroinferior corner fracture ("teardrop") fragment: (a) the isolated fracture, which is usually not associated with permanent neurologic sequelae, and (b) the three-part, two-plane fracture (in which there is a sagittal vertebral body fracture and fractures of the posterior neural arch) that is usually associated with permanent neurologic sequelae, specifically, quadriplegia.

3. Axial load is the mechanism of injury for both fracture patterns.

4. The predominant level of involvement is at C5 (74%), then C4 (16%), and then C6 (10%).

5. In football the majority (73%) of these fractures occur while attempting a tackle.

6. A complete radiologic examination includes (a) a lateral view to determine the extent of posterior displacement and angulation of the posterior vertebral body fragment and (b) an AP view, with computed tomography or tomography as necessary to determine the presence of a sagittal vertebral body, and the integrity of the posterior neural arch is essential in evaluating patients after cervical spine trauma in whom either type of lesion is suspected.

REFERENCES

1. Adelstein W, Watson P: Cervical spine injuries. *J Neurosurg Nursing* 1983; 15:65–71.

2. Aebi M, Mohler J, Zach GA, et al: Indication, surgical technique, and results of 100 surgically-treated fractures and fracture-dislocations of the cervical spine. *Clin Orthop Rel Res* 1986; 203:244–257.

3. Albrand OW, Corkill G: Broken necks from diving accidents: A summer epidemic in young men. *Am J Sports Med* 1976; 4:107–110.

4. Albrand OW, Walter J: Underwater deceleration curves in relation to injuries from diving. *Surg Neurol* 1975; 4:461–465.

5. Allen BL Jr, Ferguson RL, Lehman TR, et al: A mechanistic classification of closed, indirect fractures and dislocations of the lower cervical spine. *Spine* 1982; 7:1–27.

6. Apley AG: Fractures of the spine. *Ann R Coll Surg Engl* 1970; 46:210–223.

7. Babcock JL: Cervical spine injuries. *Arch Surg* 1976; 111:646–651.

8. Bailey RW: Observations of cervical intervertebral disc lesions in fractures and dislocations. *J Bone Joint Surg [Am]* 1963; 45:461–470.

9. Bauze RJ, Ardran GM: Experimental production of forward dislocation in the human cervical spine. *J Bone Joint Surg [Br]* 1978; 60B:239–245.

10. Beatson TR: Fractures and dislocations of the cervical spine. *J Bone Joint Surg [Br]* 1963; 45:21–35.

11. Bohlman HA: Acute fractures and dislocation of the cervical spine. *J Bone Joint Surg [Am]* 1979; 61:1119–1142.

12. Bohlman HA, Boada E: Fractures and dislocations of the lower cervical spine, in Bailey RW (ed): *The Cervical Spine.* Philadelphia, JB Lippincott, 1983.

13. Braakman R, Penning L: The hyperflexion sprain of the cervical spine. *Radiol Clin Biol* 1968; 37:309–320.

14. Bradford DS: Spinal instability: Orthopedic perspective and prevention. *Clin Neurosurg* 1979; 27:591–609.

15. Burke DC: Hyperextension injuries of the spine. *J Bone Joint Surg [Br]* 1971; 53:3–12.

16. Carvell JE, Fuller DJ, Duthrie RB, et al: Rugby football injuries to the cervical spine. *Br Med J* 1983; 286:49–50.

17. Ciccone R, Richman R: The mechanism of injury and the distribution of three thousand fractures and dislocations caused by parachute jumping. *J Bone Joint Surg [Am]* 1948; 30:77–100.

18. Cloward RB: Acute cervical spine injuries. *Clin Symp* 1980; 32:2–32.

19. Coin CG, Pennink Menna, Ahmad WD, et al: Diving-type injury of the cervical spine: Contribution of computed tomography to management. *J Comput Assist Tomogr* 1979; 3:362–372.

20. Dalinka M, Kessler H, Weiss M: The radiologic evaluation of spinal trauma. *Emerg Med Clin North Am* 1985; 3:475–490.

21. Dall DM: Injuries of the cervical spine. *S Afr Med J* 1972; 46:1048–1056.

22. Dolan KD: Radiological determination of cervical spine fracture and stability. *Clin Neurosurg* 1979; 27:368–384.

23. Dolan KD, Feldick HG, Albright JP, et al: Neck injuries in football players. *Am Fam Phys* 1975; 12:86–91.

24. Door LD, Harvey JP Jr: The traumatic lesions in fatal acute spinal column injuries. *Clin Orthop* 1981; 157:178–190.

25. Dorwart R, LeMasters DL: Application of computed tomographic scanning of the cervical spine. *Orthop Clin North Am* 1985; 16:381–393.

26. Durbin FC: Fracture-dislocations of the cervical spine. *J Bone Joint Surg [Br]* 1957; 39:23–38.

27. Edeiken-Monroe B, Wagner LK, Harris JH Jr: Hyperextension dislocation of the cervical spine. *Am J Radiol* 1986; 146:803–808.

28. Evans DK: Anterior cervical subluxation. *J Bone Joint Surg [Br]* 1976; 58:318–321.

29. Experimental investigations of spinal injuries. *J Bone Joint Surg [Br]* 1959;41:855.

30. Fielding JW, Hawkins RJ: Roentgenographic diagnosis of the injured neck. American Academy of Orthopaedic Surgeons Instructional Course Lectures. St Louis, Mosby–Year Book, 1976, pp 149–170.

31. Forsyth HF: Extension injuries of the cervical spine. *J Bone Joint Surg [Am]* 1964; 46:1792–1797.

32. Forsyth HF, Alexander E, Davis C, et al: The advantages of early spine fusion in the treatment of fracture-dislocation of the cervical spine. *J Bone Joint Surg [Am]* 1959; 41:17–36.

33. Frykman G, Hilding S: Hop pa studsmatta kan orska allvarliga skador. [Trampoline jumping can cause serious injury.] *Lakartidningen* 1970; 67:5862–5864.

34. Fuentes J-M, Bloncourt J, Vlahovitch B: La tear drop fracture: Contribution a l'etude du mecanisme et des lesions osteo-disco-ligamentaires. *Neurochirurgie* 1983;29:129–134.

35. Funk FJ Jr, Wells RE: Injuries of the cervical spine in football. *Clin Orthop* 1975; 109:50–58.

36. Garger WN, Fisher R, Halfmann HW: Vertebrectomy and fusion for "tear drop fracture" of the cervical spine: Case report. *J Trauma* 1969; 9:887–893.

37. Gehweiler JH, Clark WM, Schaaf R, et al: Cervical spine trauma: The common combined conditions. *Radiology* 1979; 130:77–86.

38. Gosch HH, Gooding E, Schneider RC: An experimental study of cervical spine and cord injuries. *J Trauma* 1972; 12:570–575.

39. Haines JD: Occult cervical spine fractures. *Postgrad Med* 1986; 80:73–77.

40. Hammer A, Schwartzbach AL, Darre E, et al: Svaere neurologiske skader some folge af trampolinspring. [Severe neurologic damage resulting from trampolining. *Ugeskr Laeger* 1981; 143:2970–2974.

41. Harris JH Jr: Radiographic evaluation of spinal trauma. *Orthop Clin North Am* 1986; 17:75–86.

42. Harris JH Jr, Edeiken-Monroe B, Kopaniky DR: A practical classification of acute cervical spine injuries. *Orthop Clin North Am* 1986; 17:15–30.

43. Hodgson VR, Thomas LM: *Mechanisms of Cervical Spine Injury During Impact to the Protected Head.* Twenty-Fourth Stapp Car Crash Conference, 1980, pp 15–42.

44. Holdsworth F: Fractures, dislocations, and fracture-dislocations of the spine. *J Bone Joint Surg [Am]* 1970; 52: 1534–1551.

45. Horlyck E, Rahbek M: Cervical spine injuries. *Acta Orthop Scand* 1974; 45:845–853.

46. Huelke DF, Nusholtz G: Cervical spine biomechanics: A review of the literature. *J Orthop Res* 1986; 4:232–245.

47. Jackson DW, Lohr FT: Cervical spine injuries. *Clin Sports Med* 5:373–386.

48. Jacobs B: Cervical fractures and dislocations (C3–7). *Clin Orthop Rel Res* 1975; 109:18–32.

49. Kazarian L: Injuries to the human spinal column: Biomechanics and injury classification. *Exercise Sport Sci Rev* 1981; 9:297–352.

50. Kewalramani LS, Taylor RG: Injuries to the cervical spine from diving accidents. *J Trauma* 1975; 15:130–142.

51. Kim KS, Chen HH, Russell EJ, et al: Flexion teardrop fracture of the cervical spine: Radiographic characteristics. *AJR Am J Roentgenol* 1989; 152:319–326.

52. King DM: Fractures and dislocations of the cervical spine. *Aust NZ J Surg* 1967; 37:57–64.

53. Lee C, Kim KS, Rogers LF: Triangular cervical body fragments: Diagnostic significance. *AJR Am J Roentgenol* 1982; 138:1123–1132.

54. Lee C, Kim KS, Rogers LF: Sagittal fracture of the cervical vertebral body. *AJR Am J Roentgenol* 1982; 139:55–60.

55. Lewis VL, Manson PN, Morgan RF, et al: Facial injuries associated with cervical fractures: Recognition, patterns and management. *J Trauma* 1985; 25:90–93.

56. Maiman DJ, Sances A, Myklebust JB, et al: Compression injuries of the cervical spine: A biomechanical analysis. *Neurorsurgery* 1983; 13:254–260.

57. Mansfield CM: A vertical fracture of the fifth cervical vertebra without neurologic symptoms. *AJR Am J Roentgenol* 1961; 86:277–280.

58. Marar BC: Hyperextension injuries of the cervical spine. *J Bone Joint Surg [Am]* 1974; 56:1655–1662.

59. Mawk JR: C7 burst fracture with initial "complete" tetraplegia. *Minnesota Med* 1983; 66:135–138.

60. McCoy GF, Piggot J, Macafee AL, et al: Injuries of the cervical spine in schoolboy Rugby football. *J Bone Joint Surg [Br]* 1984; 66-B:500–503.

61. McCoy SH, Johnson KA: Sagittal fracture of the cervical spine. *J Trauma* 1976; 16:310–312.

62. Mennen U: Survey of spinal injuries from diving: A study of patients in Pretoria and Cape Town. *South Afr Med J* 1981; 59:788–790.

63. Mertz HJ, Hodgson VR, Murray TL, et al: An assessment of compressive neck loads under injury-producing conditions. *Phys Sportsmed* 1978; 6:95–106.

64. Mori S, Ohiro N, Ojima T, et al: Observation of "tear-drop" fracture-dislocation of the cervical spine by computerized tomography. *J Jpn Orthop Assoc* 1983; 57:373–378.

65. Nielsen PB: Asymptomatic vertical fracture of a cervical vertebra. *Acta Orthop Scand* 1965;36:250–256.

66. Oliveira JC: Anterior plate fixation of traumatic lesions of the lower cervical spine. *Spine* 1987; 12:324–329.

67. Petrie JG: Flexion injuries of the cervical spine. *J Bone Joint Surg [Am]* 1964; 46-A:1800–1806.

68. Richman S, Friedman R: Vertical fracture of cervical vertebral bodies. *Radiology* 1954; 62:536–542.

69. Roaf R: A study of the mechanics of spinal injuries. *J Bone Joint Surg [Br]* 1960; 42-B:810–823.

70. Roaf R: International Classification of Spinal Injuries. *Paraplegia* 1972; 10:78–84.

71. Rogers WA: Fractures and dislocations of the cervical spine: An end-result study. *J Bone Joint Surg [Am]* 1957; 39-A:341–376.

72. Sances AJ, Myklebust JB, Maiman DJ, et al: Biomechanics of spinal injuries. *Crit Rev Biomed Eng* 1984; 11:1–76.

73. Scher AT: "Crashing" the Rugby scrum—an avoidable cause of cervical spinal injury. *South Afr Med J* 1982; 61:919–920.

74. Scher AT: Diversity of radiological features in hyperextension injury of the cervical spine. *S Afr Med J* 1980; 58:27–30.

75. Scher AT: Diving injuries to the cervical spinal cord. *South Afr Med J* 1981; 59:603–605.

76. Scher AT: The high Rugby tackle—an avoidable cause of cervical spinal injury? *South Afr Med J* 1978; 53:1015–1018.

77. Scher AT: Injuries to the cervical spine sustained while carrying loads on the head. *Paraplegia* 1978–1979; 16:94–101.

78. Scher AT: Radiographic indicators of traumatic cervical spine instability. *South Afr Med J* 1982; 62:562–565.

79. Scher AT: "Tear-drop" fractures of the cervical spine—radiologic features. *South Afr Med J* 1982; 61:355–359.

80. Schneider RC: A syndrome in acute cervical spine injuries for which early operation is indicated. *J Neurosurg* 1951; 8:360–367.

81. Schneider RC, Kahn EA: Chronic neurologic sequelae of acute trauma to the spine and spinal cord. Part I. The significance of the acute-flexion or "tear-drop" fracture dislocation of the cervical spine. *J Bone Joint Surg [Am]* 1956; 38-A:985–997.

82. Schneider RC: The syndrome of acute anterior spinal cord injury. *J Neurosurg* 1955; 12:95–123.

83. Silver JR: Injuries of the spine sustained in Rugby. *Br Med J* 1984; 288:37–43.

84. Silver JR: Rugby injuries to the cervical cord. *Br Med J* 1979; 1:192–193.

85. Stauffer ES: Cervical spine: Trauma, in American Academy of Orthopaedic Surgeons: *Orthopaedic knowledge update I. Home study syllabus,* 1984, pp 199–208.

86. Stauffer ES, Kaufer H: Fractures and dislocations of the spine, in Rockwood, CA Jr, Green DP: *Fractures,* vol 2, chap 12. Philadelphia, JB Lippincott, 1975.

87. Steel HH: Personal communication.

88. Steinbruck J, Paeslack V: Trampolinspringen—ein gefahrlicher Sport? [Is trampolining a dangerous sport?] *Munchen Med Wochenschr* 1978; 120:985–988.

89. Tator CH, Edmonds VE, and New ML: Diving: Frequent and potentially preventable cause of spinal cord injury. *Can Med Assoc J* 1981; 124:1323–1324.

90. Tator CH, Ekong CEU, Rowed DA, et al: Spinal injuries due to hockey. *Can J Neurol Sci* 1984; 11:34–41.

91. Tator CH, Edmonds VE: National survey of spinal injuries to hockey players. *Can Med Assoc J* 1984; 130:875–880.

92. Thomas JC: Plain roentgenograms of the spine in the injured athlete. *Clin Sports Med* 1986; 5:353–371.

93. Torg JS, Das M: Trampoline-related quadriplegia: Review of the literature and reflections on the American Academy of Pediatrics' position statement. *Pediatrics* 1984; 74:804–812.

94. Torg JS, Vegso JS, Yu A, et al: *Cervical Quadriplegia Resulting from Axial Loading Injuries: Cinematographic, Radiographic, Kinetic, and Pathologic Analysis.* Proceedings, Interim Meeting, American Orthopaedic Society for Sports Medicine. Feb 9, 1984, Atlanta.

95. Torg JS, (ed): Athletic injuries to the head, neck and face. *Mechanisms and Pathomechanics of Athletic Injuries to the Cervical Spine.* Philadelphia, Lea & Febiger, 1982.

96. Torg JS, Vegso JJ, Sennett B, et al: The National Football Head and Neck Injury Registry. 14 year report on cervical quadriplegia, 1971 through 1984. *JAMA* 1985; 254:3439–3443.

97. Torg JS, Vegso JJ, O'Neill MJ, et al: The epidemiologic, pathologic, biomechanical, and cinematographic analysis of football-induced cervical spine trauma. *Am J Sports Med* 1990; 18:50–57.

98. Torg JS, Vegso JJ, Torg E: Cervical quadriplegia resulting from axial loading injuries: Cinematographic, radiographic, kinetic and pathologic analysis. American Academy of Orthopaedic Surgeons Audio-Visual Library, 1987.

99. Walter J, Doris P, Shaffer MA: Clinical presentation of patients with acute cervical spine injury. *Ann Emerg Med* 1984; 13:512–515.

100. Watkins RG: Neck injuries in football players. *Clin Sports Med* 1986; 5:215–246.

101. White AA III, Punjabi MM: *Clinical Biomechanics of the Spine.* Philadelphia, JB Lippincott, 1978.

102. Whitley JE, Forsyth HF: The classification of cervical spine injuries. *AJR* 1960; 83:633–644.

103. Williams CF, Bernstein TW, Jalenko C III: Essentiality of the lateral radiograph. *Ann Emerg Med* 1981; 198–204.

104. Williams JPR, McKibbin B: Cervical spine injuries in Rugby Union football. *Br Med J* 1978; 2:1747.

105. Woodford MJ: Radiography of the acute cervical spine. *Radiography* 1987; 53:3–8.

106. Wu WQ, Lewis RC: Injuries of the cervical spine in high school wrestling. *Surg Neurol* 23:143–147.

CHAPTER 36

Cervical Spinal Stenosis With Cord Neurapraxia and Transient Quadriplegia

Joseph S. Torg, M.D.

Colleen M. Fay, M.D.

The purpose of this chapter is to define as a distinct clinical entity the syndrome of neurapraxia of the cervical spinal cord with transient quadriplegia.

Characteristically, the clinical picture involves an athlete who sustains an acute transient neurologic episode of cervical cord origin with sensory changes that may be associated with motor paresis involving either both arms, both legs, or all four extremities after forced hyperextension, hyperflexion, or axial loading of the cervical spine.[39] To be emphasized, the findings are always bilateral and should not be confused with those associated with root or plexus neurapraxia, which are always unilateral.

Routine roentgenograms of the cervical spine are negative for fractures or dislocations in all cases. However, roentgenographic findings include developmental cervical spinal narrowing, either as an isolated finding or associated with congenital fusions, ligamentous instability, or intervertebral disk disease.[39]

A review of the literature has revealed few reported cases of transient quadriplegia occurring in athletes. Attempts to establish the occurrence rates indicate that the problem is more prevalent than expected. Specifically, in the population of 39,377 exposed football participants, the reported incidence rate for transient paresthesia in all four extremities was 6 per 10,000, while the incidence rate reported for paresthesia associated with transient quadriplegia was 1.3 per 10,000 in one season surveyed.[39] From these data it appears that the prevalence of this problem is relatively high, and an awareness of the etiology, manifestations, and appropriate management principles is warranted.

There is sparse documentation in the literature of the syndrome we call cervical spinal cord neurapraxia. Grant and Puffer[17] reported a case of quadriplegia that occurred in an 18-year-old football player with developmental cervical stenosis. Stratford[37] published an account of a professional football player who had a minimal transient neurologic deficit after a hyperextension injury to his cervical spine. Funk et al.[15] presented two cases of temporary quadriplegia occurring in football players. One, who had suffered two episodes of generalized numbness and paralysis that lasted only a few seconds after hyperextension of his neck, had reportedly normal findings on roentgenographic, myelographic, and neurologic examination. The second, a professional player, was temporarily rendered quadriplegic after neck hyperflexion.

Narrowing of the sagittal diameter of the cervical spinal canal may occur as either a diffuse developmental variation or as an acquired stenosis resulting from spondylolytic changes. Several investigators have observed that symptoms may be associated with both types of stenosis.*

Multiple investigators have reported the measurement of the sagittal diameter of the cervical spinal canal as a means of diagnosing spinal stenosis. These reports have resulted in inconsistencies in "normal" and "abnormal" values for the sagittal diameter of the cervical spine. Of the various techniques and measurements reported, the most commonly employed method for determining the sagittal spinal canal diameter utilizing the lateral roentgenographic view of the cervical spine measures the distance from the middle of the posterior surface of the vertebral body to the nearest point of the corresponding spinal laminar line, which Wilkinson et al.[42] called the preexisting sagittal diameter (PSD)* The actual millimeter measurement of the sagittal diameter as determined by the conventional method is misleading, both as reported in the literature and in actual practice, because of variations in the target distances used in obtaining the roentgenogram and the landmarks used for obtaining the measurement.

Boijsen[2] investigated the cause of variation in the reported radiographic measurements of the sagittal diameter of the cervical spinal canal and evaluated the effects of the following two factors: (1) the focus to film (F/F), that is, the target distance, and (2) the object to film (O/

F), that is, the cervical spine to cassette, the object distance. He reported that the effect of a difference between a 1 m and 1.5 m F/F distance on the resultant sagittal canal measurement is 0.5 mm. To evaluate the effects of the O/F distance, he calculated that the average difference in shoulder breadth between men and women is 10 cm, or approximately a 5 cm difference in the O/F distance. The effect of a 5 cm difference in the O/F distance on the resultant sagittal canal measurement is 1.2 mm at a F/F distance of 1.0 m and 0.7 mm at a F/F distance of 1.5 m.

The ratio method for determining the sagittal spinal canal diameter was devised by Pavlov[29, 39] and compares the standard measurement of the canal with

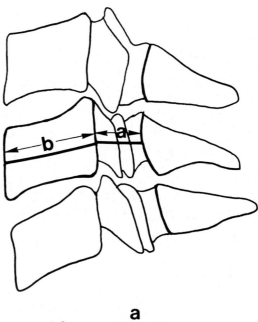

$$\text{ratio} = \frac{a}{b}$$

FIG 36–1.
The spinal canal/vertebral body ratio is the distance from the midpoint of the posterior aspect of the vertebral body to the nearest point on the corresponding spinolaminar line *(a)* divided by the anteroposterior (AP) width of the vertebral body *(b)*. Pavlov's ratio is a/b. *(From Torg JS, Pavlov H, Genuario S, et al: J Bone Joint Surg [Am] 1986: 68-A:1354–1370. Used with permission.)*

*References 2, 3, 6, 9, 12, 18, 25, 26, 31, 42, 43.
*References 2, 18, 25, 31, 41, 43.

the anteroposterior width of the vertebral body at the midpoint of the corresponding vertebral body (Fig 36–1).

The ratio method of determining cervical spinal canal narrowing is independent of magnification factors caused by differences in F/F distance, O/F distance, or body type because the sagittal diameter of the spinal canal and that of the vertebral body are in the same anatomic plane and are similarly affected by magnification. There is normally a one-to-one relationship between the sagittal diameter of the spinal canal and that of the vertebral body, regardless of sex (Fig 36–2,A). A spinal canal:vertebral body ratio of less than 0.82 was recorded at one or more levels in all patients who experienced cervical cord neurapraxia (Fig 36–2,B).

Torg et al.[39] reported a retrospective review of 32 patients in whom an acute transient neurologic episode resulted from forced hyperextension, hyperflexion, or axial loading of the cervical spine. The patients were all male, 15 to 32 years of age (mean age, 20 years). Twenty-nine were injured while playing football, 1 while playing ice hockey, 1 while playing basketball, and one was a professional boxer. Of the 29 patients who played football, 4 were professional, 16 were college, and 9 were high school players. All had reported experiencing

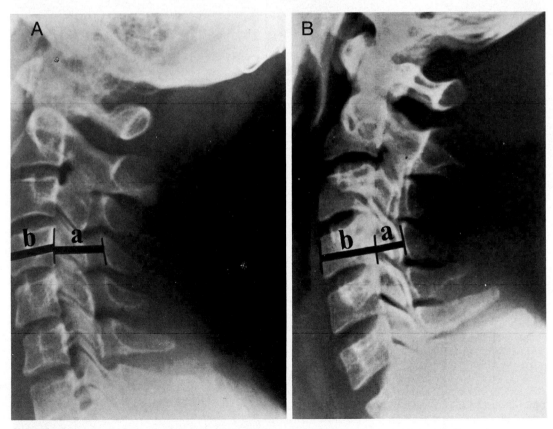

FIG 36–2.
Comparison between the ratio of the spinal canal to the vertebral body of a "normal" control subject with that of a stenotic patient demonstrated on lateral-view roentgenograms of the cervical spine. Pavlov's ratio is 1:1 (1.00) in the control subject **(A)** compared with 1:2 (0.50) in the stenotic patient **(B).** *From Torg JS, Pavlov H, Genuario S, et al: J Bone Joint Surg [Am] 1986; 68-A:1354–1370. Used with permission.)*

one or more episodes of cervical spinal cord neurapraxia.

Lateral cervical spine roentgenograms were reviewed for congenital anomalies, instability, disk disease, and spinal stenosis. Measurements for the determination of spinal stenosis were made at the level of the third through the sixth cervical vertebrae on the lateral view of the cervical spine. The presence of spinal stenosis was determined by two methods. The first was the standard method and

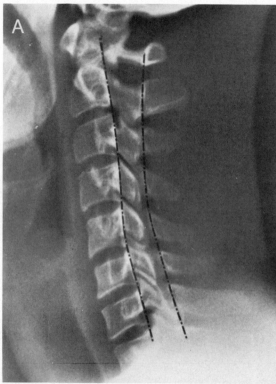

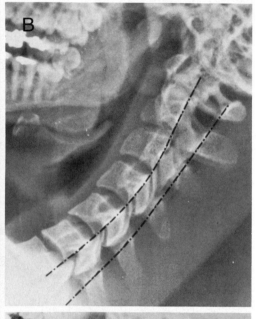

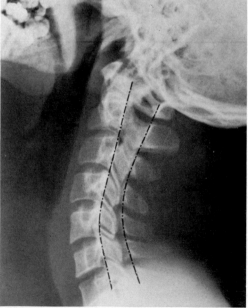

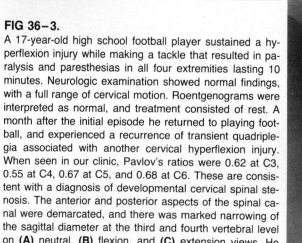

FIG 36–3.
A 17-year-old high school football player sustained a hyperflexion injury while making a tackle that resulted in paralysis and paresthesias in all four extremities lasting 10 minutes. Neurologic examination showed normal findings, with a full range of cervical motion. Roentgenograms were interpreted as normal, and treatment consisted of rest. A month after the initial episode he returned to playing football, and experienced a recurrence of transient quadriplegia associated with another cervical hyperflexion injury. When seen in our clinic, Pavlov's ratios were 0.62 at C3, 0.55 at C4, 0.67 at C5, and 0.68 at C6. These are consistent with a diagnosis of developmental cervical spinal stenosis. The anterior and posterior aspects of the spinal canal were demarcated, and there was marked narrowing of the sagittal diameter at the third and fourth vertebral level on **(A)** neutral, **(B)** flexion, and **(C)** extension views. He was advised to discontinue participation in football and other contact sports and had had no recurrence at 8-year follow-up. *(From Torg JS, Pavlov H, Genuario S, et al: J Bone Joint Surg [Am] 1986; 68-A:1354–1370. Used with permission.)*

the second that devised by Pavlov, the ratio method.[29] Lateral-view cervical spine roentgenograms of 49 male patients of similar age, but without neurologic complaints, were used as a control group, and measurements for spinal stenosis were performed at the third through the sixth cervical vertebral level by both the standard and ratio methods.

Evaluation of the medical records, including radiographic reports, revealed that all of the 32 individuals in this group who sustained cervical spinal cord neurapraxia could be subdivided into the following four subgroups: (1) developmental stenosis, (2) ligamentous instability, (3) intervertebral disk disease, and (4) congenital cervical anomalies. None of these patients had "normal" cervical spines.

DEVELOPMENTAL STENOSIS

Seventeen of the subjects had roentgenographic evidence of developmental stenosis of the spinal canal (Fig 36–3). In this group the mechanism of injury was hyperflexion in 5 cases, hyperextension in 8 cases, and axial loading in 4 cases. All 17 had experienced sensory manifestations. Eleven had had paralysis, 3 had had weakness in four extremities, 1 had had weakness in both lower extremities, and 2 had had no motor involvement.

LIGAMENTOUS INSTABILITY

Four patients had roentgenographic evidence of ligamentous instability: one between the first and second (Fig 36–4),

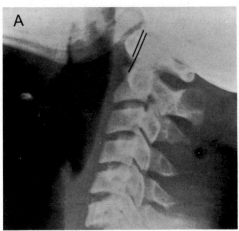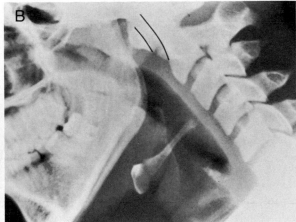

FIG 36–4.
A 20-year-old university football player sustained an injury to his cervical spine when he "lowered his head and hit an opposing carrier head on." He suffered a period of unconsciousness and 10 to 15 minutes of inability to move his arms and legs. Initial x-ray films, which did not include flexion and extension views, were interpreted as normal. He was discharged from the hospital after 2 days of observation; however, he complained of "excruciating pain" in his neck for 2 weeks. He was treated in a cervical collar for 6 weeks. Subsequently, he experienced intermittent neck pain. Six months after the injury he had repeat roentgenograms, including flexion and extension views, which demonstrated C1–C2 instability. In neutral position, the ADI (atlantodens interval) measured within the normal limits of 2.5 mm between the posterior aspect of the anterior arch of C1 and the anterior aspect of the odontoid process **(A)**. In flexion the ADI increased beyond the normal limits, indicating an atlantoaxial subluxation **(B)**. Pavlov's ratios were 0.74 at C3, 0.72 at C4, 0.74 at C5, and 0.84 at C6, consistent with the diagnosis of developmental stenosis. Because of instability, he underwent a C1–C3 cervical wiring fusion. He has not had recurrence of motor and sensory symptoms. *(From Torg JS, Pavlov H, Genuario S, et al: J Bone Joint Surg [Am] 1986; 68-A:1354–1370. Used with permission.)*

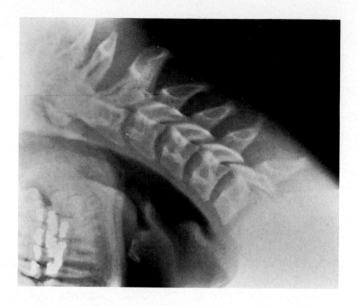

FIG 36–5.
A 15-year-old high school football player had two episodes of paresthesias throughout his body after having been struck on the top of the head while tackling. There was no history of paralysis. Cervical spine roentgenograms taken after the first injury were interpreted as normal. Subsequently the youngster participated in high school wrestling, and had several episodes of total body numbness associated with hyperflexion of the cervical spine. When seen in our clinic he had full range of cervical motion, and neurologic examination revealed normal findings. However, lateral-view roentgenograms of the cervical spine made in flexion demonstrated laxity and instability of the posterior ligamentous complex at the fifth and sixth cervical levels. Laxity is identified by a "fanning" increase in the intraspinous distance, loss of parallelism between the facet joints on the lateral view (the inferior aspects of the apophyseal joints diverge as opposed to being parallel), widening of the posterior aspect of the intervertebral disk space, and narrowing of the anterior intervertebral disk space at this level. There was no evidence of anterior subluxation. Pavlov's ratios were 0.75 at C3, 0.75 at C4, 0.75 at C5, and 0.55 at C6. These were compatible with the diagnosis of the developmental spinal stenosis associated with the described laxity. The patient was advised to discontinue both football and wrestling, and had not had a recurrence of symptoms at 3-year follow-up. *(From Torg JS, Pavlov H, Genuario S, et al: J Bone Joint Surg [Am] 1986; 68-A:1354–1370. Used with permission.)*

one between the second and third, and two between the fifth and sixth cervical vertebrae (Fig 36–5). In three cases the initial insult was reported to result from axial loading of the spine. One case followed a hyperextension injury. In one younger patient with instability between the fifth and sixth cervical vertebrae, the symptoms followed a hyperflexion injury, however. Two of the patients in this group had paralysis of all four extremities, while two had no motor impairment. All four had sensory manifestations, one having upper extremity paresthesias and the remainder having involvement in all four extremities.

INTERVERTEBRAL DISK DISEASE

Intervertebral disk disease was demonstrated in six patients, one having a myelogram (Fig 36–6) and another a magnetic resonance imaging (MRI) scan compatible with an acute disk herniation (see Fig 36–13), while the remaining four had chronic changes manifested by intervertebral disk space narrowing and posterior osteophyte formation (Fig 36–7). Both subjects with acute disk herniation had a stenotic canal at the involved level. Axial loading of the spine was the mechanism identified in two patients, hyperflexion in one, and hyperextension in the remaining three. Five of the six subjects

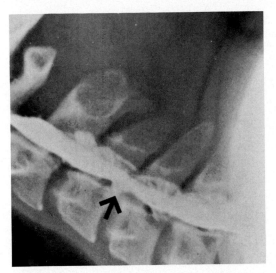

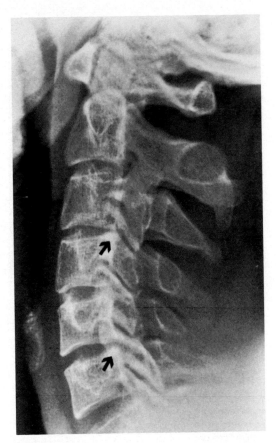

FIG 36–6.
A 19-year-old university football player injured his neck in spring practice while "engaged in spearing." Apparently he was involved in a blocking exercise and struck the dummy with the top of his head. He was unconscious for a few seconds; when he awoke, he had total quadriplegia without breathing difficulty that lasted for 5 minutes. The paralysis gradually subsided; however, weakness and paresthesias in a shawl-like distribution persisted for several days. He was admitted to the hospital, placed in traction for 3 weeks, and had a cervical myelogram that demonstrated an anterior extradural defect at the C3–C4 intervertebral disk space consistent with a herniated nucleus pulposus. Pavlov's ratios were 0.71 at C3, 0.64 at C4, 0.66 at C5, and 0.66 at C6, indicating significant spinal stenosis. Because of persistent limitation of cervical spinal motion and pain, the patient underwent an anterior C3–C4 diskectomy and interbody fusion 1 month after the injury. His postoperative course was uncomplicated, and he had no recurrence of symptoms at 14-year follow-up. *(From Torg JS, Pavlov H, Genuario S, et al: J Bone Joint Surg [Am] 1986; 68-A:1354–1370. Used with permission.)*

FIG 36–7.
A 21-year-old intercollegiate player sustained a hyperextension injury to his cervical spine and experienced four-extremity motor and sensory loss for 5 minutes. There are small hypertrophic spurs and sclerosis in the posterior corner between the fourth and sixth cervical vertebrae. The intervertebral disk spaces are narrowed at these locations, and the spurs extend beyond the posterior border of the vertebral bodies, decreasing the sagittal diameter of the spinal canal. Pavlov's ratios were 0.84 at C3, 0.79 at C4, 0.75 at C5, and 0.78 at C6. *(From Torg JS, Pavlov H, Genuario S, et al: J Bone Joint Surg [Am] 1986; 68-A: 1354–1370. Used with permission.)*

had motor paralysis, one had weakness in four extremities, and five had sensory manifestations in all four extremities, while one had bilateral upper extremity sensory manifestations only.

CONGENITAL CERVICAL ANOMALIES

There were five patients with congenital cervical anomalies. Two patients had failure of segmentation involving the second and third cervical vertebrae (Fig 36–8), one of the third and fourth cervical vertebrae (Fig 36–9), and one between the second, third, and fourth cervical vertebrae (Fig 36–10). The fifth patient had marked proliferative changes of the anterior aspect of the fourth, fifth, and sixth vertebral bodies characteristic of diffuse idiopathic skeletal hyperosto-

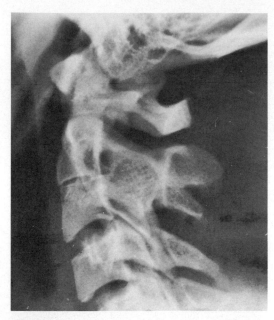

FIG 36−8.
A 21-year-old university football player sustained a hyperextension injury to his cervical spine. He had upper extremity weakness for 10 seconds and paresthesias that lasted for 48 hours. At the time of injury he was hospitalized. A lateral-view roentgenogram of the upper cervical spine demonstrated a congenital fusion between the apophyseal joints at C2 and C3 and a partial interbody fusion between C2 and C3, especially posteriorly. The intervertebral disk space was markedly reduced and obliterated in the posterior aspect. Pavlov's ratios were 1.75 at C3, 0.070 at C4, and 0.68 at C5. He was treated conservatively with head halter traction for 2 days. With full return of motor and sensory function, he was released from the hospital. At 6-year follow-up he had remained asymptomatic, but had not returned to contact sports. *(From Torg JS, Pavlov H, Genuario S, et al: J Bone Joint Surg [Am] 1986; 68-A:1354−1370. Used with permission.)*

and the twenty-four cases in the patient group in which lateral views of the cervical spine were available for review were divided into the following subgroups:

- Group A: Controls N = 49
- Group B: Developmental spinal stenosis N = 12
- Group C: Instability, disk disease, congenital anomalies N = 12
- Group D: Entire patient group N = 24

The cervical sagittal canal diameter measurements of "C3 through C6 in the symptomatic patients are summarized: for group B, the mean sagittal diameter was 14.0 mm (8.5−17.0 mm) and the mean sagittal ratio was 0.65 (0.31−0.81). For group C, the mean sagittal diameter

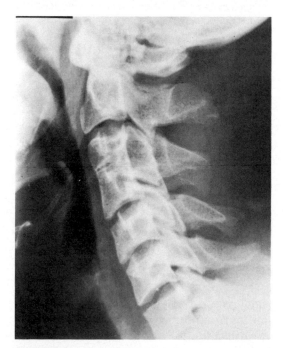

FIG 36−9.
Lateral-view roentgenogram of the cervical spine of a 29-year-old collegiate ice hockey player who experienced paresthesias of both upper extremities lasting 24 hours after hyperextension injury. In addition to the narrow canal, there is a congenital anterior interbody fusion between the third and fourth cervical vertebrae with associated fusion of the apophyseal joints. Of note, he returned to competitive ice hockey without a recurrence of symptoms.

sis[33] (Fig 36−11). Hyperextension was the precipitating mechanism in all five cases. Sensory manifestations, consisting of burning pain, numbness, and paresthesias, were limited to the upper extremity in four cases and were present in all four extremities in one case. One patient had weakness in the upper extremities, and one had paralysis of all four extremities. Three patients had no motor involvement.

For statistical purposes, the controls

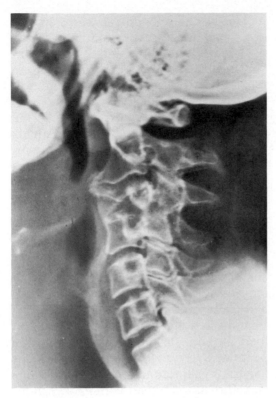

FIG 36–10.
Former high school football player first seen 33 years after an episode of transient quadriplegia that persisted in his upper extremities for 2 weeks and in his lower extremities for a month. Lateral-view roentgenogram demonstrates malformation involving the second, third, and fourth cervical vertebrae, including congenital fusions at these levels.

was 16.6 mm (12.0–23.5 mm) and the mean sagittal ratio was 0.75 (0.55–1.18). For the overall symptomatic patient population, group D, the mean sagittal diameter was 15.2 mm and the mean sagittal ratio was equal to 0.69.

The Mann-Whitney U test was used to compare each subgroup with the controls and the entire patient group with the controls. There was statistically significant spinal stenosis at $P < .001$ at each level C3 through C6 in each subgroup and in the entire symptomatic patient group, compared with the male control group A by both the "conventional" and "ratio" methods.

With use of the standard method, the actual millimeter measurement of the canals in the symptomatic patients was occasionally within the "acceptable normal" range. With use of the ratio method, the ratios were abnormal and indicated significant narrowing in all symptomatic patients. The ratio method compensates for variations in x-ray technique because the sagittal diameters of both the canal and the vertebral body are affected similarly by magnification factors. The ratio method is independent of technique variations, and the results were statistically significant. With use of the ratio method of determining the canal dimension, a spinal canal:vertebral body ratio of less than 0.80 is indicative of developmental cervical spinal narrowing.

Statistical analysis was performed comparing the spinal canal sagittal diameter between male and female patients as measured by the conventional method, and a statistical difference was identified.

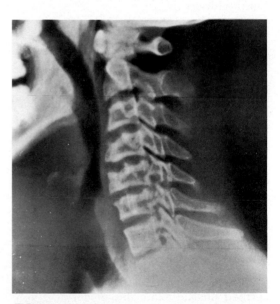

FIG 36–11.
Lateral-view roentgenogram of a 17-year-old high school football player who related bilateral "burning" paresthesias after forced hyperextension of his neck. There are anterior proliferative changes involving the fourth, fifth, and sixth cervical vertebrae, with a markedly decreased anteroposterior diameter of the spinal canal at these levels.

It was also determined that the sagittal diameter of the canal was proportional to the sagittal diameter of the vertebral body, and the vertebral bodies enlarge proportionally with the canals. No statistical difference was identified in the respective spinal canal:vertebral body ratios between the male and female control groups.[29]

Also reported were the results of a telephone survey of 223 known patients with quadriplegia listed with the National Football Head and Neck Injury Registry, in which 117 individuals were contacted personally. None of these patients recalled any episodes of transient motor paresis before their permanent lesion. When asked about any sensory episodes, 115 said they had had none, one was equivocal but described unilateral numbness lasting for one minute, and one was positive with numbness and tingling involving all four extremities and lasting for 1 minute.[39]

In an attempt to determine the nature and incidence of cervical spinal cord neurapraxia during the 1984 collegiate football season, a mail survey of the National Collegiate Athletic Association's 503 schools participating in football was conducted. Three hundred forty-four schools (68%) responded, representing 39,377 football players. Two distinct groups were identified: group I (N = 5) had experienced transient quadriplegia with paresthesia, while group II (N = 24) had experienced transient paresthesia in either the upper or the lower extremities, or both.

Group I, who had experienced both transitory paresis and paresthesia, described classic examples of cervical spinal cord neurapraxia. Numbness was reported as lasting from 1 minute to 12 hours. Tingling in all four extremities persisted anywhere from 30 minutes to several weeks. Paralysis in this group ranged from 1 minute to 24 hours, with five patients reporting quadriparesis. The incidence rate for group I was 5/39,377, or 1.3 per 10,000 participants.[39]

Group II reported only sensory involvement. Numbness and tingling were reported as lasting from 30 seconds to 48 hours. The sensory symptoms were confined to the upper extremities in the majority of cases, and only seven patients reported paresthesia in all four extremities. The incidence rate for group II was 24/39,377, or 6.0 per 10,000 participants.[39]

An attempt was made to establish recurrence patterns in the 32 patients in the study. Of the 17 individuals with developmental cervical stenosis, 9 did not attempt to return to their activity after the one episode. Three did return to football, had a second episode, and withdrew from the activity. One patient returned to football, and, despite a second episode, continued to play without further problems at 3-year follow-up. Three individuals returned to football without any problems at 2-year follow-up. A professional boxer had a cervical laminectomy after two episodes of transient quadriplegia, continues to box, and has had no further problems at 5-year follow-up.[39]

Of the five patients with congenital fusion of the upper cervical spine, four withdrew from football after the one episode. One has continued to play collegiate ice hockey without a problem at 3-year follow-up.[39]

Of the four individuals with cervical instability, two withdrew from football. One of the younger patients with ligamentous instability between the fifth and sixth cervical vertebrae had three episodes of whole body numbness precipitated by cervical spine hyperflexion while wrestling. He stopped wrestling, and is asymptomatic at 2-year follow-up. One younger patient with instability between the second and third cervical vertebrae was allowed to return to football with the use of a neck roll and keeping his head up while tackling. He has had no further problem at 1-year follow-up.[39]

Three of the six patients with degenerative disk disease withdrew from football after the initial episode. A professional football player discontinued his activity after one recurrence and was lost to follow-up. Two patients with acute intervertebral disk herniation, one basketball player and one football player, underwent anterior diskectomy and interbody fusion. Both are without recurrence; however, neither returned to his sport.[39]

Evaluations of the lateral roentgenograms available for review in 24 of the 32 cases of cervical spinal cord neurapraxia reported here have revealed, when compared with a series of 49 controls, statistically significant decreases in the anteroposterior diameter of the spinal canal between the third and the sixth cervical vertebrae. Because of the aforementioned variation in radiographic technique and differences in target distances, the ratio of the anteroposterior diameter of the spinal canal to the anteroposterior diameter of the vertebral body is the more reliable method of determining cervical spinal stenosis. With use of this method, it has been demonstrated in all symptomatic patients that the ratio was less than 0.80 for those with developmental spinal stenosis, congenital fusions, posttraumatic instability, and acute and chronic degenerative changes, and that these were significantly different from the ratios in the control group. Specifically, the mean ratio for the control group from the third through the sixth cervical vertebrae was 0.98.

On the basis of these observations, it was concluded that the factor identified that explains the described neurologic picture of cervical spinal cord neurapraxia is diminution of the anteroposterior diameter of the spinal canal either as an isolated observation or associated with intervertebral disk herniation, degenerative changes, posttraumatic insta-

bility, or congenital anomalies. In instances of developmental cervical stenosis, forced hyperflexion, or hyperextension of the cervical spine, a further decrease in the caliber of an already stenotic canal occurs as explained by the "pincers mechanism" of Penning (Fig 36–12). In those patients with stenosis associated with osteophytes or a herniated disk, direct pressure can occur, again with the spine forced in the extremes of flexion or extension. This phenomenon of mechanical compression of the cervical cord with flexion is vividly demonstrated by a MRI scan of one patient with an acute herniated pulposus at the C4–C5 level (Fig 36–13).

It is postulated that with an abrupt but brief decrease in the anteroposterior diameter of the spinal canal, the cervical spinal cord is mechanically compressed, causing transient interruption of either its motor or sensory function, or both, distal to the lesion. The neurologic aberration that results is transient and completely reversible in all instances.

Characteristically, after an episode of cervical spinal cord neurapraxia with or without transient quadriplegia, the first question raised concerns the advisability for activity restrictions. In an attempt to address this problem, 117 young athletes who sustained cervical spine injuries associated with complete permanent quadriplegia while playing football between the years 1971 and 1984 were interviewed. None of these patients recalled a prodromal experience of transient motor paresis. Conversely, none of the patients in this series who had experienced transient neurologic episodes subsequently sustained an injury that resulted in permanent neurologic injury. On the basis of these data it is concluded that the young patient who has had an episode of cervical spinal cord neurapraxia with or without transient quadriplegia is not predisposed to permanent neurologic injury because of it.

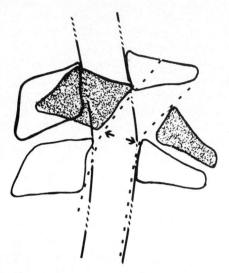 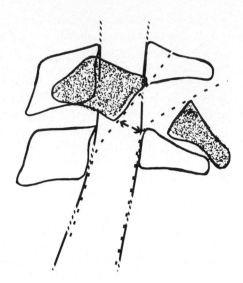

FIG 36–12.
The pincers mechanism, as described by Penning,[32] occurs when the distance between the posteroinferior margin of the superior vertebral body and the anterosuperior aspect of the spinolaminar line of the subjacent vertebra decrease with hyperextension, with compression of the cord occurring. With hyperflexion, the anterosuperior aspect of the spinolaminar line of the superior vertebra and the posterosuperior margin of the inferior vertebra would be the "pincers."

With regard to activity restrictions, no definite recurrence patterns have been identified to establish firm principles in this area. However, athletes who have this syndrome associated with demonstrable cervical spine instability or acute or chronic disc disease or degenerative changes should not be allowed further participation in contact sports. Those athletes with developmental spinal stenosis or spinal stenosis associated with congenital abnormalities should be treated on an individual basis. As indicated, of the six youngsters with obvious cervical stenosis who returned to football, three had a second episode and withdrew from the activity, and three returned without any problems at 2-year follow-up. The data appear to indicate that those with developmental spinal stenosis are not predisposed to more severe injuries with associated permanent neurologic sequelae.

The significance and implications of cervical spinal stenosis and transient cord neurapraxia have required further delineation. We have collected and analyzed a significant body of appropriate data to:

1. Determine the occurrence of cervical spinal stenosis as defined by a spinal canal/vertebral body ratio of less than 0.8 in a larger control group and among various subsets of football players.

2. Ascertain whether there is a relationship between cervical spinal stenosis and quadriplegia after an injury.

3. Further clarify the status of athletes with stenosis of the cervical spine with or without a history of transient neurapraxia in regard to the advisability of continued participation in contact sports.

Four populations of football players, as well as a control group of 105 nonathletes, were studied. Spinal canal: vertebral body ratios were determined at the C3, C4, C5, and C6 levels according to the technique described by Pavlov. Cervical spinal stenosis was defined by a spinal

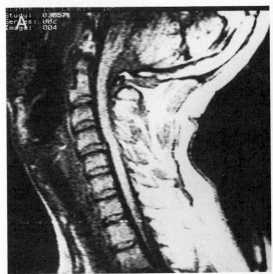
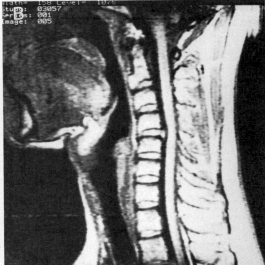
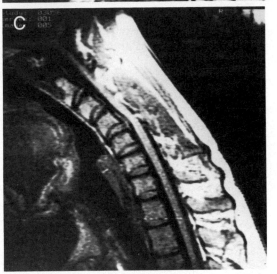

FIG 36–13.
A, a 29-year-old recreational basketball player was rebounding and experienced a forced hyperflexion injury when elbowed. He had a sudden onset of transient numbness and weakness in all four extremities. He resumed play, and at the end of the game experienced paresthesias in both upper extremities. Findings on evaluation at the emergency room, including roentgenograms of the cervical spine, were considered normal. His paresthesias improved after several days. Two weeks after the initial injury, while spotting a weight lifter, the paresthesias returned. His family physician prescribed Indocin (indomethacin) and rest. At 1 month postinjury, he was evaluated at our clinic. He had full range of motion, normal muscle tone, and normal reflexes. Roentgenograms obtained at the time of injury were reviewed. Pavlov's ratios were 0.85 at C3, 0.79 at C4, 0.75 at C5, and 0.78 at C6, indicating developmental spinal stenosis. **A,** MRI scan of the midsagittal cervical spine showed a herniated disk at the C4–C5 level. Further flexion of the cervical spine demonstrated cord compression due to limited anteroposterior diameter at the C4–C5 level. After a course of conservative treatment, consisting of anti-inflammatory drugs and a collar, the paresthesias still persisted. The patient subsequently underwent a C4–C5 anterior diskectomy and fusion. **B,** MRI with mild flexion of the cervical spine demonstrates herniation of the disk with displacement of the posterior longitudinal ligament and compression of the cord, with a decrease in its anteroposterior diameter at the fourth and fifth cervical vertebrae. **C,** MRI made with a greater flexion of the cervical spine demonstrates an additional decrease in the anteroposterior diameter of the cord or tenting over the herniated nucleus pulposus. *(From Torg JS, Pavlov H, Genuario S, et al: J Bone Joint Surg [Am] 1986; 68-A:1354–1370. Used with permission.)*

canal:vertebral body ratio of less than 0.8.

Cohort I consisted of 227 asymptomatic elite collegiate football players.

Cohort II were 97 asymptomatic professional football players.

Cohort III consisted of 45 high school, college, and professional players who had sustained at least one episode of transient cervical cord neurapraxia. All had recovered completely and were presently asymptomatic.

Cohort IV were 77 high school and college athletes who had been rendered quadriplegic as a result of a football injury.

These were derived from a listing of athletes registered with the National Football Head and Neck Injury Registry.[40]

Cohort V, the control group, consisted of 105 nonathletic male subjects aged 15 to 38 years. None of these had a history of significant cervical spine injury, transient neurapraxia, or neurologic complaints.

The mean, median, and range of ratios of each level, C3 through C6, were determined for each cohort. With use of a computerized statistical software package (Minitab), the following were performed:

1. One-way analysis of variance of the mean ratios between levels of each cohort.
2. The graphic distribution of combined ratios of all levels of each cohort.
3. One-way analysis of variance of the mean ratios between cohorts.

In order to determine whether transient cord neurapraxia is associated with increased risk of permanent quadriplegia, the telephone survey was expanded to include 177 permanently quadriplegic athletes. Each individual was questioned as to whether he had ever experienced an episode of transient neurapraxia before his catastrophic injury.

A follow-up of the patients with transient neurapraxia initially reported on was also done to determine if any had subsequently sustained a permanent neurologic injury.

A one-way analysis of variance of mean ratios between the levels C3–C6 within each cohort revealed no statistical difference between these levels within each cohort. Therefore, all levels C3–C6 for each cohort were combined and used to determine both graphic distributions of the combined ratios and a one-way analysis of variance of the pooled ratios between cohorts.

One-way analysis of variance of the combined ratios between cohorts demonstrated (1) no statistical difference between the college and professional subgroups, (2) no statistical difference between the quadriplegic and control subgroups, and (3) a statistically significant difference between the transient quadriplegic group and all four cohorts ($P < .0001$) (Fig 36–14).

Graphic distribution of the combined ratios for all levels C3–C6 for each cohort demonstrated a chance distribution in each instance (Figs 36–15 to 36–19).

```
ANALYSIS OF VARIANCE
SOURCE      DF        SS        MS            F
FACTOR       4     2.5463    0.6366        57.35
ERROR      546     6.0602    0.0111
TOTAL      550     8.6065
```

```
                                     INDIVIDUAL 95 PCT CI'S FOR MEAN
                                     BASED ON POOLED STDEV
LEVEL       N      MEAN    STDEV    --+---------+---------+---------+----
COL MEAN   227    0.8784   0.1050                       (-*)
PRO MEAN    97    0.8563   0.1005                     (-*-)
CON MEAN   105    0.9760   0.0980                              (-*-)
QUA MEAN    77    0.9517   0.1088                         (-*--)
TRA MEAN    45    0.7177   0.1263      (--*--)
                                     --+---------+---------+---------+----
POOLED STDEV =     0.1054           0.70      0.80      0.90      1.00
```

ALL COHORTS – MEAN RATIOS

$p < .0001$

FIG 36–14.
One-way analysis of variance of the combined ratios between the five cohorts.

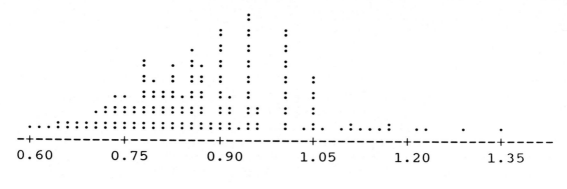

227 COLLEGE PLAYERS   EACH LEVEL (C3–C6)

FIG 36–15.
Graphic distribution of the combined ratios for levels C3–C6 for cohort I, the 227 asymptomatic college players, demonstrates a chance distribution. Each dot represents six points, with seventeen points missing or out of range.

The rationale for establishing a canal/body ratio of 0.8 or less as indicative of developmental spinal canal narrowing (stenosis) is predicated on the findings in the group who experienced episodes of cervical cord neurapraxia. Specifically, each subject, whether a high school, college, or professional player, had one or more levels with a ratio of 0.82 or less. Also, as a group, they were significantly different from the other four groups. Although the pooled means and standard deviations for the college (0.88 ± 0.11) and professional (0.86 ± 0.10) groups are statistically different from the transient group (0.72 ± 0.13), their mean ratios are less than that of the control (0.98 ± 0.10) and quadriplegic (0.95 ± 0.13) groups, with a certain percentage having one or more levels below 0.80 (Fig 36–14). This observation is explained by a comparison of the measurements of the anteroposte-

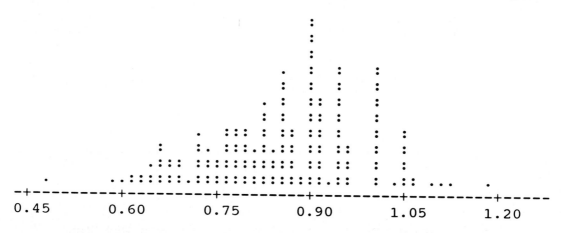

97 PROFESSIONAL PLAYERS   EACH LEVEL (C3–C6)

FIG 36–16.
Graphic distribution of the combined ratios for levels C3–C6 for cohort II, the 97 asymptomatic professional players, demonstrates a chance distribution. Each dot represents three points, with thirteen points missing or out of range.

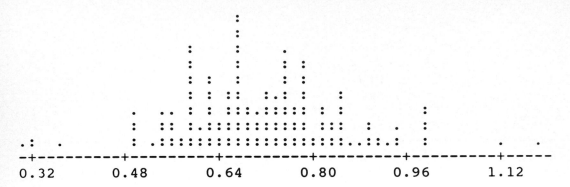

```
                        :
                        :
              :         :           .
              :         :        :  :
              :  :      :        :  :
              :  :   ::  :     :.: :       :
        .   ..  :  ::.:::::::::::  : :           :
        :   ::  :.:::::::::::::::: :::   :  .   :
  .:  .     : .::::::::::::::::::::::::..::.:   :        .     .
  -+---------+---------+---------+---------+---------+-----
  0.32      0.48      0.64      0.80      0.96      1.12
```

45   TRANSIENT CERVICAL CORD NEURAPRAXIA
EACH LEVEL (C3-C6)

FIG 36–17.
Graphic distribution of the combined ratios for levels C3–C6 for cohort III, the 45 high school, college, and professional players who sustained an episode of transient cervical cord neurapraxia, demonstrates a chance distribution. Each dot represents one point, with four points missing or out of range.

rior diameters of the spinal canal and vertebral bodies of the control, college, professional, and transient groups (Table 36–1).

Specifically, an analysis of variance of the pooled mean measurements of the anteroposterior diameters of the spinal canal C3–C6 demonstrated those of the college, professional, and control groups to be similar, whereas the diameters of all three were statistically larger than the diameter of the transient group (Fig

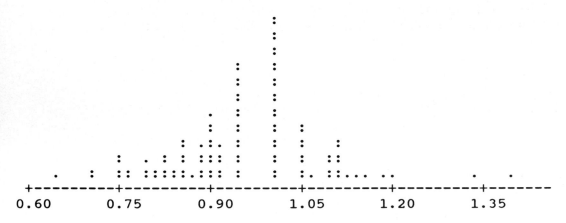

```
                         :
                         :
                         :
                 :       :
                 :       :
                 :       :
             .   :       :
                 :       :   :
           : ..:. :       :   :      :
       . : : ::: :       :   :    ::
    .   : :: ::::::.::: :     :   :. :: ... ..      .    .
  +---------+---------+---------+---------+---------+-------
  0.60      0.75      0.90      1.05      1.20      1.35
```

77   QUADRIPLEGIC HIGH SCHOOL AND COLLEGE PLAYERS
EACH LEVEL (C3-C6)

FIG 36–18.
Graphic distribution of the combined ratios for levels C3–C6 for cohort IV, the 77 high school and college athletes who were rendered quadriplegic, demonstrates a chance distribution. Each dot represents 3 points, with ninety-nine points missing or out of range.

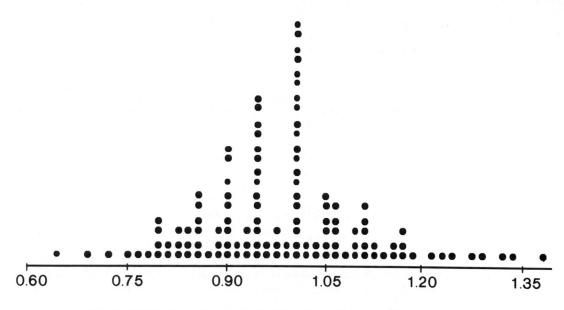

105 CONTROL MALE PATIENTS – EACH LEVEL (C3–C6)

FIG 36–19.
Graphic distribution of the combined ratios for levels C3–C6 for cohort V, the 105 asymptomatic controls, demonstrates a chance distribution. Each dot represents four points, with one point missing or out of range.

36–20). The pooled mean measurements of the vertebral bodies C3–C6, on the other hand, demonstrated their antero-posterior diameters in the college, professional, and transient groups to be similar but statistically larger than their diameter in the control group (Fig 36–21). Clearly, the relatively lower ratios observed in the elite college and professional groups are due to the larger vertebral bodies rather than to smaller canals.

Of the 177 quadriplegic athletes contacted by telephone, none reported an episode(s) of transient quadriplegia before their major injury. Also, none of those with symptoms of transient neurapraxia suffered a subsequent injury resulting in permanent neurologic injury.

On the basis of these data, the following is concluded:

1. An individual with cervical canal narrowing as defined by a spinal canal/vertebral body ratio of less than 0.8 is no more susceptible to neurologic injury than individuals in the general population.

2. Episodes of transient cervical cord

TABLE 36–1.

Conventional Measurements of the Pooled Anteroposterior Diameter C3–C6 of the Spinal Canal and Vertebral Bodies in Millimeters

	N	Spinal Canal Mean (Range)	Vertebral Body Mean (Range)
Control	105	18.8 (14.5–23.5)	19.3 (15.9–25)
College	227	18.7 (14.8–25.5)	21.5 (15.7–29)
Professional	97	18.7 (13.6–28.4)	22.0 (17.5–30)
Transient	45	15.3 (9.3–21.0)	21.5 (17.5–28)

```
ANALYSIS OF VARIANCE
SOURCE        DF          SS         MS         F
FACTOR         3       485.74     161.91      42.96
ERROR        470      1771.59       3.77
TOTAL        473      2257.34
                                        INDIVIDUAL 95 PCT CI'S FOR MEAN
                                        BASED ON POOLED STDEV
LEVEL          N        MEAN       STDEV    --------+---------+---------+--------
COLL CAN     227      18.742       1.882                                 (-*-)
PRO CAN       97      18.696       2.104                               (--*--)
CONT CAN     105      18.758       1.700                               (--*--)
TRAN CAN      45      15.283       2.364     (---*----)
                                          --------+---------+---------+--------
POOLED STDEV =        1.941                   15.6      16.8      18.0
```

ALL COHORTS - SPINAL CANAL

$p < 0.0001$

FIG 36–20.
Analysis of variance of the pooled mean measurements of the AP diameters of the spinal canal C3–C6 demonstrates those of the college, professional, and control groups to be statistically larger than the diameter of the transient group.

neurapraxia are not a harbinger of more severe neurologic injury. Conceptually, an exception to this would be individuals with concomitant instability or intervertebral disk disease.

3. Due to anthropomorphic differences, the characteristics of the cervical spine, that is, larger vertebral bodies rather than smaller canals, of individuals with the physical habitus of the profes-sional and elite college football player re-sult in uniformly lower ratios. This fact should not adversely influence any decision regarding apparent risks and continued participation for these two groups of individuals.

Specific criteria for activity participation for individuals with developmental spinal narrowing with and without his-

```
ANALYSIS OF VARIANCE
SOURCE        DF          SS         MS         F
FACTOR         3       455.82     151.94      31.32
ERROR        470      2279.86       4.85
TOTAL        473      2735.68
                                        INDIVIDUAL 95 PCT CI'S FOR MEAN
                                        BASED ON POOLED STDEV
LEVEL          N        MEAN       STDEV    --+---------+---------+---------+----
COLL VB      227      21.502       2.322                          (--*--)
PRO VB        97      21.979       2.410                            (----*---)
CONT VB      105      19.308       1.705     (---*---)
TRAN VB       45      21.492       2.139                      (------*-----)
                                          --+---------+---------+---------+----
POOLED STDEV =        2.202               19.0      20.0      21.0      22.0
```

ALL COHORTS - VERTEBRAL BODY

$p < 0.0001$

FIG 36–21.
Analysis of variance of the pooled mean measurements of the AP diameters of the vertebral bodies C3–C6 demonstrates the diameters of the college, professional, and transient groups to be statistically larger than the diameter of the control group.

tory of an episode(s) of cervical cord neurapraxia are delineated in Chapter 39.

BIBLIOGRAPHY

1. Alexander E, Davis CH, Field CH: Hyperextension injuries of the cervical spine. *Arch Neurol Psychiatry* 1958; 79:146–157.

2. Boijsen E: Cervical spinal canal in intraspinal expansive processes. *Acta Radiol* 1954; 42:101–115.

3. Brain L, Wilkinson M (eds): *Cervical Spondylolysis and Other Disorders of the Cervical Spine*, ed 1. Philadelphia, WB Saunders Co, 1967.

4. Breig A: *Biomechanics of the Central Nervous System*. Stockholm, Almqvist and Wiksell, 1961.

5. Buetti-Bauml C: *Funktionelle Röntgendiagnostik der Halswirbelsaule*. Stuttgart, Thieme, 1954.

6. Burrows EH: The sagittal diameter of the spinal canal in cervical spondylolysis. *Clin Radiol* 1963; 17:77–86.

7. Burrows EH: Sagittal diameter of the spinal canal and cervical spine stenosis. *Clin Radiol* 1963; 14:777–786.

8. Chrispin AR, Lees F: The spinal canal in cervical spondylosis. *J Neurol Neurosurg Psychiatry* 1963; 26:166–170.

9. Countee RW, Vijayanathan T: Congenital stenosis of the cervical spine: Diagnosis and management. *J Natl Med Assoc* 1979; 71:257–264.

10. Di Chiro G, Fisher RL: Contrast radiography of the spinal cord. *Arch Neurol* 1964; 11:125–143.

11. Ehni G: *Cervical Arthrosis: Diseases of Cervical Motion Segments (Spondylosis Disk Rupture, Radiculopathy, and Myelopathy)*. St Louis, Mosby–Year Book, 1984, pp 26–43.

12. Epstein JA, Carras R, Epstein VS, et al: Myelopathy in cervical spondylolysis with vertebral subluxation and hyperlordosis. *J Neurol Sci* 1970; 32:421.

13. Epstein NE, Epstein JA, Zilkha A: Traumatic myelopathy in a seventeen year-old child with cervical spinal stenosis (without fracture or dislocation) and a C2–C3 Klippel-Feil fusion. A case report. *Spine* 1984; 9:344.

14. Epstein VA, Epstein JA, Jones MD: Cervical spinal stenosis. *Radiol Clin North Am* 1977; 15:215–281.

15. Funk FJ, Wells RE: Injuries of the cervical spine in football. *Clin Orthop Rel Res* 1975; 109:50–58.

16. Gonsalves CG, Hudson AR, Horsey WJ, et al: Computed tomography of the cervical spine and spinal cord. *Comput Tomog* 1978; 2:279–293.

17. Grant T, Puffer J: Cervical stenosis: A developmental anomaly with quadriparesis during football. *Am J Sports Med* 1976; 4:219–221.

18. Hinck VC, Hopkins CE, Savara BS: Sagittal diameter of the cervical spinal canal in children. *Radiology* 1962; 79:97–108.

19. Hinck VC, Sachdev NS: Developmental stenosis of the cervical spinal canal. *Brain* 1966; 89:27–36.

20. Kehilnani MT, Wolf BS: Transverse diameter of cervical spinal cord on pantopaque myelography. *J Neurol Surg* 1963; 20:660–664.

21. Kessler JT: Congenital narrowing of the cervical spinal canal. *J Neurol Neurosurg Psychiatry* 1975; 38:1218–1224.

22. Lowman RM, Finkelstein A: Air myelography for demonstration of cervical spinal cord. *Radiology* 1942; 39:700–706.

23. Maroon JC: "Burning hands" in football spinal cord injuries. *JAMA* 1977; 238:2049–2051.

24. Metz CE: ROC methodology in radiologic imaging. *Invest Radiol* 1986; 21:720–733.

25. Moiel RH, Raso E, Waltz TA: Central cord syndrome resulting from congenital narrowing of the cervical canal. *J Trauma* 1970; 10:502–510.

26. Nugent GR: Clinico-pathologic correlations in cervical spondylolysis. *Neurology* 1959; 9:273–281.

27. Pallis C, Jones AM, Spillane JD: Cervical spondylolysis: Incidence and implications. *Brain* 1954; 77:274.

28. Paul LW, Chandler A: Myelography in expanding lesions of the cervical spinal cord. Exhibit, 45th Annual Meeting of the Radiologic Society of North America. Chicago, Nov 15, 1959.

29. Pavlov H, Torg JS, Robie B, et al: Spinal canal: Vertebral body ratio for determining cervical spinal stenosis. *Radiology* 1987; 164:771–775.

30. Payne EE: The cervical spine and spondylolysis. *Neurochirurgi* 1959; 1:178–136.

31. Payne EE, Spillane JD: The cervical spine: An anatomico-pathological study of 70 specimens (using special technique) with particular reference to problems of cervical spondylolysis. *Brain* 1957; 80:571–596.

32. Penning L: Some aspects of plain radiography of the cervical spine in chronic myelopathy. *Neurology* 1962; 12:513–519.

33. Resnick D, Niwayama G: Diffuse idiopathic skeletal hyperostosis (DISH) or ankylosing hyperostosis of Forestier and Rotes-Querol, in Resnick D, Niwayama G (eds): *Diagnosis of Bone and Joint Disorders With Emphasis on Articular Abnormalities.* Philadelphia, WB Saunders Co, 1981, pp 1416–1452.

34. Schneider RC, Cherry GR, Pantek H: Syndrome of acute central cervical spinal cord injury with special reference to mechanisms involved in hyperextension injuries of cervical spine. *J Neurosurg* 1954; 11:546.

35. Sheridan TB, Farrell WB: *Man-Machine Systems: Information, Control and Decision Models of Human Performance.* MIT Press, Cambridge, Mass, 1981, pp 355–382.

36. Stoltmann HF, Blackward W: The role of the ligamentum flavum in the pathogenesis of myelopathy in cervical spondylolysis. *Brain* 1974; 87:45.

37. Stratford J: Congenital cervical stenosis: A factor in myelopathy. *Acta Neurochir* (Wien) 1978; 41:101–106.

38. Taylor AR: The mechanism of injury to spinal cord in the neck without damage to the vertebral column. *J Bone Joint Surg [Br]* 1951; 33-B:543–546.

39. Torg JS, Pavlov H, Genuario SE, et al: Neurapraxia of the cervical spinal cord with transient quadriplegia. *J Bone Joint Surg [Am]* 1986; 68A:1354–1370.

40. Torg JS, Vegso JJ, Sennett B, et al: The National Football Head and Neck Injury Registry, 14-year report on cervical quadriplegia, 1971 through 1984. *JAMA* 1985; 254:3439–3443.

41. Wells CE, Spillane JD, Bligh AS: The cervical spinal canal in syringomyelia. *Brain* 1959; 82:23–40.

42. Wilkinson HA, LeMay ML, Ferris EJ: Roentgenographic correlation in cervical spondylolysis. *AJR* 1969; 105:370–374.

43. Wolf BS, Khilnani M, Malis L: Sagittal diameter of the bony cervical canal and its significance in cervical spondylolysis. *J Mt Sinai Hosp* 1956; 23:283–292.

CHAPTER 37

Exercise Conditioning of the Spinal Cord–Injured Patient Via Functional Electrical Stimulation

Roger M. Glaser, Ph.D.

Spinal cord injury (SCI) typically results in skeletal muscle paralysis that limits one's ability to exercise voluntarily. This condition frequently leads to a sedentary life-style and a marked loss of physical fitness, as well as to an increased incidence of secondary health and medical complications, including cardiovascular diseases, muscle atrophy, osteoporosis, and decubitus ulcers. During the past 17 years a major goal of our research effort has been to develop specialized exercise techniques and to evaluate their effectiveness for improving the physical fitness of SCI individuals. The purpose of this chapter is to introduce functional electrical stimulation (FES) concepts and techniques for exercise conditioning of SCI patients, as well as to present some recently developed FES exercise modes and protocols that have been shown to be effective via physiologic studies.

Patients with paralyzed legs usually compensate by using their functional arms for manual wheelchair locomotion and exercise conditioning. However, because of the limited exercise capability of the relatively small arm musculature, paraplegics cannot develop the high levels of physical fitness (cardiopulmonary,

or aerobic fitness) that can be achieved by able-bodied individuals through leg exercise.[1, 17, 19, 24, 52] In this situation the muscles of the upper part of the body tend to fatigue because of peripheral factors (i.e., inadequate muscle fiber function) before the cardiovascular and pulmonary systems are driven to sufficiently high output levels for long enough durations to stimulate central training effects.[2, 5, 18] Quadriplegics have a substantially lower cardiopulmonary fitness development capability because of their upper extremity muscle paralysis.

During the past 25 years FES (sometimes referred to as functional neuromuscular stimulation, FNS) research has been conducted with the goal of restoring purposeful movements to paralyzed muscles.[3, 7, 20, 36] This technique uses electrical impulses from a stimulator, in conjunction with appropriately placed electrodes, to directly induce tetanic muscle contractions of controlled intensity. Although much of this research has been focused on enabling the performance of skilled activities (e.g., ambulation by paraplegics, hand function by quadriplegics), this technique can also enable paralyzed lower limbs to be used for exercise.

Therefore, FES-induced exercise of the paralyzed legs has the potential of utilizing a large muscle mass that otherwise would be dormant, while augmenting the circulation of blood. Ultimately this may lead to exercise modes that can improve the health, physical fitness, and rehabilitation potential of SCI patients to levels higher than can be achieved with arm exercise alone. Quadriplegics will most likely find this involuntary exercise mode to be particularly advantageous. However, it should be understood that FES exercise *does not* "cure" paralysis, and, similar to voluntary exercise training, any health and fitness benefits derived from FES exercise training will most likely be lost several weeks after this activity is terminated. Thus FES exercise should become part of one's lifestyle if beneficial effects are to be maintained.

Although much of the instrumentation for FES exercise described in the research literature was especially designed and constructed, the availability of commercial stimulators for clinical and home use is increasing. These range from single-channel, patient-operated units that are hand-held to multichannel, computer-controlled systems that incorporate closed-loop, feedback control. For exercise applications, skin surface electrodes typically are used.

CONSIDERATIONS FOR FUNCTIONAL ELECTRICAL STIMULATION USE

A primary requirement for FES use is that the muscles to be exercised are paralyzed as a result of upper motor neuron damage and that the motor units (lower motor neurons and the skeletal muscle fibers they innervate) are intact and functional. The presence of the functional stretch reflex and spasticity indicate that the individual is a potential candidate for this form of exercise. But if the patient retains some degree of sensory function (as is typical with incomplete SCI), FES may be uncomfortable or painful, and the high levels of stimulation that are needed to induce forceful contractions may not be tolerated. Therefore actual patient testing is usually required to determine if FES is usable, tolerable, and safe. Evaluation of one's FES response may be achieved by using a portable (battery-powered) neuromuscular stimulator and skin surface electrodes placed over motor points (where the motor nerve enters the muscle).[3] Motor points may be located by placing an indifferent (common) electrode over one end of the muscle (or muscle group) and moving the active electrode around the muscle belly while applying short stimulation pulses (e.g., 0.25 second) at an intensity that is just above the contraction threshold level. At motor points there will be a lower threshold for contraction, and a greater contraction force will be observed for a given stimulation level. For individuals who respond well, gradual increases in stimulation current (within limits) will result in recruitment of more muscle fibers and smooth generation of greater contraction force.

Special Precautions

For patient safety, a thorough medical examination is essential before initiating an FES exercise program. This should include radiographs of the paralyzed limbs, range of motion testing, neurologic examination, an electrocardiogram, and, possibly, evaluation of psychologic status. The patient should be informed of the potential benefits and risks of FES exercise and should clearly understand that it *will not* regenerate damaged nerves and restore voluntary function.

Since the paralyzed lower limbs of

SCI individuals usually have deteriorated muscles, bones, and joints, FES-induced contractions should be kept as smooth as possible to prevent injury. In some individuals this may be difficult to achieve because FES may trigger severe spasms in various muscles. Therefore it is important to monitor the quality of the FES-induced contractions closely to be certain that they are not hazardous. On the other hand, if patients take muscle relaxant medications to alleviate spasms, this may cause rapid muscle fatigue during FES exercise.[20] It is prudent to limit the maximal contraction force generated to a safe level, since it may be possible to enhance muscle strength with chronic training to levels that cannot be withstood by the bones and joints.[20, 30] Our laboratory has used an arbitrary limit of 15 kg for knee extension resistance exercise with no observable adverse effects. Safe force limits for other joint actions have not yet been established. A major difficulty in accomplishing this is that standard radiographs are not sensitive enough to quantify osteoporosis precisely, and a 30% to 50% change in bone mass can occur before it is detected.[31, 33] There currently is no convincing evidence that FES exercise training can either prevent or reverse osteoporosis.[20]

Inasmuch as FES exercise is induced peripherally, it effectively bypasses central nervous system (CNS) control. Thus autonomic sympathetic outflow may be deficient (because of insufficient stimulation and/or CNS damage), and cardiovascular adjustments that usually accompany voluntary exercise may not occur to the same extent.[6, 16, 20, 30] This can result in the rapid onset of fatigue because of limited cardiac output (lower heart rate and stroke volume [SV] capability) and deficient blood flow to the exercising muscles. It is also possible that active muscles can be overheated during prolonged FES exercise because thermoregulatory mechanisms for heat dissipation (e.g., altering patterns of blood flow and sweat secretion) may be inoperative.[20, 30] Some patients (especially those with high-level SCI) may exhibit autonomic dysreflexia during FES exercise, which can result in dangerously high blood pressure.[20, 30] Therefore, it is recommended that blood pressure be monitored periodically, especially during initial FES exercise sessions. If any response is observed that places the patient at risk, exercise should be discontinued immediately.

EXERCISE TRAINING WITH FUNCTIONAL ELECTRICAL STIMULATION

As indicated, prolonged immobilization due to muscle paralysis typically causes muscle atrophy, osteoporosis, and loss of cardiopulmonary fitness. Other medical problems that may be encountered include edema and deep venous thrombosis (and the potential development of oftentimes fatal pulmonary embolism) due to pooling and stasis of venous blood in the lower extremities, as well as decubitus ulcers due to prolonged pressure on tissues. FES exercise training hypothetically can prevent or reverse some of these problems. Potential health and fitness benefits that may be derived from FES exercise encompass improvement of muscle strength and endurance (see references 11, 30, 34, 38, 40, 43, 44, 50), cardiopulmonary function,[13, 14, 18, 25, 42] circulation in the active limbs (see references 8–10, 12–14, 18, 27), self-image,[24, 30] and temporary alleviation of muscle spasms.[35, 40] The following FES exercise modes appear to be usable for patients with lower limb paralysis due to upper motor neuron damage.

Training for Muscle Strength and Endurance

FES-Induced Resistance Exercise.— Early FES exercise training studies reported only limited improvements in muscle performance characteristics.[34, 38] This may have been due to inadequate loading of the muscles and the use of inappropriate stimulation patterns and intensities, as well as training protocols that were not highly effective. However, recent studies indicated that many of the same principles established for voluntary resistance training (i.e., weight training) can be adapted for FES applications, including dynamic contractions through a large range of motion, progressive overload, and exercise sets of relatively low number of repetitions at relatively high load resistance.[11, 30, 40] In addition, it appears that stimulation patterns of gradually ramped intensity are more effective and safer than abrupt on-off (square wave) patterns of stimulation.[22, 23] It is currently clear that FES-induced resistance exercise can markedly improve muscle strength and endurance (for FES activity).[11, 30, 40] Physiologic mechanisms for this enhanced performance appear to be localized within the muscles (peripheral) rather than central circulatory in nature. These adaptations possibly include muscle hypertrophy, conversion of fast- to slow-twitch fiber characteristics, increased concentration of metabolic enzymes, and higher capillary density (see references 4, 29, 37, 39, 42, 45–49, 51).

Figure 37–1 illustrates a laboratory-constructed device for knee extension

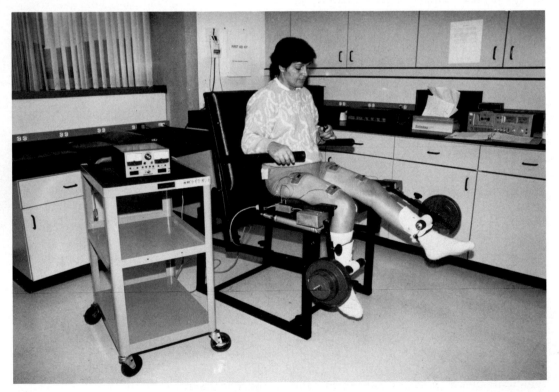

FIG 37–1.
FES-induced knee extension weight training exercise being performed by a person with SCI. The instrumentation illustrated was especially designed and constructed for this purpose. *(From Glaser RM: Spinal cord injuries and neuromuscular stimulation, in Torg JS (ed):* Current Therapy in Sports Medicine. *Toronto, BC Decker [in press]. Used with permission.)*

FES weight training.[21] A two-channel, battery-powered stimulator is used to induce contractions of gradually ramped intensity of the quadriceps muscle groups via surface electrodes. However, commercial, battery-powered stimulators (which provide ramped output current) in conjunction with ankle weights may also be effective. Protocols designed for this FES weight training incorporate 10 to 30 repetitions per set at a rate of three to five lifts per minute, two to three sets per session, and two to four sessions per week.[11, 30, 40, 44] As performance improves with training, a weight load progression of 0.5 kg appears to be suitable. When the maximal limit is achieved (e.g., 15 kg), the number of repetitions may be increased to improve endurance. Several weeks of this exercise have been reported to result in greater muscle strength and resistance to fatigue, as well as quadriceps hypertrophy.[11, 30, 40] Figure 37–2 depicts the load weight progression that was used by Gruner et al.[30] for knee extension training of six SCI individuals during a 12-week period. Similar techniques and protocols can be used to exercise other muscles.

Training for Cardiopulmonary Fitness

FES-Induced Cycle Ergometry.—Although FES resistance exercise training may cause peripheral adaptations to increase muscle strength and endurance, it does not elicit metabolic (aerobic) and cardiopulmonary responses of sufficient magnitudes and for long enough durations to stimulate central circulatory training effects.[6] In an effort to enable SCI patients to

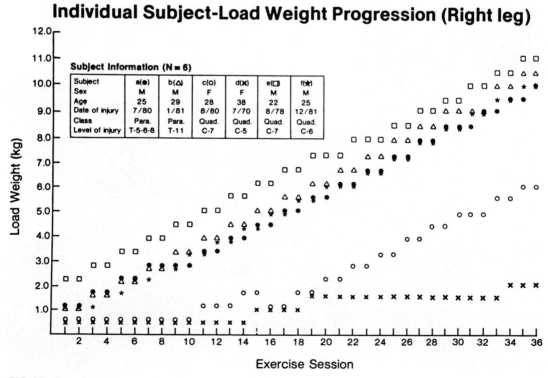

FIG 37–2.
Individual subject load weight progression data (right leg) during 12 weeks (three times each week) of FES-induced knee-extension exercise conditioning. *(Modified from Gruner JA, Glaser RM, Feinberg SD, et al: J Rehabil Res Dev 1983; 20:21–30.)*

develop higher levels of cardiopulmonary fitness, a cycle ergometer that can be operated by the paralyzed legs was designed and constructed by Petrofsky et al.[41] This device uses computer-controlled FES of the quadriceps, hamstring, and gluteus maximus muscle groups to induce contractions at appropriate angles during the pedal cycle. In 1984 Therapeutic Technologies Inc. (Ft Lauderdale, Fla) began manufacturing sophisticated versions of this FES cycle ergometer for clinical and home use. The ERGYS I, which was designed for home use, is illustrated in Figure 37–3.[21] During operation at the target pedal rate of 50 rpm, these cycle ergometers induce 50 contractions of each contralateral muscle group each minute (a total of 300 muscle contractions per minute), with the cyclic stimulation pattern and intensity controlled by a microprocessor. Thus this ex-

ercise mode utilizes more muscle mass than weight training, and the muscles are stimulated to contract at a substantially higher rate. Exercise is automatically terminated when the pedal rate falls below 35 rpm. FES cycle ergometry appears to be well suited for endurance, rather than strength training. Many SCI patients can pedal continuously for 30 minutes.

During the typical training protocol, the patient initially pedals the FES cycle ergometer at 0 W (no load resistance) for up to 30 minutes. If fatigue occurs, three bouts are given in an attempt to achieve 30 minutes of exercise (exercise bouts are followed by 10 minutes of rest). When 30 minutes of continuous exercise can be achieved, subsequent sessions use higher load resistance to increase power output (PO) to 6.1 W. Once pedaling at this higher PO can be accomplished for 30

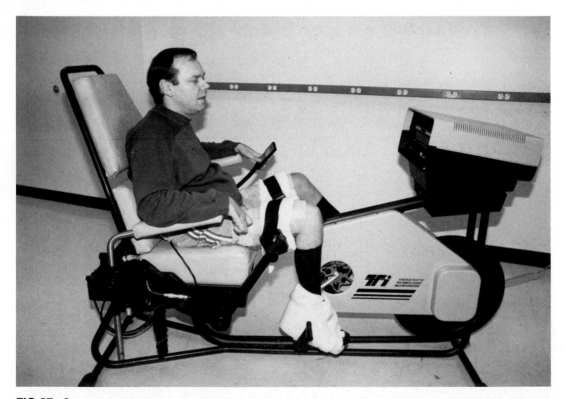

FIG 37–3.
FES cycle ergometer exercise being performed by a person with SCI on an ERGYS I. *(From Glaser RM: Spinal cord injuries and neuromuscular stimulation, in Torg JS (ed): Current Therapy in Sports Medicine. Toronto, BC Decker, 1990. Used with permission.)*

minutes, the PO is further increased by 6.1 W. This progressive intensity protocol is repeated as performance improves, to a maximum PO of 42.7 W. Exercise usually is scheduled three times per week.

Physiologic studies conducted on SCI individuals suggest that this mode of exercise may provide more effective cardiopulmonary fitness training (especially for quadriplegics) than arm exercise.[13, 14, 25, 43] This is because of the relatively high magnitudes of aerobic and cardiopulmonary responses that are elicited and the more advantageous central and peripheral hemodynamic responses.

Figure 37–4 provides steady-state data from Glaser et al.[25] depicting oxygen uptake ($\dot{V}O_2$), pulmonary ventilation ($\dot{V}E$), and heart rate (HR) responses of 12 SCI patients during progressive intensity FES cycle ergometry. Near-linear relationships between PO and $\dot{V}O_2$, $\dot{V}E$, and HR were found. The range of PO for this relatively untrained group was 0 to 30 W. One patient who could pedal at 30 W had a peak $\dot{V}O_2$ of 1.77 L/min, $\dot{V}E$ of 45 L/min, and HR of 135 beats/min. These data suggest that if a well-trained individual could pedal at the maximum PO of 42.7 W, then FES cycle ergometry may elicit a peak $\dot{V}O_2$ of about 2.0 L/min with propor-

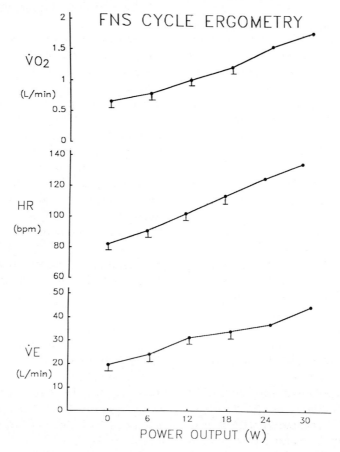

FIG 37–4.
Steady-state $\dot{V}O_2$, $\dot{V}E$, and HR responses of patients with spinal cord injury in relation to PO for FES cycle ergometry. (n = 12 at 0 W, 10 at 6.1 W, 9 at 12.2 W, 4 at 18.3 W, and 1 at 24.4 W and 30.5 W). *(Modified from Glaser RM, Figoni SF, Collins SR, et al: Physiologic responses of SCI subjects to electrically induced leg cycle ergometry. Proceedings of the 10th Annual Conference of Engineering in Medicine and Biology Society, 1988, pp 1638–1640.)*

tionally higher $\dot{V}_E$ and HR responses. Considering that able-bodied individuals typically jog at $\dot{V}_{O_2}$ levels of 1.5 to 2.0 L/min (50% to 60% of their maximal $\dot{V}_{O_2}$), FES cycling offers a potential means for SCI patients to achieve a similar metabolic rate while training. It is doubtful that this magnitude of $\dot{V}_{O_2}$ can be attained by arm exercise for a sufficient duration (e.g., 30 minutes) to elicit marked cardiopulmonary adaptations. However, SCI individuals need to be well trained to achieve such high PO and $\dot{V}_{O_2}$ levels for long durations, and most patients tend to perform cycle ergometry at levels that are equivalent to walking (e.g., $\dot{V}_{O_2}$ of about 1.0 L/min).

It is interesting to note that the PO levels used to achieve the relatively high $\dot{V}_{O_2}$ levels for FES cycle ergometry by SCI individuals are quite low compared with the PO levels used during voluntary cycling by able-bodied individuals. For example, SCI patients who can perform FES cycling at 42.7 W may have a $\dot{V}_{O_2}$ of about 2.0 L/min, whereas able-bodied individuals pedaling voluntarily at this same PO would usually have a $\dot{V}_{O_2}$ of less than 0.9 L/min. This mechanical *inefficiency* for FES exercise may be due to the nonphysiologic activation of the muscles, histochemical changes in the paralyzed muscles, and inappropriate joint biomechanics.[25, 26] However, for exercise applications, this inefficiency seems advantageous since higher levels of metabolic and cardiopulmonary responses can be elicited by SCI patients with lower stress to their paralyzed muscles, bones, and joints.

FES cycle ergometry may also offer superior central hemodynamic responses to SCI individuals compared with voluntary arm cranking. In a study by Figoni et al.,[13] six quadriplegic men performed FES cycle ergometer exercise and, on another occasion, arm cranking exercise at POs that elicited a $\dot{V}_{O_2}$ of approximately 1.0 L/min (11 and 38 watts, respectively).

It was found that the FES cycling elicited a 59% greater SV (92 vs. 58 mL/beat) and a 20% greater CO (8.01 vs. 6.66 L/min). The mechanism for these responses may be that FES-induced contractions of the paralyzed leg muscles activate the venous muscle pump and promote return of venous blood to the heart. In addition, the 25% lower HR (87 vs. 116 beats/min) and 19% lower rate-pressure product during FES cycling indicate that the higher cardiac volume load was achieved with lower myocardial oxygen demands. Thus it appears that FES cycling may be more effective and cause lower cardiovascular risk than arm cranking for the aerobic training of quadriplegics.

Hybrid FES Cycling and Voluntary Arm Cranking Exercise.—It may be possible to enhance cardiopulmonary fitness training capability for SCI patients by using a hybrid form of exercise consisting of simultaneous FES cycling and voluntary arm cranking. This setup is illustrated in Figure 37–5.[21] Recent physiologic data indicated that this hybrid exercise (and other combination FES–voluntary exercise modes) will most likely provide superior training than either mode of exercise performed separately.[9, 18, 28] This is because of the greater muscle mass utilized, the higher levels of metabolic and cardiopulmonary responses elicited, and possibly better circulation of blood to muscles of both the upper and lower parts of the body. Figure 37–6 illustrates data reported by Glaser[18] depicting additive effects of this hybrid exercise for aerobic metabolism. The $\dot{V}_{O_2}$ of a T8 male paraplegic is given at rest (0.25 L/min), during FES cycling at 6.1 W (0.75 L/min), voluntary arm cranking at 25 W (0.75 L/min), and hybrid exercise at a total of 31.1 W (1.25 L/min). Thus a higher $\dot{V}_{O_2}$ of 0.5 L/min could be achieved with this combined exercise mode. Hooker et al.[32] had eight quadriplegics perform this hybrid exercise

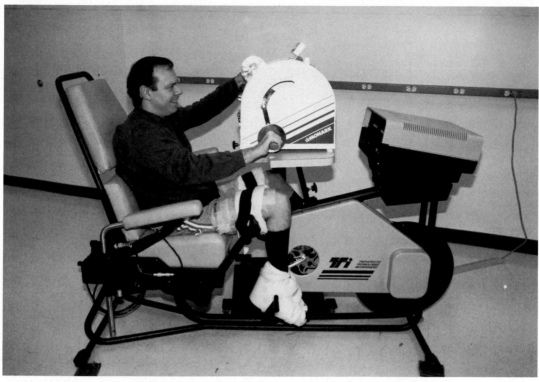

FIG 37–5.
Hybrid (simultaneous FES-induced cycle ergometer and voluntary arm-crank ergometer) exercise being performed by a person with SCI. The adjustable stand supporting the arm-crank ergometer was especially designed and constructed. *(From Glaser RM: Spinal cord injuries and neuromuscular stimulation, in Torg JS (ed):* Current Therapy in Sports Medicine. *Toronto, BC Decker, 1990. Used with permission.)*

and found significantly higher peak $\dot{V}O_2$, $\dot{V}E$, HR, and CO ($\dot{Q}$), and significantly lower total peripheral resistance than for performing either arm cranking or FES cycling alone. Figoni et al.[15] had nine quadriplegic subjects combine 0 W (unloaded) FES cycling with maximal effort arm cranking and observed significant increases in peak levels of $\dot{V}O_2$ (by 0.3 L/min, +35%), SV (by 11 mL/beat, +26%), $\dot{Q}$ (by 2.7 L/min, +46%), and HR (by 11 beats/min, +18%). It is common for this hybrid exercise to elicit peak $\dot{V}O_2$ levels of more than 1.5 and 2.0 L/min from nonathletic quadriplegic and paraplegic persons, respectively. Considering that most of the reported peak $\dot{V}O_2$ data for aerobically trained wheelchair athletes during maximal effort arm exercise is in the 2 to 3 L/min range,[19] this hybrid exercise technique seems to be advantageous since similar peak $\dot{V}O_2$ values can be elicited from the general population of SCI individuals. Since hybrid exercise involves a relatively large muscle mass, it appears likely that *central* circulatory factors, rather than *peripheral* factors, limit exercise capacity. Therefore hybrid exercise may provide the optimal levels of physiologic responses for aerobic conditioning of SCI individuals, while providing training benefits to the musculature of both the upper and lower part of the body. It is doubtful that arm exercise training by itself has any effect on alleviating the deterioration of the lower part of the body. More research is needed to establish optimal hybrid exercise training protocols and to quantify cardiopulmonary fitness changes with long-term training.

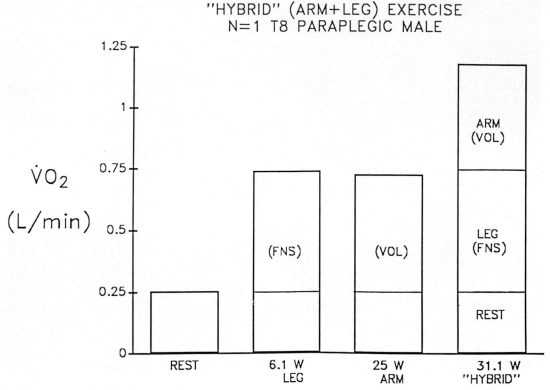

FIG 37–6.
$\dot{V}O_2$ of a T8 paraplegic male subject at rest, during FES cycle ergometer at 6.1 W, during voluntary arm-cranking at 25 W, and during hybrid exercise at a total power output of 31.1 W. Note the additive effect upon $\dot{V}O_2$. *(From Glaser RM: Spinal cord injuries and neuromuscular stimulation, in Torg JS (ed): Current Therapy in Sports Medicine. Toronto, BC Decker, 1990. Used with permission.)*

SUMMARY

The purpose of this chapter is to present currently researched techniques to permit FES exercise of paralyzed leg muscles. It seems clear that FES-induced resistance-training (i.e., weight-training) exercise can markedly improve the strength and endurance of the paralyzed muscles for this exercise mode. Studies also suggest that FES-induced cycle ergometer exercise can elicit aerobic metabolic and cardiopulmonary responses of sufficient magnitudes and durations to stimulate cardiopulmonary training effects. These responses may be superior to those elicited by voluntary arm crank exercise. We believe, however, that FES leg exercise should be used in conjunction with arm exercise (separately and combined) to optimize fitness of the upper and lower parts of the body and cardiovascular fitness. Thus hybrid-type exercise appears to be a promising technique for promoting effective and efficient development of aerobic fitness in paraplegic and quadriplegic individuals. Ultimately FES exercise may contribute to improved health, physical fitness, and rehabilitation potential of SCI individuals. More research is needed, however, to develop safe and effective FES exercise techniques and protocols, and to document the physiologic responses and training benefits.

Acknowledgments

The author wishes to thank the Dayton Veterans Affairs Medical Center and the Rehabilitation Institute of Ohio at Miami Valley Hospital for enabling implementation of this research project on FES. Most of the research projects from the author's laboratory were supported by the Rehabilitation Research and Development Service of the U.S. Department of Veterans Affairs.

REFERENCES

1. Åstrand P-O, Saltin B: Maximal oxygen uptake and heart rate in various types of muscular activity. *J Appl Physiol* 1961; 16:977–981.

2. Bar-Or O, Zwiren LD: Maximal oxygen consumption test during arm exercise—reliability and validity. *J Appl Physiol* 1975; 38:424–426.

3. Benton LA, Baker LL, Bowman BR, et al: *Functional Electrical Stimulation: A Practical Clinical Guide.* Downey, Calif, Professional Staff Association of the Rancho Los Amigos Hospital.

4. Buchegger A, Nemeth PM, Pette D, et al: Effects of chronic stimulation on the metabolic heterogeneity of the fibre population in rabbit tibialis anterior muscle. *J Physiol* 1984; 350:109–119.

5. Clausen JP, Klausen K, Rasmussen B, et al: Central and peripheral circulatory changes after training of the arms or legs. *Am J Physiol* 1973; 225:675–682.

6. Collins Sr, Glaser RM: Comparison of aerobic metabolism and cardiopulmonary responses for electrically-induced and voluntary exercise. *Proceedings of the Eighth Annual RESNA Conference on Rehabilitation Engineering*, 1985; pp 391–393.

7. Cybulski GR, Penn RD, Jaeger RJ: Lower extremity functional neuromuscular stimulation in cases of spinal cord injury. *Neurosurgery* 1984; 15:132–146.

8. Davis GM, Figoni SF, Glaser RM, et al: Cardiovascular responses to FNS-induced isometric leg exercise during orthostatic stress in paraplegics. *Proceedings of the International Conference of Associations for Advancement of Rehabilitation Technology*, 1988, pp 326–327.

9. Davis GM, Servedio FJ, Glaser RM, et al: Hemodynamic responses during electrically-induced leg and voluntary arm exercise in lower-limb disabled males. *Proceedings of the 10th Annual RESNA Conference on Rehabilitation Engineering*, 1987, pp 591–593.

10. Davis GM, Williamson JW, Pawelczyk JA, et al: Cardiovascular responses to FNS-induced isometric leg exercise during lower body negative pressure. *Proceedings of the 12th Annual RESNA Conference on Rehabilitation Engineering*, 1989, pp 95–96.

11. Fahr PD, Glaser RM, Figoni SF, et al: Feasibility of using two FNS exercise modes for spinal cord injured patients. *Clin Kinesiol* 1989; 43:62–68.

12. Figoni SF, Davis GM, Glaser RM, et al: FNS-assisted venous return in exercising SCI men. *Proceedings of the International Conference of Associations for Advancement of Rehabilitation Technology*, 1988, pp 328–329.

13. Figoni SF, Glaser RM, Hendershot DM, et al: Hemodynamic responses of quadriplegics to maximal arm-cranking and FNS leg cycling exercise. *Proceedings of the 10th Annual Conference of Engineering in Medicine and Biology Society.* 1988, pp 1636–1637.

14. Figoni SF, Glaser RM, Hooker SP, et al: Peak hemodynamic responses of SCI subjects during FNS leg cycle ergometry. *Proceedings of the 12th Annual RESNA Conference on Rehabilitation Engineering*, 1989, pp 97–98.

15. Figoni SF, Glaser RM, Rodgers MM, et al: Hemodynamic responses of quadriplegics to arm, ES-leg, and combined arm and ES-leg ergometer. *Med Sci Sports Exerc* 1989; 21(suppl):S96.

16. Freyschuss U, Knuttson E: Cardiovascular control in man with transverse cervical cord lesions. *Life Sci* 1969; 8:421–424.

17. Glaser RM: Arm exercise training for wheelchair users. *Med Sci Sports Exerc* 1989; 21(suppl):149–157.

18. Glaser RM: Central and peripheral etiology of fatigue for the disabled. *1988 American Association EMG Electrodiagnosis Didactic Program*, 1988, pp 21–26.

19. Glaser RM: Exercise and locomotion for the spinal cord injured, in Terjung RL (ed): *Exercise and Sport Sciences Reviews*, vol 13. New York, Macmillan Publishing Co, 1985, pp 263–303.

20. Glaser RM: Physiologic aspects of spinal cord injury and functional neuromuscular stimulation. *Cen Nerv Syst Trauma* 1986; 3:49–62.

21. Glaser RM: Spinal cord injuries and neuromuscular stimulation, in Torg JS (ed): *Current Therapy in Sports Medicine.* Toronto, BC Decker 1990.

22. Glaser RM, Collins SR, Horgan HR: An electrical stimulator for exercising paralyzed mus-

cles. *Proceedings of the 8th Annual Conference on Rehabilitation Technology*, 1987, pp 597–599.

23. Glaser RM, Collins SR, Strayer JR, et al: A closed-loop stimulator for exercising paralyzed muscles. *Proceedings of the 8th Annual Conference on Rehabilitation Technology*, 1985, pp 388–390.

24. Glaser RM, Davis GM: Wheelchair-dependent individuals, in Franklin BA, Gordon S, Timmis GC (eds): *Exercise in Modern Medicine: Testing and Prescription in Health and Disease.* Baltimore, Williams & Wilkins, 1988, pp 237–267.

25. Glaser RM, Figoni SF, Collins SR, et al: Physiologic responses of SCI subjects to electrically-induced leg cycle ergometry. *Proceedings of the 10th Annual Conference of Engineering in Medicine and Biology Society*, 1988, pp 1638–1640.

26. Glaser RM, Figoni SF, Hooker SP, et al: Efficiency of FNS leg cycle ergometry. *Proceedings of the 11th Annual Conference of Engineering in Medicine and Biology Society*, 1989.

27. Glaser RM, Rattan SN, Davis GM, et al: Central hemodynamic responses to lower-limb FNS. *Proceedings of the 9th Annual Conference of Engineering in Medicine and Biology Society*, 1987; pp 615–617.

28. Glaser, RM, Strayer JR, May KP: Combined FES leg and voluntary arm exercise of SCI patients. *Proceedings of the 7th Annual Conference of Engineering in Medicine and Biology Society*, 1985, pp 308–313.

29. Green HF, Reichmann H, Pette D: Fiber type specific transformations in the enzyme activity pattern of rat vastus lateralis muscle by prolonged endurance training. *Pflugers Arch* 1983; 399:216–222.

30. Gruner JA, Glaser RM, Feinberg SD, et al: A system for evaluation and exercise-conditioning of paralyzed leg muscles. *J Rehabil Res Dev* 1983; 20:21–30.

31. Health and Public Policy Committee, American College of Physicians: Radiologic methods to evaluate bone mineral content. *Ann Intern Med* 1984; 100:908–911.

32. Hooker SP, Glaser RM, Figoni SF, et al: Physiologic responses of simultaneous voluntary arm crank and electrically-stimulated leg exercise in quadriplegics. *Proceedings of the 12th Annual RESNA Conference on Rehabilitation Engineering*, 1989; pp 99–100.

33. Kaplan FS: *Osteoporosis.* West Caldwell, NJ, Ciba Clinical Symposia, 1983.

34. Kralj A, Bajd T, Turk R: Electrical stimulation providing functional use of paraplegic patient muscles. *Med Prog Technol* 1980; 7:3–9.

35. Kralj A, Bajd T, Turk R, et al: Gait restoration in paraplegic patients: A feasibility study using multi-channel surface electrode FES. *J Rehabil Res Dev* 1983; 20:3–20.

36. Mortimer JT: Motor prostheses, in Brookhart JM, Mountcastle VB, Brooks VB, et al (eds): *Handbook of Physiology. The Nervous System II.* Bethesda, Md, American Physiological Society, 1981, pp 155–187.

37. Munsat TL, McNeal D, Waters R: Effects of nerve stimulation on human muscle. *Arch Neurol* 1976; 33:608–617.

38. Peckham PH, Mortimer JT, Marsolais EB: Alteration in the force and fatigability of skeletal muscle in quadriplegic humans following exercise induced by chronic electrical stimulation. *Clin Orthop* 1976; 114:326–334.

39. Peckham PH, Mortimer JT, Van Der Meulen JP: Physiologic and metabolic changes in white muscle of cat following induced exercise. *Brain Res* 1973; 50:424–429.

40. Petrofsky JS, Phillips CA: Active physical therapy: A modern approach to rehabilitation therapy. *J Neurol Orthop Surg* 1983; 4:165–173.

41. Petrofsky JS, Phillips CA, Heaton HH III, et al: Bicycle ergometer for paralyzed muscles. *J Clin Eng* 1984; 9:13–19.

42. Pollack SF, Axen K, Spielholz N, et al: Aerobic training effects of electrically induced lower extremity exercises in spinal cord injured people. *Arch Phys Med Rehabil* 1989; 70:214–219.

43. Ragnarsson KT: Physiologic effects of functional electrical stimulation–induced exercise in spinal cord injured individuals. *Clin Orthop* 1988; 233:53–63.

44. Ragnarsson KT, Pollack S, O'Daniel W Jr, et al: Clinical evaluation of computerized functional electrical stimulation after spinal cord injury: A multicenter pilot study. *Arch Phys Med Rehabil* 1988; 69:672–677.

45. Reddanna P, Moorthy CVN, Govindappa S: Pattern of skeletal muscle chemical composition during in vivo electrical stimulation. *Indian J Physiol Pharmacol* 1981; 25:33–39.

46. Rhagnar M, Hudlicka O: Capillary growth in chronically stimulated adult skeletal muscle as studied by intravital microscopy and histologi-

cal methods in rabbits and rats. *Microvasc Res* 1978; 16:73–90.

47. Riley DA, Allin EF: The effects of inactivity, programmed stimulation and denervation on the histochemistry of skeletal muscle fiber types. *Exp Neurol* 1973; 40:391–413.

48. Salmons S, Gale DR, Steter FA: Ultrastructural aspects of the transformation of muscle fiber type by long term stimulation: Changes in Z discs and mitochondria. *J Anat* 1978; 127:17–31.

49. Salmons S, Vrbova G: The influence of activity of some contractile characteristics of mammalian fast and slow muscles. *J Physiol* 1969; 201:535–549.

50. Servedio FJ, Servedio A, Davis GM, et al: Voluntary strength gains in paretic muscle after hybrid (FNS-VOLUNTARY) exercise training. *Proceedings of the 10th Annual RESNA Conference on Rehabilitation Engineering*, 1987, pp 594–596.

51. Vrbova G: Factors determining the speed of contraction of striated muscle. *J Physiol* 1966; 185:17–18.

52. Zwiren LD, Bar-Or O: Responses to exercise of paraplegics who differ in conditioning level. *Med Sci Sports* 1975; 7:94–98.

CHAPTER 38

Rehabilitation of Cervical Spine, Brachial Plexus, and Peripheral Nerve Injuries

Joseph J. Vegso, M.S.

The cervical spine is placed at risk of injury in a number of athletic activities. Football, diving, wrestling, ice hockey, equestrian events, and gymnastics are those in which injuries to the cervical spine occur most frequently. Rehabilitation can be efficacious either as treatment itself or as follow-up to other modalities, traction, or surgery. The injuries for which therapeutic exercises are appropriate include acute cervical sprain syndrome, brachial plexus neurapraxia, brachial plexus axonotmesis, vertebral body end plate fractures, wedge compression and other stable fractures, and peripheral nerve injuries. In addition to being a recommended treatment of injury, exercise is a valuable preventive measure. It is important to understand the principles and methods of therapeutic and rehabilitative exercises both to prepare the athlete for the demands each sport will place on his or her body and to return the injured athlete to activity safely.

General principles of rehabilitation are reviewed, followed by a discussion of the clinical entities of concern and descriptions of the specific rehabilitation exercises for each injury.

REVIEW OF REHABILITATION PRINCIPLES

The first step in the rehabilitation process is the initiation of a set of exercises to increase range of motion and flexibility. There are several methods of stretching a joint to increase motion. The simplest and most effective is a slow, steady stretch that places the joint or the muscle, or both, in the extreme range of available motion. This position is then maintained for between 10 and 30 seconds or more depending on patient tolerance. It can be done actively or passively. The amount of force used to stretch the joint or muscle is dependent on several factors: length of time since injury or surgery, severity of injury, surgical procedure, the joint involved, length of immobilization, and patient tolerance.

Range-of-motion exercises may be preceded by moist heat in the form of whirlpools, hydrocollator steam packs, or warm showers when the injury is past the acute inflammatory stage.[7]

The general guidelines for static stretching and range of motion are as follows:

1. The athlete must be relaxed.

2. Enter the motion or stretch position slowly.

3. The stretch should produce a comfortable sensation.

4. The stretch position should be maintained for 10 to 30 seconds and repeated ten or more times.

Strength

Muscular strength is the single most important factor in athletic performance. After injury or surgery, a significant portion of the rehabilitation program must be devoted to regaining strength in the muscle groups that have been injured or immobilized.

In recent years there has been tremendous growth in the variety of equipment available for strengthening muscles. Despite the overabundance of equipment, the basic principles of strengthening muscle remain unchanged. The following review of terminology and techniques is coupled with recommendations for applying these techniques to a rehabilitation program.

Muscle strength is defined as the maximum force that a muscle can exert in a single contraction. Strength can be further defined as being static or dynamic. Static strength is commonly associated with a muscular contraction without joint movement (i.e., isometric), whereas dynamic strength involves a contraction with associated joint movement. Furthermore, a muscular contraction can be concentric or eccentric in nature. Concentric muscular contraction occurs when a muscle is contracted against resistance and the muscle shortens in length, whereas eccentric muscular contraction refers to a contraction of a muscle against a resistance while the muscle lengthens.

An important aspect of the eccentric contraction is that a muscle can produce more force during this phase of contraction than during the concentric phase. This has implications during the rehabilitation program if an athlete cannot produce enough force to complete a concentric workout. Eccentric workouts can be used effectively to increase strength in the early phases of rehabilitation. Methods of strengthening muscles fall into these main areas: isometric, isotonic, and isokinetic.

Isometric Exercise.—Isometric exercise is typically defined as being a muscular contraction without associated movement of the joint or limb upon which the muscle(s) act. Simply put, the force a muscle generates is less than, or equal to, the resistance being applied. The effectiveness of isometric exercise in increasing strength first gained notoriety in the 1950s as a result of Hettinger and Muller's work.[4] The number of repetitions can be varied depending on the phase of rehabilitation and muscle condition.

There are several implications for the use of isometric strengthening exercises in a rehabilitation setting. Isometric strengthening is most effective in the very early stages of rehabilitation when joint motion is limited or not advisable, when the force that a muscle produces is not sufficient to utilize weights or other resistance equipment, and in athletes or patients who have conditions that do not allow for strengthening through an isotonic method.

Isometric exercise is convenient because it requires minimal equipment and supervision.

Isotonic Exercise.—Isotonic exercise is usually defined as a strengthening exercise in which a joint moves through a range of motion against a constant resistance or weight. This is easily accomplished through the use of a barbell, sandbag, weight bench, or more sophisticated equipment such as a Universal gym.

As the weight is lifted, the muscle fatigues. After a period of time, the muscle adapts and increases in strength. When this occurs, it becomes easier to lift the weight. Additional weight is added to overload the muscle(s). This cycle is referred to as progressive resistance exercise (PRE); it is the hallmark of muscle-strengthening programs and was developed by DeLorme in the 1940s. Since that time many variations on the theory have been introduced, but the basic principle remains unchanged. One must progressively increase the amount of weight one lifts in order to increase muscle strength. Typically, a minimum of three sets of six to ten repetitions of each exercise is performed during each rehabilitation session. In many instances injured athletes can perform their strength exercises every day to maintain their rehabilitation.

When isotonic exercises are used for rehabilitation, it is important to monitor the patient on a regular basis, daily if possible, to be sure that the exercise program is not aggravating the injury. Swelling, discomfort, pain, effusion, and loss of motion are important warning signs that indicate the athlete is not ready for an isotonic strengthening program or that he or she is progressing too rapidly.

Variable Resistance.—A variation of the isotonic strengthening method that has become readily available in recent years is variable resistance exercise. Simply stated, like isotonics, the joint(s) or muscle groups(s) move(s) through a range of motion against resistance. Unlike isotonics, however, the resistance varies to mimic or reproduce the mechanical advantages of the muscle and joint so that the muscle must work at a near maximum force throughout the range of motion.

Common examples of variable resistance equipment are Nautilus, Universal-DVR, and CAM 2. Variable resistance equipment is normally used in the same manner as isotonic equipment in a rehabilitation setting.

Isokinetic Exercise.—Isokinetic exercise is dynamic in nature, as is isotonic variable resistance. The aspect of isokinetic exercise that distinguishes it from other forms of dynamic exercise is maximum accommodating resistance. The equipment provides maximum resistance to the muscle throughout the entire range of motion for every repetition. This is accomplished by controlling the speed at which the exercise is performed, usually through a hydraulic system. The Cybex and the Orthotron were the first pieces of equipment to utilize the isokinetic method of exercise.

The advantage of isokinetic exercise over isotonics and variable resistance is speed of exercise. A joint or muscle group can be exercised at slow speeds (30 to 60 degrees per second) to stimulate strength gains along the lines of isotonic exercises, or at higher speeds (up to 300 degrees per second) to stimulate strength gains at more functional rates of muscle contraction.

Manual Resistance.—Often overlooked, manual resistance is a very effective method for strengthening muscles in a rehabilitative setting. It requires no equipment, is excellent for use in isolating specific muscles, and can produce isokinetic or near maximum accommodating resistance. Typically, exercise regimens follow a pattern similar to isokinetics, namely, three sets of six to ten repetitions. However, this may vary with the speed of the exercise. At faster rates of speed, more repetitions are performed to provide a sufficient workload.

This general review of rehabilitative principles allows for the discussion of specific injuries to the neck and the specific rehabilitative exercises for each.

CERVICAL SPINE INJURIES

Acute "Cervical Sprain" Syndrome

An acute cervical sprain is an injury frequently seen in contact sports; the patient complains of having "jammed" his or her neck, with subsequent pain localized to the cervical area. Characteristically, the patient is first seen with limitation of cervical spine motion without radiation of pain or paresthesia. Neurologic and roentgenographic examinations show negative findings.

In the absence of findings other than pain and limitation of neck motion, identifying the exact nature of the injury may be difficult or impossible. It is assumed, however, that the intervertebral disk structures, ligamentous supporting structures, or the joints between the articular processes have been injured.

In general, treatment of athletes with "cervical sprains" should be tailored to the degree of severity. Immobilizing the neck in a soft collar and using analgesics and anti-inflammatory agents until there is a full, spasm-free range of neck motion are appropriate. If the patient has severe pain and muscle spasm of the cervical spine, hospitalization and the head halter traction may be indicated. It should be emphasized that individuals with a history of collision injury, pain, and lack of normal range of cervical motion should have a routine cervical spine roentgenographic study. Also, lateral flexion and extension roentgenograms are indicated after the acute symptoms subside.[9]

BRACHIAL PLEXUS INJURIES

Grade I Brachial Plexus Neurapraxia[1, 3]

These injuries are characterized by a sharp, burning pain in the shoulder and arm on the side of the body where the injury occurred. Pain can be felt in the neck, and it sometimes radiates to the shoulder, arm, and hand. Associated weakness and paresthesia are additional symptoms. The key to the nature of the lesion is its short duration and persistence of full, pain-free range of neck motion.[8] There may be motor and sensory loss, which is usually regained within 5 to 10 minutes.[4]

Grade II Brachial Plexus Injuries (Brachial Plexus Axonotmesis)[1, 3]

These injuries are caused by a stretching of the plexus as the head and cervical spine are forced laterally away from the symptomatic arm and shoulder, usually as a result of a shoulder tackle or fall. Paralysis or weakness, numbness, and burning sensations in the hands are experienced.[2] Additional characteristics include tenderness in the trapezius muscle, usually in the upper middle portion.[4] This can last for a few days. Motor and sensory function may not return to normal for 2 weeks to several months.

Loss of strength is a major problem resulting from this injury. Grade II injuries are characterized by weakness of shoulder abduction, elbow flexion, and external humeral rotation, due to weakening of the deltoid, biceps, and infraspinatus muscles.[2, 8] Weakness of triceps and wrist extensor muscles and grip strength also may be present.[2] Strength loss in grade II injuries persists longer than in grade I brachial plexus injuries; 80% to 90% strength may not be seen for 3 weeks, and full strength may take as long as 6 months to be regained.[4]

Treatment should include a light isotonic strengthening program, with gradual progression to a full shoulder rehabilitation program, and eventual return to activity. Neck rehabilitation exercises, as well as biceps, triceps, and wrist strengthening exercises, are described subsequently. Individuals with these injuries should not be permitted to compete until full strength returns.[8] This can be assessed by comparing weight lifting ability with the preseason baseline measurements, or by comparing the strength of the injured extremity with that of the uninjured extremity.

Preventive measures can be implemented to avoid these injuries. Among such measures are (1) allowing individuals to participate only in sports appropriate for their height and weight, (2) performing neck exercises, and (3) using the proper equipment, padding, and techniques, as well as neck collars.[2] Manual resistance exercises and Nautilus exercises should be performed on a year-round basis.

PERIPHERAL NERVE INJURIES

These injuries may involve the spinal accessory nerve (trapezius muscle), the suprascapular nerve (the supraspinatus, the infraspinatus, and the teres major muscles), the axillary nerve (deltoid and teres minor muscles), and the long thoracic nerve (serratus anterior muscles).

The spinal accessory nerve is vulnerable anteriorly, just proximal to its entrance into the undersurface of the trapezius muscle, approximately 1 in. above the clavicle. It can be injured by a direct blow from a hockey or a lacrosse stick, or a shoulder pad could be forced against it. With significant trauma, there may be weakness when lifting the arm or shrugging the shoulders, and there may be a rotary winging of the scapula. This injury should be diagnosed by electromyography. If there is no recovery within 6 months, the nerve should be explored.

The suprascapular nerve may be injured by a direct blow to the base of the neck. This causes shoulder weakness, which is noticeable at 90 degrees of abduction. This injury must be differentiated from a resolving grade II brachial plexus injury. In follow-up of grade II brachial plexus injuries, we have noted that the biceps and deltoid functions return to normal significantly faster than the supraspinatus and infraspinatus. Hence a grade II plexus injury, if seen late, may readily appear as an isolated suprascapular nerve injury. Careful questioning and electromyographic evaluation often help differentiate between the two. This differential diagnosis is particularly important because suprascapular nerve injury without significant return of strength after 6 months may warrant surgical exploration. An axillary nerve injury is an uncommon injury without a concomitant shoulder dislocation.

Several months after the injury it may be difficult to distinguish between a partially recovered brachial plexus injury and a peripheral nerve injury. An awareness of the clinical manifestations and the electromyographic findings at serial intervals may help to differentiate between the two entities.[9]

Rehabilitation should be directed toward strengthening the muscle group(s) involved.

REHABILITATION PROGRAM

Rehabilitation for Cervical Spine Injuries

Whether it is used initially as part of a conservative course or postoperatively, the aim of the rehabilitation program is usually the same: to restore range of motion and adequate strength.

The rehabilitation program can begin with range-of-motion exercises and isometric strengthening, followed by manual resistance through the pain-free range of motion, and finally progressing to isotonic exercises as the physician sees fit.

Range of Motion

Range-of-motion exercises include neck flexion, neck extension, lateral bending (right and left), and lateral rotation (right and left).

Neck Flexion.—While standing or sitting, flex the neck forward and attempt to touch the chin to the chest. Hold this position for 10 to 15 seconds, relax, and repeat six to ten times (Fig 38–1, A).

Neck Extension.—While standing or sitting, extend the neck backward and attempt to touch the back of the head to the upper part of the back. Hold for 10 to 15 seconds, relax, and repeat six to ten times (Fig 38–1, B).

Lateral Bending (Right).—While standing or sitting, look straight ahead. Bend the neck to the right and attempt to touch the right ear to the top of the right shoulder. There should be a stretch on the left side of the neck. Hold the stretch for 10 to 15 seconds, relax, and repeat six to ten times (Fig 38–1, C).

Lateral Bending (Left).—Begin sitting or standing and look straight ahead. Bend the neck to the left and attempt to touch the left ear to the top of the left shoulder. There should be a stretch on the right side of the neck. Hold the stretch for 10 to 15 seconds, relax, and repeat six to ten times (Fig 38–1, D).

Lateral Rotation (Right).—Begin standing or sitting. Rotate the head to the

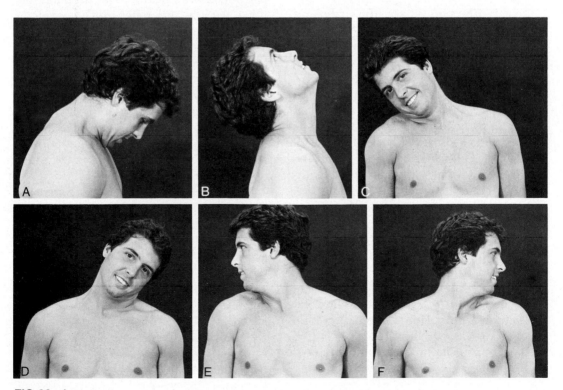

FIG 38–1.
Range-of-motion exercises. **A,** neck flexion. **B,** neck extension. **C,** lateral bending (right). **D,** lateral bending (left). **E,** lateral rotation (right). **F,** lateral rotation (left). *(From Torg JS, Vegso JJ, Torg E:* Rehabilitation of Athletic Injuries: An Atlas of Therapeutic Exercise. *St Louis, Mosby-Year Book, 1987. Used with permission.)*

right and try to touch the chin to the right shoulder. Hold the stretch for 10 to 15 seconds, relax, and repeat six to ten times (Fig 38–1, *E*).

Lateral Rotation (Left).—Begin standing or sitting. Rotate the head to the left and try to touch the chin to the left shoulder. Hold the stretch for 10 to 15 seconds, relax, and repeat six to ten times (Fig 38–1, *F*).

Isometric Strengthening

Once range of motion has been regained, strength can be improved initially with isometric resistance exercises. These exercises help to strengthen the muscles of the neck without moving it through the range of motion.

Neck Flexion.—Place the palms of both hands on the forehead. While providing resistance with the hands, press the forehead forward. Hold for 6 seconds, relax, and repeat ten times (Fig 38–2, *A*).

Neck Extension.—With the head flexed slightly forward, place the palms of the hands against the back of the head. While providing resistance with the hands, try to push the head backward without actually moving it. Hold for 6 seconds, relax, and repeat ten times (Fig 38–2, *B*).

Lateral Bending.—Place the right hand against the side of the head. While providing resistance with the hand, try to move the head to the right shoulder. Resist actual motion. Hold the position for 6 seconds, relax, and repeat ten times (Fig 38–2, *C*). Repeat this same exercise for the opposite side (Fig 38–2, *D*).

Lateral Rotation (Right).—Place the right hand against the temple. While applying pressure with the right hand, rotate the head to the right and try to touch the chin to the right shoulder. Resist actual motion. Hold the position for 6 seconds, relax, and repeat ten times (Fig 38–2, *E*).

Lateral Rotation (Left).—Place the left hand against the temple. While applying pressure with the left hand, rotate the head to the left and try to touch the chin to the left shoulder. Resist actual motion. Hold the position for 6 seconds, relax, and repeat ten times (Fig 38–2, *F*).

Isotonic Exercise

An isotonic exercise program can often follow the isometric or manual resistance program. Wall pulleys can be used, as can Universal and Nautilus equipment.[5] Among the exercises that can be performed are flexion, extension, and oblique flexion and extension, as well as shoulder shrugs and high pulls.[5]

Nautilus strength training may be necessary for athletes participating in certain sports, such as football and wrestling, but this level of training is not required for all individuals. This kind of rehabilitation program should be performed following the recommendation of a physician or certified athletic trainer.

Nautilus Four-Way Neck Extension (Back of the Neck).—With the seat properly adjusted, sit in the machine so that the back of the head is touching the pads. The neck will be flexed forward so that the chin is touching the chest. Cross both arms in front and grasp both handles to either side (Fig 38–3).

Nautilus Four-Way Neck Lateral Contraction (Side of Neck).—Sit in the machine with the left ear to the center of the pads. The neck will be laterally contracted fully to the right. Cross both arms in front and grasp the handles on either side (Fig 38–4, *A*).

From the starting position, move the

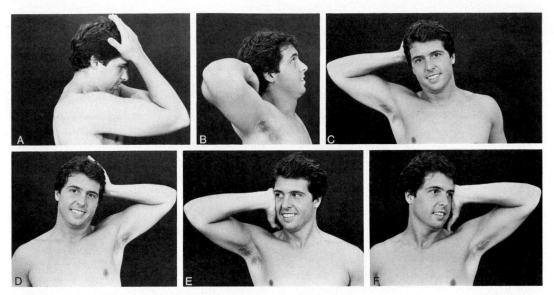

FIG 38–2.
Isometric exercises. **A,** neck flexion. **B,** neck extension. **C,** lateral bending (right). **D,** lateral bending (left). **E,** lateral rotation (right). **F,** lateral rotation (left). *(From Torg JS, Vegso JJ, Torg E:* Rehabilitation of Athletic Injuries: An Atlas of Therapeutic Exercise. *St Louis, Mosby-Year Book, 1987. Used with permission.)*

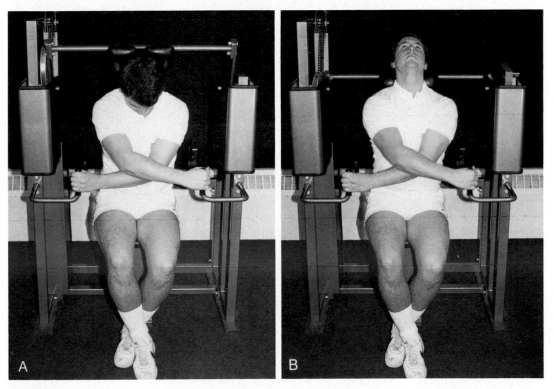

FIG 38–3.
Nautilus four-way neck extension (back of the neck). **A,** starting position for posterior extension on the Nautilus four-way machine. **B,** full posterior extension. *(From Torg JS, Vegso JJ, Torg E:* Rehabilitation of Athletic Injuries: An Atlas of Therapeutic Exercise. *St Louis, Mosby-Year Book, 1987. Used with permission.)*

head from right to left against the pads, until the left ear is as close as possible to the left shoulder. Hold this position for 2 seconds. Keep the shoulders square (Fig 38–4, *B*). Slowly return to the count of four to the starting position, relax, and repeat eight to twelve times.

REHABILITATION FOR BRACHIAL PLEXUS INJURIES

Dumbbell weights are used to perform shoulder exercises in an isotonic program; these include shoulder flexion, shoulder abduction, and shoulder extension. Shoulder circles are also performed, and a broomstick is used for internal and external rotation exercises.

Shoulder Exercises

Shoulder Flexion (Supraspinatus, Infraspinatus, Teres Minor, Subscapularis Muscles).—Standing with the arm at the side and the elbow fully extended, raise the arm up in front of the body until it is parallel with the floor. Hold this position for 1 to 2 seconds and then slowly return the arm to the starting position (Fig 38–5, *A* and *B*).

Shoulder Abduction (Deltoid, Supraspinatus Muscles).—Standing with the arm at the side and the elbow fully extended, raise the arm away from the side of the body until it is parallel to the floor. Hold this position for 1 to 2 seconds and then slowly return to starting position (Fig 38–5, *C*).

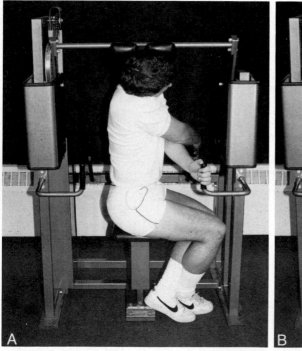 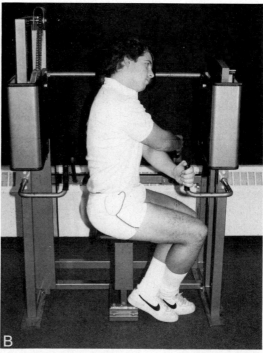

FIG 38–4.
Nautilus four-way neck lateral contraction (side of neck). **A,** starting position for lateral contraction to the left on the Nautilus four-way neck machine. **B,** full lateral contraction to the left. *(From Torg JS, Vegso JJ, Torg E: Rehabilitation of Athletic Injuries: An Atlas of Therapeutic Exercise. St Louis, Mosby-Year Book, 1987. Used with permission.)*

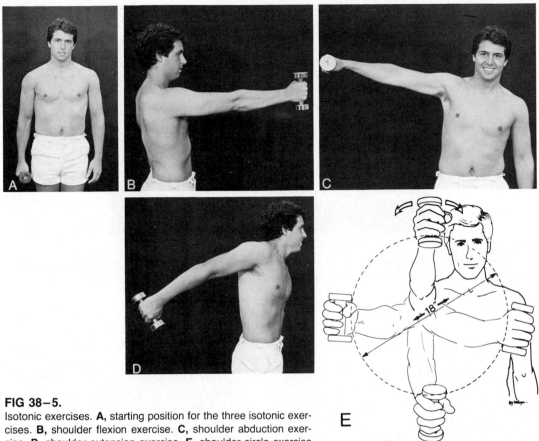

FIG 38–5.
Isotonic exercises. **A,** starting position for the three isotonic exercises. **B,** shoulder flexion exercise. **C,** shoulder abduction exercise. **D,** shoulder extension exercise. **E,** shoulder circle exercise with 18 in. diameter. *(From Torg JS, Vegso JJ, Torg E:* Rehabilitation of Athletic Injuries: An Atlas of Therapeutic Exercise. *St Louis, Mosby-Year Book, 1987. Used with permission.)*

Shoulder Extension (Deltoid, Teres Minor Muscles).—Standing with the arm at the side and the elbow fully extended, extend the arm straight back as far as possible without bending at the waist. Hold this position for 1 to 2 seconds and then slowly return to the starting position (Fig 38–5, *D*).

Shoulder Circles.—Standing with the arm at the side and the elbow fully extended, extend the arm in front of the body until it is parallel with the floor. Make an 18 in. diameter circle in the clockwise position and then an 18 in. diameter circle in the counterclockwise direction (Fig 38–5, *E*).

Internal Rotation.—Standing with upper arms against the side of the chest, bend the elbows to 90 degrees, palms up. Grasp a broomstick with the hands 18 in. apart. Try to push the hands together for 10 seconds, but do not allow the hands to slip along the stick. Repeat with the hands 12 in. apart, and then repeat with the hands 6 in. apart (Fig 38–6).

External Rotation.—Standing with upper arms against the side of the chest, bend elbows to 90 degrees, palms up. Grasp a broomstick with hands 6 in. apart. Try to pull hands apart for 10 seconds; do not allow hands to slip. Repeat

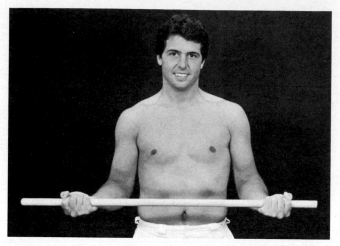

FIG 38−6.
Internal and external rotation isometrics with the broomstick. *(From Torg JS, Vegso JJ, Torg E:* Rehabilitation of Athletic Injuries: An Atlas of Therapeutic Exercise. *St Louis, Mosby-Year Book, 1987. Used with permission.)*

with hands 12 in. apart, and then repeat with hands 18 in. apart.

The following program should be done: shoulder flexion, ten repetitions; shoulder abduction, ten repetitions; shoulder extension, ten repetitions; shoulder circles counterclockwise, ten repetitions; shoulder circles clockwise, ten repetitions. Repeat this sequence two more times for a total of three sets.

Next, the following sequence is performed: external rotation, ten repetitions; internal rotation, ten repetitions; wrist flexion, ten repetitions; elbow flexion, ten repetitions; elbow extension, ten repetitions (see Figs 38−14 to 38−19). Apply ice to shoulder for 20 minutes.

It is important to remember that good form must always be maintained in order to achieve the full benefit of these exercises. Try to increase the amount of weight lifted by 2½ pounds every 7 to 14 days.

Nautilus Exercises

Super Pullover Machine (Latissimus Dorsi Muscle and Other Torso).—Adjust the seat so that the tops of the shoulders are aligned with the axes of the cams. Check to make sure that the appropriate weight is set. Sit in the seat, adjust the seatbelt, and depress the foot pedal with both feet. This will raise the elbow pads in front of you. Place the elbows on the pad and the palms of the hands on the curved portion of the bar. Provide resistance with the elbows and release the foot pedal. Allow the weight to gently pull the arms backward. Drive with the elbows and lower the bar to the count of two, until it touches the hips/thighs. Hold the position for the count of two. To the count of four, slowly allow the bar to return to the starting position. Repeat the exercises again, eight to twelve times (Fig 38−7).

Double Chest Machine/Arm-Cross Machine (Pectoralis Major, Deltoid Muscles).—Adjust the seat so that, when in the position illustrated in Figure 38−8,*B*, the shoulders are aligned with the cams of the machine overhead. Check to make sure that the appropriate weight is set. Fasten the seatbelt. With the back straight and the head back, put the forearms behind the pads and place the palms of the

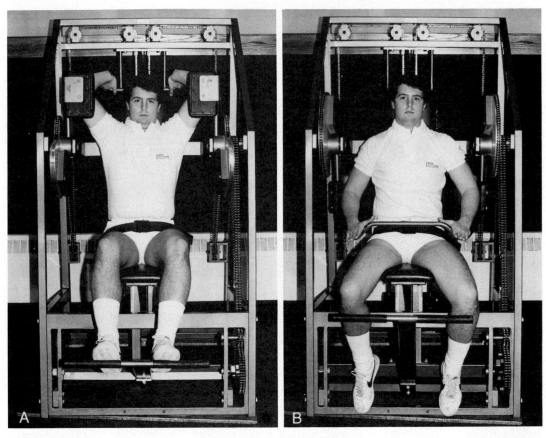

FIG 38–7.
Super pullover machine (latissimus dorsi muscle and other torso). **A,** starting position for the pullover exercise. **B,** the bar is lowered to the count of 2 to the hip/thigh, where it is held for two counts. *(From Torg JS, Vegso JJ, Torg E: Rehabilitation of Athletic Injuries: An Atlas of Therapeutic Exercise. St Louis, Mosby-Year Book, 1987. Used with permission.)*

hands against the handle. Apply pressure against the pads with the forearms and push forward, to the count of two, until the arms come together in front of you. Hold this position for two counts. To the count of four, slowly return the arms to the starting position. Repeat eight to twelve times (Fig 38–8). Then proceed to the next exercise.

Nautilus Decline Press (Chest, Shoulder, Triceps).—Leave the seat adjusted as for the arm-cross exercise. Raise the handles into the starting position by depressing the footpad with both feet. Place the palms of the hands behind the handles.

Keep the back straight and flat against the back of the machine, and keep the head back. Press the bars forward, to the count of two, until the arms are almost but not completely extended. Keep the elbows up while doing this. Hold this position for two counts. To the count of four, return slowly to the starting position. Repeat eight to twelve times (Fig 38–9).

Behind the Neck Machine.—Adjust the seat so that the shoulders are aligned with the cams of the machine. Sit straight, with the back flat against the back of the machine, and fasten the seatbelt. Cross the forearms over the head

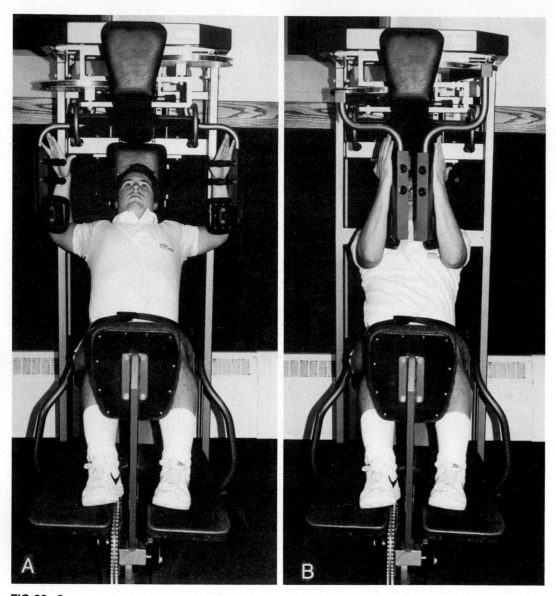

FIG 38–8.
Double chest machine/arm-cross machine (pectoralis major, deltoid muscles). **A,** starting position for the arm-cross exercise. **B,** apply pressure against the pads with the forearms and push forward to the count of 2, until reaching the position shown. *(From Torg JS, Vegso JJ, Torg E: Rehabilitation of Athletic Injuries: An Atlas of Therapeutic Exercise. St Louis, Mosby-Year Book, 1987. Used with permission.)*

and place the backs of the upper arms between the rollers. Apply pressure with the arms against the rollers, lowering them to the count of two, until they touch the torso. Keep the elbows flexed to 90 degrees and the forearms parallel to the wall behind. Hold this position for two counts. Slowly return to the starting position, taking four counts to do so. Repeat eight to twelve times at the appropriate weight (Fig 38–10).

Rowing (Deltoid and Trapezius Muscles).—Enter the machine and sit with the back straight and flat against the back of the machine. Use additional pads be-

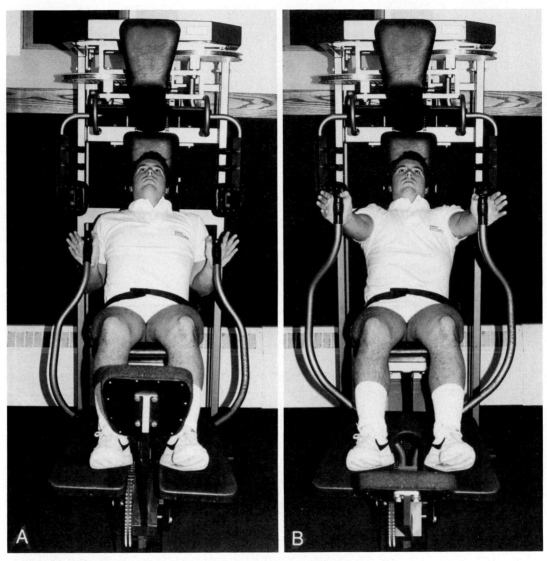

FIG 38–9.
Decline press (chest, shoulders, triceps muscle). **A,** starting position for the decline press. **B,** extended position.
(From Torg JS, Vegso JJ, Torg E: Rehabilitation of Athletic Injuries: An Atlas of Therapeutic Exercise. *St Louis, Mosby-Year Book, 1987. Used with permission.)*

tween the torso and the front padding if necessary. Place the arms between the rollers, cross one over the top of the other, and flex the elbows to 90 degrees. Drive with the elbows and apply pressure against the pads, pushing them backward as far as possible. Keep the elbows flexed to 90 degrees and the forearms parallel to the floor. Hold this position for two counts. Slowly return to the starting posi-

tion, taking four counts to do so. Repeat eight to twelve times (Fig 38–11).

Double Shoulder Machine Lateral Raise (Deltoid Muscles).—Adjust the seat so that the tops of the shoulders are aligned with the cams of the machine. Sit up straight, keep the head back, and fasten the seatbelt. Place the hands behind the pads and rest the palms on the han-

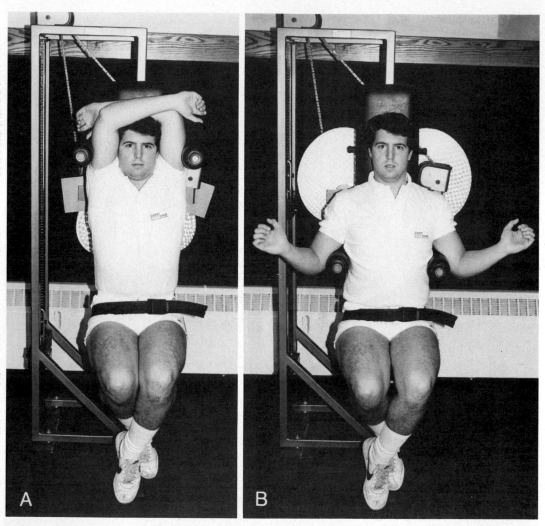

FIG 38–10.
Behind neck machine (latissimus dorsi muscle). **A,** starting position. **B,** apply pressure with the arms against the rollers, lowering them to the count of 2, until they touch the sides of the torso. *(From Torg JS, Vegso JJ, Torg E: Rehabilitation of Athletic Injuries: An Atlas of Therapeutic Exercise. St Louis, Mosby-Year Book, 1987. Used with permission.)*

dles. Abduct the arms away from the body, leading with the elbows. Raise the arms to the count of two, until the arms are parallel to the floor. Hold this position for two counts. To the count of four, slowly lower the arms to the starting position. Repeat eight to twelve times (Fig 38–12).

Overhead Press (Deltoid and Trapezius Muscles).—With the seat adjusted as for the lateral raise, and with the back straight, head back, and seatbelt fastened, grasp the handles located just above either shoulder. Press the handles up over the head until the arms are extended. This should take two counts. Hold this position for two counts. Keep the back pressed flat against the back pad while performing this exercise. Do not arch! To the count of four, slowly lower the handles to the starting position. Repeat eight to twelve times (Fig 38–13).

The shoulder should not be placed in a compromised position if surgery has not been performed.[10] Progress will be

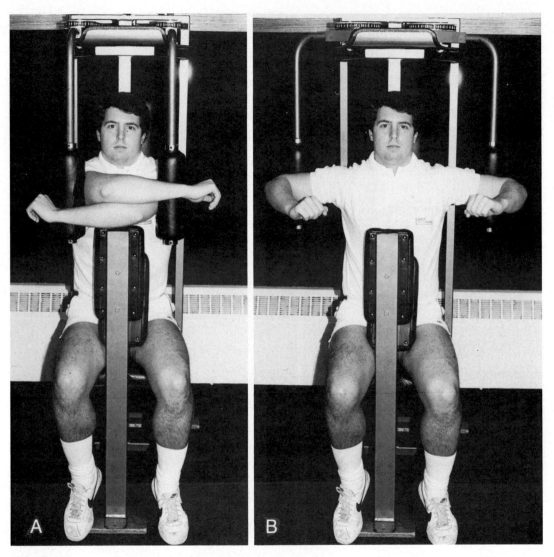

FIG 38–11.
Rowing machine (deltoid and trapezius muscles). **A,** starting position for rowing. **B,** driving with the elbows, apply pressure against the pads, pushing them as far back as possible. *(From Torg JS, Vegso JJ, Torg E:* Rehabilitation of Athletic Injuries: An Atlas of Therapeutic Exercise. *St Louis, Mosby-Year Book, 1987. Used with permission.)*

slower, atrophy will be greater, and range of motion will be more limited if there has been extensive damage.

Elbow Exercises

Elbow Flexion Exercises/Biceps Curls (Standing).—With the elbow extended and the upper extremity by the side, grasp a dumbbell weight. Keeping the el-bow and upper arm close to the body, flex the arm, lifting the weight through the range of motion to the fully flexed position. Hold in this position for 2 seconds, and then lower slowly to the starting position. Repeat eight to twelve times (Fig 38–14).

Elbow Extension Exercises—Biceps Curls (Standing).—With the arm fully ab-

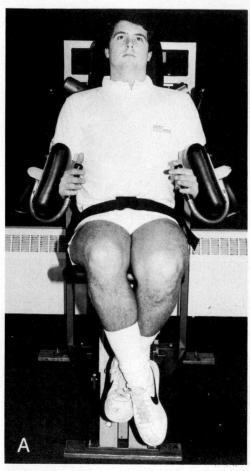
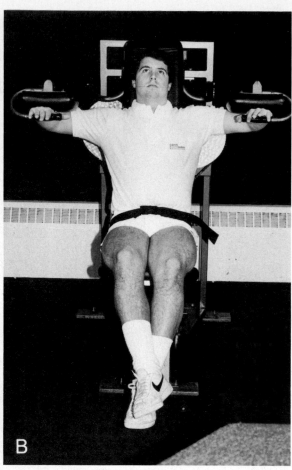

FIG 38–12.
Double shoulder machine lateral raise (deltoid muscle). **A,** starting position for the lateral raise. **B,** fully abducted position. *(From Torg JS, Vegso JJ, Torg E:* Rehabilitation of Athletic Injuries: An Atlas of Therapeutic Exercise. *St Louis, Mosby-Year Book, 1987. Used with permission.)*

ducted and externally rotated and the elbow flexed, isotonic triceps contraction results in elbow extension. Hold this position for 2 seconds, then lower slowly to the starting position. Repeat 8 to 12 times (Fig 38–15).

Nautilus Biceps/Triceps Machine— Biceps Curls.—Adjust the weight. Sit in the seat and align the elbows with the cams of the machine. Use extra padding if necessary. Keep the back straight. With palms up, grasp the bar with both hands at the curved portion (Fig 38–16, A).

Raise the weight by pulling the bar to

the chin. Hold this position for 2 seconds, and then slowly lower to the count of four to the starting position. Keep the back straight while doing this exercise. Concentrate on pulling with the arms, not the shoulder and back. Repeat eight to twelve times (Fig 38–16, B).

Nautilus Biceps/Triceps Machine— Triceps Extension.—Set the appropriate weight. Sit in the seat and place the elbows on the pads in front, aligning them with the cams of the machine. Place the hands behind the pads at the shoulders so that the fingers touch the pads and the

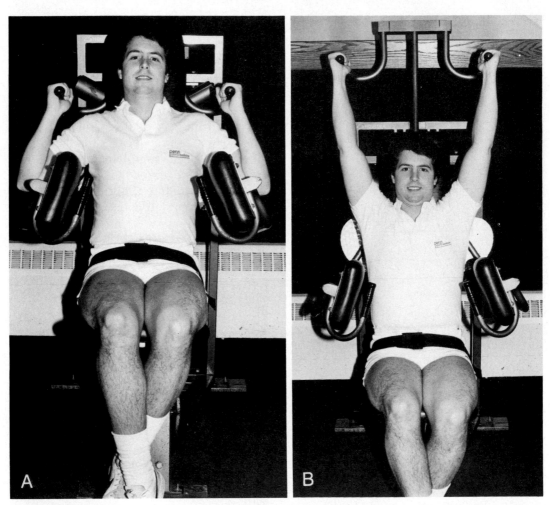

FIG 38–13.
Overhead press (deltoid and triceps muscles). **A,** starting position for the overhead press. **B,** fully extended position. *(From Torg JS, Vegso JJ, Torg E: Rehabilitation of Athletic Injuries: An Atlas of Therapeutic Exercise. St Louis, Mosby-Year Book, 1987. Used with permission.)*

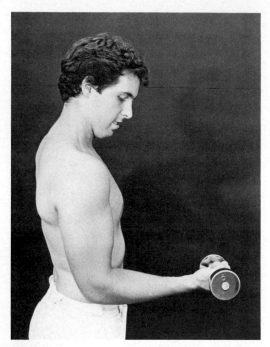

FIG 38–14.
Elbow flexion/biceps curls. *(From Torg JS, Vegso JJ, Torg E:* Rehabilitation of Athletic Injuries: An Atlas of Therapeutic Exercise. *St Louis, Mosby-Year Book, 1987. Used with permission.)*

thumbs are toward the shoulders. Adjust the padding so that the elbows are slightly higher than the shoulders (Fig 38–17, A).

Extend the arms, pushing against the pads with the hands, moving through the range of motion until full extension is reached. Hold this position for 2 seconds, and then return slowly to the count of four to the starting position. Concentrate on keeping the elbows on the pad. Repeat eight to twelve times (Fig 38–17, B).

Wrist Exercises

Wrist Extension.—Place the forearm on a flat surface, palm down. Bend the elbow to 90 degrees. Grasp a dumbbell weight and allow it to pull the wrist into the fully flexed position. Slowly extend the wrist until it is fully extended. Hold

this position for 1 second, and then slowly return to the starting position (Fig 38–18).

Wrist Flexion.—Place the forearm on a flat surface, palm up. Bend the elbow to 90 degrees. Grasp a dumbbell weight and allow it to pull the wrist into the fully extended position. Slowly flex the wrist until it is fully flexed. Hold this position for 1 second, and then slowly return to the starting position (Fig 38–19).

Do ten repetitions of wrist flexion and then ten repetitions of wrist extension, continuing to alternate sets until three sets of ten repetitions for each exercise have been completed. Once three sets have been completed, rest for 5 minutes. Then do three more sets of each, once again alternating between extension

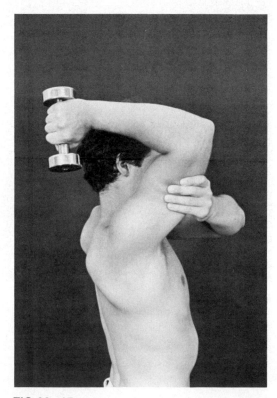

FIG 38–15.
Elbow extension/triceps curls. *(From Torg JS, Vegso JJ, Torg E:* Rehabilitation of Athletic Injuries: An Atlas of Therapeutic Exercise. *St Louis, Mosby-Year Book, 1987. Used with permission.)*

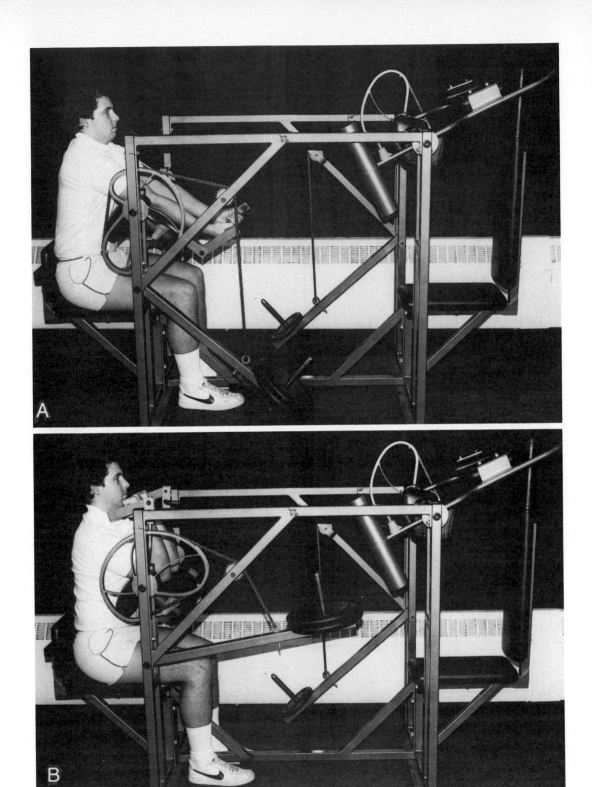

FIG 38–16.
Nautilus biceps/triceps machine. **A,** starting position for the biceps curl. **B,** full biceps extension. *(From Torg JS, Vegso JJ, Torg E:* Rehabilitation of Athletic Injuries: An Atlas of Therapeutic Exercise. *St Louis, Mosby-Year Book, 1987. Used with permission.)*

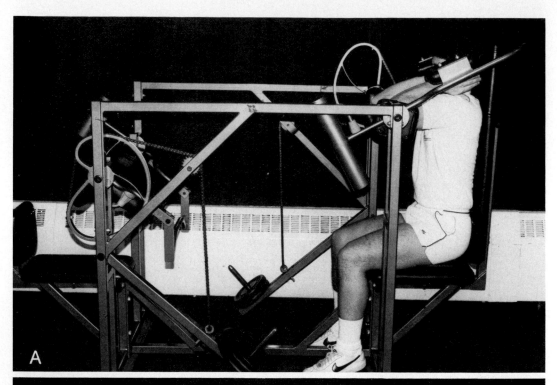

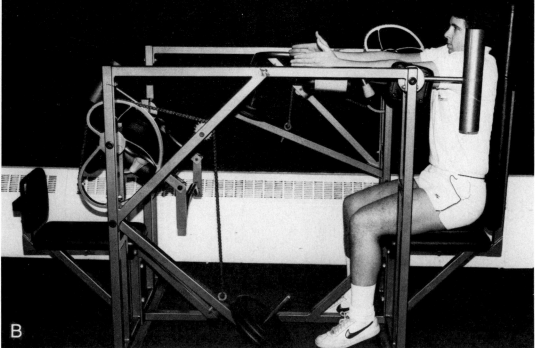

FIG 38–17.
Nautilus biceps/triceps machine. **A,** starting position for the triceps extension. **B,** full triceps extension. *(From Torg JS, Vegso JJ, Torg E:* Rehabilitation of Athletic Injuries: An Atlas of Therapeutic Exercise. *St Louis, Mosby-Year Book, 1987. Used with permission.)*

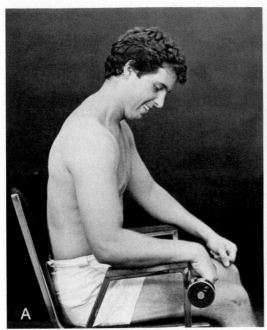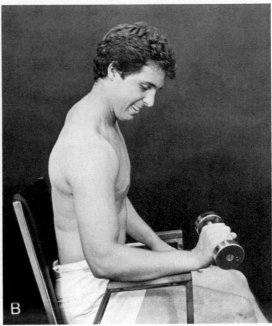

FIG 38–18.
Isotonic strengthening–wrist extension. **A,** starting position for the wrist extension exercise. **B,** fully extended position. *(From Torg JS, Vegso JJ, Torg E: Rehabilitation of Athletic Injuries: An Atlas of Therapeutic Exercise. St Louis, Mosby-Year Book, 1987. Used with permission.)*

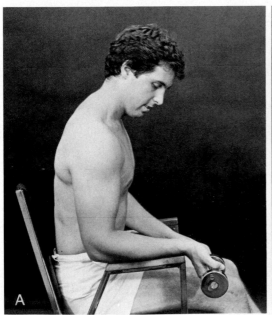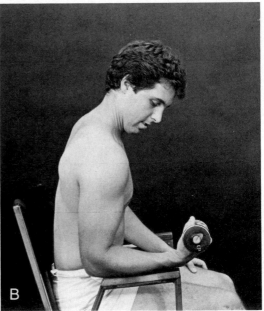

FIG 38–19.
Isotonic strengthening–wrist flexion. **A,** starting position for the wrist flexion exercise. **B,** fully flexed position. *(From Torg JS, Vegso JJ, Torg E: Rehabilitation of Athletic Injuries: An Atlas of Therapeutic Exercise. St Louis, Mosby-Year Book, 1987. Used with permission.)*

and flexion. Place ice on the wrist for 15 to 20 minutes. This exercise should be repeated once per day. Try to increase the number of pounds per week according to the specifications of the physician or certified athletic trainer.

REFERENCES

1. Archembault JL: Brachial plexus stretch injury. *J Am Coll Health* 1983; 31:256–260.

2. Basmajian JV (ed): *Therapeutic Exercise*, ed 3. Baltimore, Williams & Wilkins, 1978, p 127.

3. Clancy WG: Brachial plexus and upper extremity peripheral nerve injuries, in Torg JS (ed): *Athletic Injuries to the Head, Neck, and Face.* Philadelphia, Lea & Febiger, 1982, pp 215–220.

4. Hettinger T, Muller EA: Muskelleistung und Muskel Training. *Int Z Angew Physiol Einschl Arbeitsphys* 1953; 15:111–126.

5. Kuprian W (ed): *Physical Therapy for Sports.* Philadelphia, WB Saunders Co, 1981, p 106.

6. Roy S, Irvin R: *Sports Medicine—Prevention, Evaluation, Management, and Rehabilitation.* Englewood Cliffs, NJ, Prentice-Hall, 1983.

7. Sapega AA, Quedenfeld TC, Moyer RA, et al: Biophysical factors in range of motion exercise. *Phys Sportsmed* 1981; 9:57–65.

8. Torg JS: Athletic injuries to the cervical spine. *Surg Rounds* Nov 1978, pp 40–50.

9. Torg JS, Wiesel SW, Rothman RH: Diagnosis and management of cervical spine injuries, in Torg JS (ed): *Athletic Injuries to the Head, Neck, and Face.* Philadelphia, Lea & Febiger, 1982, pp 181–209.

10. Vegso JV: Modalities, in Torg JS, Vegso JV, Torg E: *Rehabilitation of Athletic Injuries: An Atlas of Therapeutic Exercise.* St Louis, Mosby–Year Book, 1987.

CHAPTER 39

Criteria for Return to Contact Activities After Cervical Spine Injury

Joseph S. Torg, M.D.

Steven G. Glasgow, M.D.

Injury to the cervical spine and associated structures as a result of participation in competitive athletic and recreational activities is not uncommon. It appears that the frequency of these various injuries is inversely proportional to their severity. Whereas Albright et al.[1] have reported that 32% of college football recruits sustained "moderate" injuries while in high school, catastrophic injuries with associated quadriplegia occur to less than 1/100,000 participants per season at the high school level. As indicated in Chapter 30, the variety of possible lesions is considerable and the severity variable. The literature dealing with diagnosis and treatment of these problems is considerable. However, conspicuously absent is a comprehensive set of standards or guidelines for establishing criteria for permitting or prohibiting return to contact sports (boxing, football, ice hockey, lacrosse, Rugby, wrestling) after injury to the cervical spinal structures. The explanation for this void appears to be twofold. First, the combination of a litigious society and the potential for great harm should things go wrong makes "no" the easiest, and perhaps most reasonable advice. Second and perhaps most important, with the exception of the matter of transient quadriplegia, is the lack of credible data pertaining to post-injury risk factors. Despite a lack of credible data, this chapter attempts to establish guidelines to assist the clinician as well as the patient and his parents in the decision making process.

Cervical spine conditions requiring a decision as to whether participation in contact activities is advisable and safe can be divided into two categories: (1) congenital or developmental and (2) post-traumatic. Each condition has been determined to present either (1) no contraindication, (2) relative contraindication, or (3) an absolute contraindication on the basis of a variety of parameters. Information compiled from more than 1,200 cervical spine injuries documented by the National Football Head and Neck Injury Registry has provided insight into whether various conditions may or may not predispose to more serious injury.[7-10] A review of the literature in several instances provides significant data for a limited number of specific conditions. Analysis of many conditions predicated on an understanding of recognized injury mechanisms has permitted categorization on the basis of "educated" conjecture. And, lastly, much reliance has been placed on personal experience that must be regarded as anecdotal.

The structure and mechanics of the cervical spine enable it to perform three important functions. First, it supports the head as well as the variety of soft tissue structures of the neck. Second, by virtue of segmentation and configuration, it permits multiplanar motion of the head. Third, and most important, it serves as a protective conduit for the spinal cord and cervical nerve roots. A situation that would impede or prevent the performance of any of the three functions in a pain-free manner either immediately or in the future is unacceptable and contraindicated.

CURRENT CONCEPTS

In an attempt to "categorize and prognosticate athletic spinal injuries," Bailes et al.[2] defined the following classification:

- Type I injury: Involves the spinal cord.
- Type II injury: Cord-type symptoms.
- Type III injury: Radiographic abnormalities without neurologic signs or symptoms

More specifically, a type I injury is one that occurs to the spinal cord. Although symptoms are either minor or resolved and despite a normal neurologic examination, spinal cord involvement is demonstrated by magnetic resonance imaging (MRI). Bailes et al. believe that if a radiographically demonstrable spinal cord injury has been documented, the athlete should not be allowed to return to contact sports.

Type II injuries at initial presentation show neurologic symptoms or findings referable to the spinal cord, but the patient has a normal neurologic and radiographic examination. In this group are found those described as having had an episode of neurapraxia. Also, a similar phenomenon is frequently witnessed in those youngsters experiencing brachial plexus neurapraxia. Bailes et al.[2] state,

In the absence of a neurologic deficit, radiologic demonstrable injury, and congenital cervical spinal anomaly, these patients may return to full participation in contact sports. If the athlete becomes a repeat offender with multiple episodes suggestive of cord origin of the symptoms, he or she is at a higher risk of catastrophic injury and thought should be given for withholding further participation.

Type III injuries include those patients who have a radiographic abnormality[2]:

In those who have a fracture or a fracture dislocation which is unstable and requires stabilization either by surgical means or external bracing, they would not be candidates for further participation. In those who have a bony injury that is stable on flexion/extension radiographs, it must be discerned whether this lesion is stable only during a physiologic range of motion or whether the injury would indeed be stable under stress. The latter would be considered for isolated lamina, spinous process or minor vertebral body fracture. A more difficult issue involves those bony injuries which have healed, are stable on physiological range of motion testing (lateral flexion and extension radiographs), but exist in an area of the spine which normally conveys a significant contribution to spinal column stability.

Bailes et al.[2] acknowledge,

"There are little experimental or clinical data to use in assessing the degree of stability following a healed fracture or ligamentous injury of the cervical spine when it is placed under extreme degrees of stress. It is known that the cervical posterior ligamentous structures contribute more to stability in flexion, while the anterior ligaments are most important in extension . . . . In the absence of reliable data, and with no objective measurement of the degree of dynamic stress stability, any healed fracture of the spinal column, with the exception of healed, isolated minor vertebral body, lamina and spinous process fractures, probably should be considered to be unsuitable to safely withstand further challenges from impact sports.

They further state,[2]

Other Type III injuries having a radiographic abnormality other than fracture are considered in two groups. The first is those patients who have evidence of spinal cord contusion manifested by an intrinsically widened cord shadow on myelography in the absence of bony compression, herniated disc or epidural hematoma. More recently, MRI has for the first time directly imaged this lesion, best seen on intermediate images as a high intensity lesion within the cord. Another lesion is that which has evidence of spinal motion on dynamic radiographs implying ligamentous injury, which requires halo brace or surgical stabilization. In both of these types of patients, we would not recommend further participation in contact sports as a likelihood of injury would be considered to be significantly higher than normal.

Watkins[11] categorizes those with congenital and traumatic cervical spine problems into three risk groups:

1. Minimal risks: Those with a very small increased chance of risks compared with his or her situation before the injury. Example of the minimal-risk category are:
   a. Asymptomatic bone spurs.
   b. Certain healed facet fractures.
   c. Brachial plexus and neurapraxia.
   d. Healed disk herniation.
   e. Healed lamina fractures.
   g. Spinous process fractures.
2. Moderate risk: Those where there is a reasonable percentage chance that the patient will have a recurrence of symptoms and a chance that he is at risk for some permanent injury. Examples of moderate-risk category are:
   a. Facet fractures.
   b. Lateral mass fractures.
   c. Nondisplaced healed odontoid fractures.
   d. Nondisplaced healed ring of C1 fractures.

   e. Acute lateral disk herniations.
   f. Cervical radiculopathy due to foraminal spur.
3. Extreme risk: The patient who runs a high risk of occurrence of symptoms and permanent damage. Examples of the high risk category are:
   a. Os odontoideum.
   b. Ruptured transverse ligament C1–C2.
   c. Occipitocervical dislocation.
   d. Odontoid fracture.
   e. Total ligamentous disruption of a neuromotor segment of the lower cervical spine.
   f. An unstable fracture dislocation.
   g. Unstable Jefferson's fracture.
   h. Cervical cord anomaly.
   i. Acute large central disk herniation.

White et al.[12] recognized that the literature is "neither always clear or consistent in describing what constitutes an unstable cervical spine." Using fresh cadaver specimens, they performed load displacement studies on sectioned and unsectioned two-level segments to determine the horizontal translation and rotation in the sagittal plane after each ligament was transected. The experiments constituted a quantitative biomechanical analysis of the effects of destroying ligaments and facets on the stability of the cervical spine below C2 in an attempt to determine cervical stability. The express purpose of this study was to establish indications for treatment methods to stabilize the spine. Although the intent of the study was to define clinical instability to formulate treatment standards and was not intended to establish criteria for return to contact athletics, it does appear that their findings are relevant to this latter issue.

White et al.[12] described "clinical stability as the ability of the spine to limit its patterns of displacement of physiologic loads so as not to damage or irritate the spinal cord or the nerve roots."

Basically, the authors delineated several important findings. First, in sectioning the ligaments, there were small increments of change followed without warning by sudden, complete disruption of the spine. Second, removal of the facets alters the motion segment such that in flexion there is less angular displacement and more horizontal displacement. Third, the anterior ligaments contribute more to stability in extension than the posterior ligaments, and in flexion the posterior ligaments contribute more than the anterior ligaments.

The fourth and most relevant findings from the standpoint of parameters for return to contact sports as follows. The adult cervical spine is unstable, on the brink of instability, when any of the following conditions are present:

1. All the anterior or all the posterior elements are destroyed or unable to function.

2. More than 3.5 mm horizontal displacement of one vertebra in relationship to an adjacent vertebra measured on lateral roentgenograms (resting or flexion-extension) (Fig 39–1).

3. More than 11 degrees of rotation difference to that of either adjacent vertebra measured on a resting erect lateral or flexion-extension roentgenogram (Fig 39–2).

Evaluation of the cervical spine for the purpose of determining suitability for participation in contact activities involves consideration of the history, physical examination, and roentgenographic findings, including computed tomographic (CT) and MRI scans. Albright et al.[1] have reported a lack of correlation between these three parameters in a study involving pre-season examination of 104 active high school football players and 75 college freshman as candidates. Of those who reported a positive history for neck injury, only one-half demonstrated roentgenographic changes, and of the 32 subjects with abnormal x-ray find-

ings only two demonstrated abnormal physical findings. Abnormal roentgenographic findings among the 75 college freshman included 8 compression fractures, 7 with abnormal motion, 5 with narrow disk spaces, and 4 with neural large fractures. Interestingly, only 10, or 13%, of the 75 gave a positive history for injury.

The following proposed criteria for return to contact activities in the presence of cervical spine abnormalities or af-

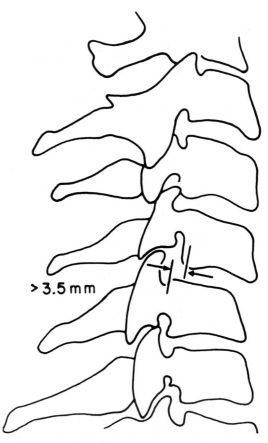

FIG 39–1.
The method for determining translatory displacement, as described by White et al. With use of the postero-inferior angle of the superior vertebral body as one point of reference and the posterosuperior angle of the vertebral body below, the distance between the two in the sagittal plane is measured. A distance of 3.5 mm or greater is suggestive of clinical instability. *(From White AA, Johnson RM, Panjabi MM, et al: Clin Orthop 1975; 109:85. Used with permission.)*

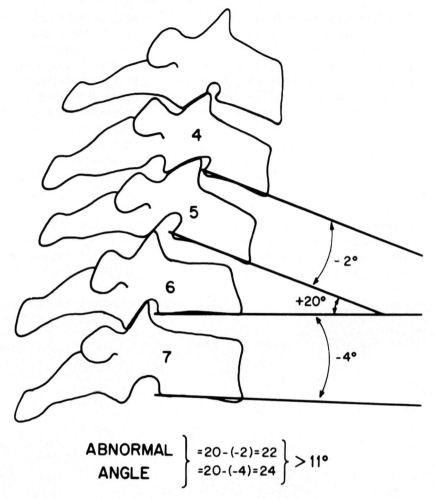

$$\left.\begin{array}{l} \text{ABNORMAL} \\ \text{ANGLE} \end{array}\right\} \left.\begin{array}{l} =20-(-2)=22 \\ =20-(-4)=24 \end{array}\right\} > 11°$$

FIG 39–2.
Abnormal angulation between two vertebrae at any one interspace is determined by comparing the angle formed by the projection of the inferior vertebral body borders with that of either the vertebral body above or the vertebral body below. If the angle at the interspace in question is 11 degrees or greater than either adjacent interspace, this is considered by White et al. as clinical instability. *(From White AA, Johnson RM, Panjabi MM, et al: Clin Orthop 1975; 109:85. Used with permission.)*

ter injury are intended only as guidelines. It is fully acknowledged that for the most part they are, at best, predicated on the antidotal, and no responsibility can be assumed for their implementation.

Critical to the application of these guidelines is the implementation of coaching and playing techniques that preclude the use of the head as the initial point of contact in a collision situation. Exposure of the cervical spine to axial loading is an invitation to disaster and relegates any and all safety standards as meaningless.

CRITERIA

I. Congenital conditions
   A. Odontoid anomalies: Hensinger[4] has stated that "patients with congenital anomalies of the odontoid are leading a precarious exist-

ence. The concern is that a trivial insult superimposed on already weakened or compromised structure may be catastrophic." This concern became a reality during the 1989 football season when an 18-year-old high school player was rendered a respiratory-dependent quadriplegic while making a head tackle that was vividly demonstrated on the game video. Post-injury roentgenograms revealed an os odontoideum with marked C1–C2 instability (Fig 39–3). Thus the pres-

ence of odontoid agenesis, odontoid hypoplasia, or os odontoideum is an absolute contraindication to participation in contact activities.

B. Spina bifida occulta: A rare, incidental roentgenographic finding that presents no contraindication.

C. Atlanto-occipital fusion: A rare condition characterized by partial, or complete, congenital fusion of the bony ring of the atlas to the base of the occiput. The onset of signs and symptoms, referable to the posterior columns be-

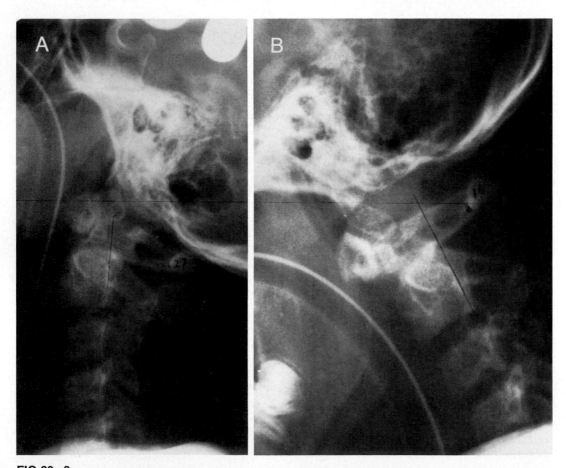

FIG 39–3.
A and **B,** inherent instability at C1 in a patient with an os odontoideum, resulting in respiratory-dependent quadriplegia after a spear tackle by this 18-year-old high school football player. The reduction in the space available for the cord (SAC) is vividly demonstrated by the lateral extension and flexion views post-injury. (From Torg JS, Glasgow SG: *Clin J Sports Med* 1991; 1:12–27. Used with permission.)

cause of cord compression by the posterior lip of the foramen magnum, usually occurs in the third or fourth decade. Signs and symptoms usually begin insidiously and progress slowly, but sudden onset or instant death has been reported. Atlanto-occipital fusion as an isolated entity or coexisting with other abnormalities constitutes an absolute contraindication to participation in contact activities.

D. Klippel-Feil syndrome: The eponym applied to congenital fusion of two or more cervical vertebrae. For purposes of this discussion, the variety of abnormalities can be divided into two groups: type I, mass fusion of the cervical and upper thoracic vertebrae (Fig 39–4), and type II, fusion of only one or two interspaces (Fig 39–5). To be noted, a variety of associated congenital problems have been identified to be associated with congenital fusion of the cervical vertebrae and include pulmonary, cardiovascular, and urogenital problems. Pizzutillo[5] has pointed out that "children with congenital fusion of the cervical spine rarely develop neurologic problems or signs of instability." However, he further states that "the literature reveals more than 90 cases of neurologic problems . . . that developed as a consequence of occipital cervical anomalies, late instability, disc disease, or degenerative joint disease." These reports included cervical radiculopa-

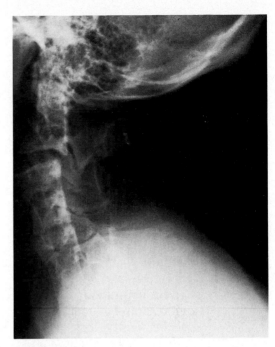

FIG 39–4.
Type I Klippel-Feil deformity with multiple-level fusions and deformities as demonstrated on the lateral-view roentgenogram. (From Torg JS, Glasgow SG: *Clin J Sports Med* 1991; 1:12–27. Used with permission.)

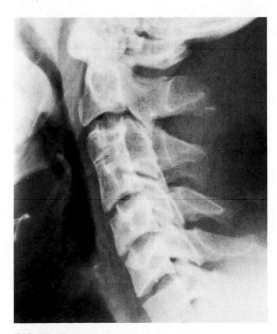

FIG 39–5.
Type II Klippel-Feil deformity with a one-level congenital fusion at C3–C4 involving both the vertebral bodies and the lateral masses. (From Torg JS, Glasgow SG: *Clin J Sports Med* 1991; 1:12–27. Used with permission.)

thy, spasticity, pain, quadriplegia, and sudden death. Also, "more than two thirds of the neurologically involved patients had single level fusion of the upper area, whereas many cervical patients with extension fusions of five to seven levels had no associated neurologic loss."[5] Despite this, the type I lesion, a mass fusion, constitutes an absolute contraindication to participation in contact sports. As well, a type II lesion with fusion of one or two interspaces with associated limited motion or associated occipitocervical anomalies, instability, disk disease, or degenerative changes also constitutes absolute contraindication to participation. On the other hand, type II lesions involving fusion of one or two interspaces at C3 and below in an individual with full cervical range of motion and an absence of occipitocervical anomalies, instability, disk disease, or degenerative changes should present no contraindication.

II. Developmental conditions
   A. Developmental narrowing (stenosis) of the cervical spinal canal and its association with cervical cord neurapraxia and transient quadriplegia has been well defined (Chapter 36).[9] Defining narrowing or stenosis as a cervical segment with one or more vertebrae having a canal/body ratio of 0.8 or less is predicated on the fact that 92% of all reported clinical cases have fallen below this value at one or more levels. To be noted, 12% of asymptomatic controls also fell below the 0.8 level, as did 48% of asymptomatic professional and 45% of asymptomatic college players. In the group of reported symptomatic players, there was in every instance complete neurologic return, and in those who continued with contact activities, recurrence was not predictable.

Clearly, the presence of developmental narrowing of the cervical spinal canal does not predispose permanent neurologic injury. Eisman et al.[3] have indicated, on the basis of experience with cervical fractures/dislocations resulting from automobile accidents, that the degree of neurologic impairment was inversely related to the anteroposterior diameter of the canal. Due to the all-or-nothing pattern of axial load football spine injuries, this phenomenon has not been observed in athletic-related injuries.

The presence of a canal/vertebral body ratio of 0.8 or less is no contraindication to participation in contact activities in asymptomatic individuals. We further recommend against pre-participation screening roentgenograms in asymptomatic players. Such studies will not contribute to safety, are not cost effective, and will only contribute to the hysteria surrounding this issue.

In those individuals with a ratio of 0.8 or less who experience either motor or sensory manifestations (or both) of cervical cord neurapraxia, there is a relative contraindication to return to contact activities (Fig 39–6). In these instances, in each case the decision must be determined on an individual basis, depending on the understanding of the player and his parents and their willingness to accept any presumed theoretic risk.

Absolute contraindications to continued participation apply to those individuals who experience a documented episode of cervical cord neurapraxia associated with any of the following:

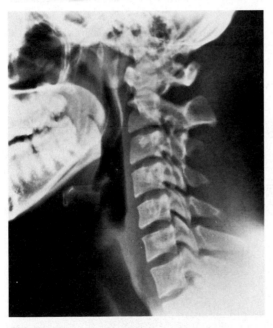

FIG 39–6.
Lateral-view roentgenogram of a 20-year-old intercollegiate player who had one episode of transient quadriplegia that lasted 10 minutes after a hyperflexion injury. The canal/vertebral body ratios are narrow from C3 through C7. Specifically, the ratio at C4 measures 0.6. This player returned to his activity, playing for two seasons without a recurrence. (From Torg JS, Glasgow SG: *Clin J Sports Med* 1991; 1:12–27. Used with permission.)

1. Ligamentous instability.
2. Intervertebral disk disease.
3. Degenerative changes.
4. MRI evidence of cord defects or swelling.
5. Symptoms of positive neurologic findings lasting more than 36 hours.
6. More than one recurrence.

B. *"Spear tacklers' spine"*: Analysis of material recently received by the National Football Head and Neck Injury Registry has allowed for the description of *"spear tacklers' spine,"* an entity that consists of developmental narrowing, reversal of normal cervical lordosis or kyphosis, and subtle torticollis in an individual who employs spear tackling techniques (Fig 39–7). In two players with pre-injury roentgenograms as well as video documentation of axial loading of the spine due to spear tackling, a bilateral C3–C4 facet dislocation resulted in one instance and C4–C5 fracture dislocation in the other, with both being rendered quadriplegic. Whether the straightened "segmented column" alignment of the spine or the headfirst tackling technique, or a combination of the two, predisposes those with "spear tacklers' spine" to catastrophic injury is not clear. This combination of factors constitutes an absolute contraindication to further participation in contact sports.

III. Traumatic conditions of the upper cervical spine (C1–C2)
As indicated in Chapter 32, the anatomy and mechanics of C1–C2 segment of the cervical spine

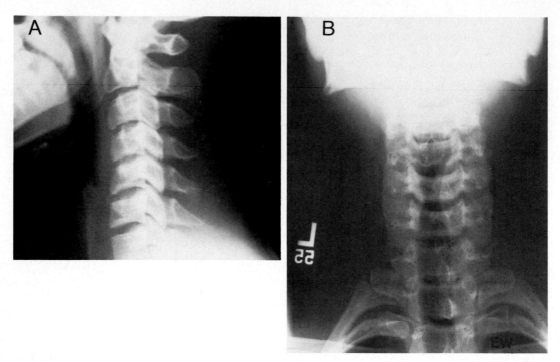

FIG 39–7.
A and **B,** roentgenographic characteristics of *"spear tacklers' spine"* include developmental narrowing, reversal of the normal cervical lordosis in the erect, neutral position on the lateral views, and suggestion of a wryneck attitude, with tilt of the cervical spine to the left on the anteroposterior views. This particular 18-year-old high school football player's cervical CT and MRI scans were normal. He was precluded from further participation in contact sports. (From Torg JS, Glasgow SG: *Clin J Sports Med* 1991; 1:12–27. Used with permission.)

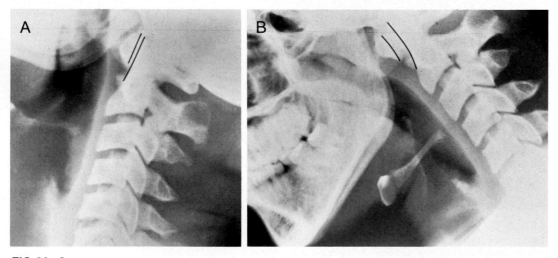

FIG 39–8.
A and **B,** the atlantodens interval (ADI) is the distance on the lateral-view roentgenogram between the anterior aspect of the dens and the posterior aspect of the anterior ring of the atlas. In children, the ADI should not exceed 4.0 mm, whereas the upper limit in the normal adult is less than 3.0 mm. C1–C2 instability is vividly demonstrated in the extension and flexion views shown here. (From Torg JS, Glasgow SG: *Clin J Sports Med* 1991; 1:12–27. Used with permission.)

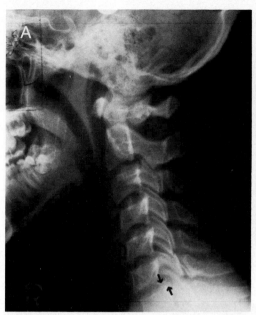
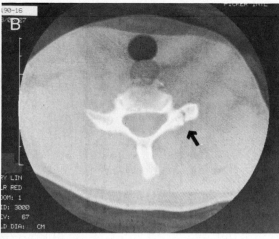

FIG 39–9.
A, lateral-view roentgenogram of the cervical spine in the erect neutral position of a 21-year-old college football player demonstrates anterior translation of C6 on C7 of more than 3.5 mm *(dark arrows).* **B,** a CT scan of C6, in the sagittal plane demonstrates a fracture through the lateral mass *(arrow).* Persistent displacement despite healing of the fracture constitutes an absolute contraindication to further participation in contact sports. (From Torg JS, Glasgow SG: *Clin J Sports Med* 1991; 1:12–27. Used with permission.)

differ markedly from the middle or lower segments. Lesions with any degree of occipital or atlantoaxial instability portend a potentially grave prognosis. Thus any injury involving the upper cervical segment that involves a fracture or ligamentous laxity is an absolute contraindication to further participation in contact

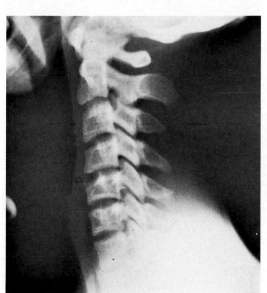

FIG 39–10.
Lateral-view roentgenogram of the cervical spine taken in the erect neutral position demonstrates an anterosuperior compression defect in the vertebral body of C5 *(open arrow).* There is no evidence of angulation, displacement, or subluxation indicating adherent stability of the spine. Such a radiographic finding would not constitute a contraindication to further participation. (From Torg JS, Glasgow SG: *Clin J Sports Med* 1991; 1:12–27. Used with permission.)

activities (Fig 39–8). Healed, nondisplaced Jefferson fractures, healed types I and II odontoid fractures, and healed lateral mass fractures of C2 constitute a relative contraindication providing the patient is pain free, has a full range of cervical motion, and has no negative neurologic findings.

Because of the uncertainty of the results of cervical fusion, the gracile configuration of C1, and the importance of the alar and transverse odontoid ligaments, fusion for instability of the upper segment constitutes an absolute contraindication regardless of how successful the fusion appears roentgenographically.

IV. Traumatic conditions of the middle and lower cervical spine
A. Ligamentous injuries: The criteria of White et al.[12] for defining clinical instability were intended to help establish indications for surgical stabilization. However, although the limits of displacement and angulation correlated with disruption of known structures, no one determinant was considered absolute. In view of the observations of Albright et al.[1] that

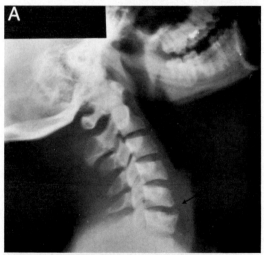

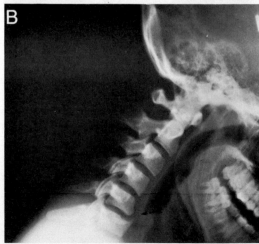

FIG 39–11.
A and **B,** lateral flexion and extension views of a healed, stable end plate fracture involving the superior aspect of C6 in a 22-year-old intercollegiate football player. The injury had occurred 4 years previously while participating in high school sports. He relates having had a sore neck, missing two games, but not having been examined roentgenologically. There were no subsequent problems despite participation in high school and college varsity football. (From Torg JS, Glasgow SG: *Clin J Sports Med* 1991; 1:12–27. Used with permission.)

10% (7/75) of the college freshman in his study demonstrated "abnormal motion," as well as on the basis of our own experience, it appears that in many instances some degree of "minor instability" exists in populations of both high school and college football players without apparent adverse effects. The question, of course, is, What are the upper limits of "minor" instability? Unfortunately there are no available data to relate this to the clinical situation that allow reliable standards.

Clearly, however, lateral-view roentgenograms demonstrating more than 3.5 mm of horizontal displacement of either one vertebra in relationship to another or more than 11 degrees of rotation than either adjacent vertebra represent an absolute contraindication to further participation in contact activities (Fig 39–9). With regard to lesser degrees of displacement and rotation, further participation enters the realm of "trial by battle," and such situations can be considered a relative con-

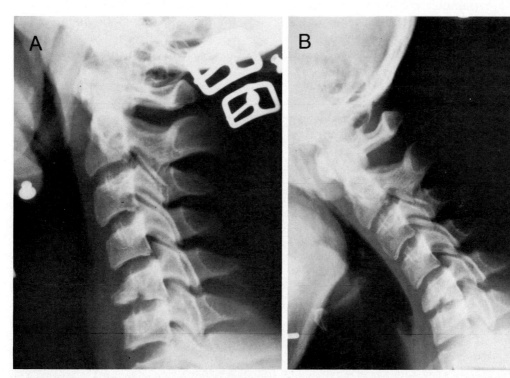

FIG 39–12.
A, lateral-view roentgenogram of the cervical spine taken while in a cervical brace demonstrates a displaced compression fracture of the vertebral body of C5. Of note is the fact that there is no associated angulation, displacement, intervertebral disk space narrowing, facet incongruity, nor fanning of the spinous processes. **B,** lateral flexion view demonstrates pathologic angulation as defined by White et al.[12] There is no translation, disk space narrowing, facet incongruity, nor fanning of the spinous processes, suggesting a stable lesion. The increased angulation is attributed to the deformity of the vertebral body. Assuming that there was no progression of the deformity, evidence of instability, and the patient had a pain-free neck with normal range of motion, this would constitute a relative contraindication to participation in contact activities depending on the player's level, position, and willingness to accept risk of re-injury. (From Torg JS, Glasgow SG: *Clin J Sports Med* 1991; 1:12–27. Used with permission.)

traindication depending on factors such as level of performance, physical habitus, or position played (e.g., interior lineman vs. defensive backs).

B. Fractures: An acute fracture of either the body or posterior elements with or without associated ligamentous laxity constitutes an absolute contraindication to participation.

The following healed, stable fractures in an asymptomatic patient who is neurologically normal and has full range of cervical motion can be considered to have no contraindication to participation in contact activities;

1. Stable compression fractures of the vertebral body without a sagittal component on anterior/posterior roentgenogram and without involvement of either the posterior ligamentous or bony structures (Fig 39–10).

2. A healed stable end plate fracture without a sagittal component on anterior/posterior roentgenograms or involvement of the posterior ligamentous or bony structure (Fig 39–11).

3. Healed spinous process "clay shoveler" fractures.

Relative contraindications apply to the following healed stable fractures in individuals who are asymptomatic, neurologically normal, and have a full pain-free range of cervical motion:

1. Stable displaced vertebral

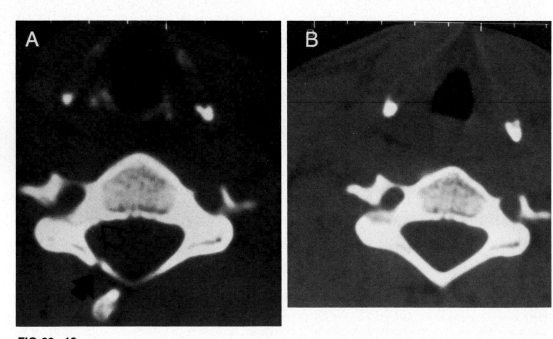

FIG 39–13.
A, CT scan of a vertebral neural arch in the coronal plane, demonstrating a hairline fracture through the lateral mass *(open arrow)* as well as a more evident nondisplaced fracture through the ipsilateral lamina *(closed arrow).* **B,** patient was treated in a halo brace with satisfactory evidence of healing. After immobilization and the return of normal pain-free motion, he was permitted to return to contact activity once rehabilitation was effected with full, pain-free cervical range of motion and paravertebral muscle strength. (From Torg JS, Glasgow SG: *Clin J Sports Med* 1991; 1:12–27. Used with permission.)

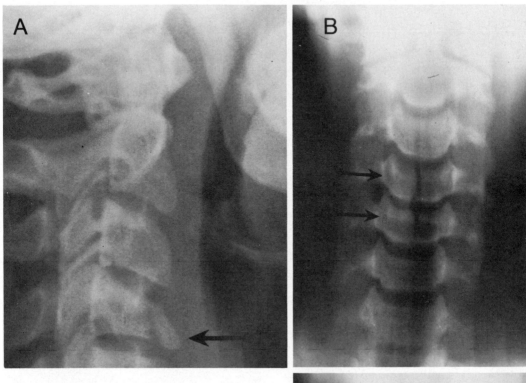

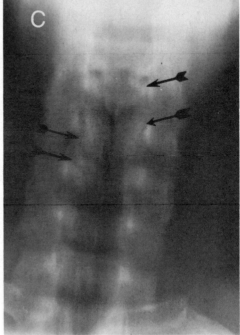

FIG 39–14.
A, lateral view of the cervical spine of a 17-year-old high school football player who was struck on the top of his head with a spring-loaded tackling device demonstrates a so-called "teardrop" fracture of C4 *(arrow)*. **B,** antero-posterior view demonstrates sagittal fractures through the body of C4 and C5 *(arrows)*. **C,** laminagram in the anteroposterior projection through the neural arch demonstrates concomitant fractures through the posterior structures *(arrows)*. Although the youngster remained neurologically intact and went on to successful healing of the fractures, return to contact activities was absolutely contraindicated because of involvement of both anterior and posterior elements. In keeping with Steel's rule of the ring, a sagittal fracture through the vertebral body is associated with a disruption of the neural arch. (From Torg JS, Glasgow SG: *Clin J Sports Med* 1991; 1:12–27. Used with permission.)

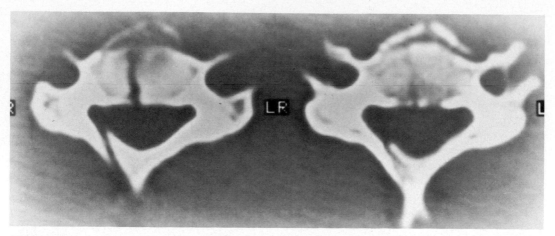

FIG 39–15.
CT scan in the coronal plane of a cervical vertebra of a high school football player injured while spear tackling. Although there was no neurologic involvement, this axial load "teardrop" fracture vividly demonstrates involvement of both the anterior and posterior vertebral structures and constitutes an absolute contraindication to further participation in contact activities. (From Torg JS, Glasgow SG: *Clin J Sports Med* 1991; 1:12–27. Used with permission.)

body compression fractures without a sagittal component on anterior/posterior roentgenograms. The propensity for these fractures to settle with increased deformity must be considered and carefully followed (Fig 39–12).

2. Healed stable fractures involving the elements of the posterior neural ring in individuals who are asymptomatic, neurologically normal, and have a full pain-free range of cervical motion. In evaluating radiographic and imaging studies to find the location and subsequent healing of posterior neural large fractures, it is important to understand that, as pointed out by Steel,[6] a rigid ring cannot break in one location. Thus healing of paired fractures of the ring must be demonstrated (Fig 39–13).

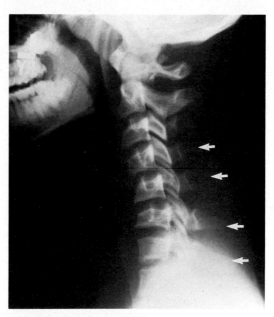

FIG 39–16.
Lateral-view roentgenogram of the cervical spine in the erect neutral position demonstrates an anterosuperior compression defect in the vertebral body of C6 *(large arrow)*. In addition, there is fanning of the C5–C6 spinous process, indicating posterior instability due to disruption of the intraspinous and posterior longitudinal ligaments *(small arrows)*. This situation constitutes an absolute contraindication to contact sports. (From Torg JS, Glasgow SG: *Clin J Sports Med* 1991; 1:12–27. Used with permission.)

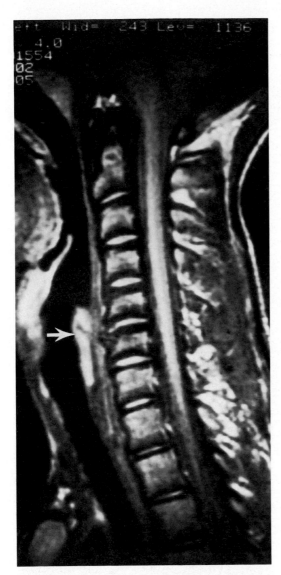

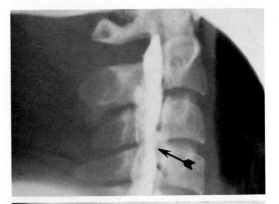

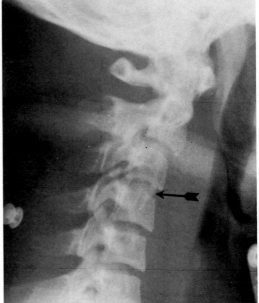

FIG 39–17.

MRI (sagittal) of the cervical spine in a 17-year-old high school football player with a history of prior neck injury. An anterior intervertebral disk herniation with disk space changes at the C5–C6 level is visualized *(arrow)*. At the time of follow-up examination, the youngster was asymptomatic, neurologically negative, and had a pain-free full range of cervical motion. He was permitted to return to contact activities. (From Torg JS, Glasgow SG: *Clin J Sports Med* 1991; 1:12–27. Used with permission.)

FIG 39–18.

A, myelogram demonstrates a herniated nucleus pulposus at C3–C4 *(arrow)* in a 21-year-old college football player who was injured when he struck a blocking dummy with his head. **B,** C3–C4 anterior diskectomy and interbody fusion were performed because of persistent symptoms. Lateral-view roentgenogram 1 week after surgery demonstrated excellent graft placement *(arrow)*. Normally a solid one-level interbody fusion in an individual who was asymptomatic, neurologically negative, and had a full range of motion will allow the individual to return to contact activities. In this particular case, however, the youngster has a congenital narrowing (stenosis) of his cervical canal, had an episode of transient quadriplegia, and demonstrates reversal of the normal cervical lordosis. Because of this he was excluded from further contact activities. (From Torg JS, Glasgow SG: *Clin J Sports Med* 1991; 1:12–27. Used with permission.)

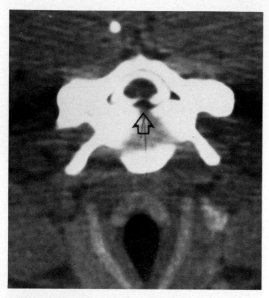

FIG 39–19.
Coronal section of a CT myelogram through the C5–C6 interspace *(arrow)* demonstrates a small central herniation without pressure on the spinal cord. The patient, a high school football player, had had an episode of cervical cord neurapraxia associated with congenital narrowing (stenosis) of the cervical canal. Lateral-view roentgenograms demonstrated reversal of the normal cervical lordosis. In addition, he had a wryneck attitude and decreased neck motion. His situation represents an absolute contraindication to participation in contact activities. (From Torg JS, Glasgow SG: *Clin J Sports Med* 1991; 1:12–27. Used with permission.)

Absolute contraindication to further participation in contact activities exists in the presence of the following fractures:

1. Vertebral body fracture with a sagittal component (Figs 39–14 and 39–15).
2. Fracture of the vertebral body with or without displacement, with associated posterior arch fractures or ligamentous laxity, or both (Fig 39–16).
3. Comminuted fractures of the vertebral body with displacement into the spinal canal.
4. Any healed fracture of either the vertebral body or posterior components with associated pain, neurologic findings, and limitation of normal cervical motion.
5. Healed displaced fractures involving the lateral masses, with resulting facet incongruity.
6. Any injury or lesion with associated MRI evidence of cord defects or swelling.

V. Intervertebral disk injury
There is no contraindication to participation in contact activities in individuals with a healed anterior or lateral disk herniation treated conservatively (Fig 39–17) or those requiring an inter-

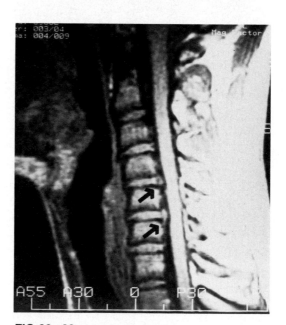

FIG 39–20.
MRI (sagittal) of cervical spine of a 17-year-old high school football player who complained of posterior neck pain while butt blocking, as well as a right unilateral transient radiculopathy or "burner." Visualized are intervertebral disk herniations at C4–C5 and C5–C6, which are indenting the spinal cord at both levels *(arrows)*. Although neurologic examination showed normal findings, the presence of a wryneck attitude, limited neck extension, congenital canal narrowing (stenosis), and reversal of a normal cervical lordosis on roentgenographic examination precluded the youngster from participation in contact sports. (From Torg JS, Glasgow SG: *Clin J Sports Med* 1991; 1:12–27. Used with permission.)

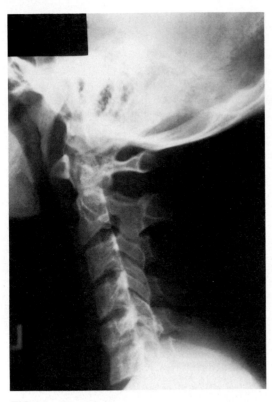

FIG 39–21.
Lateral-view roentgenogram of a 28-year-old professional ice hockey player who underwent a successful one-level interbody fusion at C5–C6 for instability. He subsequently played 2 years without a problem. (From Torg JS, Glasgow SG: *Clin J Sports Med* 1991; 1:12–27. Used with permission.)

vertebral diskectomy and interbody fusion for a lateral or central herniation who have a solid fusion (Fig 39–18), are asymptomatic, neurologically negative, and have a full pain-free range of motion.

A relative contraindication exists in those individuals with either conservatively or surgically treated disk disease with residual facet instability.

An absolute contraindication exists in the following situations:

1. Acute central disk (Fig 39–19).
2. Acute or chronic "hard disk" herniation with associated neurologic findings, pain, or significant limita-

tion of cervical motion (Fig 39–20).
3. Acute or chronic "hard disk" herniation with associated symptoms of cord neurapraxia due to concomitant congenital narrowing "stenosis" of the cervical canal.

VI. Status postcervical spine fusion
   A. A stable one-level anterior or posterior fusion in a patient who is asymptomatic, neurologically negative, pain free, and has a normal range of cervical motion presents no contraindication to continued participation in contact activities (Fig 39–21).
   B. Individuals with a stable two- or three-level fusion who are asymptomatic, neurologically

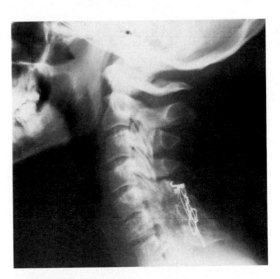

FIG 39–22.
Lateral-view roentgenogram of the cervical spine of a 28-year-old former professional football player who had undergone a C4–C5–C6 posterior fusion for a posttraumatic instability. He subsequently returned to play 2 years of professional football; however, he developed stiffness, neck discomfort, and limited motion. The individual who elects to return to contact activities after more than a two-level fusion must understand that the probability of symptoms resulting from degenerative changes at the articulations above and below the fusion must be considered. (From Torg JS, Glasgow SG: *Clin J Sports Med* 1991; 1:12–27. Used with permission.)

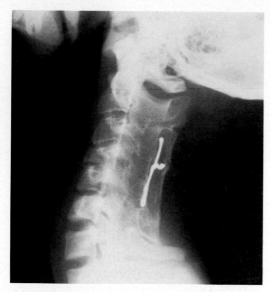

FIG 39–23.
Lateral-view roentgenogram of an 18-year-old patient who had injured his neck playing football at the age of 13. At that time, a three-level posterior fusion and wiring was performed; however, it appears that periosteal stripping of adjacent vertebrae above and below resulted in a five-level fusion. Such a situation is an absolute contraindication to participation in contact activities. (From Torg JS, Glasgow SG: *Clin J Sports Med* 1991; 1:12–27. Used with permission.)

negative, and have a pain-free full range of cervical motion present a relative contraindication (Fig 39–22). Because of the presumed increased stresses at the articulations of the adjacent uninvolved vertebrae and the propensity for the development of degenerative changes at these levels, only rarely should this type of patient be permitted to continue contact activities.

C. In those individuals with more than a three-level anterior or posterior fusion, an absolute contraindication exists as far as continued participation in contact activities (Fig 39–23).

REFERENCES

1. Albright JP, Moses JM, Feldich HG, et al: Nonfatal cervical spine injuries in interscholastic football. *JAMA* 1976; 236:1243–1245.

2. Bailes JE, Hadley MN, Quigley MR: Management of athletic cervical spine and spinal cord injuries. *J Neurosurg* (in press).

3. Eismont FJ, Clifford S, Goldberg M, et al: Cervical sagittal spinal canal size in spine injuries. *Spine* 1984; 9:663–666.

4. Hensinger RN: Congenital anomalies of the odontoid, in The Cervical Spine Research Society Editorial Committee: *The Cervical Spine*, ed 2. Philadelphia, JB Lippincott Co, 1989, pp 248–257.

5. Pizzutillo PD: Klippel-Feil syndrome, in The Cervical Spine Research Society Editorial Committee: *The Cervical Spine*, ed 2. Philadelphia, JB Lippincott Co, 1989, pp 258–271.

6. Steel HH: Rule of the ring. Personal communication.

7. Torg JS, Truex R, Quedenfeld TC: The National Football Head and Neck Injury Registry: Report and conclusions. *JAMA* 1979; 241:1477–1479.

8. Torg JS, Vegso JJ, Sennett B: The National Football Head and Neck Injury Registry; 14 year report on cervical quadriplegia, 1971 through 1985. *JAMA* 1985, 254:3439–3443.

9. Torg JS, Pavlov H, Genuario SE, et al: Neurapraxia of the cervical spinal cord with transient quadriplegia. *J Bone Joint Surg [Am]* 1988; 68A:1354–1370.

10. Torg JS, Vegso JJ, O'Neill J: The epidemiologic, pathologic, biomechanical and cinematographic analysis of football-induced cervical spine trauma. *Am J Sports Med* 1990; 18:50–57.

11. Watkins R: Personal communication.

12. White AA, Johnson RM, Panjabi MM, et al: Biomechanical analysis of clinical stability in the cervical spine. *Clin Orthop* 1975; 109:85.

PART FIVE

Facial, Oral, and Eye Injuries

CHAPTER 40

Diagnosis and Management of Maxillofacial Injuries

Steven D. Handler, M.D.

Sports-related activities account for approximately 12% of maxillofacial injuries seen in large trauma centers.[2, 6] Despite the increased use of face guards and masks, facial and cervical trauma continue to present significant problems in diagnosis and treatment.

GENERAL PRINCIPLES

There are important factors that are common to the management of significant maxillofacial injuries. While these injuries most often occur as isolated trauma, one must be aware of the possibility of associated injuries. Trauma to the chest, abdomen, eye, musculoskeletal system, or the central nervous system may be present in the injured athlete. Attention to these problems often takes priority over the management of the maxillofacial injuries.

Infection is an important factor influencing the ultimate healing of maxillofacial injuries. Antibiotics are frequently given on a prophylactic basis because of the contamination of the wound with intraoral or sinonasal flora and the risk of perichondritis in injuries of the cartilaginous nose and ear.

If the skin has been broken in an injury, protection against tetanus should be assessed. Tetanus toxoid is given if the last immunization was more than 10 years previously (5 years if the wound is deep and contaminated), or if the status of tetanus immunization is unknown. In the latter case, tetanus antitoxin may also be required.

Dental occlusion is an important concept in evaluating jaw fractures and dislocations. In normal occlusion (neutroclusion) (Fig 40–1), the anterior upper incisors are slightly anterior to the lower incisors. The midlines (spaces between central incisors) of the maxillary and mandibular dental arches line up with each other. The outer or buccal cusps of the upper molars are slightly lateral to their lower counterparts. While deviations from these relationships may be normal for any one individual, they may indicate a misalignment resulting from a jaw fracture or a dislocation.

SOFT TISSUE INJURY

Contusions, abrasions, and lacerations comprise the majority of soft tissue injuries of the face and neck. Facial con-

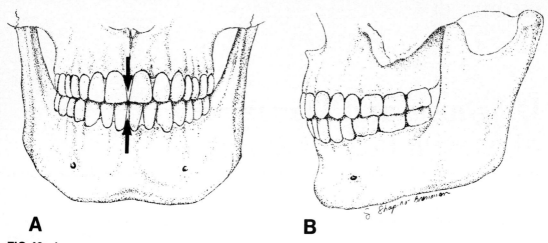

A **B**

FIG 40–1.
Normal occlusion. **A,** frontal view. **B,** lateral view. The midlines of the upper and lower dental arch *(arrows)* line up with each other. The outer cusps of the upper molars are more lateral than those of the mandibular arch, and the maxillary incisors are anterior to the mandibular incisors.

tusions usually resolve spontaneously. However, they must be differentiated from the facial edema associated with a hematoma or underlying facial fracture, which requires further attention and treatment.

Abraded skin surfaces are gently cleansed and antibiotic ointment is applied; the wound is covered with a small protective bandage. Injuries resulting from falls on asphalt or gravel surfaces may cause small foreign bodies to become embedded in the dermal layers. These must be removed to prevent permanent tattooing of the skin. A surgical scrub brush can be helpful in removing these particles. A local or, occasionally, a general anesthetic is necessary to permit adequate cleansing of the area. Grease or oil embedded in the wound may be dissolved and removed with small amounts of ether or acetone.

Linear lacerations, puncture wounds, and avulsion injuries are caused by contact with sharp objects such as ice-skate blades or shoe cleats. Blunt trauma to the cheek or forehead may cause a burst type of laceration, which is frequently stellate in appearance. In evaluating the facial lacerations, one must be certain that

there has not been damage to the deeper structures, such as the parotid duct, facial nerve, vascular structures of the neck, or facial skeleton.

If the laceration is small, superficial, and uncomplicated, the player may continue playing after application of a sterile dressing. Prepare the skin with tincture of benzoin so that the tape will adhere, taking care to protect the eyes and nasal mucous membrane.

Extensive lacerations may require immediate suturing before the player returns to the playing field. Bleeding can usually be stopped with simple pressure on the wound. Ligation of bleeding vessels is rarely required. Injection of 1% lidocaine (Xylocaine) with 1:100,000 epinephrine solution can be used, if necessary, to control bleeding. After adequate cleansing with saline and bland soap, full-thickness lacerations should be reapproximated by suture. Use of small adhesive strips is contraindicated in the definitive treatment of lacerations because the athlete will be expected to practice and play before wound healing occurs. A definitive "plastic" closure using 5-0 nylon suture is preferred in managing facial lacerations. To a large extent suture removal should be determined by the athlete's activity schedule. Care should be taken to avoid premature removal of all sutures and risking the chance of the wound separating. As a general rule, remove every other suture at 4 days and the remainder at 7.

Large or complicated injuries require more immediate attention. The presence of damage to underlying neural, vascular, and bony structures must be determined before definitive repair of these wounds is begun. Any avulsed or loosely pedicled tissue should be preserved and protected for possible inclusion in the final repair. The wound is usually covered with a sterile gauze dressing until the repair can be undertaken. Wound closure should be accomplished with use of standard sterile plastic surgical techniques. Depending on the depth of the injury, a one- or two-layer closure is performed. Lacerations through cartilage require careful approximation of the cartilage edges (trimmed, if necessary) and the overlying perichondrium. This is especially important when reattaching avulsed portions of the nose or ear (Fig 40–2). In large, deep wounds, a small rubber drain may be required to prevent blood accumulation under the skin closure.

If avulsed or pedicled portions of skin cannot be incorporated into the repair, a skin defect can be closed by wide undermining of the wound edges, local flaps, or skin grafts. Skin sutures are generally removed in 5 days to prevent formation of suture track marks. Plastic revision of an unsightly scar may be performed at any time after the injury, but it is usually best to wait at least 1 year to allow for maximal normal healing to occur.

Hematomas of the subcutaneous tissue of the face occur as a result of blunt trauma. Swelling, pain, and discoloration are the common signs of a hematoma. If the hematoma is small and stable, it usu-

ally resolves spontaneously. Larger hematomas often require a drainage procedure. Soon after the injury, a small incision can be made in the skin overlying the hematoma; the jellylike hematoma is then manually expressed from the wound. If one waits until the hematoma liquefies (5 to 7 days), the blood can be aspirated with a syringe and needle. After evacuation of the hematoma, a pressure dressing is usually applied to the wound to prevent reaccumulation of the blood or serum in the hematoma cavity. Progressively enlarging hematomas indicate persistent vascular damage, which may require angiography and surgical exploration.

Hematoma of the Auricle

Hematomas of the auricle pose a special problem that requires prompt attention (Fig 40–3). They result from blunt trauma to the exposed auricle in activities such as wrestling or boxing. The hematoma forms between the perichondrium and the cartilage of the ear. This compromises the blood supply to the cartilage, which is derived from the perichondrium. The hematoma should be aspirated as soon as possible to prevent a cosmetic deformity of the auricle. After aspiration, a contoured pressure dressing of cotton impregnated with mineral oil is applied to the auricle and held in place with a snug head dressing. This forces the perichondrium back against the underlying cartilage, prevents reaccumulation of the hematoma, and reestablishes the blood supply to the cartilage. Alternatively, a cotton ball conforming to the shape of the concha can be held in place by through-and-through bolster sutures. This avoids the use of the more cumbersome head dressing.

During this time of healing, the hematoma is prone to redevelop if repeated trauma occurs.

If the hematoma is not evacuated, the

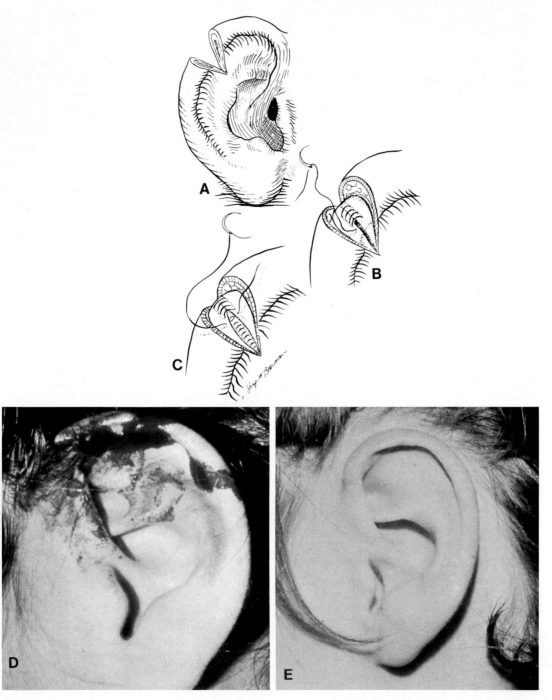

FIG 40–2.
A, auricular cartilage laceration. **B,** careful reapproximation of the cartilage edges. **C,** the overlying perichondrium is closed over the cartilage repair. **D,** acute laceration of ear cartilage. **E,** result of careful reapproximation, 6 weeks later.

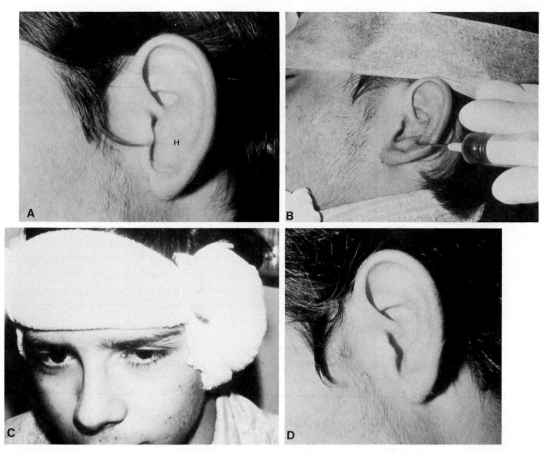

FIG 40–3.
A, hematoma *(H)* of auricle caused by wrestling injury. **B,** hematoma being aspirated. **C,** contoured head dressing to force perichondrium back against auricular cartilage. **D,** good result 4 weeks postinjury.

blood begins to organize, and fibrosis of the overlying skin and pressure necrosis of the auricular cartilage occur. The end result is the "cauliflower ear" (Fig 40–4), in which the delicate cartilaginous contours of the auricle are lost. Treatment of this complication of an auricular hematoma is difficult and usually unsatisfactory.

Intraoral Trauma

Intraoral trauma is usually the result of a self-inflicted bite of the tongue or buccal mucosa. If there has been no damage to any intraoral structures, intraoral lacerations may be managed conservatively. Large, gaping lacerations should be reapproximated to restore normal functional anatomy and to aid the healing process. Through-and-through lacerations of the cheek should be carefully reapproximated with at least a two-layer closure. Large lacerations may require a small rubber drain for 24 hours. Antibiotics are given to prevent infection from intraoral flora.

Significant bleeding may occur with intraoral trauma. In the extreme case in which direct pressure or suture ligature is unsuccessful in stopping the bleeding, ligation of the external carotid artery may be necessary. If the mouth is filled with blood or packing, respiratory embarrassment can occur.

Patients with lacerations of the phar-

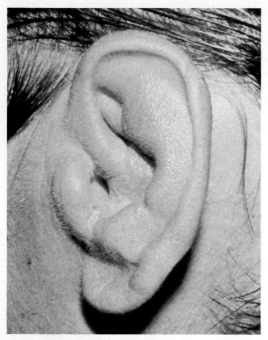

FIG 40–4.
"Cauliflower ear." Thickened and fibrotic ear as a result of cartilage necrosis caused by an untreated auricular hematoma.

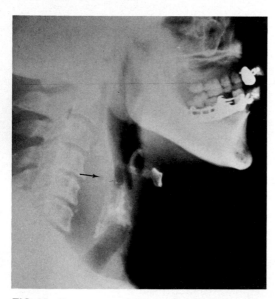

FIG 40–5.
Lateral-view radiograph of neck demonstrating retropharyngeal abscess *(arrow)* that occurred as a complication of a pharyngeal injury.

ynx should be examined for signs of perforation. Odynophagia (pain on swallowing) and cervical crepitus are early signs of a perforated viscus. Lateral-view radiographs of the neck will show free air in the soft tissues. The patient with crepitus is placed on antibiotics and observed in the hospital. While cervical free air often resolves spontaneously, endoscopy and repair of larger perforations may be required. Spiking fevers, dysphagia, and increasing respiratory distress may indicate the development of a lateral or posterior pharyngeal abscess. Lateral-view radiographs of the neck (Fig 40–5) or computed tomography (CT) scans can help to identify and localize the abscess site. Treatment consists of surgical drainage of the abscess, usually by an external approach.

FACIAL FRACTURES

Nasal Trauma

The most common sequela of blunt nasal trauma is epistaxis (nosebleed). This usually occurs from a mucosal laceration in the interior of the nose. Bleeding most often originates from Kiesselbach's plexus, a network of prominent superficial blood vessels on the anterior nasal septum. Most instances of epistaxis stop spontaneously. Pressure applied by squeezing the nostrils together often stops persistent bleeding. Topical vasoconstrictors such as 0.5% phenylephrine hydrochloride (Neo-Synephrine) nose spray may also be useful. Cauterizing the bleeding site or packing the nasal cavity with cotton or petrolatum-impregnated gauze is rarely required for the treatment of any but the most profuse nosebleeds. When the bleeding has stopped and there is no sign of a more serious nasal injury, the player may return to the game.

Nasal fractures account for more than 50% of all maxillofacial fractures that occur from sports-related injuries.[6] While face masks and guards have decreased the incidence of nasal injuries, fractures continue to occur in significant numbers. Direct-blunt trauma may cause a nasal contusion with swelling and ecchymosis, or a fracture of the nasal skeleton. In most instances the diagnosis of nasal fracture is obvious on clinical examination. The nasal bones are deviated to one side or depressed onto the face. Stepoffs (bony irregularities) may be palpated at the fracture site (Fig 40–6). Because of the edema common to facial injuries, however, it may be difficult to determine the presence of a nasal fracture or the degree of nasal deformity at the initial clinical examination. In cases in which a fracture is not clinically apparent, radiographs may be useful in determining the existence of a fracture and the amount of displacement of the nasal bones. Lateral and basal views of the nasal bones and the upright Waters' view of the facial

bones demonstrate the nasal skeleton most effectively (Fig 40–7). However, since many nasal fractures cannot be identified on plain films, diagnosis and treatment of suspected nasal fractures must be made on the basis of clinical examination.

If a nasal fracture is suspected, a complete examination of the nose and surrounding structures must be performed. If present, associated injuries to the orbit must be identified and treated. The epistaxis that often accompanies these injuries usually stops spontaneously or with compression of the anterior nares; rarely is nasal packing necessary. The interior of the nose should be examined to evaluate the nasal septum. The trauma may have caused a fracture or dislocation of the septum, which must be recognized and treated together with any external deformity. If a septal hematoma has occurred, prompt treatment (de-

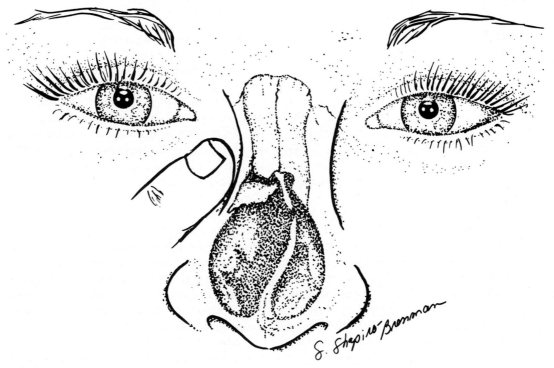

FIG 40–6.
Bony irregularities (stepoffs) can often be palpated at the site of a nasal fracture.

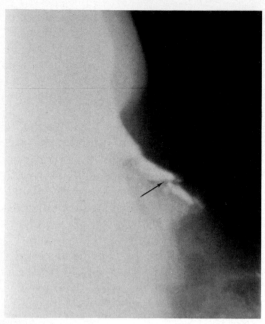

FIG 40–7.
Lateral-view radiograph of the nasal bones demonstrating a nasal fracture *(arrow)*.

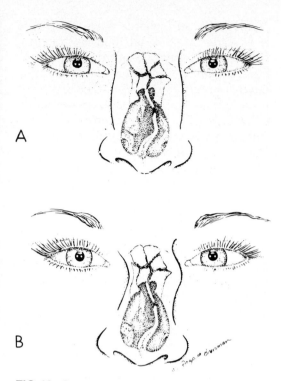

FIG 40–8.
Nasal fracture. **A,** marked edema associated with the injury may mask the deviation of the nasal bones. **B,** deviation of the nasal skeleton becomes manifest when edema subsides, approximately 5 to 7 days.

scribed in a later section in this chapter) must be instituted to prevent permanent damage to the nasal structures. External lacerations can be sutured or taped as necessary.

Reduction of a displaced nasal fracture should be performed within 7 days after the injury. After this time the fibrosis that has occurred makes it difficult to manipulate the fracture fragments. Severely comminuted or compound fractures are repaired as soon as possible. Open reduction with interosseous wires, external splints, and intranasal packing may be necessary to restore normal anatomy in severely injured noses. If the nasal bones are obviously deviated on the initial evaluation and if there is minimal edema of the overlying soft tissue, the reduction can be performed at any time. If there is sufficient edema that the presence of a fracture or the degree of deformity is masked, it is best to wait several days before making a decision regarding the necessity for a nasal reduction (Fig 40–8). If, after the edema subsides, the

fracture appears nondisplaced and has not caused any external deformity, no further treatment is required. If there is a visible external deformity, reduction of the fragments should be undertaken. A local anesthetic is required to permit the instrumentation necessary to replace the nasal bones and septum back into their normal anatomic positions (Fig 40–9). Nasal packing is inserted if there has been significant hemorrhage associated with the reduction, or if internal support is required for the nasal bones. A protective cast of plaster or metal is applied for 1 week, and the athlete should avoid contact sports for 2 to 3 weeks to allow proper healing to occur.

Nasal deformities that persist after the initial reduction, or those that have not been treated within 10 days after the injury, require a formal elective rhinoplastic procedure for their correction.

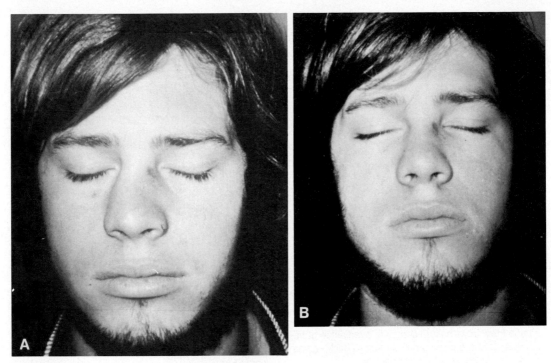

FIG 40–9.
Nasal fracture. **A,** prereduction with obvious deformity of nasal bones. **B,** postreduction showing good cosmetic results.

While this can be performed at any time after the injury, most surgeons prefer to wait at least 6 weeks to allow for complete stabilization of the nasal skeleton.

Septal Hematoma.—Septal hematomas are usually associated with nasal fractures, but they may occur as isolated injuries. The patient is seen initially with unilateral or bilateral collections of blood between the septal cartilage and its overlying mucoperichondrium (Fig 40–10). If a septal hematoma occurs as a result of nasal trauma, it must be recognized early and treated promptly to prevent permanent deformity of the nose (Fig 40–11). Incisions should be made through the mucosa overlying the hematoma, and the clot should be evacuated as soon as possible. A small drain is placed in the wound, and the nasal cavity is packed to force the mucoperichondrium back against the septal cartilage. The packing remains in place 3 to 5 days. If the he-

matoma is not evacuated, necrosis of the septal cartilage with abscess formation can develop. The loss of this portion of the support to the external area of the nose results in a saddlenose deformity

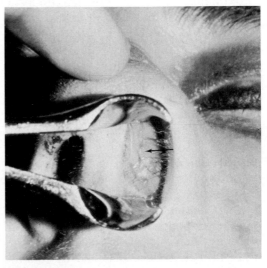

FIG 40–10.
Septal hematoma *(arrow)* must be recognized when evaluating nasal trauma.

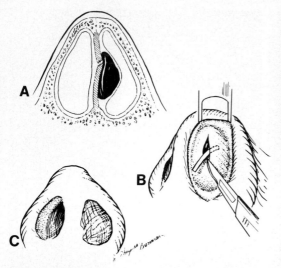

FIG 40–11.
Septal hematoma. **A,** blood collects between the cartilage and overlying mucoperichondrium. **B,** incision in nasal mucosa to drain hematoma. Often a drain is inserted to assure complete evacuation of hematoma. **C,** the perichondrium is forced back against the septal cartilage, with nasal packing.

(Fig 40–12). Late correction of this problem is difficult and often unsatisfactory.

Maxillary Trauma

Zygoma Fractures.—Fractures of the zygoma (or malar bone) account for approximately 10% of the maxillofacial fractures seen in sports injuries. These occur as a result of direct-blunt trauma to the malar eminence or cheekbone. The zygoma usually fractures at its attachments to the temporal, frontal, and maxillary bones (Fig 40–13,A). Because of the three commonly identified fracture sites, this injury is often called a tripod or trimalar fracture. Depending on the type of mechanism of injury, a varying degree of rotation and inward displacement of the fragment is present. While the resultant facial asymmetry and depression of the malar eminence can often be seen on viewing the front of the face, the deformity is usually best detected by looking at both cheeks from the top of the patient's head (Fig 40–13,B).

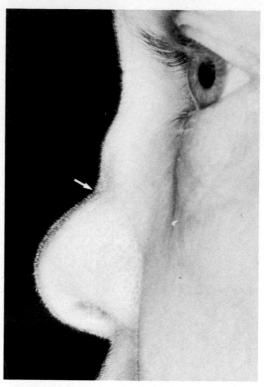

FIG 40–12.
Saddle nose deformity *(arrow)* that occurred as a result of loss of septal cartilage support because of septal hematoma and abscess.

Stepoffs can often be palpated over the fracture sites at the frontozygomatic suture line and at the inferior orbital rim. Intraorbital hypesthesia is usually present after injury to the infraorbital nerve as it exits on the anterior wall of the maxillary sinus. If the orbital floor has been fractured and orbital soft tissue has become entrapped, restriction of ocular mobility may be present.

The edema of the cheek, common in these injuries, may often mask the presence of a facial deformity and prevent recognition of a zygoma fracture. In these cases, radiographs are indispensable in detecting or confirming the presence of a fracture. The sites of fractures and the degree of displacement can be determined best on the Waters' and Caldwell views (Fig 40–14). The maxillary sinus is often opacified, with blood on the side of the

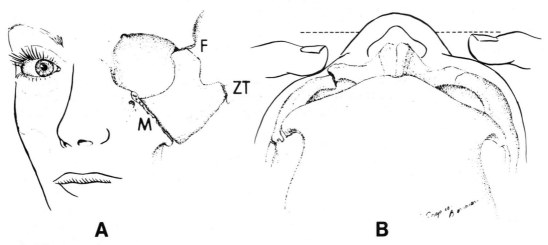

FIG 40–13.
Zygoma (trimalar) fracture. **A,** the zygoma fractures at its attachments to the maxilla *(M)*, frontal bone *(F)*, and the zygomatic process of the temporal bone *(ZT)*. **B,** the best way to evaluate a zygoma fracture is to view both cheeks from the top of the patient's head as one is palpating to determine presence and degree of depression.

injury. This usually indicates that the orbital floor has been fractured, but does not necessarily mean that there is a defect in the floor with herniation of orbital tissue (a blowout fracture). CT scans are usually necessary to demonstrate the bony defect and soft tissue herniation into the sinus that occur in a blowout fracture.

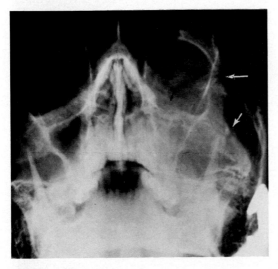

FIG 40–14.
Upright Waters view radiograph demonstrating the three fracture sites *(arrows)* characteristic of a zygoma fracture.

Immediate treatment of these injuries includes assessing the condition of the affected eye and an ophthalmologic consultation, if necessary. Antibiotics are given routinely, because the blood in the maxillary sinus is an excellent culture medium. The decision to explore the fracture may have to be delayed for several days to allow edema to subside so that an accurate determination of the cosmetic deformity can be made. If there is depression of the malar eminence greater than 1 cm, enophthalmos, or restriction of ocular mobility, the fracture should be explored. The fracture is reduced and fixed with interosseous wires or antral packing. The orbital floor is examined and any herniation of orbital soft tissue is reduced. Bony defects should be repaired with bone, alloplastic, or gelatin film implants.[1] The procedure can be performed through external incisions (lower lid and eyebrow), or by means of a sublabial (Caldwell-Luc) approach. The patient should refrain from sports activities for 3 to 4 weeks to allow adequate healing.

Some zygoma injuries may involve fracture of only the zygomatic arch. If these fragments are displaced inwardly, they can impinge on the mandible, resulting in trismus (inability to open the jaw). Depression of the arch may be masked by post-injury edema, and radiographs are often necessary to make the diagnosis. The submental-vertex view is the most suitable for evaluating the zygomatic arch (Fig 40–15). Reduction of this fracture is performed through an incision in the brow or in the buccal mucosa. The arch may require packing for 7 to 10 days to maintain its reduction.

Orbital Blowout Fractures.—Direct trauma to the eye can result in the transmission of the force of the blow through the globe to fracture the bony walls of the orbit. The orbital floor or, less commonly, the medial wall of the orbit, fractures,

leaving the orbital rim intact. Herniation of orbital fat or muscle through the bony defect results in the classic blowout fracture. Enophthalmos, diplopia, and restriction of ocular mobility are the common findings. The management of these injuries is discussed in detail in Chapter 42.

Le Fort Fractures.—Significant force is required to create the maxillary fractures described by René Le Fort in the early 1900s. Because of this, they are uncommon in sports-related injuries. High-velocity impact to the midportion of the face can cause fractures of the maxilla, with varying degrees of deformity and mobility of the maxilla with respect to

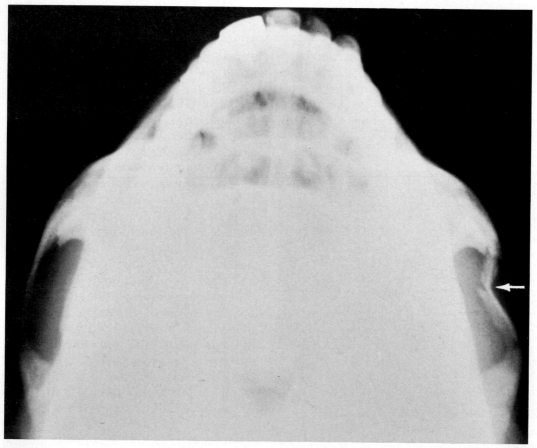

FIG 40–15.
Depressed zygomatic arch fracture *(arrow)* is best seen on a submental-vertex view.

the cranium and upper part of the face (Fig 40–16). The least severe fracture (Le Fort I) is a fracture above the alveolar ridge, thus mobilizing the palate from the face. The more severe fractures (Le Fort II and III) involve more complete craniofacial dissociations. Patients with these injuries at initial examination usually have obviously depressed or mobile facial fragments. They may be in respiratory distress from associated intraoral bleeding and tissue edema. Mobility of the maxilla with respect to the upper part of the face is pathognomonic of a Le Fort fracture (Fig 40–17). Malocclusion is also a common finding on physical examination. In the more severe injuries, cerebrospinal fluid (CSF) rhinorrhea may result from disruption of the cribriform plate.

After the initial evaluation and stabilization of the patient, radiographs (plain and CT scans) are taken to determine the fracture sites and the degree of deformity. Reduction and fixation of the fractures are usually undertaken within the first 7 days. Intermaxillary fixation is maintained for 6 weeks, and during this period the player should avoid contact sports. The CSF rhinorrhea associated with Le Fort III fractures usually resolves with conservative treatment. The player is hospitalized and placed at bed rest with his head elevated. Persistent leaks require formal exploration and repair of cribriform plate defects.

Sinus Fractures

Fractures of the facial bones that extend into the paranasal sinuses present special problems in diagnosis and management. Fractures of the walls of the maxillary sinus can occur as isolated entities or as a part of a maxillofacial injury

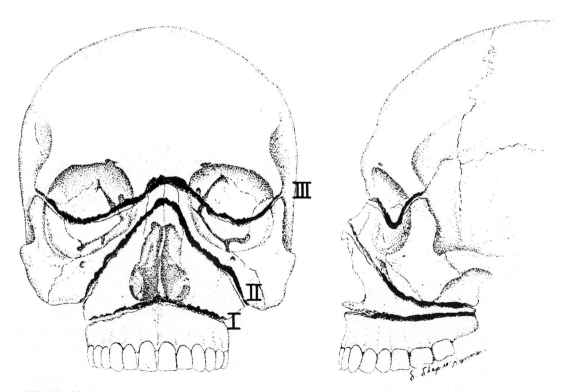

FIG 40–16.
Le Fort maxillary fractures are classified by type and severity: *I*, involves separation of palate from midportion of face; *II*, fracture extends above nasal pyramid; *III*, complete craniofacial dissociation.

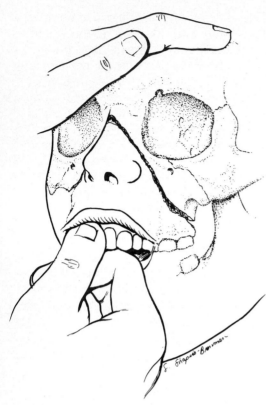

FIG 40–17.
With the head stabilized mobility of the maxilla is
pathognomonic of a Le Fort fracture.

discussed previously, for example, zygomatic or blowout fractures. Blunt or penetrating trauma to the cheek can fracture
the anterior or lateral walls of the maxillary sinus. The patient is seen initially
with pain and swelling of the anterior aspect of the cheek. Crepitus may be
present in soft tissue overlying the sinus.
Radiographs are usually needed to confirm the diagnosis and to rule out other
injuries. Fractures of the maxillary sinus
walls are best seen on the Waters', Caldwell, or lateral views of the face. The
maxillary sinus usually appears opacified, because it is filled with blood. Often
air can be seen in the soft tissues of the
cheek or orbit.

If there has been no damage to surrounding structures such as the orbit or
the zygoma, treatment is conservative.

Antibiotics are given to prevent infection
in the blood-filled sinus. The patient is
observed for signs of increasing swelling
or tenderness that could indicate development of a facial abscess. Under normal
circumstances the athlete can resume his
activities within a week, depending on
the degree of his discomfort. Long-term
complications of these fractures, such as
chronic sinusitis with obstruction of the
maxillary sinus or osteomyelitis of the
maxilla, are uncommon.

Fractures of the frontal sinus often
present significant immediate and long-
term problems. Blunt or sharp trauma to
the forehead can fracture the anterior or
posterior sinus walls. Pain and swelling
of the forehead are the most common
findings on physical examination. The
deformity of the forehead caused by a depressed frontal sinus fracture may be
masked by the immediate postinjury
edema. Epistaxis frequently accompanies
these injuries. Clear fluid draining from
the nose may be CSF, indicating a fracture of the posterior table of the frontal
sinus or the cribriform plate. Initial evaluation should involve inspection for associated cranial or orbital injuries. Radiographs are usually necessary to make the
diagnosis of a frontal sinus fracture. Posteroanterior and lateral views in the upright position are the most helpful (Fig
40–18). In addition to the bony fractures,
opacification of the sinus or an air fluid
level is usually seen.

Management of these fractures depends on the degree of cosmetic deformity and the presence of associated injuries.[5] A fracture through the posterior
wall of the frontal sinus allows communication between the sinus and the anterior cranial fossa, and should be treated
as a compound skull fracture. The patient
should be hospitalized and kept at bed
rest, with his head elevated, to decrease
CSF rhinorrhea. He is then observed for
signs of meningitis or other intracranial
problems. The sinus should be explored

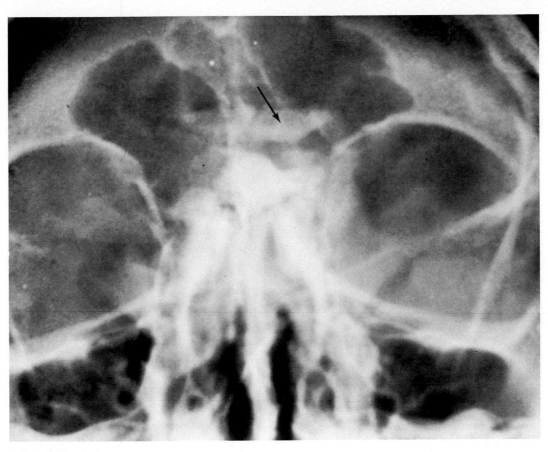

FIG 40–18.
Caldwell view of the face demonstrating frontal sinus fracture *(arrow)*.

if there is a cosmetic deformity of the forehead, a posterior table fracture, or possible injury to the nasofrontal duct. Exploration can be undertaken through a brow incision or by elevating a large scalp flap downward from above. The bony fragments are reduced and held in place with interosseous wires, if necessary, and dural lacerations are repaired. If the fracture has damaged the nasofrontal duct, thus impairing drainage of the sinus, the sinus should be stripped of all mucosa and the cavity obliterated with abdominal wall fat. This is done to prevent late complications of nasofrontal duct obstruction, such as chronic sinusitis, osteomyelitis of the frontal bone, or mucocele formation.

The ethmoid sinuses are spared from direct trauma by their relatively protected position on the face. However, they can be injured by forces transmitted through more exposed structures, such as the orbit and the nasal bones. The presenting signs of ethmoid fractures are swelling and palpable crepitus in the medial portion of the orbit (Fig 40–19). This results from escape of air from the ethmoid sinuses into the adjacent soft tissues of the orbit and face. If there has not been any associated injury to the nose or eye, fractures of the ethmoid sinus are managed conservatively. The patient is placed on antibiotics and observed for signs of orbital infection. He should be cautioned not to blow his nose until the crepitus resolves (about 5 to 7 days). By blowing his nose he could force more air

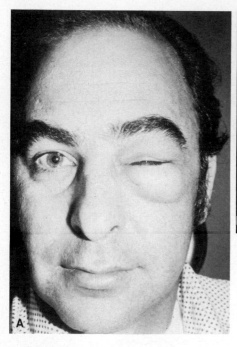

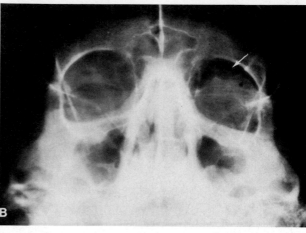

FIG 40–19.
A, patient with swelling and palpable crepitus in orbit caused by ethmoid sinus fracture. **B,** Waters' radiograph demonstrating air *(arrow)* in the orbit as a sign of this patient's ethmoid fracture.

and bacteria-laden sinus secretions into the facial soft tissues, thus increasing the risk of an orbital infection. Contact sports should be avoided for about the same length of time.

Mandibular Trauma

Fractures.—Mandibular fractures account for approximately 10% of maxillofacial fractures seen in sports-related accidents.[6] Most commonly the athlete falls and strikes the mandible against a hard playing surface. Occasionally the fracture results from contact with another player or equipment. Pain and swelling of the lower part of the face are the usual presenting symptoms. If the fracture extends through the intraoral mucosa, as almost all of them do, bleeding may occur from the mouth. The patient complains that his bite feels uncomfortable and that he has pain when attempting to move his jaw. Malocclusion and abnormal mobility of the mandible are the most common findings on physical examination.

If a mandibular fracture has occurred, airway management is the most impor-

tant aspect of the immediate treatment. Blood, avulsed teeth or fragments of teeth, and saliva should be carefully cleared from the mouth. Prolapse of the tongue with airway obstruction often oc-

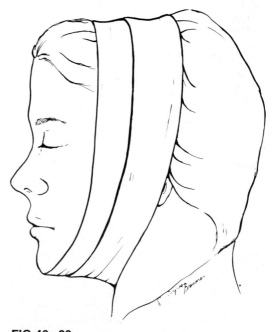

FIG 40–20.
Circumferential head dressing (Barton bandage) is helpful in restricting jaw movement and minimizing pain associated with mandibular fractures.

curs as a result of mandibular arch instability. The mobile jaw fragments may require support either manually or with a snug head dressing (Barton bandage) (Fig 40–20). This dressing also helps to reduce the pain associated with these frac-tures by restricting jaw movement. Radiographs are extremely useful in evaluating these fractures. Plain mandibular views show most fractures well, but panoramic dental films (Fig 40–21) may be necessary to evaluate the position of the frag-

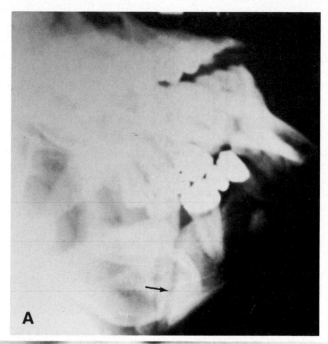

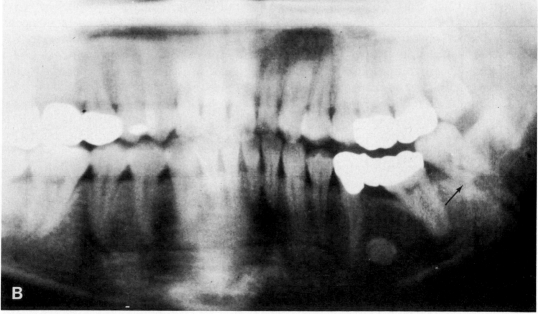

FIG 40–21.
A, angle fracture of mandible *(arrow)* is well seen in standard view of mandible. **B,** panoramic dental film is necessary to detect fractured tooth root *(arrow)*, necessitating extraction before reduction of fracture.

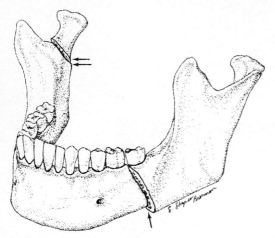

FIG 40–22.
The arch-shaped structures of the mandible are responsible for the common occurrence of two fracture sites in traumatic injuries. This figure illustrates one such injury with a body fracture *(arrow)* and contralateral subcondylar fracture *(double arrows).*

ments and the status of the involved teeth.

The parts of the mandible most frequently fractured are the subcondylar area (40%), body (20%), angle (20%), and symphysis (15%).[3] Because of the structure of the mandibular arch, fractures often occur at two sites. Therefore, when a mandibular fracture has been identified, it is important to search for a second fracture site (Fig 40–22).

If there is no compromise of the airway, the patient can be managed initially with a liquid diet. Since these fractures almost always extend through the oral mucosa or the periodontal ligament surrounding a tooth root, and are therefore compound fractures, antibiotics are given routinely. Simple, uncomplicated fractures of the subcondylar area may be managed with soft diet alone if the patient has good occlusion (Fig 40–23). This continues for about 6 weeks until the patient can move his jaw normally

without pain. If fragments are displaced by their attached muscles or if there is evidence of malocclusion, stabilization of the fracture by open or closed reduction and placement of intermaxillary fixation becomes necessary (Fig 40–24). Fractured or devitalized teeth in the fracture line are removed. Dental splints can be utilized to provide better fixation in occlusion, especially in patients with poor dentition. Fixation is maintained for 6 weeks. The athlete can resume sports activities once he is out of fixation and there is good evidence that the fracture has healed.

Mandibular trauma may transmit significant forces through the condylar joint and into the external auditory canal. Patients with mandibular fractures should have a thorough examination of the external ears to determine if the bony ear canal has been fractured. Packing of the ear canal may be required to stabilize the bony fragments and to keep the canal patent.

Dislocation of the Mandible.—If the mandible is suddenly depressed in a sports activity, dislocation can occur. The mandibular condyle comes to rest anterior to the articular eminence of the glenoid fossa and is held there by spasm of the masticatory muscles. The chin tends to deviate to the side opposite the dislocation, and the patient is unable to close his mouth (open bite deformity) (Fig 40–25,A). Radiographs are necessary to differentiate this condition from a fractured mandible or to determine if a fracture has accompanied a traumatic dislocation.

The mandible should be repositioned as soon as possible (Fig 40–25,B). Postinjury edema and muscle spasm may make

FIG 40–23 (facing page).
A, subcondylar fracture *(arrow)* in a patient with good occlusion. **B,** fracture site healed after 6 weeks on a soft diet.

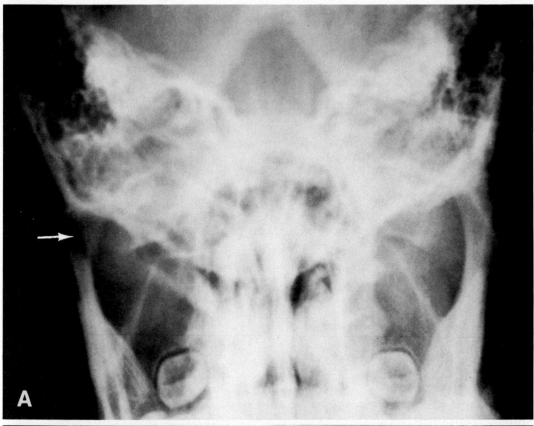

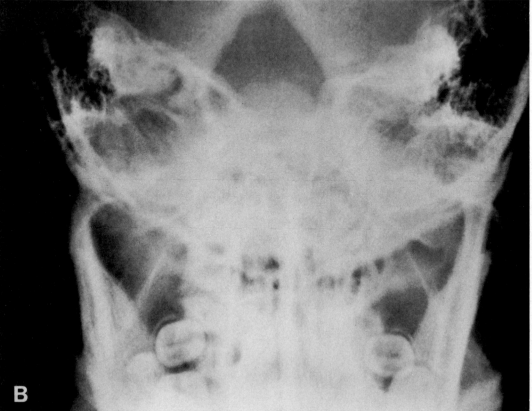

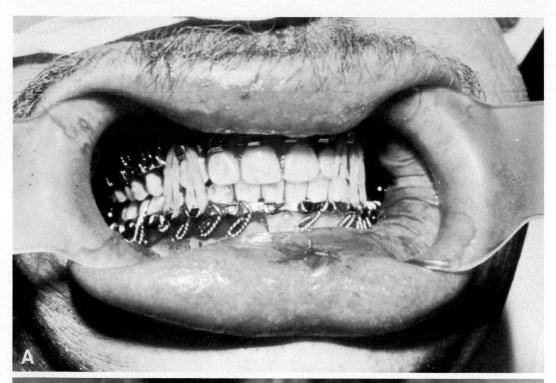

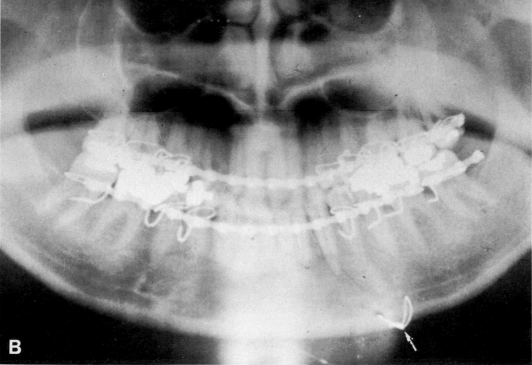

FIG 40–24.
A, arch bars and rubber bands are used to provide intermaxillary fixation. **B,** radiograph showing intermaxillary fixation and interosseous wire *(arrow)*.

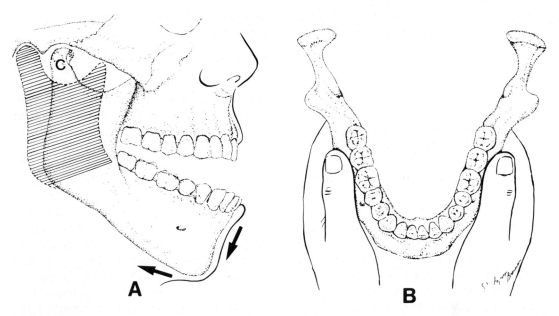

FIG 40–25.
Dislocation of mandible. **A,** mandibular condyle *(C)* is displaced anteriorly from its normal position *(striped lines)*. **B,** to replace mandible, physician's hands are placed on mandible as shown, and downward and backward forces are exerted (indicated in **A**) to allow the condyle to slip back into its normal position.

this difficult to perform without some form of muscle relaxant, sedative, or, occasionally, a general anesthetic. The patient is usually in the sitting position with his head supported. The physician's thumbs are placed on the mandibular body lateral to the lower molars, and his fingers grasp the mandibular body. Wrapping the physician's thumbs with cloth helps to prevent injury to his hand. The posterior portion of the mandible is depressed downward and posteriorly so that the condyle can slip under the articular eminence and return to the glenoid fossa. Once the reduction is accomplished, the patient is placed on a soft diet and should refrain from contact sports for 2 to 3 weeks to allow healing of the muscles and ligaments that were stretched during the dislocation. Chronic or recurrent dislocations may require formal surgical procedures, such as placement of intermaxillary fixation or exploration of the temporomandibular joint.

NECK TRAUMA

Blunt Trauma

Blunt trauma can cause a hematoma in the soft tissues of the neck. When first seen by the physician, the patient has a painful, ecchymotic swelling that appears soon after the injury. Initially, one should evaluate the size, location, and progression of the hematoma and the patency of the airway. Small, stable hematomas are usually caused by venous tears and are self-limited. They resolve spontaneously as the blood is resorbed. Larger hematomas may require evacuation to aid in their resolution. The clot can be expressed out through a small incision made over the hematoma, or the hematoma can be aspirated after the clot has liquefied. Progressively enlarging hematomas may endanger the airway, and usually require surgical intervention. After arteriography to determine the source of the hemorrhage, neck exploration and ligation of the bleeding vessel are indicated. An anteriovenous fistula may occur as a late complication of large vascular injuries if they are not recognized and repaired early.

Lacerations

Lacerations of the neck may range from small superficial cuts to large, gaping wounds. They are often caused by contact with sharp playing equipment such as ice skates. The diagnosis is usually obvious on initial examination. The initial evaluation should include a search for associated injuries of the cervical spine, upper airway, and underlying vascular and neural structures. Hemorrhage is usually mild in nature and stops spontaneously, or with mild pressure. Rarely is the bleeding so brisk that surgical exploration and ligation of a small vessel are required. If the laceration is small and uncomplicated, the wound edges may be reapproximated with Steri-Strips, and the player can resume his activities. Larger lacerations may require formal repair as described in the section on soft tissue injury.

Any laceration or puncture wound that penetrates the platysma muscle can potentially produce an associated neural, vascular, or aerodigestive tract injury. While some authors recommend routine surgical exploration of these wounds, I believe that each case should be individually evaluated and treated.[4] If the injury is not associated with neural deficits, absent or diminished pulses, expanding hematoma, or signs of injury to the aerodigestive tract, it may be repaired without formal surgical exploration. If any of the conditions mentioned are present, further evaluation by angiography, endoscopy, and neck exploration may be indicated. The wounds are generally closed in layers, and a small rubber drain is utilized. Unless the wound is in continuity with the aerodigestive tract, antibiotics are not given.

INJURIES TO THE UPPER AERODIGESTIVE TRACT

Blunt Trauma

Blunt trauma to the aerodigestive tract occurs most frequently in high-velocity sports such as hockey. Direct trauma to the exposed neck can crush the larynx and upper part of the trachea and cause airway embarrassment. The esophagus is rarely involved in these injuries. At initial presentation, the athlete with significant injury to the larynx has neck pain, odynophagia (pain on swallowing), and dyspnea. Hemoptysis usually accompanies laryngeal trauma. The voice can be normal, hoarse, or absent (aphonia). The severity of respiratory obstruction is dependent on the type and extent of the injury. Ecchymosis and crepitus are usually noted over the anterior aspect of the neck. The absence of the normal prominence of the thyroid cartilage ("Adam's apple") indicates a significant crush injury of the larynx (Fig 40–26). In severe injuries in which airway obstruction is complete, endotracheal intubation and even emergency tracheostomy may become lifesaving maneuvers in the first few minutes after the injury.

Once the diagnosis of blunt trauma to the larynx or trachea has been made, the patient should be transferred to a medical facility for further evaluation and treatment. Radiographs (plain films and CT) are useful in detecting the presence and degree of injuries to the larynx or esophagus (Fig 40–27). Otolaryngologic consultation should be obtained to evaluate the status of the airway and vocal cord function. Nondisplaced laryngeal fractures or small hematomas of the vocal cords may not require any further intervention. The patient should be hospitalized and observed for development of respiratory distress. Intubation or tracheostomy may become necessary because post-injury edema can obstruct the upper airway. More severe injuries require en-

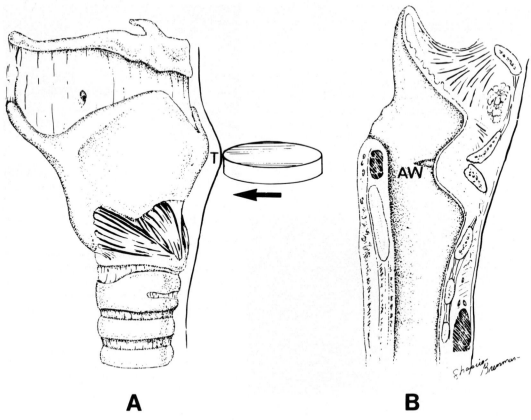

A   **B**

FIG 40–26.
Blunt trauma to the larynx. **A,** normal anterior prominence of the thyroid cartilage *(T)* before trauma. **B,** acute trauma with laryngeal fracture. Note depression of cartilage and absence of thyroid prominence. Airway *(AW)* is markedly decreased.

doscopy to evaluate the integrity of the larynx and the upper part of the trachea. Formal neck exploration and fixation of laryngeal fragments may be necessary in the more comminuted or depressed fractures. The patient is placed on antibiotics, and the neck wounds are routinely drained. While many with mild injuries may return to activities within 6 to 8 weeks, those with a history of severe laryngeal injuries should probably refrain from contact sports in the future.

Penetrating Trauma

Penetrating injuries to the aerodigestive tract in the neck are uncommon. They are freak accidents, such as when a player is "speared" in the neck by a sharp piece of sports equipment. The player with this injury complains of neck pain, dysphagia, and, occasionally, dyspnea. Physical examination reveals crepitus in the soft tissues of the neck, and the player often has hemoptysis. Changes in the voice, such as hoarseness or aphonia, are indicators of laryngeal trauma. Patency of the upper airway is the prime concern, and intubation or tracheostomy may be required. Secretions should be gently cleared from the mouth and pharynx, and the player is transferred to a medical facility for observation and treatment. Lateral-view radiographs of the neck often demonstrate free air in the soft tissues, indicating perforation of the aero-

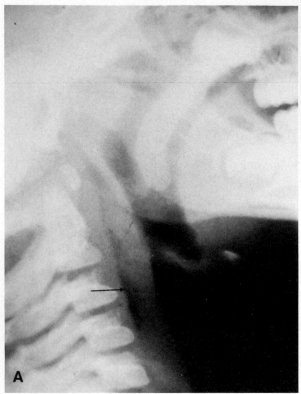

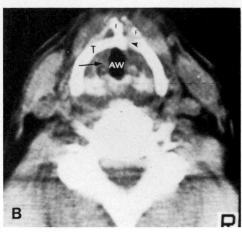

FIG 40–27.
Laryngeal injury. **A,** lateral-view radiograph of neck demonstrating free air in the neck *(arrow)* as a result of laryngeal disruption. **B,** horizontal CT scan of same patient showing fracture of the thyroid cartilage *(T)* with multiple fragments *(f).* Airway *(AW)* is markedly compromised by the edema and hemorrhage caused by this injury. (CT scan courtesy of Anthony Mancuso, M.D., and William Hanafee, M.D., University of California, Los Angeles Department of Radiology.)

digestive tract. The severity of the injury determines the treatment, which may consist of close observation, endoscopy, or surgical exploration and repair of the perforation.

REFERENCES

1. Canalis RF, et al: Complications of orbital floor implants. *Transactions of the Pacific Coast Otoophthalmolic Society* 1978; 61:81.

2. Converse JM: *Surgical Treatment of Facial Injuries,* ed 3. Baltimore, Williams & Wilkins, 1974.

3. Dingman RO, Natvig R: *Surgery of Facial Fractures.* Philadelphia, WB Saunders Co, 1964.

4. May M: Penetrating neck wounds. *Laryngoscope* 1975; 85:57.

5. Newman MH, Travis LW: Frontal sinus fractures. *Laryngoscope* 1975; 85:1.

6. Schultz RC: *Facial Injuries,* ed 2. St Louis, Mosby–Year Book, 1977.

CHAPTER 41

Diagnosis and Management of Oral Injuries

Martin S. Greenberg, D.D.S.
Philip S. Springer, D.M.D.

DENTAL INJURIES

Injuries to the teeth are common in sports. The picture of a smiling face devoid of maxillary anterior teeth has become synonymous with hockey, although elbows in basketball, high-bouncing ground balls in baseball, fists, knees, hardwood floors, and pavements are all common contributors to dental injury and malformation. Approximately 15% of school-children have significant dental injuries before the age of 18.[3] The major causes of these injuries are sports, games, and bicycle riding. Horseback riding is also a significant cause of dental injuries in areas where this activity is common. Studies performed to date show that these injuries occur twice as often in male individuals.[4] However, with the recent increase in female participation in sports, including contact sports, one can expect an increase in the number of women receiving dental injuries.

In Hawke and Nicholes'[11] study of rugby players, 62% interviewed had a history of oral injury. The most common, which occurred in 50% of all rugby players, was injury to the lip. The second most common, which occurred in 26% of the players, was dental injury requiring the services of a dentist. About one half of these dental injuries were accompanied by lip injuries. Tongue injuries occurred in about 21% of the players.

Depending on the direction of the trauma, injuries to the teeth can be divided into two categories. Direct trauma to the teeth by a stick, ball, or bat frequently fractures the maxillary anterior teeth. Direct trauma to the lip reduces the frequency of tooth fracture by cushioning the blow, but increases the incidence of luxation of the tooth.

Indirect trauma is caused by upward force on the mandible. This occurs in boxing or sports in which falling is frequent, such as football, lacrosse, or hockey. In these instances, the mandibular teeth are suddenly forced into the maxillary teeth, causing injury to the posterior teeth, which support the bite. Teeth with large fillings or previous root canal treatment are particularly susceptible to fractures from indirect trauma.

Dental injuries can occur alone or in conjunction with other injuries to the maxillofacial region. Multiple injuries are particularly common in high-speed sports, such as hockey, skiing, or auto racing.

The physician or dentist attending

635

the injured athlete with an obvious dental injury must consider other maxillofacial injuries. Limitation in opening the mandible or malocclusion may indicate a fracture of the mandible, maxilla, zygomatic arch, or injury to the temporomandibular joint. The patient should be examined for anesthesia or paresthesia of the lip or cheek and mobility of jaw fragments. Examination for a maxillary fracture should include placing a finger in the middle of the hard palate and pressing it in all directions while looking for both intraoral and extraoral mobility. The presence of diplopia often indicates a fracture involving the orbit. Mobility of a single tooth may indicate a root fracture or avulsion of the tooth. Adjacent teeth moving together suggest a fracture of the alveolar bone. If a tooth fracture is accompanied by an adjacent laceration of the lip, the fragments of the tooth should be accounted for. If this cannot be done, a roentgenogram of the lip should be taken to look for fragments.

Avulsed Teeth

Avulsed teeth that have been completely extruded from the socket because of trauma can often be found lying in the patient's mouth or on the ground (Fig 41–1). These teeth can be saved, but speed is an important factor. Studies of reimplantation of avulsed teeth conclude that the sooner the tooth is reimplanted, the higher the success rate, and that teeth not reimplanted within 2 hours of avulsion have little chance for successful reimplantation.[4] The team physician or trainer should institute treatment immediately by replacing the tooth in the socket instead of waiting for a dentist.

If a tooth has been out of the socket for less than 2 hours, wash the tooth with cool saline and attempt to replace it in its normal position in the socket. If the tooth has been positioned properly, the patient should be able to close his teeth normally. If the patient's teeth close on the reimplanted tooth first, it has not been completely seated in the socket. Avoid touching the roots. If the tooth cannot be replaced by gentle pressure, place it under the patient's tongue and take him to a dentist skilled in emergency dental procedures as soon as possible. While waiting, do not allow the tooth to dry since this decreases the chance of a successful result.

Recent evidence indicates that root canal therapy should not be attempted until 1 to 2 weeks after the tooth has been reimplanted in the socket. Root canal therapy performed in the dentist's hands before reimplantation reduces the chance of success. Studies also indicate that rigid fixation of avulsed teeth for more than 1 week increases root resorption. Therefore, wire or acid etch resin splints should be removed 7 days after reimplantation, and root canal therapy should be started within the next week.

In young patients whose teeth have opened, developing apices, normal circulation may be restored after implantation, and root canal treatment may not be necessary (Fig 41–2). In older patients root canal treatment is done, in most cases, to prevent root resorption and periapical abscesses.

Luxated Teeth

A luxated tooth is one that has been displaced from its normal position within the socket. The tooth may be intruded, extruded, or laterally displaced (Fig 41–3). Extruded teeth are those that have been partially displaced outward from the socket. If this occurs during a sporting event in which a team dentist is not present, the team trainer or physician should not wait for a dentist to perform initial treatment. An immediate attempt should be made to place the tooth into its normal position in the socket with firm finger pressure. The patient should then

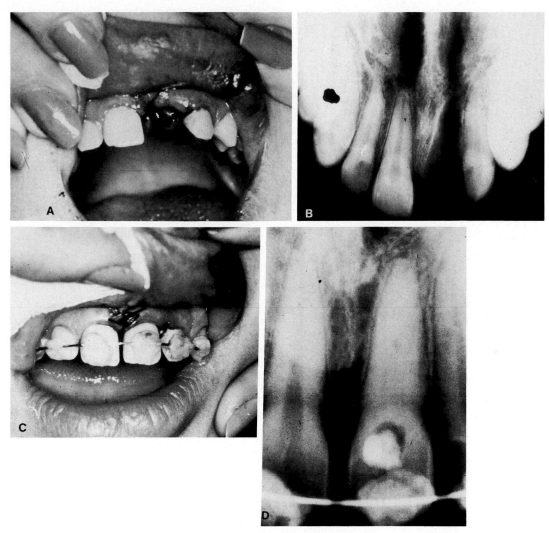

FIG 41–1.
A, a 9-year-old girl tripped while playing softball. She avulsed a maxillary central incisor and sustained lacerations of her lip and gingiva. **B,** radiograph of avulsion site. **C,** incisor reimplanted and stabilized with wire and acid etch resin. **D,** radiograph of reimplanted incisor.

be taken to the dentist for final treatment. The dentist should take a dental radiograph to ensure that the tooth has been completely replaced, and then firmly splint the tooth to the surrounding teeth with acid etch resin. If personnel administering dental first aid are unable to replace the tooth in the socket completely, firmer pressure requiring local anesthesia may be necessary. Occasionally a blood clot forms between the apex of the tooth

and the alveolar bone. In these cases the tip of the root may be removed or a surgical vent may be cut in the gingiva and the alveolar bone to the apex of the tooth. This releases the blood clot, enabling the tooth to be pushed back to its normal position. The tooth should then be splinted in place. Luxated teeth that are not accompanied by an alveolar fracture should be splinted for 2 to 3 weeks, while luxated teeth complicated by alveolar bone

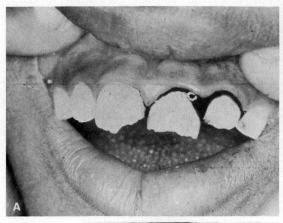

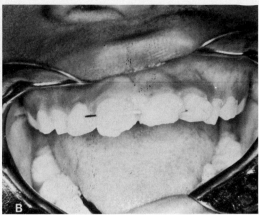

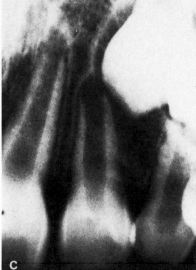

FIG 41–2.
A 9-year-old boy was hit in the mouth with a ball while playing baseball. The right maxillary central and lateral incisors were avulsed and chipped. The left maxillary central incisor was chipped. **A,** avulsed teeth reimplanted with finger pressure. **B,** wire and resin splint placed. **C,** radiograph of root canal with wide-opened apex. Reimplanted quickly, these teeth may not require root canal treatment.

fractures should be splinted for 4 to 8 weeks, depending on the extent of the fracture. During this time, the tooth should be completely out of occlusion, even if it is necessary to relieve the bite on the opposing tooth with a dental stone or bur.

The same principles apply to laterally luxated teeth. The teeth should be replaced into their normal position in the dental arch, splinted in place, and ground away from direct biting forces.

Teeth that are intruded, or driven further into the socket by injury, should be treated in a different manner. No immediate treatment is necessary at the time of injury. No attempt should be made to suddenly pull intruded teeth into their correct position. This maneuver often results in the permanent loss of the tooth. Some intruded teeth will reerupt on their own with no treatment. If several weeks pass and no movement of the tooth is noted, slow movement with orthodontic appliances should be considered.

Patients with a history of luxated teeth should be examined clinically and radiographically at 3-month intervals for at least 2 years after the injury to ensure that there is no evidence of pulpal necrosis or root resorption. Teeth with pulpal necrosis or root resorption require endodontic therapy.

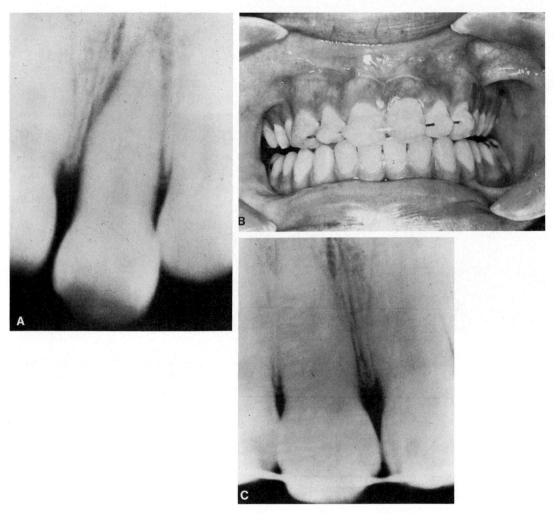

FIG 41–3.
A 19-year-old man with an extruded, subluxated maxillary central incisor. **A,** radiograph of extruded incisor. **B,** clinical photograph of tooth stabilized with wire and resin. **C,** radiograph of proper placement of tooth.

Alveolar Fractures

Alveolar fractures can be diagnosed clinically. The diagnosis is obvious when two or more adjacent teeth move as a unit. Proper treatment for alveolar fracture is early reduction of the fracture by manual pressure on the displaced teeth and bone and immediate rigid splinting of the teeth with wires or acid etch resin for 4 weeks (Fig 41–4). Unsuccessful treatment is directly related to delay in stabilizing the fragments. Continued mobility of the fragments compromises the blood supply to the teeth, and causes necrosis. Andreasen[2] studied a large series of alveolar fractures; pulpal necrosis requiring root canal treatment was necessary in 75% of the cases. Pulpal necrosis did not occur in those patients in whom the fragment was immediately reduced and rigidly splinted. Root resorption occurred in a little more than 10% of the cases of alveolar fracture. Unlike root resorption resulting from avulsion, root resorption in patients with alveolar fractures appears to be self-limiting and superficial.

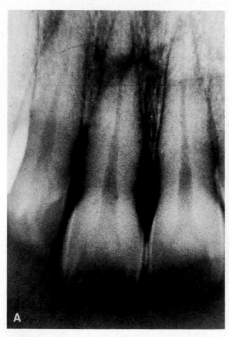
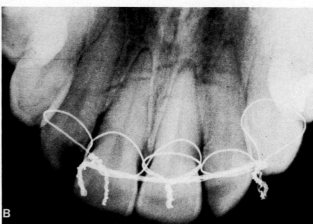

FIG 41–4.
A 35-year-old woman was hit in the mouth by a ball while a spectator at a baseball game. **A,** radiograph demonstrating alveolar fracture of maxillary anterior region and fracture of apical one third of maxillary central incisor root. **B,** teeth and fragment stabilized with ligation wire and quick-cure acrylic.

Tooth Trauma Without Fracture or Displacement

When a tooth is traumatized without fracture, check for mobility to rule out subluxation or alveolar fracture. If the findings in the examination are negative, no immediate treatment is necessary, but the patient should be referred to a dentist skilled in managing these injuries for adequate follow-up. Trauma to the tooth may lead to bleeding into the pulp chamber, and result in necrosis. This problem may not become apparent for several weeks or even months. Signs and symptoms of pulpal necrosis resulting from trauma are increased sensitivity of the tooth to heat or cold, and sensitivity to percussion, discoloration, and swelling above the apex of the tooth.

There are several radiographic signs of pulpal necrosis. Radiolucency at the apex of the tooth indicates granuloma or cyst formation. In younger patients there

occurs interruption of normal root development. An increase in odontoblastic activity in response to inflammation results in obliteration of the pulp. External root resorption is caused by traumatic stimulation of osteoclastic activity in the periodontal membrane. Internal root resorption, on the other hand, is caused by osteoclastic activity within the pulp chamber.

Proper treatment for external and internal root resorption after trauma is repeated treatment with calcium hydroxide into the root canal at monthly intervals followed by careful completion of root canal therapy with a gutta-percha filling.

Crown Fractured, Pulp Not Exposed

Fractures of the enamel cause few or no symptoms; however, sharp edges of the tooth should be smoothed to prevent further injury to the lips and oral mucosa. Fractures that involve the dentin cause pain and should be referred to a dentist. Proper treatment consists of placing a sedative dressing over the exposed dentin. This dressing consists of a zinc oxide and eugenol paste.

Aesthetic restoration of fractured anterior teeth is now possible. Tolerating untreated fractured anterior teeth until one becomes "old enough" for a full crown is no longer necessary. Materials are now available that can aesthetically repair the teeth before, or instead of, insertion of a permanent full crown. Among the most important of these materials is a composite resin, which physically bonds to the tooth after the surrounding enamel is etched with a dilute acid.

Crown Fractured With Pulp Exposure

Teeth with pulp exposures should not be extracted, and the patient should be referred to a dentist immediately. Reducing the contamination of the exposed pulp by the oral flora improves the prognosis.

Pulp exposures can be treated by one of three techniques. If the pulp exposure is small, a pulp capping procedure may be attempted. This procedure should be attempted within 2 to 3 hours of the injury. It involves the placement of calcium hydroxide on the area of the exposure. This medication stimulates the formation of a new odontoblastic layer, which bridges the exposed portion of the pulp chamber. If this treatment is successful, it eliminates the necessity for root canal treatment.

The second treatment that can be used for teeth with exposed pulp is pulpotomy. This involves removing the vital pulp tissue in the coronal portion of the root canal, leaving the vital uninjured pulp present in the root. This is a particularly good form of treatment in young patients whose roots have not fully formed. If successful, it maintains the vitality of the pulp tissue until root formation is complete.

The third treatment for an exposed pulp is complete pulpectomy, the removal of the entire pulpal contents of both the crown and the root. In uncomplicated cases with vital pulps, the entire root canal treatment can be completed in one visit. If the root canal has been contaminated, two or more visits may be necessary.

One treatment that has recently been studied in the management of vital pulp-exposed teeth is the technique of partial pulpotomy. This consists of removing only part of the vital pulp tissue near the injury and placing calcium hydroxide over the exposed area. In a study by Cuek,[6] 80 traumatized teeth were treated with partial pulpotomy. He reported successful healing requiring no further treatment in 96% of the cases.

Subgingival Coronal Fractures

In the past, teeth fractured below the gingiva were usually extracted. This is no longer necessary. These teeth can now be restored in one of two ways. In the first technique, sufficient gingiva and bone are removed to expose the root. Standard root canal treatment is performed on the tooth and the tooth is restored with a full crown with use of a post into the root canal to increase retention. A newer technique involves the use of an orthodontic appliance, which can extrude the tooth before root canal treatment and restoration.[7, 14] This technique is preferable in a cooperative patient since surgery is not necessary, aesthetics are improved, and the prognosis for the long-term retention of the tooth is improved.

Root Fractures

Root fractures are commonly seen in male adolescents who are active in sports

(Fig 41–5). The chief clinical sign of root fracture is mobility. The clinician should also examine the teeth adjacent to the obviously mobile tooth because root fractures are often associated with alveolar bone fractures.

Remember that routine jaw films may not show root fractures. If a root fracture is suspected, periapical dental films should be taken of the area. Dental films taken too soon after the injury may not show the fracture clearly, and these films may have to be repeated in 1 or 2 days when inflammation separates the fragments. Teeth with vertical fractures involving the entire length of the crown and root require extraction. More frequently, the root fracture is horizontal.

Some clinicians automatically extract these teeth, although many can be saved by proper management. If the horizontal fracture is in the apical one half of the tooth, the prognosis is good. The tooth may remain vital, with healing of the root fragments. Roots, like bone, may heal with deposition of new dentin or connective tissue. The proper treatment for a horizontal fracture consists of splinting the tooth in its proper position. Splinting can be successfully accomplished with use of arch bars, orthodontic bands, wires, acrylic, or composite resin (Fig 41–6). A splint should remain in place for approximately 6 weeks. If infection or sensitivity of the tooth occurs during this period, the tooth should not be removed,

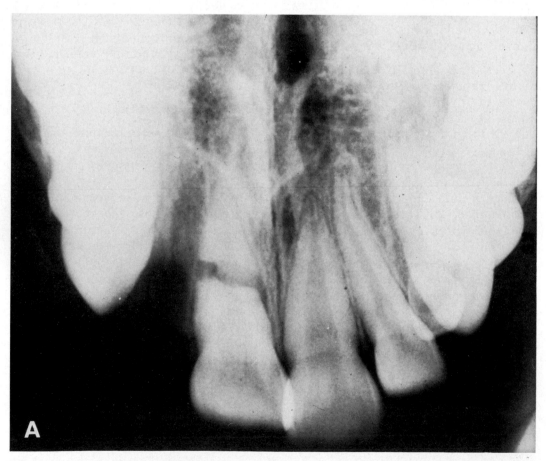

FIG 41–5.
A 10-year-old boy sustained a horizontal root fracture during a neighborhood football game. **A,** pretreatment radiograph showing midroot fracture. (*Continued.*)

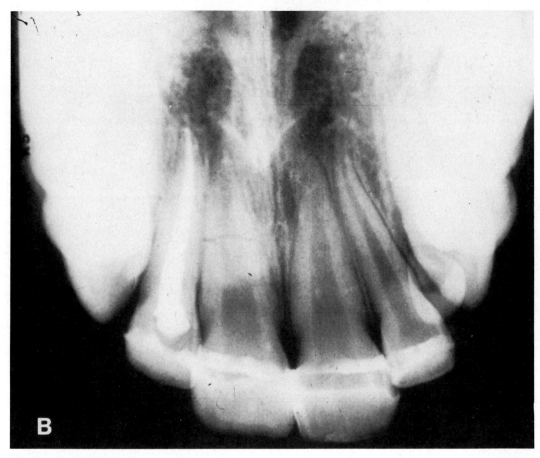

FIG 41–5 (cont.).
B, proper reduction of root fracture with use of arch bar and resin.

but should be treated with endodontic therapy. If root healing does not take place, the apical fragment of the root may have to be removed surgically. These procedures are preferable to removing the tooth and replacing it with a fixed or removable bridge.

TEMPOROMANDIBULAR JOINT INJURIES

Pain and limitation of jaw movement are common sequelae associated with trauma to the mouth, chin, or side of the face. These symptoms may result from injury to the temporomandibular joint (TMJ) or the muscles of mastication. Common trauma-induced TMJ injuries include traumatic arthritis, ankylosis, condylar fracture, dislocation, and displacement of the articular disk.

Traumatic Arthritis

A patient with mild, acute traumatic arthritis of the TMJ has pretragus pain, limitation of mandibular opening, difficulty chewing, and a deviation of the mandible to the affected side. The involved joint is also tender to palpation and may appear swollen. Radiographically, limited movement of the condyle on tomograms (opened and closed views) is apparent. A widening of the space between the condyle and the temporal bone may reflect edema.

The use of aspirin or nonsteroidal

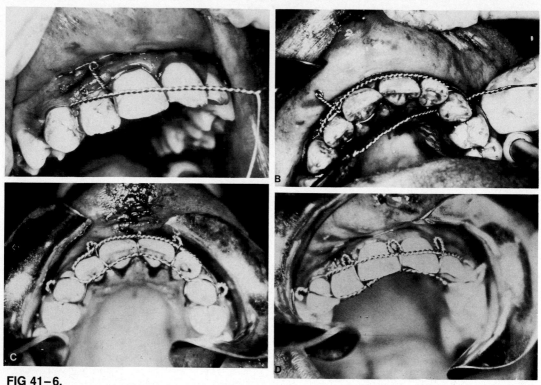

FIG 41–6.
Wire ligation technique used to stabilize alveolar fractures, avulsed teeth, or subluxated teeth. **A,** double-twisted wire placed across labial surface of involved to uninvolved teeth. **B,** same wire placed through the interproximal space and across the lingual surfaces of the teeth. **C,** interproximal wires placed between each tooth and twisted around labial and lingual wire. **D,** completed splint in place.

anti-inflammatory medications is beneficial in the treatment of mild, acute traumatic arthritis. Cold compresses to the TMJ during the first 24 hours after injury and a relative decrease in joint function for 2 or 3 days are also helpful. Most symptoms resolve in 1 to 2 weeks.

Symptoms may be more severe when extensive damage to the joint occurs. An intraoral acrylic occlusal splint (i.e., a maxillary night guard) may help unload the affected joint and permit more rapid healing. The use of interarticular steroids may be indicated in the treatment of moderate to severe, acute traumatic arthritis.

Chronic TMJ pain or dysfunction, or both, after trauma should be evaluated by tomography. Magnetic resonance imaging or arthrography is also beneficial in as-

sessing possible soft tissue derangements of the joint. Arthroscopy has become a conservative technique in evaluating and treating traumatic arthritis of the TMJ. Fibrotic adhesions that may form between the disk and the bone can be severed during arthroscopic procedures.

Ankylosis

Bony or fibrous ankylosis of the condyle to the temporal bone is a possible complication of trauma to the TMJ. Limited movement of the condyle and deviation of the mandible to the affected side on opening are characteristic. Because of increased osseous and fibrotic activity, ankylosis is more likely to be seen in injuries to children. If the growth center of the condyle is disturbed, asymmetry may result. Surgery is indicated when bony ankylosis occurs.

Spasm of the Muscles of Mastication

Myofascial pain caused by spasm of the muscles of mastication is a finding often observed after injuries to the mandible. Classically, the patient complains of unilateral dull preauricular pain and limitation of mandibular movement. The muscles most often noted to be in spasm are the lateral pterygoid and masseter muscles. The key to making the diagnosis is detecting tenderness on palpation of these muscles. No radiographic evidence of changes in the TMJ is apparent in myofascial pain.

Conservative therapy is usually successful in relieving the symptoms. First the patient should be reassured that the problem appears to be only muscle spasm and not something more serious. Applying ice, having the patient slowly stretch, and then, after 10 to 15 minutes of repetition, applying hot, moist compresses are beneficial. Following a relatively soft diet and taking aspirin or nonsteroidal anti-inflammatory medications are advised. The topical application of fluoromethane refrigerant spray helps anesthetize the affected muscles and allows the patient to stretch out and break up muscle spasms. Similarly, injection of the muscles with a local anesthetic not containing epinephrine (e.g., 2% lidocaine or 0.5% bupevacaine [Marcaine]) can also be helpful. It should be noted that clenching and grinding of the teeth, caused by stress, are the principal causes of myofascial pain in the general population.

Condylar Fractures

Condylar fractures often result from a blow to the chin. These injuries include fractures of the condylar head and neck, in addition to fractures of the subcondy-

lar region. The patient with a condylar fracture usually shows limitation and deviation of the mandible to the injured side on opening. A traumatic arthritis, with edema and pain, is also evident. Bilateral condylar fractures can result in an anterior open bite. Radiographs provide the definite diagnosis.

Intracapsular, nondisplaced fractures of the condylar head are usually left untreated. Early mobilization of the mandible is emphasized to prevent a bony or fibrotic ankylosis. The indication for surgical intervention increases as the site of the fracture occurs further below the condylar head and as the extent of displacement of the fractured segment increases.

Dislocation

Acute dislocation of the mandible usually results from excessive opening of the mandible during eating or yawning and, less commonly, from truama. In dislocation, the condyle is positioned anterior to the articular eminence and cannot return to its normal position without assistance. Dislocations of the mandible may be unilateral or bilateral in presentation. The signs and symptoms associated with dislocations include the inability to close the mouth, acute pain due to muscle fatigue and ligament stretch, a deep facial depression in the pretragus area, and deviation of the mandible with unilateral dislocation. The condyle can usually be repositioned without the use of muscle relaxants or general anesthetics. If muscle spasms are severe and reduction is difficult, the use of intravenous diazepam (Valium) can be beneficial.

The practitioner who is repositioning the mandible should stand in front of the seated patient. He then should place his thumbs lateral to the mandibular molars on the buccal shelf of bone; the remaining fingers of each hand should be placed under the chin. The condyle is repositioned by a downward and backward movement. This is achieved by simultaneously pressing down on the posterior part of the mandible while raising the chin. As the condyle reaches the height of the eminence, it can usually be guided posterior to its normal position.

Postreduction management consists of decreasing mandibular motion and use of aspirin or nonsteroidal medications to lessen inflammation. The patient should be cautioned not to open wide in eating or yawning, because recurrence is common. Long periods of immobilization, however, are not advised because of the possibility of ankylosis.

Disk Displacement

Trauma to the chin or side of the mandible may cause an abrupt posterior and superior movement of the condyle, with stretching of the posterior attachment of the articular disk. This may result in an anterior displacement of the disk. Clicking of the TMJ after trauma is usually related to an anteriorly displaced disk that reduces on condylar movement. Signs and symptoms of anterior disk displacement without reduction may include pain, limited mandibular opening, deviation of the mandible to the affected side on opening, and limited lateral mandibular range of motion to the opposite side. Secondary myofacial pain of the muscles of mastication may also be evident. Magnetic resonance imaging or arthrography help confirm the clinical impression of TMJ articular disk displacement.

Slight clicking of the TMJ without pain or dysfunction usually does not need to be treated. Significant pain and dysfunction related to an anterior displaced disk with or without reduction usually can be relieved by acrylic occlusal splints, which help unload the TMJ and sometimes temporarily anteriorly reposition the mandible to improve

function. Nonsteroidal anti-inflammatory medications are also used. Chronic pain and dysfunction related to a displaced articular disk may require surgery to reposition the disk.

PREVENTION OF ORAL INJURIES

Mouth injuries were once considered to be an inevitable by-product of participation in many sports. Missing teeth and oral lacerations were accepted risks of athletic competition, with the mouth being the most frequently injured area of the body in contact sports. Today, however, there exists the technology to produce mouth protectors that can prevent or lessen injuries to teeth, lacerations of the lips, gingiva, and mucosa, trauma to the TMJ, and concussions. Mouth protectors were used initially in boxing in the early part of this century. Besides their acceptance by amateur and professional boxers, mouth protectors have gained popularity in football, rugby, and, to a lesser extent, in ice hockey.

Since 1974 it has been mandatory for all college and high school football players in the United States to wear mouth protectors. Dental and oral injuries comprised 50% of all football injuries before face guards and mouth protectors were employed. The use of face guards reduced these injuries by half, and mouth protectors have almost eliminated them. A conservative estimate is that 100,000 to 200,000 oral injuries are prevented each year in football with the use of mouth guards. There is a high frequency of oral trauma in other sports; however, more than half of the oral injuries and one third of the concussions are reported in sports other than organized football.

The results of studies conducted during the 1960s implied that mouth protectors provide more than just protection against injuries to the oral tissues. Stenger et al.[19] provided mouth protectors to the Notre Dame football team for 5 years. In addition to the expected decrease in dental injuries, they observed a significant reduction in the number of concussions and neck injuries experienced by the players. A British study conducted in 1969 found that mouth protectors reduced the incidence of fractured jaws in rugby players.

Hickey et al.[12] studied the effect of a blow to the chin on intracranial pressure and bone deformation. They found that such an injury can cause deformation of the bones of the skull, an increase in intracranial pressure, and an acceleration of the head itself. They noted that each of these changes was capable of producing brain damage. They then demonstrated that the amplitude of the intracranial pressure wave was significantly reduced and bone deformation was also moderately decreased by using custom-made mouth protectors. They concluded that some mouth protectors can prevent concussions by decreasing the shock transmitted through the TMJ to the skull.

A properly constructed mouth protector should provide maximum protection of the lips, teeth, and gums by absorbing energy, spreading impact, cushioning contacts between the upper and lower teeth, and keeping the upper lip away from the incisal edges of the teeth. The appliance should also be durable, retentive, resilient, inexpensive, easy to fabricate, tasteless, odorless, and not bulky. It must not encroach on the airway, affect speech, or be uncomfortable.

An external type of mouth protector is widely used in amateur ice hockey, especially in the junior levels. The apparatus attaches to the helmet in place of the chin strap. The advantages to this piece of equipment are its strength, malleability, and lack of odor and taste. Also, no impressions need to be taken. The external type of mouth protector has been recommended for children less than 13 years of age. Rapid changes in dentition and bone growth in children make a custom-fitted intraoral appliance impractical. An external mouth protector, when used by itself, does not provide protection against concussions resulting from a blow to the chin.

The most commonly used devices for preventing oral injuries are intraoral mouth protectors. There are three basic types of intraoral mouth protectors: stock, mouth-formed, and custom fitted. Any type of mouth guard will provide some degree of protection and lessen the incidence of oral injuries.

Stock mouth protectors are usually made of latex rubber. They are available at most sporting goods stores in small, medium, and large sizes. These protectors are ready to be used, as bought, without any further preparation. Stock mouth protectors must be held in place by constant occlusal pressure and tend to interfere with speech and breathing. They are also bulky and lack retention. These disadvantages have made the stock protectors the least acceptable among athletes.

Mouth-formed protectors are also commercially available. They usually consist of a firm outer shell, which is fitted with a softer inner material. The softer material is thermally or chemically set after being molded over the individual athlete's teeth. Ideally, the liner remains resilient at mouth temperature to provide the shock-absorbing quality of the protector. Thermoplastic material, soft acrylic resins, and silicone have been used as the inner material. The thermoplastic materials have the drawback of losing their elasticity at mouth temperature, causing the protector to loosen. Mouth-formed protectors lack extension into the labial and buccal vestibules. Therefore, they do not provide adequate protection for the oral soft tissues. These devices must be centered properly over the dental arch during initial fabrication in order to be effective; they usually cannot be resoftened to make corrections.

Mouth-formed protectors also tend to be excessively bulky.

Custom-fitted mouth protectors require a fabrication by a dentist. The dentist takes an impression, usually of the maxillary teeth, of each athlete. The maxillary teeth are usually chosen for coverage because their prominence makes them more prone to damage. A model is made over which a material such as thermoplastic vinyl (i.e., polyvinyl acetate-polyethylene) is then vacuum adapted. Custom-fitted mouth protectors are retentive, tasteless, odorless, tear resistant, resilient, translucent, and of uniform thickness. Custom-fitted protectors are generally considered comfortable and have little effect on speaking, drinking, or breathing. These appliances are fabricated with extension to the mucobuccal fold to provide protection to the gingival tissues. Most custom-fitted mouth protectors last 1 to 2 years. Although the custom-fitted mouth guards are relatively inexpensive and have the desired qualities that have been noted, stock and mouth-formed protectors are used more extensively in school programs because they cost less and do not require a dentist for fabrication.

A custom-made bimaxillary mouth guard, which covers both the upper and lower dental arches, has been designed to improve orofacial protection. With this appliance, the mandible is opened to a predetermined position (the position of heavy breathing) while permitting adequate oral airflow. The bimaxillary mouth guard provides protection for the lower teeth as well as the upper, stabilizes the mandible to the head, and reduces mandibulocranial force transmission.

Although boxing, football, hockey, and rugby have been the predominant sports in which mouth protectors have been employed, participants in any activity in which there is occasional trauma to the mouth or jaws would benefit. Mouth protectors could also be used in lacrosse, wrestling, soccer, karate, judo, gymnastics, and basketball.

BIBLIOGRAPHY

1. Andreasen JO: Fractures of the alveolar process of the jaw. *Scand J Dent Res* 1970; 78:263.

2. Andreasen JO: *Traumatic Injuries of the Teeth*, vol 2. St. Louis, Mosby–Year Book, 1981.

3. Bishop BM, Davies EH, von Fraunhofer JA: Materials for mouth protectors. *J Prosthet Dent* 1985; 53:256–261.

4. Carlsson GE: Arthritis and allied diseases of the temporomandibular joint, in Zarb GA, Carlsson GE (eds): *Temporomandibular Joint-Function and Dysfunction*. St. Louis, Mosby–Year Book, 1979.

5. Chapman PJ: The bimaxillary mouthguard: A preliminary report of use in contact sports. *Aust Dent J* 1985; 31:200–206.

6. Cuek M: A clinical report on partial pulpotomy and capping with calcium hydroxide in permanent incisors with complicated crown fracture. *J Endo* 1978; 4:232.

7. Delevanes P, Delevanes H, Kuftinec MM: Endodontic-orthodontic management of fractured anterior teeth. *J Am Dent Assoc* 1978; 97:483.

8. Garon MW, Merkle A, Wright JT: Mouth protectors and oral trauma: A study of adolescent football players. *J Am Dent Assoc* 1986; 112:663–665.

9. Goho C: Prevention of dental trauma. Custom mouthguards. *Clin Prevent Dent* 1985; 7:5–6.

10. Going RE, et al: Mouthguard materials: Their physical and mechanical properties. *J Am Dent Assoc* 1974; 89:132.

11. Hawke JL, Nicholes NK: Dental injuries in rugby football. *NJ Dent J* 1969; 65:173.

12. Hickey JC, et al: The relation of mouth protectors to cranial pressure and deformation. *J Am Dent Assoc* 1967; 74:735.

13. Laskin DM: Etiology of the pain-dysfunction syndrome. *J Am Dent Assoc* 1969; 79:147.

14. Picozzi A: Mouth protectors. *Dent Clin North Am* 1975; 19:385.

15. Seals RR, Jr, Morrow RM, Kuebker WA, et al: An evaluation of mouthguard programs in

Texas high school football. *J Am Dent Assoc* 1985; 10:904–909.

16. Shira RB, Alling CC: Traumatic injuries involving the temporomandibular joint articulation, in Schwartz L, Choyes C (eds): *Facial Pain and Mandibular Dysfunction*. Philadelphia, WB Saunders Co, 1968.

17. Simon JHS, et al: Extrusion of endodontically treated teeth. *J Am Dent Assoc* 1978; 97:17.

18. Springer PS, Greenberg MS: Disorders of the temporomandibular joint and myofascial pain dysfunction syndrome, in Lynch MA (ed): *Burket's Oral Medicine*, ed 8. Philadelphia, JB Lippincott Co, 1984.

19. Stenger JM, et al: Mouthguards: Protection against shock to head, neck, and teeth. *J Am Dent Assoc* 1964; 69:273.

20. Stokes AN, Croft GC, Gee D: Comparison of laboratory and intraorally formed mouth protectors. *Endo Dent Traumatol* 1987; 3:255–258.

21. Tompson BD: Protection of the head and face. *Dent Clin North Am* 1982; 26:659.

22. Turner CT: Mouth protectors. *Br Dent J* 1977; 143:82.

23. Wehner PJ: Maximum prevention and preservation: An achievement of intraoral mouth protectors. *Dent Clin North Am* 1965; 9:493.

24. Wood AWS: Head protection: Cranial, facial, and dental in contact sports. *Oral Health* 1972; 62:23.

25. Wood AWS: Mouth protectors: 11 years later. *J Am Dent Assoc* 1973; 86:1365.

CHAPTER 42

Diagnosis and Management of Injuries to the Eye and Orbit

Alexander J. Brucker, M.D.

David M. Kozart, M.D.

Charles W. Nichols, M.D.

Irving M. Raber, M.D.

ANATOMY OF THE EYE AND ADNEXA

An awareness of the anatomy of the eye and its surrounding structures is essential to the evaluation of an ocular injury (Fig 42–1).

The front part of the eye includes the cornea, a crystal clear structure through which light passes on its path to the retina. It is continuous with the sclera, which forms the opaque, tough fibrous outer coat of the eye. The sclera is covered by a layer of loose connective tissue, Tenon's capsule, which is continuous with the dural covering of the optic nerve and the mucosal lining of the sinuses surrounding the orbit. The anterior portion of the sclera and overlying Tenon's capsule also are covered by the conjunctiva, which runs as a continuous sheet of tissue from the posterior margin of the lid to the limbus, the junction of the cornea and the sclera. The middle coat of the eye is the uveal tract, and consists of three parts: the iris, the ciliary body, and the choroid. The iris, or colored part of the eye, functions as a diaphragm regulating the amount of light that passes through the pupil. It is innervated by the third cranial nerve and the sympathetic fibers. The ciliary body produces aqueous humor and also regulates the focusing of light by the lens. The choroid furnishes the blood supply to the outer portion of the retina and to the entire macular area. The inner coat of the eye is the retina, which receives the light input and transmits it as an electric impulse through the optic nerve to the brain.

The inside of the eye is divided into three chambers: the anterior chamber, the posterior chamber, and the vitreous cavity. The anterior chamber is bound anteriorly by the cornea and posteriorly by the iris and the pupillary space. It contains aqueous humor, which drains out of the eye through the canal of Schlemm, located in the angle formed by the iris and the corneoscleral junction. The posterior chamber is limited anteriorly by the iris, posteriorly by the vitreous, and centrally by the lens. The ciliary processes (part of the ciliary body), which form the outer limit of the posterior chamber, produce the aqueous humor and give rise to the

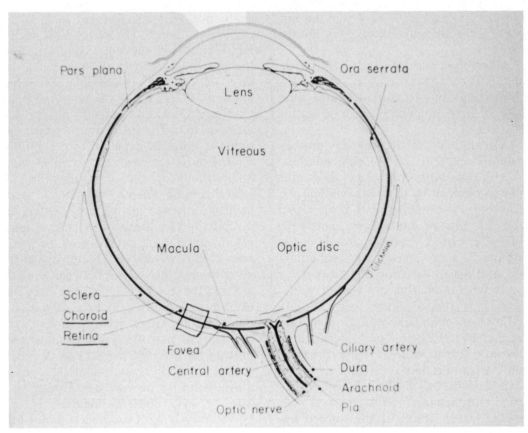

FIG 42–1.
Schematic diagram of anatomy of the eye.

zonular fibers that suspend the lens in the pupillary space. The largest cavity within the eye is the vitreous space filled by the vitreous, a clear, jellylike substance that is in close contact with the retina.

The movement of the eye is produced by six extraocular muscles that attach to the sclera. The inferior oblique and medial, inferior, and superior rectus muscles are innervated by the third cranial nerve, the lateral rectus muscle is innervated by the sixth cranial nerve, and the superior oblique muscle is innervated by the fourth cranial nerve.

The front part of the eye is protected by the lid. The lid is formed by skin and muscle (orbicularis) in its outer half and by a thick, fibrous plate (tarsus) and con-junctiva in its inner half. The tarsus provides the support of the lid and, along with the conjunctiva, produces the tears that normally wet the cornea. The nasal portion of the lids contain the lacrimal punctum and the canaliculus, which provide the drainage channel for the tears.

The eyeball is protected by the bony orbit and the cushion of orbital fat. The orbital walls separate the orbit from the sinuses and the cranium.

EXAMINATION OF THE TRAUMATIZED EYE

Although sophisticated instrumentation and expertise are necessary for a thorough eye examination, much useful information can be gleaned from the history and careful inspection of the injured eye.

Often the cause of injury will be obvious. It is important to determine whether the injury resulted from a blunt force, a sharp implement, or a projectile, however.

The patient's symptoms may provide an important clue as to the nature and extent of the injury and may determine whether referral to an ophthalmologist is indicated. Loss of all or part of the visual field in one or both eyes, persisting blurred or distorted vision, double vision (diplopia), light sensitivity (photophobia), and boring or throbbing eye pain or headache around the eye are all symptoms suggestive of severe ocular injury and dictate immediate referral to an ophthalmologist. Foreign body sensation or blurred vision, which clears intermittently with blinking, may indicate superficial corneal trauma and may be diagnosed and managed locally.

The examination of the injured eye ideally begins with an assessment of the visual function of the eye. If the lids are swollen shut and the patient cannot voluntarily open them, however, it is mandatory that no effort be made to mechanically open them. This maneuver may lead to further injury and even loss of the eye. Visual function should be evaluated by first asking the patient to compare the vision of the injured eye with that of the uninvolved eye. If the vision of the injured eye is blurred, the acuity of that eye may be assessed by noting whether the patient can see light or hand movements in all quadrants of gaze, can count fingers held at a specified distance in front of the eye, or can read print.

The nature and extent of injury should be determined by careful inspection with the aid of a penlight. Certain signs suggestive of significant injury to the eye or adenexal structures and requiring referral to an ophthalmologist for evaluation and management include the following. Tense, swollen, and ecchymotic lids that prevent visualization of the eye may indicate serious ocular injury, such as a ruptured globe. Deep lacerations of the lid, with or without involvement of the tarsal plate, and lacerations of the lid margin require meticulous surgical repair. Protrusion (exophthalmos) or posterior displacement (enophthalmos) of the globe may indicate orbital trauma, such as fractures or hemorrhage. Injection of the conjunctiva, especially in the limbal area, and a small pupil suggest the presence of an iritis. Loss of corneal clarity, shallowing of the anterior chamber, blood between the cornea and the iris (hyphema), pupillary distortion, irregularity, dilation or constriction (in comparison with the other eye), or the presence of brown tissue (uvea) protruding through the cornea or sclera are all ominous signs. Restriction of eye movement may be due to an orbital fracture or may indicate damage to the nerves supplying the extraocular muscles anywhere along their course from the brain stem to the eye.

Certain ocular findings seen in association with head trauma may indicate serious brain injury. These include loss of vision in one or both eyes in a portion of the visual field, pupillary dilatation, paralysis of eye movement in one or more directions of gaze, and papilledema. In the following sections a brief discussion of commonly seen ocular injuries and their management is presented.

TRAUMA TO THE ANTERIOR SEGMENT OF THE EYE

Subconjunctival Hemorrhage

The most common consequence of ocular trauma is a subconjunctival hemorrhage resulting from a blow to the eye (Fig 42–2). Similar hemorrhages are seen in scuba divers. Spontaneous subcon-

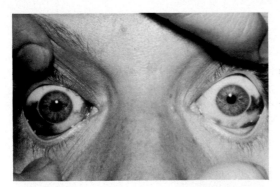

FIG 42–2.
Bilateral subconjunctival hemorrhages sustained while scuba diving.

junctival hemorrhages also can occur for no apparent reason. Subconjunctival hemorrhage requires no treatment and resolves spontaneously in 1 to 3 weeks. However, if there are associated symptoms (such as blurred vision or pain) or signs (such as limitation of movement of the eye, marked hemorrhagic chemosis of the conjunctiva, lid swelling, the presence of blood in the anterior chamber, or ocular hypotony), serious injury to the eye has occurred, and the patient should be referred to the ophthalmologist for evaluation.

Conjunctival Foreign Body

Foreign matter, such as cinders, dirt, and glass, commonly finds its way into the conjunctival sac of active athletes. There is an immediate sensation of something in the eye, followed by irritation and tearing. Frequently the profuse tearing itself will wash the foreign body out of the conjunctival sac. If symptoms persist, the eye should be examined carefully in an effort to locate and remove the foreign matter. When trying to find foreign material in the conjunctival sac, the simplest procedure is to have the patient move his eye in all directions and attempt to visualize anything on the eye. If a foreign body is found, it sometimes can be gently irrigated out with water or nor-

mal saline. If this does not work, it should be removed with a sterile cotton swab. If no foreign body is found on initial examination, a more thorough search is required. First, have the patient look in extreme upgaze and pull down his lower lid, thereby exposing the lower fornix of the conjunctiva. Then have the patient look down and evert the upper lid by grasping the lashes while applying counterpressure with a cotton swab at the upper edge of the tarsus. The patient should maintain downgaze throughout. Upon completion of the examination, the lid can be returned to its normal position merely by asking the patient to look up (Fig 42–3). Double eversion of the upper lid to expose the upper fornix of the conjunctiva may be needed to find the foreign body (Fig 42–4). If the foreign body is located, it can be wiped away with a sterile cotton applicator. Care must be taken to avoid damaging the cornea while removing the foreign body. After its removal, topical antibiotics should be used prophylactically for 24 to 48 hours.

Contact Lens–Related Problems

Athletes often wear contact lenses while participating in their activities. These normally sit on the cornea, but may become dislodged onto the conjunctiva, with a resultant diminution of vision and foreign body sensation in the eye. This occurs much more commonly with hard rather than with soft contact lenses. The subject usually will be able to tell what has happened and will reposition the lens by himself. However, he may need help in finding the lens, which can become lodged under the upper or lower lid. The lens usually can be maneuvered back into place by manipulation of the eyelid. Another method for removing displaced hard contact lenses utilizes a small, inexpensive suction cup that can be applied directly to the contact lens (Fig 42–5). Failure to locate a dis-

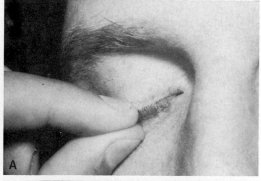

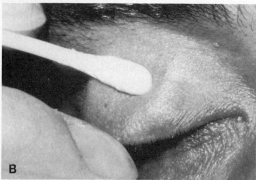

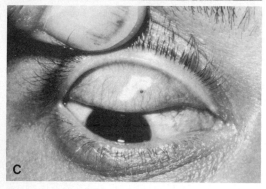

rial may get underneath the lens and damage the cornea, or the cornea may be scratched while inserting or removing the lens. If a contact lens wearer experiences eye pain or discomfort, the lens should be removed immediately. The patient usually will be able to remove the lens himself, but, if there is pain or photophobia, he may require assistance. If the pa-

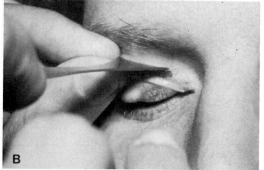

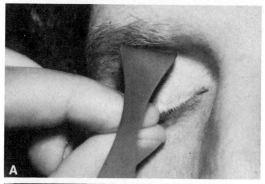

FIG 42–3.
Eversion of the upper lid. **A,** have subject look down and grasp his lashes. **B,** apply counterpressure with a cotton swab at the upper edge of the tarsus. **C,** evert upper lid by pulling lashes upward. Foreign body embedded in upper tarsal conjunctiva. Subject must maintain downgaze throughout.

lodged contact lens may be due to the lens having fallen out of the eye. Most everybody has witnessed a sporting event in which play has been interrupted by players crawling on their hands and knees in search of a lost contact lens.

Contact lenses frequently are implicated in corneal abrasions. Foreign mate-

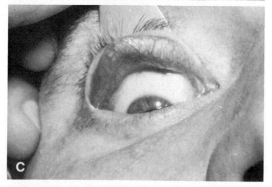

FIG 42–4.
Double eversion of the upper lid. **A,** have subject look down and grasp his lashes. Use a lid retractor to apply counterpressure. **B,** evert the upper lid over the retractor. **C,** lift up on the retractor, thereby exposing the upper fornix. Subject must maintain downgaze throughout.

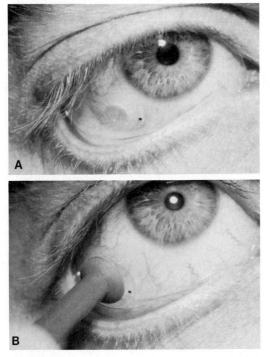

FIG 42–5.
Displaced hard contact lens. **A,** lens in lower fornix. Note the air bubble under the lens. **B,** removing lens with the aid of a suction cup. Dot on lens marked the lens for the right eye.

tient is wearing a soft contact lens, it may be removed by asking him to look up; the weight of the lens will carry it partly off the cornea onto the lower conjunctival surface. A finger is then applied against the portion of the lens off of the cornea, and the lens is then maneuvered into the lower fornix where it can be pinched between two fingers and removed (Fig 42–6). One should never try to grasp the lens while it is centered on the cornea, because this may cause a large corneal abrasion. A hard contact lens can be removed by asking the person to open his eyes widely and then grasping the outer canthus and pulling the lids temporally. This tightens the upper and lower lids against the globe. A forcible blink will then pop the lens out of the eye. A hand should be kept under the eye to catch the lens when it comes out. The entire procedure should be carried out over a table or

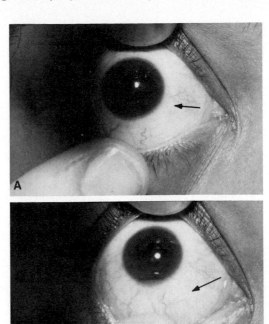

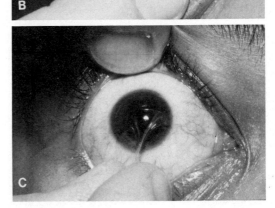

FIG 42–6.
Removal of a soft contact lens. **A,** lens in place. **B,** subject looks up and lens is maneuvered into the lower fornix. *Arrow* indicates contact lens edge. **C,** lens is pinched between two fingers and removed.

a bench to ensure that the lens will not fall on the ground where it can be damaged or lost.

Corneal Abrasion

A corneal abrasion results in sudden onset of pain, tearing, and photophobia. The discomfort is aggravated by blinking and movement of the eye. The patient inevitably complains of an intense foreign body sensation. Even though a foreign body usually is not found, careful inspection of the eye is indicated to rule out its presence.

The diagnosis of a corneal abrasion is confirmed by instilling fluorescein dye into the conjunctival sac. The fluorescein will stain any area devoid of epithelial cells. The green color of the dye is augmented by using a blue light while examining the cornea. The pattern of the fluorescein stain is noteworthy. For example, multiple linear stains in the upper half of the cornea should alert one to the possibility of a foreign body lodged under the upper lid (Fig 42–7).

Treatment of a corneal abrasion consists of a short-acting topical cycloplegic, such as cyclopentolate 1%, a broad-spectrum antibiotic ointment, and a semipressure patch for 24 to 48 hours. The cyclo-

plegic relaxes ciliary muscle spasm resulting from secondary iritis. The antibiotic is used as a prophylaxis against secondary bacterial infection. The patching makes the patient more comfortable and promotes healing of the epithelial defect by splinting the lids. When applying the patch, utmost care must be taken to ensure that the lids are closed beneath the patch and that the patch is sufficiently firm to prevent the lids from opening and closing beneath it.

Corneal Foreign Body

Superficial corneal foreign bodies frequently can be removed by irrigation or by gently wiping them away with a sterile cotton swab. However, at times foreign bodies become deeply embedded in the cornea (Fig 42–8). These are best removed under topical anesthesia with appropriate instrumentation and with the illumination and magnification of the slit lamp. After removing the foreign body, a rust ring often remains. A small amount of rust left behind is usually of no consequence. However, should it need removal, care must be taken not to be too vigorous, since the more manipulation used the greater the residual scar. After removal of the foreign body and rust ring,

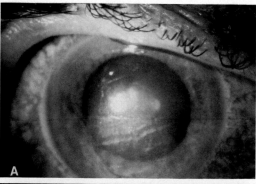

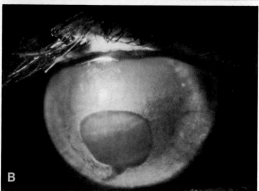

FIG 42–7.
Corneal abrasion. **A,** without fluorescein. **B,** with fluorescein.

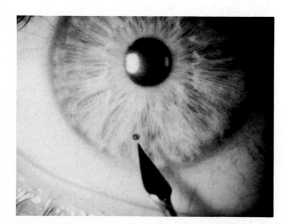

FIG 42–8.
Corneal foreign body about to be removed with a spud.

the eye is treated as a simple corneal abrasion.

Chemical Burns

Chemical burns of the athlete's eye may be caused by swimming pool chemicals such as chlorine, or from accidents with some types of lime used to line sports fields. Chemical burns constitute a vision-threatening emergency and require prompt, on-the-spot treatment. Copious irrigation of the eyes should be carried out immediately, with use of the most readily available source of water. The lids must be held open to allow access to the cornea and conjunctiva. The irrigation should be continued for 20 to 30 minutes before arranging for transfer to a medical facility where more definitive treatment is available. Any particulate chemical matter lodged in the fornices and conjunctival folds should be removed with cotton swabs. It must be emphasized that the initial prompt irrigation of the eyes is the single most important part of the management of these cases.

Hyphema

A hyphema (hemorrhage in the anterior chamber) may result from blunt trauma to the eye. Squash injuries are a frequent cause of hyphemas. Because of the relative confines of the court and the speed of the action, there exists a moderate risk of being struck in the eye by a racquet. The ball also represents a direct threat to the globe. Because of its small size, it can fit within the protective bony margins of the orbit, thereby inflicting damage directly on the eye. This is in contrast to a tennis ball, which rarely causes ocular injury because it is too large to fit within the orbital margins. Hockey is another sport in which ocular trauma is prominent. Injuries inflicted by either the stick or the puck are common and frequently result in hyphemas. Any direct blow to the eye can cause a hyphema.

The amount of blood in the anterior chamber varies from case to case and ranges from microscopic amounts to total hyphemas filling the entire chamber (Fig 42–9). Initially there is a red tinge in the anterior chamber, but within a few hours the blood will settle inferiorly. This produces a red fluid layer in the anterior chamber, usually visible with a hand light. Traumatic hyphemas may be associated with other ocular injuries such as blowout fractures of the orbital floor, iridodialysis (disinsertion of the iris from the ciliary body), vitreous hemorrhage, concussive injuries to the posterior pole, retinal detachments, and scleral rupture. A thorough ocular examination is required to rule out any associated ocular damage.

Patients with traumatic hyphemas tend to be drowsy. This is especially true in children, although the mechanism is not clear. It is essential to rule out any neurologic deficit before attributing the drowsiness to the hyphema alone.

The conventional treatment of traumatic hyphemas consists of hospitalization, bed rest with elevation of the head of the bed to 30 or 45 degrees, bilateral patching, and sedation. Analgesics are frequently required, but the use of aspirin-containing compounds is to be

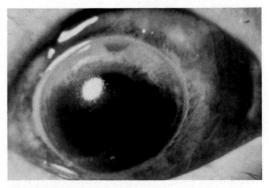

FIG 42–9.
Hyphema. Note that the blood in the anterior chamber obscures the lower half of the iris.

avoided. Aspirin prolongs the bleeding time and increases the risk of rebleeding.

Elevation of the intraocular pressure is a common problem in hyphemas. The ocular hypertension is a result of a contusion injury to the trabecular meshwork and clogging of the outflow pathways with blood. The pressure usually can be controlled with carbonic anhydrase inhibitors such as acetazolamide (Diamox), or hyperosmotic agents such as mannitol.

The initial hemorrhage usually resorbs in a few days. If the hemorrhage clears uneventfully and there is no associated ocular damage, the prognosis is good. A rebleed occurs in approximately 20% of all hyphemas. This usually occurs between 3 and 5 days after the initial trauma, and is an ominous sign with a poor visual prognosis. The intraocular pressure becomes more difficult to control after a secondary hemorrhage.

Surgical intervention is indicated in the presence of medically uncontrolled intraocular pressure and blood in the anterior chamber. Failure to control the pressure may result in blood staining of the cornea and irreversible damage to the optic nerve.

Hyphemas frequently are associated with traumatic recession of the anterior chamber angle and subsequent impairment of aqueous outflow. This predisposes the involved eye to the development of chronic glaucoma months or years after the injury. Thus any eye having sustained a hyphema must be evaluated regularly for the development of glaucoma.

Traumatic Iritis

Mild trauma to the eye can set up an inflammatory iridocyclitis. The eye becomes injected and the pupil becomes small (Fig 42–10). The injection is most

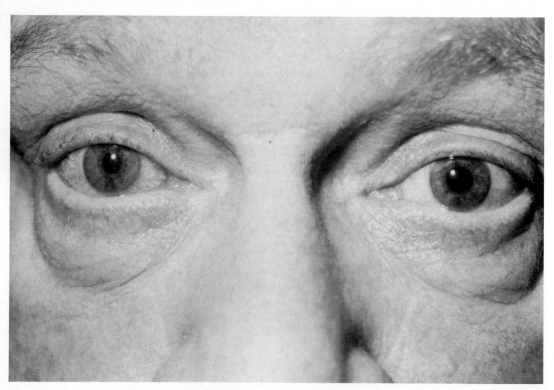

FIG 42–10.
Traumatic iritis. Note the small pupil and injection of the right eye.

intense in the perilimbal area (ciliary flush), in contrast to an infected conjunctivitis in which the reaction is most intense in the palpebral conjunctiva. Depending on the severity of the inflammatory reaction, the anterior chamber becomes cloudy and the patient complains of blurred vision and photophobia. In certain cases the pupil becomes dilated instead of miotic. This is a result of contusion injury to the iris sphincter. The pupil reacts minimally and is often slightly irregular. The mydriasis may persist for days to weeks. More severe trauma can produce a tear in the iris sphincter and a permanent pupillary deformity.

The treatment of traumatic iritis includes topical cycloplegic mydriatics to relax ciliary spasm and prevent posterior synechial formation (inflammatory adhesions between the posterior surface of the iris and the lens). Topical corticosteroids are used for their anti-inflammatory effect.

Traumatic Cataract and Dislocated Lens

Traumatic cataracts may be caused by blunt or perforating injuries. Those related to perforating injuries are dealt with in the section on corneal lacerations. In blunt trauma the characteristic lens change is the formation of a rosette-shaped opacity in the anterior or posterior subcapsular area (Fig 42–11). These opacities may be stationary or progressive. Rarely they may disappear completely with the passage of time. Other lens changes varying from minimal to total cataract may also be produced by blunt ocular trauma.

Traumatic cataracts resulting from contusion injuries frequently are associated with damage to related ocular structures. The trauma can break the zonular attachments to the lens, with resultant subluxation or dislocation of the lens (Fig 42–12). Subluxation of the lens is sus-

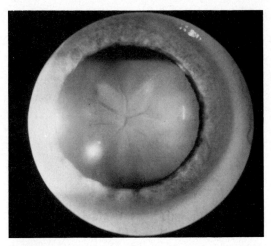

FIG 42–11.
Traumatic "rosette" cataract.

pected if there is irregularity in the depth of the anterior chamber or visible trembling of the iris, with quick movements of the eye (iridodonesis). The presence of vitreous in the anterior chamber confirms the diagnosis of a subluxated lens.

Surgical intervention for a dislocated lens is hazardous. A major indication for emergency surgery exists when the lens blocks the pupil or is situated in the anterior chamber, with secondary acute glaucoma. Surgery may be indicated at a later date if the subluxated lens becomes

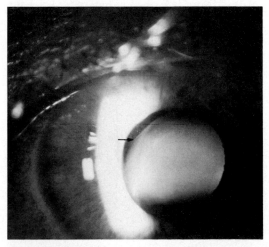

FIG 42–12.
Subluxated cataractous lens. *Arrow* indicates edge of the lens displaced into the pupillary space.

opacified and interferes with vision or causes phacolytic glaucoma. Even in the absence of a significant opacity, a subluxated lens may cause distressing symptoms such as unstable vision, distortion, and diplopia. Surgical intervention should be approached with great caution because of the attendant hazards and guarded prognosis.

Blunt Corneal Trauma

Severe direct trauma to the cornea can produce marked stromal edema with underlying folds in Descemet's membrane. This usually is seen initially as a thickened, central, disk-shaped, corneal haziness with a clear peripheral margin (diskiform edema). The edema usually clears within a few weeks, leaving little or no permanent opacification. Topical corticosteroids may hasten the recovery.

Corneal Lacerations

Lacerations of the anterior segment of the eye are caused by trauma from sharp objects such as nails, darts, skate blades, and broken glass (Fig 42–13). Superficial corneal lacerations rarely need suturing unless there is loss of substance or gaping of the wound. A pressure patch or "bandage" soft contact lens with concomitant

topical antibiotics and cycloplegics, is usually all that is required.

Any time the eye has been lacerated, pressure on the globe must be avoided to prevent extrusion of the intraocular contents. If, during an athletic event, a penetrating eye injury is suspected, the eye should be covered immediately with a protective shield. Pressure from the shield should be on the bony orbit rather than on the eyelid and globe (Fig 42–14). The athlete should be transferred to the nearest ophthalmic facility for treatment.

Lid lacerations can be associated with underlying corneal or scleral lacerations, or both. When treating a lid laceration, the physician always should check to make sure that the underlying globe is intact.

X-ray examination of all corneal lacerations is necessary to rule out any opaque intraocular foreign bodies. Conjunctival smears and cultures should be obtained, and systemic antibiotics should be started.

A corneal laceration associated with

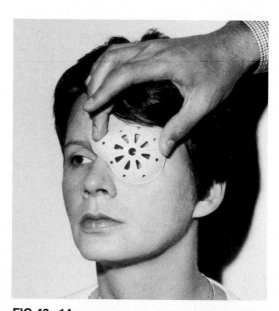

FIG 42–14.
Plastic protective shield. Care must be taken to ensure that no pressure is placed on the globe. Shield may be held in place by tape.

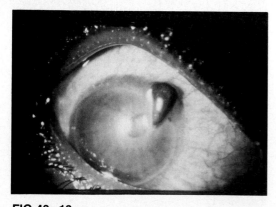

FIG 42–13.
Corneal laceration with flat anterior chamber and iris.

loss of the anterior chamber and iris prolapse requires surgical repair and should be operated on as soon as possible.

TRAUMA TO THE OCULAR ADENEXA

Periorbital Ecchymosis (Black Eye)

Black eye is a frequent and obvious consequence of blunt injury to the periorbital region. Blood from injured vessels dissects in the subcutaneous tissue and produces the violaceous appearance of the skin. Associated edema often may restrict movement of the lids.

Periorbital ecchymosis may be an accompanying manifestation of severe injury to the globe or surrounding facial bones. X-ray films of the orbit and facial bones should be obtained to rule out fractures. If the eye itself is not readily visible, no attempt should be made to force the lids apart, since, if there is a serious, coincident ocular injury such as a ruptured globe, this maneuver may result in the expulsion of intraocular contents. If injury to the globe is suspected or if the eye cannot be seen easily, the patient should be referred to an ophthalmologist for evaluation.

In the absence of associated injury to the globe or surrounding structures, the black eye, although temporarily debilitating, is of no lasting consequence. Therapy consists of ice packs to reduce swelling.

Lid Lacerations

Lid lacerations may result from blunt trauma, sharp trauma, or the impact of a projectile. Not infrequently the globe also may be injured, so a thorough examination of the eye must be performed as part of the evaluation.

Superficial lacerations of the skin of the lids may be treated with a butterfly bandage to approximate the wound edges. Deeper lacerations and lacerations involving the tarsal plate or the lid margin require meticulous surgical repair to minimize functional and cosmetic deformities.

Occasionally blunt trauma may result in minimal injury to the external surface of the lid, but produce an extensive rupture of the tarsal plate, at times including avulsion of the levator muscle. This type of injury can be detected only if the examination includes careful eversion of the lids (Fig 42–15).

Special attention should be given to puncture wounds of the lids produced by

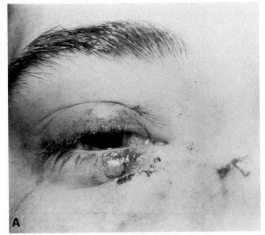

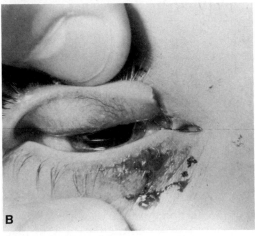

FIG 42–15.
A, laceration of right upper lid. **B,** only after lid is everted is the extent of injury evident. Laceration involves the full thickness of the lid.

a projectile or a pointed object. Depending on the trajectory of the wound, an occult penetrating injury of the globe can occur, or, especially if the path of the wound is directed upward, the orbital roof may be fractured, with injury to the frontal cortex. Careful clinical evaluation and x-ray examination to detect a fracture or foreign body must be performed.

Injury to the Lacrimal Drainage System

Traumatic injury to the nasal aspect of either the upper or lower lid may produce damage to the lacrimal drainage system. Normally the tears enter the drainage system at the punctum, a small aperture on the lid margin approximately 6 mm temporal to the medial canthus, and are carried through the canaliculi into the lacrimal sac, the bony nasolacrimal duct, and ultimately into the nose (Fig 42–16). The most common type of injury to the lacrimal drainage system involves interruption of the continuity of the canaliculus anywhere along its course. Often, in the presence of soft tissue swelling, it is difficult to determine the existence of canalicular injury by inspection alone. The diagnosis may require irrigation of the system through the punctum to establish the presence of a lacerated canaliculus. Failure to identify the existence of injury to the lacrimal system will result in obstruction of tear drainage and consequent epiphora. Treatment requires surgical reapproximation of the torn canaliculus and maintenance of a patent lumen.

Trauma to the canalicular portion of the lids often results in associated injury to the medial canthal ligament, a structure important in maintaining the proper position of the puncta in the tear lake. Failure to repair the medial canthal ligament may result in ectropion of the punctum and persisting epiphora despite adequate surgical repair of the canaliculi.

Fracture of the Orbital Floor (Blowout Fracture)

A blowout fracture is produced by the impact of a blunt force to the front of the orbit, resulting in a sudden rise in intraorbital pressure. This leads to posterior displacement of the orbital contents and transmission of the force of impact to the orbital walls. Typically, the orbital margin remains intact and the fracture occurs in the area of least resistance, namely, the orbital floor (Fig 42–17). Herniation of the inferior orbital contents through the defect in the floor may occur, with incarceration of tissue by bony fragments.

The diagnosis of an orbital floor fracture is based on clinical and x-ray findings. Clinical findings suggestive of an orbital floor fracture include diplopia, restricted movement of the globe, enophthalmos and downward displacement of the globe, and anesthesia or hypesthesia in the distribution of the infraorbital branch of the maxillary nerve. The presence of diplopia and restricted movement of the globe does not establish the diagnosis of a fracture, since soft tissue swelling and hemorrhage, with or without associated fracture, may produce these findings. In the presence of a fracture, the diplopia and restricted movement may be a consequence of herniation and incarceration of the inferior rectus muscle (and less commonly the inferior oblique muscle), damage to the inferior branch of the third cranial nerve to the inferior rectus or oblique muscle, or adhesions and scarring of the orbital tissue to the fracture site. Forced ductions may be useful in determining the presence of mechanical restriction.

Enophthalmos and downward displacement of the globe may be an early or late clinical finding. Not uncommonly, the injury initially may produce proptosis as a result of edema. With time, the edema resolves and diminution of orbital

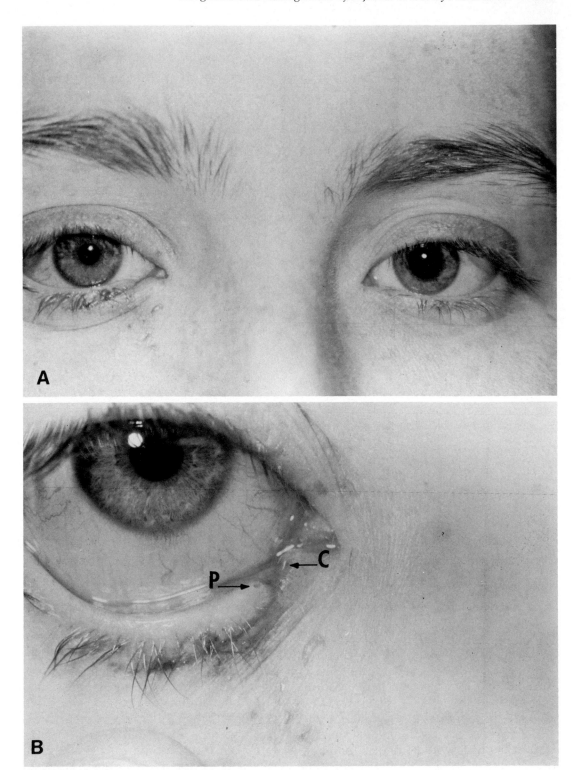

FIG 42–16.
Laceration of lower lid and canaliculus. **A,** laceration involving medial aspect of right lower lid. **B,** lid everted revealing laceration of canaliculus. Lumen of canaliculus *(C)* visible; punctum *(P)*.

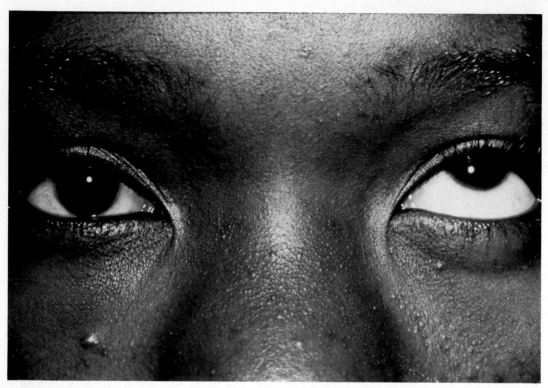

FIG 42–17.
Right orbital floor fracture with entrapment of inferior rectus muscle and inability to elevate the eye.

fat because of herniation or scarring ensues, leading to displacement of the globe backward and downward. This may produce a cosmetic deformity with or without functional derangement.

Hypesthesia or anesthesia of the skin of the malar region, upper lid, or upper gum and teeth on the involved side is often associated with an orbital floor fracture. This occurs as a consequence of trauma to the infraorbital nerve in its course through the orbital floor.

X-ray films of the orbit (stereoscopic Waters' and Caldwell views) are useful in the diagnosis of an orbital floor fracture. The presence of clouding of the maxillary sinus is suggestive of a floor fracture (Fig 42–18). However, the radiologic diagnosis can be made with certainty only with the finding of tissue herniated into the maxillary sinus. Often tomograms are necessary for this determination (Fig 42–19).

Trauma sufficiently severe to cause a fracture frequently also produces injury to the eye itself. Thus a thorough eye examination must be a part of the evaluation of the patient with a suspected fracture. The absence of diplopia in a patient with a blowout fracture may in fact be due to loss of vision in the involved eye, rather than to absence of muscle involvement!

The initial treatment of an orbital floor fracture consists of systemic antibiotics administered prophylactically to decrease the likelihood of an orbital cellulitis. (A fracture of the orbital floor provides communication between the potentially contaminated maxillary sinus and the orbit.) Some difference of opinion exists regarding the surgical repair of orbital floor fractures. Some surgeons advocate surgery for all fractures associated with herniation of soft tissue into the maxillary sinus. On the other hand, other surgeons prefer to defer surgery for 5 to

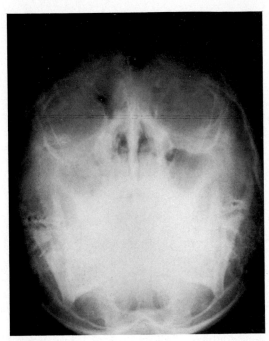

FIG 42–18.
Waters' view of patient in Fig 42–17, showing clouding of right maxillary sinus.

10 days to determine the extent of spontaneous resolution of diplopia. Surgery is then indicated for persisting, incapacitating diplopia.

Medial Wall Fracture

Blunt trauma to the orbit may result in a fracture of the medial wall, thus producing a communication between the orbit and the ethmoid sinus. In the absence of incarceration of the medial rectus muscle, diplopia usually is absent. Subcutaneous emphysema (detected by palpating the lids and noting crepitation) is a frequent finding and may be accentuated by nose blowing. The diagnosis is supported by the x-ray findings of air in the orbit and by tomographic evidence of a fracture of the ethmoid bone. Treatment consists of systemic antibiotics. Surgery is not indicated unless there is entrapment of the medial rectus muscle.

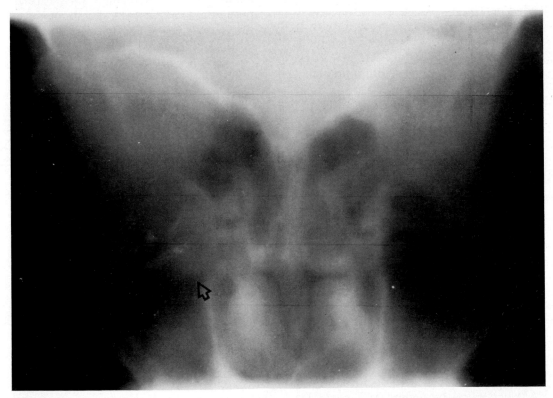

FIG 42–19.
Tomogram of patient in Fig 42–17, showing prolapse of orbital tissue *(arrows)* into right maxillary sinus.

Retrobulbar (Orbital) Hemorrhage

Hemorrhage into the orbit can occur as a consequence of fractured orbital bones or direct or indirect trauma to the orbital vessels. The bleeding may occur at the time of trauma or may be delayed for several days. If the hemorrhage is extensive, it may lead to proptosis of the globe with corneal exposure, restriction of movement of the eye, increase of intraocular pressure, and compromise of the blood supply to the optic nerve and internal structures of the eye. The patient may complain of pain, decreased vision, and diplopia. If the integrity of the eye is threatened, surgical decompression of the orbit is indicated.

TRAUMA TO THE POSTERIOR SEGMENT OF THE EYE

Damage to the posterior segment of the eye (sclera, choroid, retina, optic nerve, and vitreous) may occur with or without injury to the anterior segment. Although trauma to this part of the eye requires referral to an ophthalmologist, an understanding of the nature of these types of injuries is useful in facilitating proper management.

Retinal Edema

Blunt trauma to the eye may produce retinal edema. When the edema involves the peripheral retina, the patient may be asymptomatic. Usually the edema subsides spontaneously and without any permanent retinal damage. Occasionally, however, the edema may lead to serious retinal complications such as retinal holes and detachment.

Edema involving the macular area produces immediate symptoms of blurred or distorted vision. Although usually there is return of normal function, occasionally severe damage to the macula can occur, leading to permanent visual loss. Clinically, retinal edema produces a white appearance to the involved areas, in contrast to the orange appearance of the healthy retina. This often results in the appearance of a cherry red spot in the center of the maculae. Although systemic steroids and other anti-inflammatory agents such as indomethacin have been employed, there is no proof that they are therapeutically useful.

Retinal Breaks

Peripheral retinal tears after blunt trauma may be associated with symptoms of floaters (black dots, dust, smoke). Retinal breaks can exist with or without symptoms, and their occurrence may be a late consequence of blunt injury. For this reason the sudden onset of such symptoms requires prompt referral to an ophthalmologist. Peripheral retinal breaks after injury should be treated surgically as a prophylaxis against the development of retinal detachment. A variety of therapeutic modalities is available, which include cryotherapy, laser, and diathermy.

Macular hole formation usually occurs as a consequence of severe macular edema and produces profound, irreversible loss of central vision. Macular holes rarely lead to retinal detachment, and no treatment is indicated (Figs 42–20 and 42–21).

Retinal Detachment

Retinal detachment is a consequence of fluid seeping into a retinal break and separating the neurosensory retina from the retinal pigment epithelium. If the retinal separation extends into the macula, there will be severe loss of vision. If the macula is spared, however, central vision may be normal, but a field defect or blurred vision will be noted in the quadrant opposite from the location of the detachment. In some cases a peripheral ret-

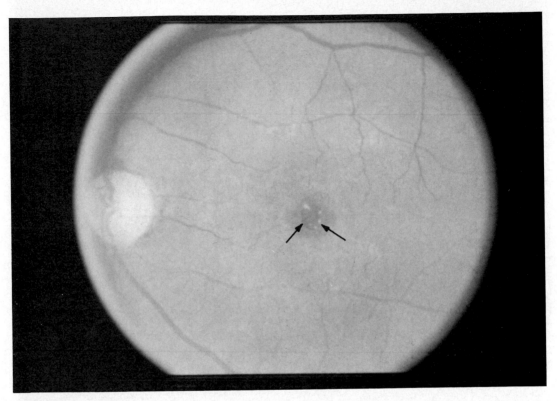

FIG 42–20.
Macular hole. Atrophic macular hole *(small arrows)* after blunt trauma and macular edema.

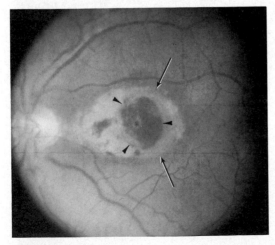

FIG 42–21.
Macular hole and pigment epithelial abnormalities. Typical macular hole *(arrowheads)* and retinal pigment epithelial changes *(arrows)* resulting from blunt trauma, with macular edema and subretinal hemorrhage.

inal detachment may be asymptomatic. The presence of light flashes or floaters may precede or accompany the development of the detachment. A retinal detachment requires surgical correction.

Vitreous Hemorrhage

Blunt trauma to the eye can produce hemorrhage from vessels in the choroid or the retina. If blood spreads into the vitreous, the patient will note floaters. Occasionally vitreous hemorrhage may be sufficiently severe to decrease vision significantly. The presence of a vitreous hemorrhage frequently indicates significant retinal damage, and a careful search for retinal breaks and detachment must be made. If the vitreous hemorrhage is so dense that it precludes direct visualization of the retina with an ophthalmoscope, ultrasonography may be used to

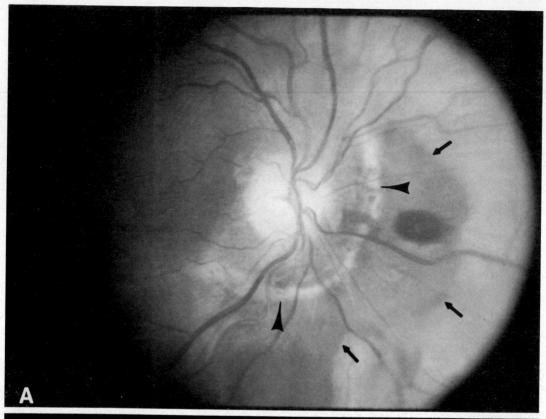

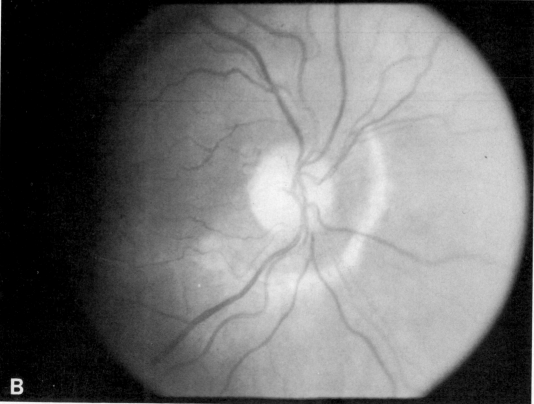

detect the presence of a retinal detachment. Vitreous hemorrhage frequently clears spontaneously during a period of weeks to months. Persisting vitreous hemorrhage is amenable to surgical correction, employing the technique of vitrectomy.

Choroidal Rupture

Blunt trauma may lead to a break in the choroid with concomitant damage to the overlying retina. Depending on the site of damage, profound, irreversible decreased vision can result. Acutely a choroidal rupture may be masked by retinal hemorrhage (Figs 42–22 and 42–23). With resolution of the hemorrhage, it appears as a white or pigmented line running concentric with the margin of the optic disk.

Ruptured Globe

Severe blunt trauma to the eye may lead to rupture of the sclera with prolapse of uveal or retinal tissue or actual loss of intraocular contents. The rupture often occurs at the thinnest part of the sclera, namely, beneath the insertion of the rectus muscles, and thus may not be directly visible. Ocular signs of a ruptured globe include a hypotonus eye, deep anterior chamber, and blood within the cavities of the eye. The patient will complain of loss of vision and pain. The immediate management consists of placing a protective shield over the eye, taking care to avoid applying pressure to the globe, and referral to an appropriate center for surgery.

Optic Nerve Injury

Severe blunt injury to the eye, head, or orbit may produce direct or indirect injury to the optic nerve. Frequently this may result in permanent visual loss. The pupillary response of the involved eye may be abnormal. Ophthalmoscopically, the nerve may appear pale, edematous, and often have splinter hemorrhages. Therapy, if indicated, consists of decompression of the nerve with the use of either osmotic agents and systemic steroids or surgery.

PREVENTION OF OCULAR INJURY

Visual acuity testing and a history dealing with ocular disease should be a routine part of an athlete's physical examination. Any athlete who does not have vision correctable to 20/20 in each eye or has a history of preexisting eye disease or previous ocular trauma should have a complete examination by an ophthalmologist. Moreover, highly myopic (nearsighted) individuals, especially if they are participating in contact sports, should have a careful examination of the retina, since myopic eyes have an increased risk of developing retinal pathology.

Adequate protective equipment should be used by athletes. Athletes who require glasses should use strong plastic or semirigid rubber frames and impact-resistant lenses. In the absence of a need for corrective lenses, in certain sports, such as squash, spectacles should work simply as a protective device. Properly designed face masks should be employed in all appropriate sports.

FIG 42–22 (facing page).
A, choroidal rupture. Right eye showing typical choroidal rupture *(arrowhead)* running concentric to the nerve head. Fresh subretinal hemorrhage *(arrows)* persists. **B,** choroidal rupture, 6 months after injury. All subretinal hemorrhage has absorbed, and concentric ring of choroidal rupture is apparent.

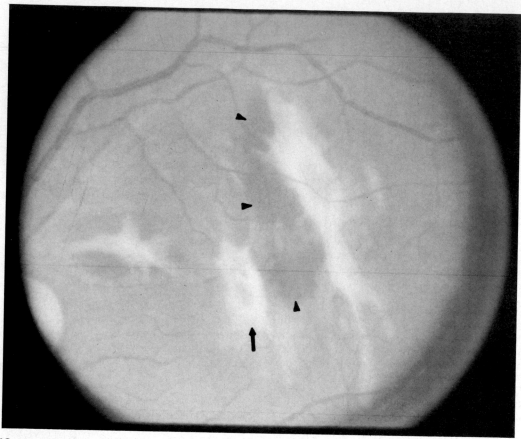

FIG 42–23.
Choroidal ruptures. Left eye showing multiple choroidal ruptures running concentric to the nerve head. Central vision is lost because of one choroidal rupture *(arrow)* running directly through the central portion of the macula. Subretinal hemorrhage *(arrowheads)* can be seen.

REFERENCES

1. Bronchoff SA (ed): Practical management of ocular injuries. *Int Ophthalmol Clin* 1974; vol 14, p 4.

2. *Ophthalmology Study Guide for Students and Practitioners of Medicine*, ed 3. American Academy of Ophthalmology and Otolaryngology, 1976.

3. Paton D, Goldberg MD: *Management of Ocular Injuries*, ed 2. Philadelphia, WB Saunders Co, 1976.

4. Zayora E: *Eye Injuries*. Springfield, Ill, Charles C Thomas, Publisher, 1970.

Index